the Health Effects of CANNABIS

Edited by

HAROLD KALANT

WILLIAM A. CORRIGALL, *Executive Editor*

WAYNE HALL

REGINALD G. SMART

Centre
for Addiction and
Mental Health
Centre de
toxicomanie et
de santé mentale

The Addiction Research Foundation is a Division of the Centre for Addiction and Mental Health.

The Health Effects of Cannabis

Canadian Cataloguing in Publication Data

Main entry under title:

The health effects of cannabis

ISBN 0-88868-325-1
Includes biographical references and index.

1. Cannabis – Toxicology. 2. Cannabis – Physiological Effect. I.Kalant, Harold, 1923- . II. Corrigall, William Alexander, 1947- . III. Centre for Addiction and Mental Health.

RA1242.C17H42 1999   615.9'52345   C98-932672-1

Printed in Canada

For information on other Addiction Research Foundation (ARF) Division products or to place an order, please contact:

Centre for Addiction and Mental Health
Marketing and Sales Services
33 Russell Street
Toronto, Ontario M5S 2S1
Canada
Tel.: 1-800-661-1111 or (416) 595-6059 in Toronto
E-mail: mktg@arf.org

Preface

In the early 1980s the World Health Organization (WHO) collaborated with the Addiction Research Foundation (ARF), a WHO Collaborating Centre for Research and Training on Alcohol and Drug Dependence Problems, to prepare a review of the health implications of cannabis use. This resulted in the publication in 1981 of the *Report of an ARF/WHO Scientific Meeting on the Adverse Health and Behavioral Consequences of Cannabis Use*. In 1993, there was a need to update this review in light of new knowledge accumulated in the intervening period and, as a result, a WHO consultation meeting was held in the same year. A group of experts was then commissioned to prepare background documents to guide the update of the review, and other experts from WHO Collaborating Centres and UN Agencies have provided feedback on this material.

On the basis of these documents and comments from more than 70 reviewers from all over the world, a summary report was produced by the WHO entitled *Cannabis: A health perspective and research agenda*, issued in December 1997.

This volume contains all the commissioned background papers, which provide a wealth of information that could not be included in the summary report. It has been compiled and edited by the Addiction Research Foundation. The opinions expressed in these papers, however, are those of the authors and do not necessarily reflect the views or the policy of WHO or of ARF.

The Addiction Research Foundation is a Division of the Centre for Addiction and Mental Health.

Editors

Harold Kalant • Addiction Research Foundation, a Division of the Centre for Addiction and Mental Health, and Faculty of Medicine, University of Toronto, Toronto, Ontario, Canada

William A. Corrigall • Addiction Research Foundation, a Division of the Centre for Addiction and Mental Health, and Faculty of Medicine, University of Toronto, Toronto, Ontario, Canada

Wayne Hall • National Drug and Alcohol Research Centre, University of New South Wales, Sydney, New South Wales, Australia

Reginald G. Smart • Addiction Research Foundation, a Division of the Centre for Addiction and Mental Health, Toronto, Ontario, Canada

Contributors

Patrick M. Beardsley • Department of Pharmacology, Medical College of Virginia, Richmond, Virginia, USA

Susan Bondy • Institute for Clinical Evaluative Sciences, Toronto, Ontario, Canada

S.M. Channabasavanna • National Institute of Mental Health and Neurosciences, Bangalore, India

Gregory Chesher • National Drug and Alcohol Research Centre, University of New South Wales, Sydney, New South Wales, Australia

Edward J. Cone • Addiction Research Centre, National Institute on Drug Abuse, Baltimore, Maryland, USA

Neil Donnelly • National Drug and Alcohol Research Centre, Newton, New South Wales, Australia

Peter A. Fried • Department of Psychology, Carleton University, Ottawa, Ontario, Canada

Wayne Hall • National Drug and Alcohol Research Centre, University of New South Wales, Sydney, New South Wales, Australia

Christine Hartel • American Psychological Association Science Directorate, Washington, DC, USA

Donald E. Hutchings • Department of Developmental Psychobiology, New York State Psychiatric Institute, New York, New York, USA

Lloyd Johnston • Institute for Social Research, University of Michigan, Ann Arbor, Michigan, USA

Thomas H. Kelly • Department of Behavioral Science, College of Medicine, University of Kentucky, Lexington, Kentucky, USA

Thomas W. Klein • Department of Medical Microbiology and Immunology, College of Medicine, University of South Florida, Tampa, Florida, USA

Donald MacPhee • Department of Microbiology, La Trobe University, Bundoora, Victoria, Australia

Billy R. Martin • Department of Pharmacology and Toxicology, Medical College of Virginia, Richmond, Virginia, USA

Laura Murphy • Department of Physiology, School of Medicine, Southern Illinois University, Carbondale, Illinois, USA

Mehdi Paes • Ar-Razi Hospital, Sale, Morocco

Robin Room • Addiction Research Foundation, a Division of the Centre for Addiction and Mental Health, Toronto, Ontario, Canada

Alison Smiley • Human Factors North Inc. and Department of Mechanical and Industrial Engineering, University of Toronto, Toronto, Ontario, Canada

Nadia Solowij • National Drug and Alcohol Research Centre, University of New South Wales, Sydney, New South Wales, Australia

Donald P. Tashkin • Division of Pulmonary and Critical Care Medicine, UCLA School of Medicine, Los Angeles, California, USA

The Health Effects of Cannabis

Table of Contents

Introduction

HAROLD KALANT, WILLIAM A. CORRIGALL, WAYNE HALL AND REGINALD G. SMART

Cannabis has a very long history of use in many parts of the world, as a medication, as a ceremonial substance and as a source of pleasure. Although there is some evidence that its intoxicating effects were known in Europe in the 17th century or earlier (Bouquet, 1912), the scientific study of its composition and pharmacological actions began relatively recently. De Sacy and Rouyer, French scholars who accompanied Napoleon's army on the expedition to Egypt in 1798, collected samples of "hashish" there and brought them back to France for study. A number of French writers, including Baudelaire (1845) and Gautier (1846), used the drug non-medically and wrote extensively about its subjective effects, including the hallucinogenic effects of very high doses. Not long afterwards, Ludlow (1857) published similar accounts in the United States. Moreau de Tours (1845), a distinguished French psychiatrist, put forward the concept of a chemically induced model psychosis, produced by high-dose cannabis, that might be used to shed light on the nature of spontaneous psychoses, but he was also enthusiastic about the possible therapeutic benefits of cannabis. O'Shaughnessy (1842), a British physician working in India, had published reports a few years earlier of the use of cannabis in treating convulsive disorders.

In the late 19th century the Indian Hemp Drugs Commission (1894), set up by the British colonial administration, conducted an exhaustive inquiry into the medical, traditional and secular use of cannabis preparations in India and produced an outstanding report that was a model of objectivity and completeness for its time. At the same time, cannabis preparations were used medically in Europe and North America, and were included in the British and United States Pharmacopoeias. However, very little scientific research was carried out on the chemical composition of these preparations, or on the identification of the active ingredients and their mechanisms of action, until several decades later.

In the 1930s and 1940s, two important monographs appeared in North America that are considered by many to be the first modern scientific studies of these questions. In New Orleans, Walton (1938) published a careful review of the literature available up to that time, together with results of his own experimental research. In New York City, a committee appointed by Mayor Fiorello LaGuardia carried out or commissioned original research on the chemistry, pharmacology and clinical effects of cannabis in regular users (Mayor's Committee, 1944). By this time, cannabis had virtually disappeared from clinical practice because of the variability of composition and potency of the extracts available at that time, and the fact that newer synthetic compounds of exact composition and greater reliability had come into general use. Therefore the Walton monograph and the Mayor's Committee report were essentially responses to growing concern about the possible adverse effects of non-medical use of cannabis, although such use was still a very minor and circumscribed phenomenon in North America at that time, confined largely to African American and Latin American groups, including jazz musicians, migrant laborers, seamen from the Caribbean and other minority groups (Walton, 1938).

The same motivation, however, became much more pressing several decades later, when non-medical use of cannabis suddenly became widespread among the majority populations in North America, and shortly afterwards in Europe and elsewhere, as part of the youth revolt against traditional values and customs that began in the 1960s and spread rapidly in the early 1970s. This phenomenon provoked bewilderment and alarm among the older generations and led to government responses that included commissions of inquiry sponsored by various authorities — including the United Kingdom (the Wootton Committee; Great Britain Advisory Committee, 1968), the World Health Organization (1971), Canada (Le Dain, Bertrand et al., 1972), and the United States (National Commission, 1972; also known as the Shafer Commission) — all within the space of five years. These commissions produced excellent reports, based on thorough reviews of the literature, original research of various types, and extensive soundings of expert and public opinion. Most importantly, they pointed out the serious gaps in scientific knowledge about cannabis that would have to be filled if the problems related to cannabis use were to be adequately identified and understood.

As a result, many western governments began to pour large amounts of money into cannabis research in response to the perceived crisis. At about the same time, the structure of tetrahydrocannabinol (THC), the major psychoactive constituent of cannabis, was ascertained and the pure compound was synthesized (Mechoulam, 1970; Mechoulam, Braun & Gaoni, 1972), making exact chemical and pharmacological studies possible for the first time. The number of scientific and clinical publications on cannabis listed in the *Index Medicus*, for example, suddenly increased from an average of less than 10 a year in the decade up to 1967, to 300–350 a year in the mid and late 1970s (Kalant, 1996). This rapid accumulation of new research findings led to a second round of reviews sponsored by official bodies, to update the reviews and conclusions reached by the various commissions of inquiry a decade earlier. One of the second-round reviews was that conducted jointly by the World Health Organization (WHO) and Ontario's Addiction Research Foundation (ARF) in 1981, that led to the publication of a volume of collected background papers and a summary report (Fehr & Kalant, 1983). Another was that conducted by the Institute of Medicine (1982) of the National Academy of Sciences of the USA the following year, chaired by Dr. Arnold Relman, then editor of the *New England Journal of Medicine*. This review covered essentially the same body of scientific evidence as the ARF-WHO review, but reached somewhat different conclusions about the magnitude of the health effects of cannabis use.

As the novelty of the use of cannabis by the youth of Western countries wore off, and the levels of use began to decrease gradually, the degree of alarm among the general populations of these countries diminished, and the funding of cannabis research by the various governments gradually decreased. This led predictably to a decrease in the numbers of scientific publications on cannabis, which fell again to less than 100 per year. However, scientific and public interest in the subject of cannabis began to increase again in the present decade as a result of two developments. The first was the discovery of cannabinoid receptors in the brain and in the periphery, followed by the discovery and characterization of the endogenous ligand for those receptors. This substance, arachidonyl ethanolamide or anandamide, like the endogenous peptide ligands for the opioid receptors discovered some years earlier, appears to have physiological roles that raise the possibility of new therapeutic uses for cannabinoids, especially for the synthetic modifications or analogues of THC that may have greater potency and selectivity of action than THC itself. The second development was the growing concern that the social and economic costs of the law enforcement measures aimed at controlling cannabis use might be greater than the costs generated by the use of the drug itself. This concern was reflected not only in scientific and professional publications (e.g., Nadelmann, 1989; Goldstein & Kalant, 1990), but also in the popular media and in political debate.

It was in this climate that the WHO decided that a new and updated review of the scientific and clinical literature on the health effects of cannabis was needed, including both adverse effects and potentially beneficial effects and therapeutic applications. In 1993, an *ad hoc* consultation was convened in Geneva to identify the main areas for review and prepare a schedule for completing it. A series of background papers was commissioned, to be prepared by independent experts in the different areas of interest, and official reviewers were chosen to prepare evaluations and commentaries on the background papers. The review was facilitated by the appearance, at about the same time, of a very thorough Australian report (Hall, Solowij & Lemon, 1994). The consultation was reconvened in May, 1995, to discuss the background papers and reviews, and prepare a summary report. This summary was circulated by the WHO secretariat to groups of external experts, whose comments were then considered by the original committee. Changes with which the committee agreed were incorporated into the final version of the summary report by an editorial subcommittee. After further consideration and some additional revisions by the WHO, the summary report was issued in December, 1997.

However, the original committee had, from the outset, urged publication of the background papers as a companion volume to the summary

report, so that interested readers could see the detailed evidence on which the summary was based. In keeping with that proposal, the authors of the background papers were asked, in the spring of 1998, to update their papers to take account of the additional scientific evidence that had accumulated since the papers were originally submitted in 1995. By agreement between WHO and ARF, the copyright for these papers was turned over to ARF, now a division of the new Centre for Addiction and Mental Health, to permit rapid publication of the papers without any implication of official endorsement of them by WHO. Accordingly, it should be understood by the reader that the contents of the present volume are the papers prepared by the original authors, as updated by them this year, with minor editorial revisions by the editorial subcommittee. They represent the best scientific judgments and interpretations by the authors, and do not represent official views or policies of either WHO, ARF or the Centre for Addiction and Mental Health.

The purpose of the book is exclusively to present the most current and scientifically valid information about health effects of cannabis. The authors and editors hope this information will be of value to a wide variety of readers in the planning of research, education, health programs and public policies.

References

Baudelaire, C. (1845). *Les paradis artificiels.* Modern reprinting 1966, Paris: Garnier-Flammarion.

Bouquet, J. (1912). *Contribution à l'étude du chanvre indien.* Lyon: Paul Legendre & Cie.

Fehr, K. O'B. & Kalant, H. (Eds.). (1983). *Cannabis and Health Hazards.* Proceedings of an ARF/WHO scientific meeting on adverse health and behavioral consequences of cannabis use. Toronto: ARF Books.

Gautier, T. (1846). Le club des hachischins. In *La Revue des Deux Mondes.*

Goldstein, A. & Kalant, H. (1990). Drug policy: Striking the right balance. *Science, 249,* 1513–1521.

Great Britain Advisory Committee on Drug Dependence (*"The Wootton Committee"*). (1968). *Cannabis.* London: HMSO.

Hall, W., Solowij, N. & Lemon, J. (1994). *The Health and Psychological Consequences of Cannabis Use* (National Drug Strategy Monograph No. 25). Canberra: Australian Government Publication Services.

Indian Hemp Drugs Commission, 1893–1894. (1894). *Report on Indian Hemp* (Vols. 1–7). Simla: Government Central Printing Office.

Institute of Medicine. (1982). *Marijuana and Health.* Washington, DC: National Academy Press.

Kalant, H. (1996). Commentary: Good report but scanty research. *Addiction, 91,* 762–764.

Le Dain, G., Bertrand, M.-A., Campbell, I.L., Lehmann, H.E. & Stein, J.P. (1972). *Cannabis. A Report of the Commission of Inquiry into the Non-Medical Use of Drugs.* Ottawa: Information Canada.

Ludlow, F.H. (1857). *The Hasheesh Eater: Being Passages from the Life of a Pythagorean.* New York: Harper & Row.

Mayor's Committee on Marihuana. (1944). *The Marihuana Problem in the City of New York.* Lancaster, PA: Jacques Cattell Press.

Mechoulam, R. (1970). Marihuana chemistry. *Science, 168,* 1159–1166.

Mechoulam, R., Braun, P. & Gaoni, Y. (1972). Syntheses of $\varnothing$-tetrahydrocannabinol and related cannabinoids. *Journal of the American Chemical Society, 94,* 6159–6165.

Moreau de Tours, J.J. (1845). *Du hachisch et de l'aliénation mentale.* Paris: Masson.

Nadelmann, E.A. (1989). Drug prohibition in the United States: Costs, consequences, and alternatives. *Science, 245,* 939–947.

National Commission on Marihuana and Drug Use. (1972). *Marihuana — A Signal of Misunderstanding.* New York: New American Library.

O'Shaughnessy, W.B. (1842). On the preparation of the Indian hemp, or gunjah (Cannabis indica): The effects on the animal system in health, and their utility in the treatment of tetanus and other convulsive diseases. *Transactions of the Medical and Physical Society of Bombay,* 421–469.

Walton, R.P. (1938). *Marihuana — America's New Drug Problem.* Philadelphia: J.B. Lippincott.

World Health Organization. (1971). *The Use of Cannabis: Report of a WHO Scientific Group* (WHO Technical Report No. 478). Geneva: WHO.

Assessing the Health and Psychological Effects of Cannabis Use

Assessing the Health and Psychological Effects of Cannabis Use

WAYNE HALL

This chapter discusses some of the difficulties in providing an authoritative assessment of the seriousness of the threat that illicit cannabis use poses to personal and public health. It begins with a brief analysis of the ways in which the debate about the legal status of cannabis has affected attempts to appraise its health effects. Some proposals are made to improve our appraisal of the personal and public health consequences of cannabis use so that more informed societal decisions can be made about policies towards cannabis use. These proposals are followed by a discussion of some of the difficulties in making causal inferences about the acute and chronic adverse health and psychological effects of cannabis use. Acute health effects are taken to be those that occur shortly after a single dose or after a small number of occasions of use. Chronic health effects are defined as those that occur after a period of regular use (e.g., daily) over a period of years or decades. Unless otherwise stated, the route of administration of cannabis is assumed to be smoking. The chapter concludes with a brief discussion of the difficulties in quantifying the personal and public health significance of the probable adverse health effects of cannabis.

The Social and Political Context of Appraisal

Appraisals of the hazards of recreational drug use are unavoidably affected by the societal approval or disapproval of the drug in question. As Room (1984) has observed, ethnographers studying the impact of alcohol on non-industrialized societies have often engaged in "problem deflation" in that they have minimized the adverse health and social impact of alcohol in these societies. This has often been in response to the "problem inflation" by missionaries and colonial authorities who wished to deny subject peoples access to alcohol. In Western cultures, the economic interests of the tobacco and alcohol industries, and the widespread social acceptance of alcohol intoxication, provide potent reasons for similar deflationary estimates of the health consequences of these drugs. Problem deflationists typically discount the adverse effects of alcohol and tobacco use, either by contesting the evidence for adverse effects, or by denying that there is a causal connection between alcohol and tobacco use and particular adverse health effects.

A favored way of discounting evidence of adverse health effects of drug use is to set such a high *standard of proof* that a case can never be made. The standard of proof reflects the degree of confidence required in an inference that there is a causal connection between drug use and harm. In courts of law, the standard of proof demanded depends upon the seriousness of the offence at issue and the consequences of a verdict. A standard of "beyond reasonable doubt" is demanded in criminal cases that may lead to imprisonment if the accused is convicted, while the "balance of probabilities" is acceptable in civil cases or those with non-custodial penalties such as fines. Although these legal standards are not directly translatable into scientific practice, biomedical scientists generally require something closer to the standard of beyond reasonable doubt than the balance of probabilities before drawing confident conclusions that a drug causes harm. That is, they demand evidence of an association and strong arguments that the association is a token of a causal relationship.

An inflationary–deflationary dialectic has also been at work in the debate about the health effects of recreational cannabis use. The symbolism of cannabis use in the late 1960s introduced a social and political dimension to the debate about the adverse health effects of cannabis, which is strongly correlated with political radicalism and conservatism. Politically conservative opponents of cannabis use, for example, justify its continued prohibition by citing evidence of the personal and social harms of its use (e.g., Nahas & Latour, 1992). When the evidence is uncertain, as it still is with many of the alleged effects of chronic cannabis use, they resolve the uncertainty by assuming that cannabis use is unsafe until proven safe.

Complementary behavior has been shown by some proponents of decriminalization. Evidence of harm is discounted, and uncertainties about the ill effects of chronic cannabis use are resolved by demanding more and better evidence. The argument is that until this uncertainty is resolved, individuals should be allowed to exercise their free choice about whether or not

they use the drug. Such approaches to the appraisal of evidence have not always been consistently applied. Both sides of the debate, for example, would (for very different reasons) not apply the approach that they use to assess the health risks of cannabis use to assessing the health hazards of alcohol, pesticides, herbicides or chemical residues in food.

There is a sense in which both problem inflation and deflation have been unnecessary. Their motivations derive from the mistaken shared view that the health effects of cannabis are decisive in social policy. According to this implicit view, cannabis should be legalized if it has few health effects and it should remain prohibited if it has adverse health effects. In fact, the health effects of cannabis are irrelevant since either side can argue its case regardless of the evidence. Proponents of legalization could argue, for example, that it is indefensible to prohibit adult cannabis use while adults are freely permitted to use alcohol and tobacco. Conversely, opponents of legalization could argue that even if cannabis is less harmful than alcohol, there are enough self-inflicted harms without adding new recreational drugs to our social repertoire, especially one that does not have a long tradition of use in our society.

Some Proposals

The following are proposals for achieving a more rational assessment of the health risks of cannabis. Their aims are: to ensure that the bases of our ignorance will be more clearly disclosed, making it easier to identify what we need to know to reduce it; to increase the chances that the debate about the health risks of cannabis use will be about issues of substance; and to make it less likely that empirical issues will be confused with moral issues and vice versa.

SEPARATE THE LEGAL AND HEALTH ISSUES

We would improve our appraisal of the health effects of cannabis and the quality of the debate about the legal status of cannabis use if we clearly separated the two issues. They are understandably connected because the adverse health effects of cannabis use are offered as the principal justification for its use remaining a criminal offence. Consequently, if there were no adverse health effects of cannabis use, a different justification would need to be found for its continued prohibition. It would be possible, for example, to argue for prohibition in the absence of adverse health effects if there was a societal consensus that it was undesirable for substantial numbers of citizens to spend a large part of their time in an intoxicated state. Such an argument would honestly acknowledge moral and political values as legitimate topics for discussion and debate. This would be a substantial improvement on moral objections to cannabis use being justified on the grounds of a threat to public health.

Even if there are adverse health effects of cannabis, the connection between the adverse health effects of cannabis and its legal status is not as simple as has often been assumed. If the existence of adverse health effects was a sufficient warrant for the legal prohibition of adult cannabis use, then consistency would demand that alcohol and tobacco use should also be prohibited. Our failure to prohibit alcohol and tobacco indicates that socially important values other than personal or public health are at stake. These include individual autonomy and personal liberty, as well as the economic and social costs of trying to prevent a substantial proportion of the adult population from doing something that they want to do, for their own good. These values must be weighed against public health in what is a political decision, albeit one that is informed by a fair appraisal of the health risks of cannabis use.

The failure to separate the health and legal issues means that the appraisers' views about the legal status of cannabis often prejudice their appraisals of its health effects. As argued above, this has operated in both directions, with opponents of its use inflating its health effects while proponents deflate their estimates, each driven by the shared assumption that the existence of adverse health effects justifies prohibition. A clear distinction between the two issues is the best way of ensuring a fair and useful discussion of both.

STOP TREATING CANNABIS AS A SPECIAL CASE

As often happens in controversies, the issues about which disagreement is fiercest distract attention from those issues on which protagonists implicitly agree. A shared assumption in the debates about the health and legal status of cannabis use is that cannabis is a "special" drug, albeit for very different reasons. According to some proponents of its use, cannabis is a "mind-expanding," "consciousness-raising" drug, which is morally superior in its effects to the more popular intoxicant alcohol and especially benign in its effects on health. To its opponents, cannabis is a "deceptively dangerous" drug in that the absence of life-threatening acute effects disguises its adverse effects on the personalities of users and the fabric of society. My proposal to reject both assumptions echoes that made earlier by Fehr and Kalant (1983): that when considering the health effects of cannabis use we should adopt the same approach as has been used to assess the health effects of other popular recreational intoxicants and stimulants such as alcohol and tobacco.

If we do so, then any inquiry into the health effects of cannabis will begin with a presumption derived from pharmacology and toxicology that cannabis is likely to harm health when used at some dose, at some frequency or duration of use, or by some methods of administration (Fehr & Kalant, 1983). This is true for all biologically active substances, water included (Barlow & De Wardener, 1959), and it is clearly the case for alcohol and tobacco. Indeed, given that cannabis is an intoxicant like alcohol, and a drug that is usually smoked like tobacco, there is thus good reason for expecting it to share at least some of the acute and chronic health effects of these two drugs.

Beginning with this presumption does not mean that one assumes that cannabis use is unsafe until proven safe. It does mean that if a *prima facie* case is made that cannabis causes a specific harm, then positive evidence of safety should be required. A *prima facie* case could be made either by presenting direct evidence that cannabis has ill effects in animals or preferably humans (e.g., from a case-control study) or by advancing some compelling argument that its use could have such an effect. An example of a compelling argument would be the following. Daily tobacco smoking is a contributory cause of cancer of the respiratory tract; cannabis and tobacco smoke are similar in their constituents; hence, it is likely that heavy cannabis smoking over many years is also a contributory cause of cancer of the respiratory tract.

USE A REASONABLE STANDARD OF PROOF

If we were to require proof beyond reasonable doubt that there are adverse health effects of cannabis, very few conclusions could be drawn about its health effects, and hence very little advice could be given on how to reduce the probable harms caused by its use. Beyond reasonable doubt is too high a standard of proof (Fehr & Kalant, 1983). Sensible, if fallible, health advice can be offered if the evidential criteria are relaxed to permit provisional conclusions to be drawn about the *probable* adverse health effects of cannabis. This standard may be taken to be satisfied by the consensus of informed scientific opinion that sufficient evidence has been provided to infer a *probable* causal connection between cannabis use and a health outcome (e.g., Fehr & Kalant, 1983; Institute of Medicine, 1982).

There will not always be consensus on the probable health effects of cannabis since opinions will differ about what sort of trade-off between relevance and rigor of evidence is acceptable. Experimental scientists have a preference for experimental rigor, whereas clinicians and epidemiologists are more impressed by observational evidence that is more relevant to conditions of human use. Most recent reviews of the literature on the health effects of cannabis have shown a preference for human evidence, both experimental and epidemiological, over animal and *in vitro* studies. In the absence of human evidence, *in vitro* and animal experiments have been taken as raising a suspicion that drug use has adverse effects on human health. The degree of suspicion raised has been assumed to be proportionate to the number of animal studies, the consistency of their results across different species and experimental preparations (Task Force on Health Risk Assessment, 1986), and the degree of expert consensus that they are based upon valid inferences from effects *in vitro* and *in vivo* to adverse effects of human use (Fehr & Kalant, 1983). The degree of consensus on the latter point is indicated by the views expressed in authoritative reviews in peer reviewed journals and in the proceedings of consensus conferences of experts (e.g., Fehr & Kalant, 1983; Institute of Medicine, 1982).

APPLY STANDARDS CONSISTENTLY

There will continue to be disagreements about standards of proof, what kinds of evidence count, and what kinds of inferences such evidence permits, but our evidential standards should be applied even-handedly. The best protection against the use of double standards in their application is for those conducting appraisals of the health effects of cannabis to be as explicit as possible about the evidential standards that they have used and as even-handed as possible in their application (e.g., Goldstein & Kalant, 1993).

Making Causal Inferences

It is easier to state the principles that are recommended for making causal inferences than it is to evaluate the degree to which the available evidence on the health effects of cannabis meets them. For example, a standard set of criteria for causal inference (e.g., Hall, 1987) requires that a number of conditions be met: that there is evidence of an association between cannabis use and an adverse health outcome; that chance is an unlikely explanation of the association; that it is clear that cannabis use preceded the health outcome; and that plausible alternative causal explanations of the association can be excluded. As will become clear, it is often difficult to satisfy all these criteria in making causal inferences about the health effects of cannabis use, especially the effects of chronic cannabis use.

Evidence of Association

Evidence of an association between cannabis use and a health outcome is provided by the observation of a relationship between cannabis use and the outcome in a case-control, cross-sectional, cohort or experimental study. These study designs differ in the ease and expense with which they can be enacted and in the strength of inference they warrant about the nature of the association between cannabis use and the particular health outcome under study.

In a case-control study, a researcher compares the history of cannabis use among persons who have been selected because they are cases (i.e., they have the disease or condition under study) and controls (persons who do not have the disease or condition) who have been matched with cases either individually or as a group. If the rate of cannabis use is higher in the cases than in the controls, then there is a relationship between cannabis use and the risk of developing the condition. Because the exposure is often assessed after the disease or condition has been identified, evidence from case-control studies is subject to various biases (e.g., in reporting or forgetting) and it can be difficult to be sure that cannabis use preceded the health outcome.

In a cross-sectional study, a sample of people is simultaneously assessed for the presence or absence of an adverse health effect and the presence or absence of cannabis use. Unlike a case-control study, the sample in a cross-sectional study is not selected because they do or do not have the disease or condition under study. The sample is often a random sample from the general population, or some subset of it (e.g., young adults). If cannabis users are overrepresented among those in the sample who have the health effect and underrepresented among those who

do not, then a relationship has been observed between cannabis use and the health outcome.

In a cohort study, samples of persons who have and have not used cannabis would be followed over time to discover whether they differed in the incidence of the adverse health effect under study. If those who used cannabis have a higher rate of the effects than those who did not, then a relationship has been found between cannabis use and the disease. Because exposure to cannabis is observed rather than arranged by the researcher, one cannot be certain that differences in the incidence of the effect are attributable to the effects of cannabis use rather than to other personal characteristics that determine who is exposed to cannabis.

In an experiment, by contrast, a sample of persons is randomly assigned (e.g., by the toss of a coin) to use cannabis or not, and then followed over time to see whether the two exposure groups differ in their health outcomes. If those who were randomly assigned to use cannabis had a higher rate of adverse health outcomes than those who did not, then there would be a relationship between the cannabis use and these health outcomes. In this case, randomization would ensure the long-run equivalence of the two groups so that we would be more confident that any difference in the incidence of the health effect was attributable to cannabis use rather than to pre-existing differences between users and non-users.

Excluding Chance

Spurious associations can arise by chance, so evidence is required that chance is an unlikely explanation of any relationship observed between cannabis use and a health outcome. Such evidence may be provided when a statistical significance test indicates that the observed association is unlikely to arise if there was no association in the population from which the sample was obtained. "Unlikely to arise by chance" is conventionally taken to mean an event that occurs less than once in 20 trials. Increasingly in the biomedical sciences, the preferred method of excluding chance is to construct a 95 per cent confidence interval around the sample value of a measure of association, such as a correlation coefficient, an odds ratio or a relative risk (Gardner & Altman, 1989). A confidence interval provides a range of values around the population estimate of the measure of association which is consistent at the 95 per cent level of confidence with the value observed in the sample. If the confidence interval does not include the value consistent with no relationship (e.g., 1.0 for an odds ratio or relative risk), then one can infer that there is an association between cannabis use and the health effect.

Ascertaining Temporal Order

If cannabis use is the cause of an adverse health effect, then there should be good evidence that cannabis use precedes (rather than follows) the health effect. Cross-sectional and case-control studies that assess cannabis use and health status concurrently often do not permit a decision to be made as to which occurred first, the cannabis use or the health outcome. This is particularly a problem when the period of risk for developing some health and psychological outcomes (e.g., school failure, schizophrenia) is in the same period when the prevalence of cannabis use is at its highest, namely, during adolescence and young adulthood. The strongest evidence that cannabis use precedes the health effects is provided by either a cohort study or an experiment. In the former the researcher observes that cannabis use precedes the health effect, whereas in the latter the experimenter ensures by design that it does so.

Deciding Between Alternative Explanations

The criterion for causal inference that is hardest to meet is that of excluding the hypothesis that the relationship between cannabis use and a health outcome is because of an unmeasured variable, which is a cause of both cannabis use and the adverse health effect. In cross-sectional surveys of high school-aged adolescents, for example, cannabis users perform more poorly at school than non-cannabis users, and the heavier their cannabis use, the poorer their school performance (Hawkins, Catalano & Miller, 1992; Kandel, 1984; Robins, Darvish & Murphy, 1970). The most "obvious" explanation of this association is that cannabis use is a cause of poor school performance. An equally plausible hypothesis, however, is that lower intellectual ability (or learning difficulties, a poor home environment and emotional conflicts) are causes of both poor school performance and cannabis use (Kandel, Davies et al., 1986; Newcombe & Bentler, 1988).

Experimental evidence provides the "gold standard" for ruling out such "third variable" or common causal explanations of associations between drug use and health outcomes. The random assignment of adolescents to use cannabis or not, for example, would ensure that cannabis users and non-users were equivalent in all relevant respects prior to their cannabis use. Hence, any subsequent differences in educational performance could be attributed to cannabis use rather than to pre-existing differences in ability. When studying anything except acute and innocuous health effects, random assignment of individuals to use cannabis or not is impossible for ethical or practical reasons. It would be unethical, for example, to force some adolescents to use cannabis, and impracticable, even if ethical, to prevent those assigned not to use the drug from doing so.

Experimentation using laboratory animals has been one way of getting around the impossibility of human experimental evaluations of the health effects of chronic cannabis use. In such studies, animals such as mice, rats, dogs or monkeys, are randomly assigned to receive either high doses of cannabis (or THC, its main psychoactive ingredient) or placebo over substantial periods of their lives. The rates of various health outcomes (e.g., cancers, immunological changes, reproductive effects) are then compared between the experimental and control animals. This has had limited application in studies of the psychological effects of chronic cannabis use. There are no suitable animal models for the most contentious psychological effects of chronic cannabis use, such as mental illness, school performance, and personal adjustment. Even when there are suitable models, there are problems in extrapolating results across species; these problems are compounded by the use of different routes of administration (e.g., oral and parenteral in animals versus smoked in humans), different forms of cannabis (pure THC in many animal studies versus smoked cannabis plant in human use), and the uncertain relevance of the very high doses of THC that are often used in animal studies to the more typical long-term low dosing of crude cannabis products smoked by humans.

When a suitable animal model does not exist, and when randomization of human subjects is impractical or unethical, a different method is needed to rule out common causal hypotheses in human studies. These involve statistical methods that attempt to estimate the effects of cannabis use on a health outcome after adjusting for the effects of other differences between cannabis users and non-users which may affect the outcome (e.g., personal characteristics prior to using cannabis and other drug use). If the relationship persists after statistical adjustment, then confidence is increased that the relationship is not attributable to the variables for which statistical adjustment has been made. This approach has been used, for example, in longitudinal studies of the effects of adolescent cannabis use on educational achievement (e.g., Kandel, Davies et al., 1986; Newcombe & Bentler, 1988).

An Overall Appraisal of Causal Hypotheses

No single research study, however well done, decides an issue; causal inferences are typically made in the light of a body of research literature. In appraising such a literature, the evidence in favor of a causal inference can be judged by the extent to which it meets the criteria outlined by Hill (1977). These criteria come with an important caveat: they are not sufficient for establishing that an association is a token of a causal relationship since it is possible for the criteria to be met and yet to be mistaken in making a causal inference. In general, however, the more of the

criteria that are met, the more likely it is that the association is a token of a causal relationship.

- *Strength of association* assumes relationships that are stronger indicate a high degree of predictability that cannabis use and a health effect will co-occur. Stronger relationships are generally more deserving of trust than weaker ones because the latter are more easily explained as artifacts of measurement or sampling.

- *Consistency* assumes relationships that are consistently observed by different investigators, studying different populations, using varied measures and research designs, are generally more credible than relationships that are not consistent. This is because the persistence of the relationship despite differences in sampling and research methods makes it unlikely that the relationship can be explained by sampling, measurement or methodological peculiarities.

- *Specificity* is a desirable but not a necessary condition. It exists when the relationship between cannabis use and a health outcome is most nearly one-to-one; that is, that cannabis use is strongly associated with the outcome and the health outcome is rare in non-cannabis users. Specificity is desirable in that if it exists we can be more confident that there is a relatively simple and direct causal relationship but its absence does not exclude the possibility of a more complex (e.g., conditional) causal relationship.

- *Biological gradient* refers to the existence of a dose-response relationship between cannabis use and the health outcome: the more heavily cannabis has been used, the greater the likelihood of the health outcome. Satisfaction of this criterion is also desirable but not necessary since there may be other patterns of relationship between exposure and disease, for example, a threshold effect, an "all or none" or a curvilinear relationship.

- *Biological plausibility* refers to the consistency of the relationship with other biological knowledge. If the relationship does not make biological sense — for example, we can think of no conceivable mechanism whereby it can happen — we may have grounds for skepticism. But in the face of compelling evidence of association from well-controlled studies, implausibility is not a compelling reason for rejecting a causal relationship: it may be a signal that existing theories are wrong, or that we need to develop new theories that explain previously unknown phenomena.

- *Coherence* means that the relationship is consistent with the natural history and biology of the disease. This too is desirable but not necessary: it is desirable if we have independent information that we can trust, but its absence is not fatal since the other knowledge with which it is inconsistent may be in error.

Acute Health Effects

The common acute health effects of any drug are easier to appraise than its chronic health effects: the temporal order of drug use and effect is clear; drug use and its effects typically occur closely together in time; and if the effect is not life-threatening or otherwise dangerous, it can be reliably reproduced in a substantial proportion of people by administering the drug under controlled conditions. All these conditions are satisfied for the most common psychoactive effects of cannabis, including those that are sought by many recreational cannabis users (such as euphoria and relaxation), as well as the more common dysphoric effects (such as anxiety, panic and depression).

Complications arise in the attribution of relatively rare acute adverse experiences (such as flashbacks and psychotic symptoms) to cannabis use. It is often difficult to decide whether these are: rare events that are coincidental with cannabis use; the effects of other drugs that are often taken together with cannabis; rare consequences of cannabis use that only occur at doses that are much higher than those used recreationally or that require unusual forms of personal vulnerability; or the results of interactions between the cannabis and other drugs.

These problems are not peculiar to cannabis use. It took around 20 years, for example, for sufficient evidence to accumulate to persuade most clinical observers that high doses of amphetamine can produce a paranoid psychosis (Connell, 1959). Even then some observers remained unconvinced until dosing studies showed that the psychotic symptoms could be reproduced by the administration of high doses of amphetamines to amphetamine users (Bell, 1973) and non-drug using volunteers (Angrist, 1983).

Chronic Effects

Causal inferences about the long-term effects of chronic cannabis use become more difficult the longer the interval between use and the occurrence of the alleged ill effects. It takes time for adverse effects to develop, and it may take a long time for suspicion to be raised about a connection between drug use and the adverse effect. In the case of chronic tobacco use, for example, it has taken more than 300 years to discover that it increases premature mortality from cancer and heart disease, and new health hazards of this drug continue to be discovered (English, Holman et al., 1995). It also typically takes considerably longer for the research technology to be developed that enables these effects to be identified and confidently attributed to drug use rather than to some other factor (Institute of Medicine, 1982). Moreover, the longer the time interval between cannabis use and the health consequence, the more numerous the alternative explanations of the association that need to be excluded.

In making causal inferences about the chronic health effects of cannabis use there is a tension between the rigor and relevance of the available evidence of an association between cannabis use and health outcomes. The most rigorous evidence is provided by laboratory investigations using experimental animals or *in vitro* preparations of animal cells and micro-organisms in which well-controlled drug doses are administered over a substantial period of the organisms' lives and related to precisely measured biological outcomes. The relevance of such laboratory research to human disease, however, is often problematic, as noted above.

Epidemiological studies of relationships between cannabis use and human disease are manifestly more relevant to evaluating the human health effects than experimental animal studies, but this relevance is purchased at the price of reduced rigor in assessing degree of exposure to cannabis and in excluding alternative explanations of observed associations between cannabis use and health outcomes. There is, consequently, some uncertainty about the interpretation of human epidemiological studies. This affects both interpretations of the causal significance of associations observed between cannabis use and health outcomes ("positive" studies) and the interpretation of studies that fail to observe such relationships ("negative" studies).

A major interpretative problem with positive epidemiological findings is that cannabis use is correlated with other drug use (e.g., alcohol and tobacco use), which is known to affect health adversely. Generally, the heavier the cannabis use, the greater the likelihood that the person uses other types of psychoactive drugs, both licit (alcohol and tobacco), and illicit (amphetamines, hallucinogens, cocaine and heroin) (Kandel, 1993; Newcombe & Bentler, 1988). The fact that these correlations can produce spurious associations between cannabis use and some health outcomes makes it difficult to attribute confidently some of these adverse health effects to cannabis (Task Force on Health Risk Assessment, 1986). This type of association has been a problem, for example, in interpreting the evidence on the role of cannabis intoxication in motor vehicle accidents, since most drivers in fatal accidents with cannabinoids in their blood are typically intoxicated with alcohol.

A different interpretative problem arises when studies fail to find adverse health effects of chronic cannabis use. In the case of immunological effects, for example, the limited epidemiological evidence suggests that there are no adverse immunological effects of chronic heavy cannabis use in humans. The animal evidence, however, suggests that large doses of THC impair cellular and humoral immunity (see Hall, Solowij & Lemon, 1994). The difficulty arises in appraising such negative evidence. Does it mean that THC has few, if any, immunological effects in humans? Have the studies lacked the sensitivity to detect any such effects in humans? The answer to these questions depends upon the likely magnitude of such effects, their relationship to dose, frequency and duration of use, and the ability of studies with small sample sizes to detect them (Hall & Einfeld, 1990).

If the magnitude of the effects is small, they may be difficult to detect in even the largest epidemiological studies. Long-term heavy cannabis use is very rare by comparison with initiation in late adolescence and discontinuation in early adulthood (Kandel, 1993). Difficulties in quantifying cannabis use compound the problem. Doses of cannabis over periods of years are difficult to quantify in the best of circumstances. The vagaries of human memory that make quantification of alcohol and tobacco consumption difficult are magnified in the case of cannabis by the unstandardized doses of THC in black-market cannabis, by the reluctance of some former users to report earlier use, and by the memory errors introduced by determining drug use retrospectively. The most likely effect of these biases is to attenuate or obscure relationships between cannabis use and rarer adverse health effects. For this reason, there has been a tendency for greater weight to be given to positive than negative findings.

Assessing the Magnitude of Risk

Ideally, once a good case has been made for a causal connection between cannabis use and an adverse health outcome, the *magnitude of risk* should be estimated so its seriousness can be quantified. For example, the consumption of large amounts of water over a short period of time can kill human beings but this is not a good reason for counselling people against drinking water. The quantities required to produce intoxication and death are so large (e.g., 30 or more litres) that only diseased or psychotic individuals consume them (Barlow & De Wardener, 1959).

The standard epidemiological measures of risk magnitude are *relative risk* and *population attributable risk*. The relative risk is the increase in the odds of experiencing an adverse health outcome among those who use cannabis compared to those who do not. This may be measured crudely by how many times greater the risk of experiencing an effect is among those who use the drug compared with those who do not. It may also be quantified as a relationship between the degree of cannabis exposure (e.g., low, medium and high) and the risk of experiencing an adverse health outcome. The population attributable risk represents that proportion of cases with an adverse outcome that is attributable to cannabis use.

The two measures of risk have different uses and implications. Relative risk is of most relevance to individuals attempting to estimate the increase in their risk of experiencing an adverse outcome if they use a drug. Attributable risk is of most relevance to a societal appraisal of the harms of drug use.

The importance of the two measures of risk depends upon the prevalence of drug use and the base rate of the adverse outcome. An exposure with a low relative risk may have a low personal significance but a large public health impact if a large proportion of the population is exposed (e.g., cigarette smoking and heart disease). Conversely, an exposure with a high relative risk may have little public health importance because very few people are exposed to it, but a major personal significance for those who are exposed. Accordingly, an appraisal of the public health importance of illicit drug use must take some account not only of the relative risk of harm, but also of the prevalence of use and the base rate of the adverse effect. As this chapter reveals, it is very difficult to estimate either relative or attributable risk of many of the probable adverse health effects of cannabis use because very few epidemiological studies that meet minimum standards have been conducted.

Ideally, it would be desirable to compare the public health significance of cannabis use with that of alcohol and tobacco. This would be measured as the product of the number of indi- viduals whose health was likely to be adversely affected by each type of drug use, and the severity of the health consequences experienced by those individuals. Such comparisons reduce the operation of double standards in the health appraisal of cannabis use by adapting a common standard when making societal decisions about the control and regulation of cannabis use. The task of comparison, however, is more difficult than it seems at first (for reasons that are discussed in detail in chapter 15).

Despite these difficulties, there is still value in making qualitative comparisons of the adverse health effects of cannabis with those of alcohol and tobacco. Such comparisons are qualitative in the sense of simply indicating whether or not cannabis shares the adverse health effects of alcohol and tobacco. The reason for selecting these drugs is that they are widely used psychoactive substances that share a route of administration with cannabis, in the case of smoking, and that are also used for intoxicating and euphoric effects, in the case of alcohol. They therefore provide a useful standard of comparison when appraising the health risks of cannabis use.

Conclusion

A fair appraisal of the health effects of cannabis has been hampered by a deflationary–inflationary dialectic between opponents and proponents of cannabis prohibition. Problem deflation has occurred because of demands for unreasonably high standards of proof, and problem inflation has resulted from a preparedness to accept the worst case interpretation of equivocal evidence that cannabis has adverse health effects. Our appraisal of the health effects of cannabis would be improved if: the health and legal and moral issues were clearly distinguished; cannabis was no longer treated as a special case; a reasonable standard of proof was used; and above all else, evidential standards were applied consistently.

Causal inferences about the adverse health effects of cannabis are complicated by: a dearth of good studies of association between cannabis use and health outcomes; uncertainty in some cases about which came first, cannabis use or the health effect; difficulties in deciding between equally plausible alternative explanations of associations that have been observed because of ethical or practical obstacles to experimental studies; and in the case of null findings, uncertainty as to whether they provide reasonable evidence of the absence of effects, or only constitute an absence of evidence. An estimation of the magnitude of the health risks of cannabis is handicapped by the absence of epidemiological studies to provide quantitative estimates of risks.

Summary

Appraisals of the hazards of cannabis are affected by the societal attitudes towards its use: those who favor it deflate estimates of its health effects while those who disapprove of its use inflate them. The following proposals aim to achieve a more rational assessment of the health risks of cannabis use.

First, we should separate the legal and health issues. A failure to do so means that appraisers' views about the legal status of cannabis may prejudice their appraisals of its health effects. Second, we should adopt the same approach to assessing the health effects of cannabis as has been used to assess the health effects of alcohol and tobacco. Third, we should use a reasonable standard of proof to arrive at provisional conclusions about the *probable* adverse health effects of cannabis. Fourth, we should apply standards consistently.

Making Causal Inferences

Causal inferences require: evidence of an association between cannabis use and an adverse health outcome; evidence that chance is an unlikely explanation of the association; evidence that cannabis use preceded the health outcome; and the exclusion of plausible alternative causal explanations of the association.

Reasonable evidence of an association between cannabis use and a health outcome is provided by the observation of a relationship between cannabis use and that outcome in a case-control, cross-sectional, cohort or experimental study.

Evidence that chance is an unlikely explanation of any relationship between cannabis use and a health outcome is provided when a statistical significance test or a confidence interval indicates that the observed association is unlikely to arise if there was no relationship in the population from which the sample was obtained. If cannabis use is the cause of an adverse health effect, then there should be good evidence that cannabis use precedes the health effect. The strongest such evidence is provided by a cohort study or an experiment.

The alternative explanation that it is hardest to exclude is that any relationship between cannabis use and a health outcome is due to an unmeasured variable that causes both cannabis use and the adverse health effect. Experimental evidence provides the "gold standard" for ruling out such explanations. The random assignment of persons to use cannabis or not, for example, ensures that cannabis users and non-users were equivalent in all relevant respects prior to their cannabis use. When studying anything except acute and innocuous health effects such random assignment is unethical.

Experiments using laboratory animals get around the ethical problems of human experiments but there are problems in extrapolating results across species which are compounded by the use of different routes of administration (e.g., oral and parenteral in animals versus smoked in humans), and by the doubtful relevance of the very high doses often used in animal studies to the more typical long-term low dosing in humans.

When an animal model does not exist, and when human experiments are unethical, statistical methods can be used to estimate the effects of cannabis use on a health outcome after adjusting for the effects of other differences between cannabis users and non-users. If the relationship persists after statistical adjustment, confidence is increased that it is not attributable to the variables for which statistical adjustment has been made.

Causal inferences are made in the light of a research literature by judging the extent to which the evidence meets widely accepted criteria. They include: strength of association, consistency of association, specificity, biological gradient, biological plausibility and coherence. These criteria are not sufficient to show that an association is causal but the more that are met, the more likely it is that the association is causal.

Acute and Chronic Health Effects

The acute health effects of a drug are easier to appraise than the chronic health effects: the temporal order of drug use and effect is clear; drug use and its effects typically occur closely together in time; and if the effects are not life-threatening or otherwise dangerous, they can be reliably reproduced by administering the drug under controlled conditions. It is more difficult to attribute relatively rare acute adverse experiences (e.g., flashbacks, psychotic symptoms) to cannabis use. It is difficult to decide whether these are: rare events that are coincidental with cannabis use; the effects of other drugs that are often taken together with cannabis; rare consequences of cannabis use that only occur at very high doses; cannabis effects that require unusual forms of personal vulnerability; or the results of interactions between the cannabis and other drugs.

Causal inferences about the long-term effects of chronic cannabis use become more difficult the longer the interval between use and the occurrence of the ill effects because the longer the interval the more numerous the alternative explanations that need to be excluded. The most rigorous evidence of chronic health effects is by laboratory studies of experimental animals in which well-controlled drug doses are administered over a substantial period of the organisms' lives. However, a great many inferences have to be made in reasoning from health effects in laboratory animals to the probable health effects of existing patterns of human use.

Epidemiological studies of relationships between cannabis use and human disease are more relevant to human health but this is at the price of reduced rigor in assessing degree of exposure to cannabis and in excluding alternative explanations of observed associations. There is uncertainty about the interpretation of both "positive" and "negative" human epidemiological evidence. In the case of positive findings cannabis use is correlated with other drug use (e.g., alcohol and tobacco use), which is known to adversely affect health. This makes it difficult to confidently attribute some of these adverse health effects to cannabis. When epidemiological studies fail to find adverse health effects of chronic cannabis use we are often uncertain whether THC has few, if any, chronic effects in humans, or we have not looked hard enough for such effects.

Assessing the Magnitude of Risk

It is difficult to estimate the relative or attributable risk of many of the probable adverse health effects of cannabis use because very few epidemiological studies have been conducted. Ideally, we would compare the public health significance of cannabis use with that of alcohol and tobacco in terms of the number of individuals whose health is adversely affected and the severity of the health consequences experienced. The comparison is made difficult because we know much more about the quantitative risks of acute and chronic tobacco and alcohol use than we know about the health risks of currently illicit drugs, and the prevalence of use of alcohol and tobacco is so different from that of cannabis that any comparison based upon existing patterns of use will make cannabis use appear innocuous. There is nonetheless still value in performing a qualitative comparison of the adverse health effects of cannabis with those of alcohol and tobacco.

Acknowledgments

I would like to thank Professor Harold Kalant and Dr. Richard Mattick for their comments on an earlier draft of this paper. Professor Kalant made very detailed comments on the draft and made substantive suggestions as to content that have greatly improved the paper. The points about the irrelevance of health effects to the debate about the legal status of cannabis and about greater value attaching to positive than negative studies were included at his suggestion.

References

Addiction Research Foundation/World Health Organization. (1981). *Report of an ARF/WHO Scientific Meeting on the Adverse Health and Behavioral Consequences of Cannabis Use.* Toronto: Addiction Research Foundation.

Andreasson, S., Allebeck, P., Engstrom, A. & Rydberg, U. (1987). Cannabis and schizophrenia: A longitudinal study of Swedish conscripts. *Lancet, 2,* 1483–1486.

Angrist, B. (1983). Psychoses induced by central nervous system stimulants and related drugs. In I. Creese (Ed.), *Stimulants: Neurochemical, Behavioral and Clinical Perspectives* (pp. 1–30). New York: Raven Press.

Barlow, E.D. & De Wardener, H.E. (1959). Compulsive water drinking. *Quarterly Journal of Medicine, 28,* 235–258.

Bell, D. (1973). The experimental reproduction of amphetamine psychosis. *Archives of General Psychiatry, 29,* 35–40.

Connell, P.H. (1959). *Amphetamine Psychosis* (Maudlsey Monograph No. 5, Institute of Psychiatry). London: Oxford University Press.

English, D., Holman, C.D.J., Milne, E., Winter, M.G., Hulse, G.K., Codde, J.P., Corti, B., Dawes, V., de Klerk, N., Knuiman, M.W., Kurinczuk, J.J., Lewin, G.F. & Ryan, G.A. (1995). *The Quantification of Drug-Caused Morbidity and Mortality in Australia.* Canberra: Commonwealth Department of Human Services and Health.

Fehr, K.O. & Kalant, H. (Eds.). (1983). *Cannabis and Health Hazards.* Toronto: Addiction Research Foundation.

Gardner, M.J. & Altman, D.G. (1989). *Statistics with Confidence*. London: British Medical Journal.

Goldstein, A. & Kalant, H. (1993). Drug policy: Striking the right balance. In R. Bayer & G.M. Oppenheimer (Eds.), *Confronting Drug Policy: Illicit Drugs in a Free Society* (pp. 78–114). Cambridge: Cambridge University Press.

Hall, W. (1987). A simplified logic of causal inference. *Australian and New Zealand Journal of Psychiatry, 21,* 507–513.

Hall, W. & Einfeld, S. (1990). On doing the "impossible": Proving the non-existence of a putative causal relationship. *Australian and New Zealand Journal of Psychiatry, 24,* 217–226.

Hall, W., Solowij, N. & Lemon, J. (1994). *The Health and Psychological Consequences of Cannabis Use* (National Drug Strategy Monograph No. 25). Canberra: Australian Government Publication Services.

Hawkins, J.D., Catalano, R.F. & Miller, J.Y. (1992). Risk and protective factors for alcohol and other drug problems in adolescence and early adulthood: Implications for substance abuse prevention. *Psychological Bulletin, 112,* 64–105.

Hill, A.B. (1977). *A Short Textbook of Statistics*. London: Hodder & Stoughton.

Husak, D.N. (1992). *Drugs and Rights*. Cambridge: Cambridge University Press.

Institute of Medicine. (1982). *Marijuana and Health*. Washington, DC: National Academy Press.

Kandel, D.B. (1984). Marijuana users in young adulthood. *Archives of General Psychiatry, 41,* 200–209.

Kandel, D.B. (1993). The social demography of drug use. In R. Bayer & G.M. Oppenheimer (Eds.), *Confronting Drug Policy: Illicit Drugs in a Free Society* (pp. 24–77). Cambridge: Cambridge University Press.

Kandel, D.B., Davies, M., Karus, D. & Yamaguchi, K. (1986). The consequences in young adulthood of adolescent drug involvement. *Archives of General Psychiatry, 43,* 746–754.

Nahas, G. & Latour, C. (1992). The human toxicity of marijuana. *Medical Journal of Australia, 156,* 495–497.

Negrete, J.C. (1989). Cannabis and schizophrenia. *British Journal of Addiction, 84,* 349–351.

Newcombe, M.D. & Bentler, P. (1988). *Consequences of Adolescent Drug Use: Impact on the Lives of Young Adults*. Newbury Park, CA: Sage.

Robins, L., Darvish, H.S. & Murphy, G.E. (1970). The long-term outcome for adolescent drug users: A follow-up study of 76 users and 146 nonusers. In J. Zubin & A.M. Freedman (Eds.), *The Psychopathology of Adolescence* (pp. 159–178). New York: Grune and Stratton.

Room, R. (1984). Alcohol and ethnography: A case of problem deflation? *Current Anthropology*, *25*, 169–191.

Task Force on Health Risk Assessment, United States Department of Health and Human Services. (1986). *Determining Risks to Health: Federal Policy and Practice*. Dover, MA: Auburn House.

Chemistry and Pharmacology of Cannabis

Chemistry and Pharmacology of Cannabis

BILLY R. MARTIN AND EDWARD J. CONE

By the early 1980s, much of our knowledge regarding the identification of cannabinoids in the plant, pyrolysis and volatilization of Ø-tetrahydrocannabinol (hereafter THC unless otherwise specified) during smoking, and the physicochemical properties of cannabinoids, had been established. In addition, considerable attention had been devoted to developing cannabinoid probes for exploring the action of cannabinoids. During the past 10 years, tremendous progress has occurred in the synthesis of highly potent and structurally diverse cannabinoids, which has enabled researchers to investigate the mechanism of action of cannabinoids. During this same period, new analytical methodologies emerged for the detection and quantification of THC and its metabolites. There are conscientious efforts underway to establish relationships between levels of cannabinoid in biological fluids and pharmacological effects. This chapter will concentrate on the progress being made in these areas.

Chemistry

The highly lipophilic nature of THC, along with its central depressant properties, led to the postulate that cannabinoids produce their behavioral effects by disruption of membrane ordering, much in the same way that had been described for general anaesthetic agents (Lawrence & Gill, 1975; Paton, Pertwee & Temple, 1972). However, structure–activity relationship (SAR) studies indicate that there were strict structural requirements for behavioral activity (Edery, Grunfeld et al., 1971). Although it was conceivable that membrane perturbation could be highly dependent on the structure of the agent, it seemed much more likely that a specific action was involved, such as interaction with a receptor. Therefore, the major emphasis on chemistry has been devoted to SARs during the past decade.

Based on the early SAR studies, it was postulated that THC interacted with a specific receptor that involved at least the following three points of attachment: (1) an appropriate substituent at the C9 position; (2) a free phenolic hydroxyl group; and (3) a lipophilic side chain as depicted in Figure 1 (Binder, Witteler et al., 1984; Howlett, Johnson et al., 1988). The structural requirements for these positions have been critically reviewed (Razdan, 1986). However, it appears that chemically distinctive subclasses of cannabinoid molecules are beginning to emerge.

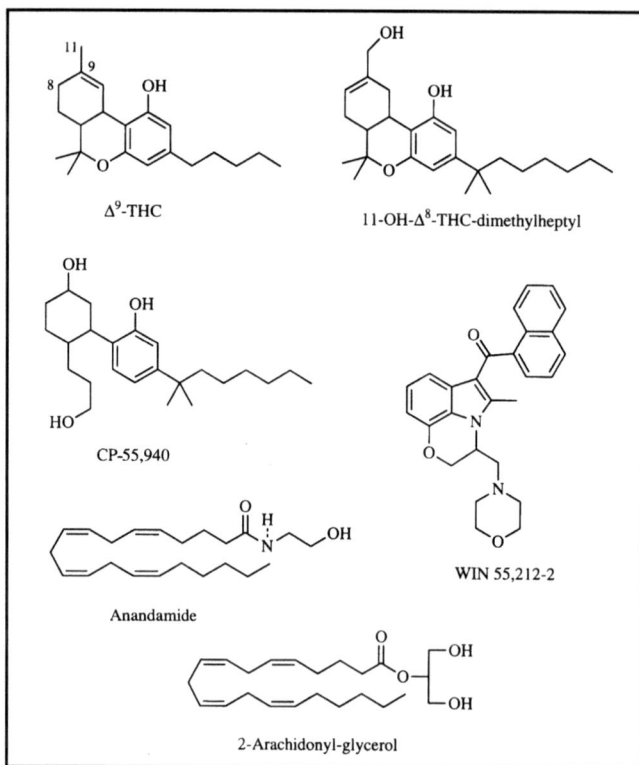

FIGURE 1.
Structures of THC, potent analogues and the endogenous ligand

Dibenzopyran Derivatives

The three-point receptor attachment described above was postulated on the basis of the notion that cannabinoids existed as dibenzopyrans that are typified by THC. A very large number of structural alterations have been made to this template and the results have been reviewed (Razdan, 1986). The most important agents to emerge from these efforts have been 11-OH-THC-dimethylheptyl (DMH) derivatives in the ∅^{8}- and ∅^{9}-THC series. Studies in the 1940s showed that substitution of a dimethylheptyl side chain for the traditional pentyl side chain resulted in a dramatic enhancement in potency (Hardman, Domino & Seevers, 1971). Numerous studies had also documented enhanced potency on hydroxylation at carbon 11 (Razdan, 1986). Therefore, both of these features were combined in the same molecule to make 11-OH-∅^{8}-THC-DMH (Mechoulam, Feigenbaum et al., 1988), as depicted in Figure 1, which was several hundred times

more potent than ∅^{8}-THC in several behavioral tests (Little, Compton et al., 1989). Razdan synthesized the corresponding 11-OH-∅^{8}-THC-DMH which exhibited similar high potency (Martin, Compton et al., 1991). More recently, the hexahydro analogue of 11-OH-THC-DMH (HU-243) was synthesized, which provided another potent analogue (Devane, Breuer et al., 1992).

A major rationale for preparing 11-OH-∅^{8}-THC-DMH was that it could be prepared with a pure stereoisomer because it is a crystalline compound. There was speculation that the relatively low stereoselectivity of THC resulted from contamination of (+)-∅^{9}-THC with the (–)-enantiomer (Mechoulam, Feigenbaum et al., 1988). As Mechoulam had predicted, almost complete stereoselectivity was achieved when highly pure enantiomers were obtained as with the case of 11-OH-∅^{8}-THC-DMH (Howlett, Champion et al., 1990; Järbe, Hiltunen & Mechoulam, 1989; Little, Compton et al., 1989; Mechoulam, Feigenbaum et al., 1988). Therefore, the preparation of 11-OH-∅^{8}-THC-DMH resulted in two important observations: first, extremely potent agonists closely resembling the structure of THC exist; and second, stereospecificity can be achieved with pure isomers. Both of these observations were supportive of a cannabinoid receptor. These results are summarized in Table 1.

Novel Bicyclic and Tricyclic Analogues

It had been assumed that an intact dibenzopyran ring system was crucial because of the fact that cannabidiol was inactive and expansion of the centre ring to a seven-member ring eliminated activity (Razdan, 1986). In an effort to develop a potent cannabinoid analgesic, a derivative of 9-*nor*-9β-hydroxyhexahydrocannabinol was synthesized that lacked the centre ring entirely and had a dimethylheptyl side chain at C3, as described above for 11-OH-Δ8-THC-DMH (Melvin, Johnson et al., 1984). One of the most significant aspects of this compound was that it led to the synthesis of a series of compounds that have a pharmacological profile similar to that of THC. CP-55,940, shown in Figure 1, is the most widely characterized compound in this series, which is 4 to 25 times more potent than THC (see Table 1). Since the development of this bicyclic series of cannabinoids represented a marked departure from the traditional dibenzo-pyran structure, considerable attention was devoted to demonstrating that this derivative is indeed THC-like. Drug discrimination in rats and monkeys revealed cross-generalization between THC and CP-55,940 (Gold, Balster et al., 1992). Furthermore, cross-tolerance developed between CP-55,940 and THC, which provided further support for a common action (Fan, Compton et al., 1994; Pertwee, Stevenson & Griffin, 1993). The contributions of the Pfizer group (Johnson & Melvin, 1986) included the demonstration that an intact dibenzopyran was not essential for cannabinoid activity and that

extremely potent agonists exist, some of which are as much as 700 times more potent than THC (Little, Compton et al., 1988).

Aminoalkylindoles

Even though the bicyclic and tricyclic novel analogues contained some unique characteristics, many of the structural features considered crucial for THC were retained in these compounds. In the search for new analgesics, it was discovered that pravadoline, an indole with non-steroidal anti-inflammatory activity, possessed greater analgesic efficacy than most NSAIDs (non-steroidal anti-inflammatory drugs). The discovery prompted a search for its mechanism of action (Ward, Childers & Pacheco, 1989; Ward, Mastriani et al., 1990). These efforts ultimately led to the synthesis of WIN 55,212 (Figure 1), a prototypic aminoalkylindole with antinociceptive properties related neither to inhibition of cyclooxygenase nor to interaction with opioid systems. Cannabinoid ligand binding studies (Pacheco, Childers et al., 1991) and extensive pharmacological characterization in mice and rats (Compton, Gold et al., 1992) revealed that

TABLE 1.

Pharmacolgical Comparison of THC, Novel Cannabinoid Analogues and Endogenous Ligands[a]

	Spontaneous activity	Tail flick	Temp.	Imm.	KI nM	Drug discri. µmols/kg	A.C. nM	MVD nM
	ED$_{50}$ (µmol/kg)							
THC	3.2[b]	4.5[b]	4.5[b]	4.8[b]	41[c]	2.2[d]	430[e]	6.3[f]
(−)-11-OH-Δ8-THC-DMH	0.01[g]	0.02[g]	0.05[g]	0.005[g]	0.073[c]	0.01[h]	1.8[e]	0.15[f]
(+)-11-OH-Δ8-THC-DMH	>80[g]	>80[g]	>80[g]	>80[g]	1990[c]	>5.0[h]	>1.000[c]	>30[f]
CP-55,940	0.11[b]	0.23[b]	0.93[b]	0.92[b]	0.92[b]	0.08[d]	25[c]	
WIN 55,212	0.1[i]	0.4[i]	12[i]	1.1[i]	6.4[i]	0.17[i]	320[j]	6[k]
Anandamide	52[l]	76[l]	18[l]	55[l]	101[l]	105[m]	540[n]	90[o]

Notes: [a] Effects on spontaneous activity, tail flick (antinociception), rectal temperature (temp.), and immobility (imm.) were measured in mice; receptor binding affinity (KI) determined by ^{3}H-CP-55,940, drug discrimination (discri.) in rats, adenylyl cyclase inhibition (A.C.) and inhibition of electrical stimulation of the mouse vas deferens (MVD); [b](Compton, Johnson et al., 1992); [c](Compton, Rice et al., 1993); [d]rat drug discrimination (Gold, Balster et al., 1992); [e](Howlett, Champion et al., 1990; Howlett, Johnson et al., 1988; [f](Pertwee, Stevenson et al., 1992); [g](Little, Compton et al, 1989); [h](Järbe, Hiltunen et al. 1989); [i](Compton, Gold et al., 1992a); [j](Pacheco, Childers et al., 1991); [k](D'Ambra, Estep et al., 1992); [l](Smith, Compton et al., 1994); [m](Wiley, Balster et al., unpublished observations); [n](Vogel, Barg et al., 1993); [o](Devane, Breuer et al., 1992).

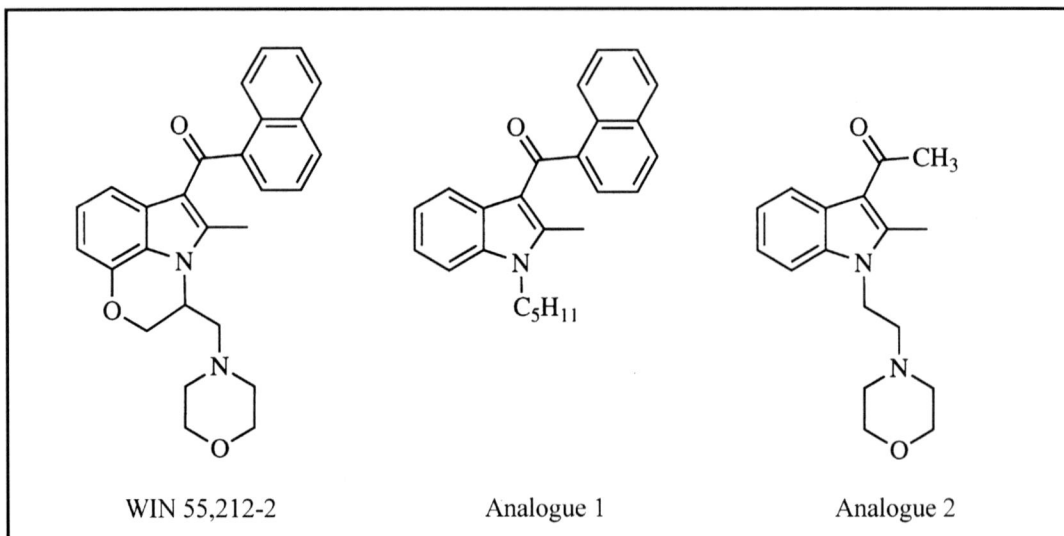

FIGURE 2.
Structure of the novel aminoalkylindole cannabinoid WIN 55,212 and structural analogues

these compounds were cannabinoids (see Table 1). The aminoalkylindoles represent the first major structural diversion in the cannabinoids. Although the bicyclic and tricyclic cannabinoids were novel, they retained several key structural features. The fact that aminoalkylindoles apparently bear little structural resemblance to THC opens a new avenue for exploring SARs. For example, a group of investigators (Huffman, Dai et al., 1994) recently showed that cannabinoid activity is retained when the morpholino group and the ring to which it is attached are removed (analogue 1, Figure 2). However, removal of the biphenyl, as depicted in analogue 2 (see Figure 2) eliminated cannabinoid activity. Further evaluation of the aminoalkylindoles should reveal new insights into the receptor pharmacophore as well as the possibility of receptor subtypes.

Arachidonic Acid Derivatives

Expanding the structural diversity of cannabinoids has not been limited to the novel bicyclic and tricyclic analogues and the aminoalkylindoles. The discovery of anandamide (see Figure 1) as an endogenous cannabinoid ligand (discussed later), revealed that a fatty acid derivative is capable of producing effects similar to those of THC (Devane, Hanus et al., 1992). Although structural commonalties between prostanoids and cannabinoids had been proposed (Milne & Johnson, 1981), it was not until the discovery of anandamide that any direct evidence was forthcoming. Three naturally occurring anandamides bind to the rat brain cannabinoid receptor (Devane, Hanus et al., 1992; Hanus, Gopher et al., 1993) and to murine Ltk⁻ cells transfected with the human cannabinoid receptor (Felder, Briley et al., 1993). The pharmacological properties of anandamide are summarized in Table 1. Additional compounds with changes in the fatty acid moiety have been evaluated (Felder, Briley et al., 1993; Mechoulam, Hanus & Martin, 1994) that allow for several tentative conclusions to be drawn regarding structural requirements in this series: (1) at least three double bonds on the fatty acid chain are required for pronounced activity; (2) reduction in activity occurs when the first double bond is on the third carbon atom from the non-acidic end of the fatty acid; (3) highest potencies are observed with the C-20 and C-22 polyunsaturated acids; and (4) bulky N-substituents eliminate activity. One of the major limitations of anandamide is its short duration of action and low potency. As a result, stable analogues have been prepared by the addition of methyl groups on either side of the amide group in anandamide (Abadji, Lin et al., 1994; Adams, Ryan et al., 1995). More importantly, recent alterations in the terminal carbon end of anandamide have yielded analogues with high potency (Ryan, Banner et al., 1997; Seltzman, Fleming et al., 1997).

The emergence of several new templates for exploring cannabinoid SARs makes it highly probable that significant progress will be made as the cannabinoid pharmacophore is re-evaluated with these structurally diverse probes. It will also be essential to evaluate anandamide in humans to verify that it is indeed behaviorally identical to THC.

Mechanism of Action

Cannabinoid Receptors

CHARACTERIZATION OF THE BINDING SITE

The highly lipophilic nature of Δ^8- and Δ^9-THC, coupled with their relatively low receptor affinities, provides the most likely explanation for the failure of earlier investigators to characterize cannabinoid receptor binding in the brain (Harris, Carchman & Martin, 1978; Roth & Williams, 1979). Attempts to circumvent lipophilicity problems with the much less lipophilic cannabinoid $[^3H]5^1$-trimethylammonium-Δ^8-THC were also unsuccessful because this ligand labelled a site that interacted with both pharmacologically active and inactive cannabinoids (Nye, Seltzman et al., 1984; 1985). However, radiolabelling the potent bicyclic CP-55,940 proved to be a successful strategy for characterizing a cannabinoid binding site in brain homogenates (Devane, Dysarz et al., 1988).

These studies were the first to provide direct evidence that a cannabinoid receptor existed. In rat brain cortical membranes, K_D values reported for CP-55,940 range from 0.13 to 5 nM, and Bmax values are on the order of 0.9 to 3.3 pmol/mg protein (Compton, Rice et al., 1993; Devane,

Dysarz et al., 1988; Westlake, Howlett et al., 1991). A selected series of analogues was reported to exhibit an excellent correlation between antinociceptive potency and affinity for this binding site (Devane, Dysarz et al., 1988). Subsequently, other investigators extended this correlation to include 60 cannabinoids and several behavioral measures (Compton, Rice et al., 1993). A high degree of correlation was found between the K_I values and *in vivo* potency in the mouse for depression of spontaneous locomotor activity, and for production of antinociception, hypothermia and catalepsy. Similarly, high correlations were demonstrated between binding affinity and *in vivo* potency in both the rat drug discrimination model and for psychotomimetic activity in humans. Therefore, these studies appear to indicate that the requirements for activation of the cannabinoid receptor are similar across different species, and that this receptor is sufficient to mediate many of the known pharmacological effects of cannabinoids. This binding site has also been characterized with $[^3H]$11-OH-hexahydrocannabinol-DMH (Devane, Breuer et al., 1992) and with $[^3H]$11-OH-Δ^8-THC-DMH (Thomas, Wei & Martin, 1992), and the findings are consistent with those reported for $[^3H]$CP-55,940.

Autoradiographic studies have shown a heterogeneous distribution in the brain that is conserved throughout a variety of mammalian species, including humans, with most of the sites being in the basal ganglia, hippocampus and cerebellum (Herkenham, Lynn et al., 1990; 1991b). Binding sites are also abundant in the cerebral cortex and striatum. It is interesting to speculate that these sites correlate with some of the pharmacological effects of marijuana, for example, cognitive impairment (hippocampus and cortex), ataxia (basal ganglia and cerebellum) and low toxicity (lack of receptors in the brainstem). Consistent results have been obtained when localization studies were conducted with $[^3H]$WIN 55,212 (Jansen, Haycock et al., 1992) and $[^3H]$11-OH-Δ^9-THC-DMH (Thomas, Wei & Martin, 1992).

Radioligand binding studies with $[^3H]$CP-55,940 in tissue homogenates and in tissue slices have shown that the receptor is localized primarily in the brain. An examination of [3H]CP-55,940 binding in all major peripheral organs of the rat resulted in detectable binding only in the immune system (Lynn & Herkenham, 1994). Binding was detected in B lymphocyte-enriched areas (marginal zone of the spleen, cortex of the lymph nodes and nodular corona of Peyer's patches), but not in T lymphocyte-enriched areas (thymus and periarteriolar lymphatic sheaths of the spleen) and macrophage-enriched areas (lung and liver). Earlier, investigators described cannabinoid receptor binding in mouse spleen that was consistent with THC inhibition of forskolin-stimulated cAMP accumulation in this tissue (Kaminski, Abood et al., 1992). Stereoselective immune modulation was observed with the enantiomers of CP-55,940 and 11-OH-Δ^8-THC-DMH. In both cases, the (–)-enantiomer demonstrated greater immunoinhibitory potency than the (+)-enantiomer, as measured by the *in vitro* sheep red blood cell antibody-forming cell response. Scatchard analysis of [3H]CP-55,940 binding demonstrated a single binding site with a KD of 910 pM and a Bmax of approximately 1,000 receptors per spleen cell.

RECEPTOR CLONING

Although receptor binding provided a compelling argument for the existence of a cannabinoid receptor, the cloning of the receptor provided the first definitive evidence (Matsuda, Lolait et al., 1990). These investigators used an oligonucleotide probe based on the G-protein-coupled receptor for substance K to isolate a clone from a rat brain library. This clone had homology with other G-protein-coupled receptors but was unique. Identification of the ligand for this "orphan receptor" involved the screening of candidate ligands until it was discovered that cannabinoids act at this site. In cells transfected with the clone, CP-55,940, THC and other psychoactive cannabinoids were found to inhibit adenylyl cyclase, whereas in untransfected cells no such response was found. Furthermore, the rank order of potency for inhibition of adenylyl cyclase in transfected cells correlated well with

cell lines previously shown to possess cannabinoid-inhibited adenylyl cyclase activity. Inactive cannabinoids failed to alter adenylyl cyclase in these transfected cells. Additionally, the distribution of the mRNA for the clone paralleled the intensity of cannabinoid receptor binding throughout the brain.

After the sequence for the cannabinoid receptor appeared, the nucleotide sequence of a human cannabinoid receptor cDNA was described (Gérard, Mollereau et al., 1990). The sequences of the rat and human cDNA's were 90 per cent identical at the nucleic acid level and 98 per cent identical at the amino acid level. These investigators subsequently expressed the human receptor in COS cells and demonstrated specific binding with [3H]CP-55,940 (Gérard, Mollereau et al., 1991). Additionally, message corresponding to this cDNA was also detected in dog, rat and guinea pig brain. Surprisingly, this message was also found in human testis. It was not found in dog stomach, spleen, kidney, liver, heart or lung, although there appeared to be traces in testis. The primary difference between localization of receptor message and previous receptor binding (Lynn & Herkenham, 1994) was the failure to detect message in spleen, an organ exhibiting receptor binding, and the failure to detect binding in testis. Species differences could account for some of these discrepancies, as well as the fact that expression of the receptor may fall below the levels of detectability.

Although multiple cannabinoid receptors have not been identified in the brain, a peripheral receptor has been identified that is structurally different from the brain receptor (Munro, Thomas & Abu-Shaar, 1993). This cloned receptor, expressed in macrophages in the marginal zone of the spleen, exhibits 44 per cent homology with the receptor reported earlier (Matsuda, Lolait et al., 1990). The homology rises to 68 per cent if only transmembrane domains are considered. These investigators examined a limited number of cannabinoids for binding properties which allowed them to draw the conclusion that this receptor was indeed cannabinoid. However, there appeared to be sufficient evidence that it differed from the receptor described by Matsuda et al. The cloning of this receptor is consistent with the findings of Kaminski et al. (1992) that spleen contains a cannabinoid binding site as well as mRNA for the cannabinoid receptor. It is too early to determine what functional role these cannabinoid receptors may play in the spleen. There is certainly the possibility that other receptor subtypes with entirely unique functional roles may exist.

Now that multiple receptor subtypes are known, it is imperative that a consistent receptor nomenclature be adopted. The receptor nomenclature committee of the International Union of Pharmacology (IUPHAR) recommends that the cannabinoid receptor be abbreviated as CB with a numerical subscript assigned according to the order of discovery. Using this nomenclature, the receptor cloned by Matsuda et al. (1990) is designated as CB_1 whereas that cloned by Munro et al. (1993) is CB_2.

Mountjoy et al. (1992) attempted to classify the CB_1 cannabinoid receptor within the category of G-protein-coupled receptors. As implied by the name, these receptors link the signal produced by receptor binding ligand to functional effect via GTP-binding or G proteins. The primary structural feature used to identify this receptor class is seven transmembrane domains. These investigators found that the cannabinoid receptors together with the recently cloned adrenocorticotropic hormone (ACTH) and melanocortin receptors, constitute a novel subgroup. This subset of receptors share the following structural similarities: (1) they lack the proline residues in the fourth and/or fifth membrane domains generally found in G-protein-coupled receptors (thought to introduce bends in the α-helical structure and participate in the binding pocket); (2) they lack one or both of the cysteine residues thought to form a disulfide bond between the first and second extracellular loops; and (3) the identity between receptors is 32 to 39 per cent. This homology is not much greater than the 20 per cent between the cannabinoid receptor and the cloned δ opioid receptor (Evans, Keith et al., 1992), the latter of which falls into the subclass consisting of peptide receptors. Therefore, assigning relevance to 30 per

cent homology must be done with caution. However, amino acids conserved between receptors that bind different ligands are targets for further investigation, such as through site-directed mutagenesis.

Second Messenger Systems

ADENYLYL CYCLASE

Typically, characterization of a receptor is followed by identification of a second messenger system. However, the opposite occurred with the cannabinoids when Howlett and Fleming (1984) first provided convincing evidence that cannabinoids inhibited forskolin-stimulated adenylyl cyclase. After ruling out the involvement of receptors traditionally found in neuroblastoma cells, they concluded that a unique cannabinoid receptor was coupled to the regulatory G-protein, G_i (Bidaut-Russell, Devane & Howlett, 1990; Howlett, 1985). The interaction of the cannabinoids with a membrane protein via ADP-ribosylation was shown to exhibit selectivity for neuroblastoma cells, but not lymphoma cells or rat sperm cytosol. The ribosylated protein was identified as the G_i protein (Howlett, Qualy & Khachatrian, 1986).

The ability of cannabinoid analogues to inhibit adenylyl cyclase correlates with their potency in several pharmacological assays, including antinociception, suggesting a cause-effect relationship (Howlett, Bidaut-Russell et al., 1990). Most of the efforts have concentrated on demonstrating a role for adenylyl cyclase in cannabinoid-induced antinociception (Howlett, Johnson et al., 1988). However, the potency of various cannabinoids to displace CP-55,940 binding and to inhibit adenylyl cyclase (Devane, Dysarz et al., 1988) has been shown to be similar in rank order to the production of not only antinociception, but also hypothermia, spontaneous activity and catalepsy by the cannabinoids (Little, Compton et al., 1988). The key link to G-proteins came when the cannabinoid receptor was cloned (Matsuda, Lolait et al., 1990). Transfection of CHO-K1 cells, which are unresponsive to cannabinoids, with the cDNA clone for the cannabinoid receptor transformed them into cells that were responsive to cannabinoid inhibition of cAMP accumulation (Matsuda, Lolait et al., 1990). Further credence to cannabinoid inhibition of adenylyl cyclase activity was provided by the findings that the aminoalkylindoles inhibited adenylyl cyclase activity in rat brain membranes (Pacheco, Childers et al., 1991) and by similar observations for anandamide (Felder, Briley et al., 1993; Vogel, Barg et al., 1993). Earlier, stable cell lines were created with both the rat and human cannabinoid receptor clones (Felder, Veluz et al., 1992). Comparison of the binding in membranes prepared from the transfected cell lines with those from rat cerebellum revealed similar affinities for $[^3H]CP-55,940$. The number of sites in the cell line expressing the human cannabinoid receptor was comparable to that of rat cerebellum (7.0 ± 0.5 pmol/mg versus 2.5 ± 0.3 pmol/mg), whereas the cell line expressing the rat receptor had a lower Bmax (0.34 ± 0.06 pmol/mg). Cannabinoid receptor-mediated inhibition of cAMP accumulation was observed in these cell lines.

Koe et al. (1997) examined the ramifications of cannabinoid attenuation of cAMP accumulation and discovered protein kinase A activity was also reduced along with suppression of transcription factor binding to cAMP-response element (CRE) sites. They concluded that the consequences of inhibition of adenylyl cyclase involved a decrease in the activation of transcription factors that bind to these CRE regulatory sites.

Monovalent cations are known for their modulatory role for G-protein/receptor coupling. In the case of cannabinoids, sodium is generally required for optimal inhibition of adenylyl cyclase by $G_{i/o}$-coupled receptors. However, Pacheco et al. (1994) found that agonists for both cannabinoid and $GABA_B$ receptors inhibited adenylyl cyclase which was sodium-independent in cerebellum but sodium-dependent in striatum. These investigators confirmed that this differential effect was not due to either the receptor or the effector. They postulated that different G-proteins could be coupled to adenylyl cyclase in these two brain regions thereby accounting for this differential cannabinoid effect.

While there is strong *in vitro* evidence for a cannabinoid receptor/adenylyl cyclase association, it has been more difficult to establish which pharmacological effects of cannabinoids are mediated through this pathway. Very early studies suggested that cannabinoid administration to rodents altered cAMP accumulation in brain; however, the effects were modest and frequently difficult to reproduce (Martin, Welch & Abood, 1994). Recently, Welch et al. (1995) demonstrated that pertussis toxin abolished the antinociceptive effects of cannabinoids in mice, and that forskolin and chloro-cAMP attenuated the antinociceptive effects of THC. These results support the involvement of adenylyl cyclase in the actions of cannabinoids, since these agents either elevate or mimic cAMP.

ION CHANNELS

There has been reasonable evidence supporting a role for cannabinoid modulation of neurotransmitter release (Dewey, 1986). Calcium is a likely mediator of this action based on its well-characterized role in neurotransmitter release and on the fact that many of the effects which have been produced by pertussis toxin could be due to G-proteins linked to either adenylyl cyclase or ion channels. Actually, there is evidence that THC decreases the release of acetylcholine presynaptically by decreasing the influx of calcium presynaptically (Kumbaraci & Nastuk, 1980). Moreover, cannabinoids decrease calcium uptake to several brain regions (Harris & Stokes, 1982). THC has also been shown to attenuate depolarization-induced rises in intracellular calcium at μM concentrations (Martin, Howlett & Welch, 1989). On the other hand, Okada et al. (1992) reported that 0.1 or 1 μM concentration of THC did not perturb calcium levels in rat brain. However, very low concentrations of THC (0.1 nM) have been shown to enhance potassium-stimulated rises in intracellular calcium, while intermediate concentrations (1 to 50 nM) of THC block potassium-stimulated rises in intracellular calcium. Electrophysiological studies in neuroblastoma cells indicated that 1 to 100 nM concentrations of several cannabinoids inhibited an omega conotoxin-sensitive, high voltage-activated calcium channel, an effect that was blocked by the administration of pertussis toxin and independent of the formation of cAMP. The cannabinoids were hypothesized to interact with an N-type calcium channel that would lead to a decrease in the release of neurotransmitters (Mackie & Hille, 1992). A similar study found that cannabinoids inhibit I_{Ca} current in neuroblastoma cells, an effect that was not dose-related, but was pertussis toxin- and omega conotoxin-sensitive (Caulfield & Brown, 1992).

Whereas several cannabinoid agonists have been shown to alter intracellular calcium, the involvement of the cannabinoid receptor has been questioned. In CHO (Chinese hamster ovary) cells, cannabinoids induced a non-specific release of intracellular calcium (Felder, Veluz et al., 1992). Both non-transfected and transfected CHO cells were able to release calcium, an effect that lacked stereoselectivity.

OTHER SECOND MESSENGERS

There is less compelling evidence for other second messenger systems. THC was reported to decrease the formation of myo-inositol trisphosphate (IP$_3$) in pancreatic islets (Chaudry, Thompson et al., 1988); however, there is no evidence that the effects of THC in brain or spinal cord are mediated through IP$_3$. While the binding of the cannabinoids in the cerebellar molecular layer co-localized with that of forskolin, protein kinase C distribution was not localized to these same areas (Herkenham, Lynn et al., 1991a). These studies support a role for cAMP rather than IP$_3$ in the actions of cannabinoids in the cerebellum. On the other hand, pituitary cGMP enhances the formation of inositol phosphates (Naor, 1990). It has been shown that the potent cannabinoid levonantradol, but not its inactive enantiomer dextronantradol, decreases basal and isoniazid-induced increases in cGMP in the cerebellum, possibly via an interaction with the release of gamma-aminobutyric acid (GABA) in the brain (Koe, Milne et al., 1985; Leader, Koe & Weisman, 1981). Thus, an interrelationship between IP$_3$ and cGMP formation could exist regarding cannabinoid action.

Bouaboula et al. (1995) have implicated mitogen-activated protein kinase in the actions of both CB$_1$ and CB$_2$ receptors. It appears that inhibition of cAMP production may be associated with CB$_2$ receptors but not with CB$_1$ receptors. Moreover, they provided some evidence that activation of both cannabinoid receptors leads to stimulation of *Knox*-24 expression.

Transfected cell lines have also been evaluated for other possible signal transduction systems (Felder, Veluz et al., 1992). Several studies suggested a role for cannabinoid agonists in arachidonic acid release and membrane phospholipid turnover. CP-55,940 was able to release [³H]arachidonic acid at concentrations greater than 100 µM, but it did so in non-transfected as well as transfected CHO cells. Furthermore, this action was not stereoselective. The investigators concluded that a cannabinoid receptor was not involved since high drug concentrations were required to stimulate release and the effect lacked stereoselectivity. On the other hand, Shivachar et al. (1996) demonstrated that both anandamide and THC were able to stimulate the release of arachidonic acid from cultured astrocytes in a concentration- and time-dependent fashion. These effects were pertussis toxin-sensitive and were attenuated by SR141716A, which implicated cannabinoid receptor involvement.

Endogenous Ligands

The isolation and characterization of anandamide as an endogenous ligand for the cannabinoid receptor represented the final component necessary for establishing the existence of a cannabinoid neurochemical system. Devane et al. (1992) reasoned that an endogenous cannabinoid should have the same physicochemical characteristics as THC and therefore sought to isolate putative ligands from lipid components of porcine brain. They succeeded in isolating anandamide which they found competed for cannabinoid receptor binding and inhibited electrically stimulated contractions of the mouse vas deferens in much the same manner as THC. In a subsequent publication, they demonstrated that anandamide administered peripherally to mice exhibited THC-like properties in producing hypomotility, hypothermia, antinociception and catalepsy (Fride & Mechoulam, 1993). Other investigators (Crawley, Corwin et al., 1993) also found a similar reduction in spontaneous activity and body temperature in mice treated with anandamide. Smith et al. (1994) conducted a thorough comparison between THC and anandamide and found anandamide to be four- to twentyfold less potent than THC, depending on the pharmacological measure, and to have a shorter duration of action. Anandamide is rapidly degraded by an amidase that can be blocked by phenylmethylsulfonyl fluoride (Deutsch & Chin, 1993).

Additional evidence that anandamide interacts with the cannabinoid G-protein-coupled receptor has emerged (Vogel, Barg et al., 1993). This group reported anandamide specifically binds to membranes from cells either transiently or stably transfected with an expression plasmid carrying the cannabinoid receptor DNA but not to membranes from control non-transfected cells. Moreover, anandamide inhibited the forskolin-stimulated adenylyl cyclase in transfected cells and in cells that naturally express cannabinoid receptors (N18TG2 neuroblastoma), but not in control non-transfected cells. These investigators also found that anandamide inhibited forskolin-stimulated adenylyl cyclase, an effect that was blocked by pretreatment with pertussis toxin. Felder et al. (1993) also found that anandamide inhibited forskolin-stimulated cAMP accumulation in CHO cells expressing the human cannabinoid receptor and that this response was blocked by pertussis toxin. N-Type calcium channels were inhibited by anandamide in N-18 neuroblastoma cells. Additionally, Mackie et al. (1993) reported that the inhibition of N-type calcium channels was voltage-dependent and N-ethylmaleimide-sensitive.

Van der Kloot (1994) reported that anandamide reversed the hypertonic gluconate-induced stimulation of the frequency of miniature endplate potentials in the frog neuromuscular junction. It was postulated that hypertonic gluconate stimulation involves activation of protein

kinase A, because Rp-cAMPS, a protein kinase A inhibitor, blocks this effect. However, increased frequency by Sp-cAMPS, a protein kinase activator, was not attenuated by anandamide. This investigator concluded that anandamide blocks adenylyl cyclase without directly altering protein kinase A and that a cannabinoid receptor is present in the frog neuromuscular junction.

Anandamide has also been reported to produce effects on the hypothalamo-pituitary-adrenal axis in the rat similar to those produced by THC (Weidenfeld, Feldman & Mechoulam, 1994). Anandamide administered intracerebroventricularly led to decreased CRF-41 levels in the median eminence and increased serum ACTH and corticosterone levels. The investigators were not able to implicate a specific mechanism for this cannabinoid action. However, it is well known that cannabinoids exhibit anxiogenic properties (Onaivi, Green & Martin, 1990), which could serve as the stimulus for CRF-41 release.

In order for anandamide to act as a neurotransmitter or neuromodulator, there should be appropriate synthetic and metabolic pathways for it. Deutsch and Chin (1993) provided the first description of the synthesis and metabolism of anandamide. They demonstrated that anandamide was readily taken up by neuroblastoma and glioma cells that rapidly degraded it. The degradative enzyme, an amidase, resides in the membranes rather than in the cytosol. Anandamide was also degraded by brain, liver, kidney and lung tissue but not heart or muscle. Synthesis was demonstrated by incubating arachidonate and ethanolamide in the presence of rat brain homogenate. Deutsch and Chin (1993) concluded that separate enzymes were responsible for synthesis and degradation since phenylmethylsulfonyl fluoride blocked degradation but not synthesis. Devane and Axelrod (1994) also found that brain (bovine) was capable of synthesizing anandamide when high concentrations of arachidonate and ethanolamide were added. Synthetic activity was greatest in hippocampus, more than twofold lower in thalamus, striatum and frontal cortex and five- to sixfold lower in cerebellum. It is noteworthy that synthetic activity is lowest in the brain area (cerebellum) with the greatest receptor density. In contrast to the finding of Deutsch and Chin (1993), Devane and Axelrod (1994) found that phenylmethylsulfonyl fluoride inhibits synthesis. There is also recent evidence that the metabolism of anandamide can be blocked by trifluoromethyl ketone, α-keto-ester and α-keto-amide analogues of anandamide by acting as transition-state inhibitors (Koutek, Prestwich et al., 1994). Based on their findings that the enzyme is CoA- and ATP-independent, Kruszka and Gross (1994) proposed that the synthesis of anandamide occurs via a novel eicosanoid pathway. While numerous questions remain regarding the synthesis and metabolism of anandamide in the brain, there is ample evidence to demonstrate that these critical biochemical events do occur.

There are two studies suggesting cellular uptake may be responsible for anandamide inactivation (Beltramo, Stella, et al., 1997; Hillard, Edgemond et al., 1997). Both studies demonstrated facilitated diffusion into cells. Beltramo et al. also demonstrated that this process involved a high-affinity transport system and that a specific anandamide analogue was capable of interfering with anandamide uptake. These observations are consistent with anandamide functioning as a neuromodulatory agent in the central nervous system.

There are several indications that endogenous cannabinoids other than anandamide may exist. Mechoulam's laboratory has isolated two other unsaturated fatty acid ethanolamides (homo-γ-linolenylethanolamide and docosatetraenylethanolamide) that bind to the cannabinoid receptor (Hanus, Gopher et al., 1993; Mechoulam, Hanus et al., 1994). Evans et al. (1994) described the calcium-stimulated release of a cannabinoid substance that differs physiochemically from anandamide. The most likely candidate for a second endogenous ligand is arachidonyl-2-glycerol (see Figure 1) that was originally isolated from canine gut (Mechoulam, Ben-Shabat et al., 1995). It was found to bind to cannabinoid receptors and produce weak cannabinoid effects *in vitro* and *in vivo*; soon thereafter, another research group detected it in brain (Sugiura, Kondo et al., 1995). Although it is not uncommon for a single endogenous substance, such as a neurotransmitter like dopamine, to interact with several receptor subtypes, there are other systems, for example, the opioids, composed of multiple endogenous ligands.

Antagonists

The search for antagonists eluded investigators until Rinaldi-Carmona et al. (1994) developed SR141716A (see Figure 3), which was found to have high affinity (Ki = 2 nM) for the CB_1 cannabinoid receptor but very low affinity for the CB_2 spleen receptor. It effectively antagonized cannabinoid-induced inhibition of adenylyl cyclase and neuronally stimulated smooth muscle contractions. More importantly, orally and intraperitoneally administered SR141716A antagonized cannabinoid-induced hypothermia, catalepsy and antinociception in mice, with high potency. It also appears that this antagonist is highly selective for the cannabinoid receptor because it failed to bind to histamine, dopamine, adrenergic, purinergic, adenosine, opioid,

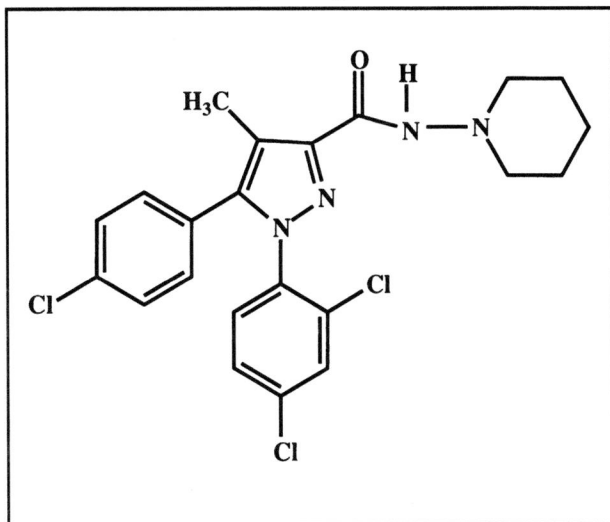

FIGURE 3.
Structure of the cannnabinoid antagonist SR141716A

neurotensin, cholecystokinin, benzodiazepine, sigma, tachykinin, serotonin or excitatory and inhibitory amino acid receptors. The discovery of this antagonist completes the basic requirements for a receptor system and provides a valuable tool for establishing the functional role of the cannabinoids in the central nervous system.

Interactions with Other Central Systems

The past 10 years of progress, as cited above, enable us to postulate that a cannabinoid neurochemical system exists. However, its role in the brain and its relationship to other neurochemical systems remains to be elucidated. In the absence of direct evidence for a primary functional role, it would seem that the cannabinoid system is largely neuromodulatory. Howlett et al. (1992) showed that adrenergic, dopaminergic, serotonergic and cholinergic agonists and antagonists do not bind directly to the CB_1 receptor. The evidence describing interactions between cannabinoids and the more traditional neurotransmitters has been discussed in several reviews (Dewey, 1986; Pertwee, 1990; 1992). Cannabinoids have been shown to enhance the formation of norepinephrine, dopamine and serotonin. They have also been reported to stimulate the release of dopamine from rat corpus striatum, nucleus accumbens and medial prefrontal cortex. Cannabinoids have also been reported to enhance the turnover of GABA. Interpretation of the actions of cannabinoids on neurotransmitter synthesis has not been straightforward because there is evidence that they also inhibit as well as stimulate neurotransmitter neuronal reuptake. Pertwee also summarized the evidence that cannabinoids can potentiate the actions of norepinephrine, acetylcholine and GABA by altering their receptors or second messenger systems. Cannabinoids reportedly interact synergistically with cholinergic agonists in the production of catalepsy, tremor, circling, salivation, lacrimation, hypothermia and drinking, and with GABA agonists in the production of catalepsy, excitement, hypothermia and antinociception (Pertwee, 1990).

It has been reported that anandamide acts in a fashion similar to that of other cannabinoids to enhance GABAergic transmission (Wickens & Pertwee, 1993). It seems that the anandamide system, like most other receptor-transmitter systems in living organisms, interacts quite extensively with other mediators. It may be more than a curious coincidence that in patients with Huntington's disease, both D_1 and cannabinoid receptors are lost in the substantia nigra (Glass, Faull & Dragunow, 1993). Dopaminergic regulation of cannabinoid receptor mRNA levels in rat caudate-putamen has also been reported (Mailleux & Vanderhaeghen, 1993a). Interactions between the dopaminergic system and the anandamide system(s) have now been documented (Chen, Marmur et al., 1993; Gardner & Lowinson, 1991; Navarro, Fernandez-Ruiz et al., 1993; Rodríguez de Fonseca, Hernandez et al., 1992).

THC can induce certain endocrine changes, such as stimulation of adrenocortical function (Dewey, 1986). Eldridge and Landfield (1990; 1992) have described the influence of cannabinoids on glucocorticoid receptors in the central nervous system. One of the most notable observations was that THC administration induced aging-like degenerative changes in rat brain similar to those resulting from elevated corticosterone (Landfield, Cadwallader & Vinsant, 1988). These investigators also demonstrated that THC competes for glucocorticoid binding in a non-competitive fashion and that chronic THC administration reduces glucocorticoid binding in the hippocampus (Eldridge & Landfield, 1992). Weidenfeld et al. (1994) have now found that intracerebroventricular injection of anandamide (50 to 150 µg/rat) significantly increases serum levels of ACTH and corticosterone in a dose-dependent manner and causes pronounced depletion of CRF-41 in the median eminence. These data suggest that anandamide parallels THC in activating the hypothalamo-pituitary-adrenal axis via mediation of a central mechanism which involves the secretion of CRF-41. It is of interest that the caudate-putamen of adrenalectomized rats contains 50 per cent higher levels of mRNA for the cannabinoid receptor than the controls. This increase could be counteracted by dexamethasone (Mailleux & Vanderhaeghen, 1993b). Taken together with the findings of Weidenfeld and colleagues, it seems possible that the corticoid and anandamide systems could be mutually regulatory. However, numerous criteria have to be satisfied before such an assumption will be acceptable.

The above discussion clearly identifies several, but not all, neuronal systems that likely play major roles in the actions of the cannabinoids. Separating the direct and indirect actions of the cannabinoids has not been easy. Given the complexity of the neuronal substrates for most behavioral effects, it is not surprising that several neurotransmitter systems have been implicated in each of the cannabinoid behavioral effects. Additional progress will be required before the interrelationships of cannabinoid and neurotransmitter systems are fully appreciated.

Relationship of Blood Concentrations of THC to Pharmacological Effects

The pharmacokinetics of THC dictates the mode of marijuana use. THC is readily absorbed when marijuana is smoked. Although oral ingestion of marijuana produces similar pharmacological effects, THC is absorbed somewhat more slowly this way compared to the smoking route. THC is metabolized in humans by a variety of oxidative routes first producing hydroxylated metabolites, followed by conversion to carboxy acids with subsequent excretion as conjugates. Figure 4 illustrates a simplified metabolic scheme for THC. The metabolite, 11-hydroxy-THC, is active (Lemberger, Weiss et al., 1972); however, it is only formed in trace amounts when marijuana is smoked. Greater amounts of 11-hydroxy-THC may be formed after oral ingestion. About 50 per cent of a dose of THC is excreted in feces and 15 per cent is excreted in urine over a period of several days (Wall, Sadler et al., 1983). The primary metabolite excreted in urine is conjugated 11-*nor*-9-carboxy-THC. Glucuronide conjugates of THC and 11-hydroxy-THC were recently identified in urine (Kemp, Abukhalaf et al., 1995). Pharmacological effects are produced rapidly and generally peak within 30 minutes of the onset of smoking. Impairment on various performance measures related to driving skills has been demonstrated immediately following marijuana usage and up to 24 hours thereafter. Generally, behavioral and physiological effects return to baseline levels four to six hours after usage. Blood concentrations of THC peak prior to drug-induced effects, leading to a counterclockwise hysteresis between blood concentrations of THC and pharmacological effects. This time discordance between blood concentrations of THC and effects has led numerous investigators, who were searching for linear correlations, to conclude that no meaningful relationships

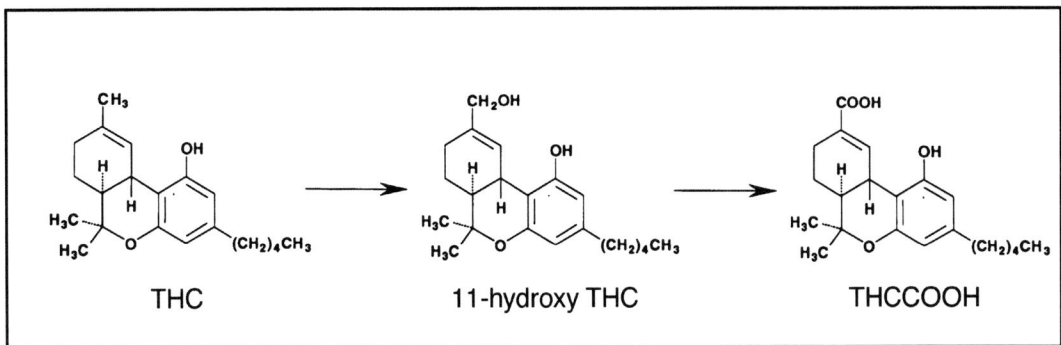

FIGURE 4.
Metabolic profile of THC

exist between blood concentrations and effects (Mason & McBay, 1985; McBay, 1986). Fortunately, the technology for measuring THC and metabolites in biological fluids and tissues has improved along with an understanding of underlying principles governing distribution of lipophilic substances, such as THC, in mammalian systems. Newly developed pharmacokinetic/pharmacodynamic models allow investigators to relate concentrations of THC in blood and other body compartments to physiological, behavioral and performance changes produced by marijuana. Mathematical models have also been developed to assist forensic toxicologists and medical examiners in the prediction of time elapsed since marijuana use based on data obtained from the analysis of a single blood sample for THC and metabolites.

Analytical Methodology

The detection and measurement of THC and metabolites in biological fluids and tissues can be performed by a variety of analytical techniques. Frequently, initial detection methods are based on thin layer chromatography (TLC) and immunoassays including radioimmunoassay (RIA), enzyme immunoassay (EIA), fluorescence polarization immunoassay (FPIA), and kinetic interaction of microparticles in solution (KIMS). Most commercial immunoassays have been developed for the detection of 11-*nor*-9-carboxy-THC in urine at cutoff concentrations of 20, 50 or 100 ng/mL; however, the antibodies employed in these assays display varying degrees of cross-reactivity with other cannabinoids. Consequently, there is sometimes a need to employ analytical techniques with greater specificity (e.g., high-performance liquid chromatography [HPLC], gas chromatography/mass spectrometry [GC/MS]) than provided by immunoassay. Reviews of laboratory methods for cannabinoids have been reported by Cook (1986) and King et al. (1987) and an excellent monograph on this topic has appeared (Hawks, 1982). A report by Gjerde (1991) advocated the use of EIA as a screening assay for THC in blood.

Blood samples obtained from impaired drivers were tested by EIA and GC/MS. When a cutoff concentration of 50 nM 11-*nor*-9- carboxy-THC (17 ng/mL) was used, 86 per cent of positive samples were confirmed for THC by GC/MS at concentrations above 1 nM (0.3 ng/mL).

More specific analytical methods for the determination of THC and metabolites in biological fluids include the use of HPLC and GC/MS. HPLC coupled with electrochemical detection was utilized for the measurement of THC in plasma and saliva (Thompson & Cone, 1987) and 11-*nor*-9-carboxy-THC in urine and plasma (Nakahara, Sekine & Cook, 1989). GC/MS has been utilized for the measurement of a wide variety of cannabinoids in biological fluids and provides excellent sensitivity and specificity (Foltz, McGinnis and Chinn, 1983). Goldberger and Cone (1994) reviewed the use of GC/MS as a confirmatory test for drugs in the workplace, and Foltz et al. (1983) reviewed methods of cannabinoid analyses by GC/MS, including specimen work-up, derivatization methods and assay performance characteristics.

THC's high potency and extensive metabolism in mammalian organisms may result in sensitivity limits below 1 ng/mL to be required in pharmacokinetic studies. One of the most sensitive GC/MS methods for the measurement of THC, 11-hydroxy-THC and 11-*nor*-9-carboxy-THC was reported by Foltz et al. (1983) who utilized negative ion chemical ionization techniques. Cannabinoid extracts were derivatized as methyl ester trifluoroacetate derivatives. Sensitivity limits of 0.2 ng/mL for THC, 0.5 ng/mL for 11-hydroxy-THC and 0.1 ng/mL for 11-*nor*-9-carboxy-THC were achieved for reliable measurement of these analytes in biological specimens. Another method utilized by Harvey et al. (1980) involved metastable ion monitoring of methylated trimethylsilyl derivatives of THC in plasma to achieve low picogram sensitivity. Biological samples containing THC as low as 5 pg/mL could be accurately measured, allowing detection of THC in plasma of marijuana users more than one week later.

Pharmaycokinetics of THC and Metabolites

APPEARANCE AND DISAPPEARANCE OF THC AND METABOLITES IN BLOOD

THC is absorbed rapidly and efficiently via the inhalation route, because each puff represents a small bolus of drug that is delivered to the circulatory system via the capillary bed surrounding the alveolar sacs of the lungs. Huestis and colleagues (1992) reported measuring detectable amounts of THC (7 to 18 ng/mL) following a single puff of marijuana smoke in individuals smoking marijuana (1.75 and 3.55 per cent THC content). Following a series of puffs, peak THC concentrations developed prior to the termination of smoking (see Figure 5). Similar findings had been reported by others (Perez-Reyes, Owens & Di Guiseppi, 1981). When experienced users smoked marijuana cigarettes containing 1.32, 1.97 and 2.54 per cent THC, peak concentrations developed in excess of 100 ng/mL (Cocchetto, Owens et al., 1981; Huestis, Sampson et al., 1992; Lemberger, Weiss et al., 1972; Ohlsson, Lindgren et al., 1980; Perez-Reyes, Di Guiseppi et al., 1982), although there was considerable intersubject variability. Obviously, the dynamics of smoking substantially influences how much drug is absorbed. The number of puffs, spacing, hold time, and lung capacity contribute to this variance. In addition, the rapid onset of effects may allow an individual to adjust subsequent puffs for greater or lesser effects as desired.

Distribution of THC begins to occur immediately on absorption. As shown in Figure 5, mean THC concentrations declined by 50 per cent approximately 10 minutes after the peak was reached following smoking marijuana. Thereafter, concentrations declined much more slowly and remained detectable for at least four hours. Much longer detection times for THC have been reported, particularly in studies in which sensitive analytical methodologies were utilized. Concentrations of deuterium-labelled THC in plasma of chronic marijuana users were detected for 13 days by GC/MS operating in the selected ion monitoring mode (Johansson, Agurell et al., 1988).

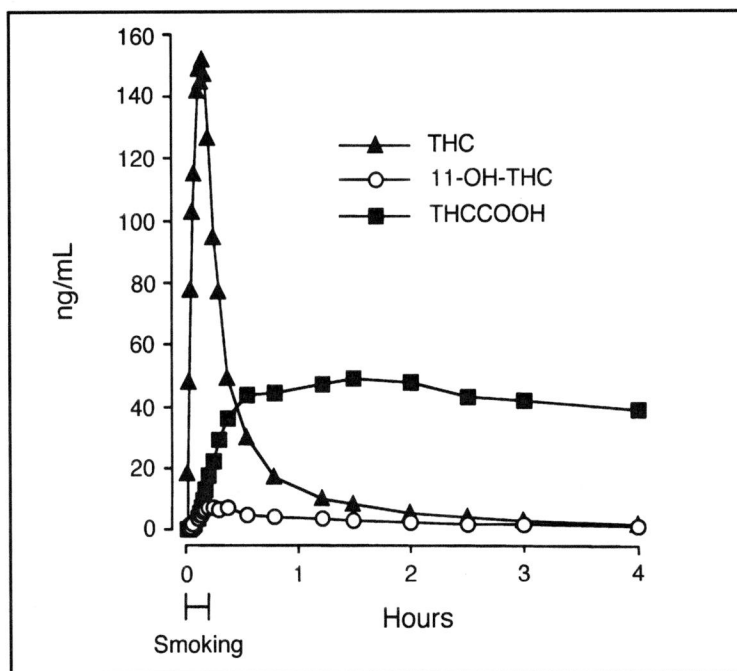

SOURCE.
From "Blood cannabinoids: II. Models for the prediction of time of marijuana exposure from plasma concentrations of Δ^9-tetrahydrocannabinol (THC) and 11-*nor*-9-carboxy-Δ^9-tetrahydrocannabinol (THCCOOH)," by M.A. Huestis, J.E. Henningfield & E.J. Cone, 1992, *Journal of Analytical Toxicology, 16,* pp. 283–290. Reprinted by permission of Preston Publications, a division of Preston Industries, Inc.

FIGURE 5.
Mean plasma concentrations of THC, 11-OH-THC and THCCOOH during and after smoking a single 3.55 per cent THC marijuana cigarette

Oral ingestion of THC or marijuana leads to the production of similar pharmacological effects as smoking, although substantial differences exist in the rate of onset of effects and in the amounts of cannabinoids appearing in blood. Oral administration of THC to women (15 mg) and men (20 mg) resulted in a gradual increase in blood levels of THC over a period of four to six hours (Wall, Sadler et al., 1983). Peak concentrations of THC were in the 10 to 15 ng/mL range. Concurrent 11-hydroxy-THC concentrations were in the range of 1 to 6 ng/mL. Concentrations of 11-*nor*-9-carboxy-THC were approximately twofold greater than those observed following intravenous dosing of THC.

Marijuana plant material cooked in brownies and consumed by male volunteers has also been studied (Cone, Johnson et al., 1988). Subjects ate the equivalent of one or two standard research grade marijuana cigarettes (2.8 per cent THC) mixed in brownies. Placebo marijuana mixed in brownies served as a control. Subjects scored significantly higher on behavioral measures after consumption of brownies containing marijuana than placebo, but the effects were slow to appear and were variable. Urinalysis by immunoassay and by GC/MS indicated that substantial amounts of 11-*nor*- 9-carboxy-THC were excreted in urine over a period of 3 to 14 days.

The metabolism of THC to 11-hydroxy-THC and to 11-*nor*-9-carboxy-THC occurs rapidly following smoking with peak blood concentrations of 11-hydroxy-THC appearing shortly after peak THC concentrations. Peak 11-*nor*-9-carboxy-THC concentrations appear later (one to two hours) and decline slowly thereafter (see Figure 5). Table 2 summarizes concentrations and times of appearance and disappearance of these analytes reported by Huestis et al. (1992b). Similar results were reported earlier following intravenous injection of THC in men and women (Wall, Sadler et al., 1983).

TABLE 2.

Mean Peak Plasma Drug Levels, Mean Time to Peak Drug Levels, Mean Detection Times for THC, 11-OH-THC, and THCOOH, and Mean Plasma Concentrations after the First Marijuana Inhalation

Analyte (% THC smoked)	Peak level (ng/mL)	Time to peak (hr)	Detection time (hr)	Levels after 1st puff (ng/mL)
THC				
1.75	84.3 (50–129)	0.14 (0.10–0.17)	7.2 (3–12)	7.0 (0–20)
3.55	162.2 (76–267)	0.14 (0.08–0.17)	12.5 (6-27)	18.1 (1.8–37.0)
11-OH-THC				
1.75	6.7 (3.3–10.4)	0.25 (0.15–0.38)	4.5 (0.54–12)	0.2 (0–1.2)
3.55	7.5 (3.8-16.0)	0.20 (0.15–0.25)	11.2 (2.2–27)	0
THCCOOH				
1.75	24.5 (15–54)	2.43 (0.8–4.0)	84.0 (48–168)	0.2 (0–1.1)
3.55	54.0 (22–101)	1.35(0.54–2.21)	52.0 (72–168)	0.2 (0–1.0)

SOURCE.

From "Blood cannabinoids: II. Models for the prediction of time of marijuana exposure from plasma concentrations of Δ^9-tetrahydrocannabinol (THC) and 11-*nor*-9-carboxy-Δ^9-tetrahydrocannabinol (THCCOOH)," by M.A. Huestis, J.E. Henningfield & E.J. Cone, 1992, *Journal of Analytical Toxicology*, *16*, pp. 283–290. Reprinted by permission of Preston Publications, a division of Preston Industries, Inc.

TABLE 3.
Pharmacokinetic Parameters of THC

Subjects	Drug/THC Dose	Route	Bioavailability (%)	Pharmacokinetic model	Half-life (hr)	Clearance (mL/min)	Reference
Men	THC/4 mg	IV	–	2-compartment	36	–	Wall, Sadler et al., 1983
	THC/20 mg	Oral	19	–	25	–	
Women	THC/2.2 mg	V	–	2-compartment	29	–	
	THC/15 mg	Oral	10.9	–	25	–	
Heavy users	THC/5 mg	IV	–	–	–	–	Ohlsson, Lindgren et al., 1982
	MJ/10 mg	Smoke	27	–	–	980	
Light users	THC/5 mg	IV	–	–	–	–	
	MJ/10 mg	Smoke	14	–	–	950	
Heavy users	THC/5 mg	IV					Lindgren, Ohlsson et al., 1981
	MJ/13 mg	Smoke	23				
Light users	THC/5 mg	IV					
	MJ/13 mg	Smoke	0				
Heavy users	THC/5 mg	IV	–		1.9	777	Kelly & Jones, 1992
Light users	THC/5 mg	IV	–		1.6	771	
Heavy users	THC/0.5 mg	IV	–	2-compartment	28	–	Lemberger, Tamarkin et. al., 1971
Non-users	THC/0.5 mg	IV	–	2-compartment	57	–	
Acute	THC/2	IV		4-compartment	19.6	–	Hunt & Jones, 1980
Chronic	THC/2	IV	–	4-compartment	18.7	651-197	
Men	THC/5 mg	IV	–	–	–	–	Ohlsson, Lindgren et al., 1980
	THC/20 mg	Oral	6	–	–	–	
	MJ/1.64% THC	Smoke	18	–	–	–	
Chronic	MJ/15 mg	Smoke	–	–	4.1 days	–	Johansson, Ohlsson et al., 1987
Acute	MJ/1% THC	Smoke	–	3-compartment	–	–	Barnett, Chiang et al., 1982

Note: THC=tetrahydrocannabinol; MJ=marijuana

SOURCE.
From "Relating blood concentrations of tetrahydrocannabinol and metabolites to pharmacologic effects and time of marihuana usage," by E.J. Cone & M.A. Huestis, 1993, *Therapeutic Drug Monitoring, 15,* pp. 527–532. Reprinted by permission of Raven Press.

PHARMACOKINETIC MODELS

Descriptive mathematical models of THC aid in the understanding of marijuana use. The initial increase in THC blood concentrations during smoking is followed by rapid redistribution to tissues. Subsequent re-entry into the circulation occurs slowly, resulting in a prolonged elimination half-life. A number of kinetic models have been proposed to describe plasma THC data, because of THC's complex distribution and elimination phases. A summary of pharmacokinetic parameters for THC following oral ingestion, intravenous infusion, and smoked marijuana is shown in Table 3. The blood curve for THC for the first six hours after smoking was described by a triexponential function (Barnett, Chiang et al., 1982). Disposition of THC was described empirically as being represented by a two-compartment model with first order input from smoking. Others have utilized two- and four-compartment models to describe the disposition of THC administered intravenously.

Plasma half-life estimates for THC range from 18 hours to 4 days. This variance in the terminal half-life of THC was likely due to a number of factors, including the variation in sensitivity of early assays and lack of extended sampling periods. When more sensitive GC/MS assays have been utilized for measurement of the terminal phase of THC elimination, the half-lives have been substantially longer. Estimates for THC clearance from blood have been less variable and ranged from 650 to 1000 mL/min. Oral bioavailability of THC appears to be lower (6.0 to 19.0 per cent) than THC from smoked marijuana (14 to 27 per cent). The low bioavailability of oral THC is likely due to extensive metabolism in its first pass through the liver prior to entering circulation. THC from smoked marijuana is lost due to an entirely different mechanism. Substantial losses occur during smoking as a result of pyrolysis, diversion via side-stream, and deposition in the cigarette butt, oral cavity and mucosa. The experience of the smoker appears to play a key role in the bioavailability of THC. For example, individuals inhaling smoke from 4.5 per cent THC marijuana cigarettes had a mean area-under-the-plasma curve (AUC) for THC of 5,515 compared to 3,127 for 1.3 per cent THC cigarettes (Perez-Reyes, 1985). The expected AUC ratio based on the relative potency of the two cigarettes was 3.6:1, whereas the observed AUC ratio was 1.8:1. This discrepancy led to speculation that the smokers could sense the rate of appearance and intensity of their "high" and titrate their intake accordingly. Ohlsson et al. (1980) reported that heavy marijuana users smoked more efficiently (23 to 27 per cent bioavailability) than light smokers (10 to 14 per cent bioavailability) and concluded that the experienced smokers utilized a more adept smoking technique, for example, deeper inhalations, than the inexperienced smokers. Two studies to assess pharmacokinetic differences between heavy and light cannabis users reported that there was a trend for heavy users to exhibit lower plasma concentrations than light users, but the differences were not statistically significant (Lindgren, Ohlsson et al., 1981; Ohlsson, Lindgren et al., 1982).

Pharmacodynamics of Marijuana

PHYSIOLOGY AND BEHAVIOR

Marijuana produces a plethora of physiological and behavioral effects in humans when administered by smoking and oral routes. Although these effects are described in detail in other chapters, a summary of prominent effects often noted following acute exposure is shown in Table 4 in approximate order associated with increasing doses of THC (Jones, 1980). Chronic effects of marijuana are also listed, but such studies are difficult to perform and much less is understood regarding long-term effects of marijuana.

TABLE 4.

Acute and Chronic Pharmacologic Effects of Marijuana

Pharmacologic effects of acute marijuana exposure

- Mood elevation
- Euphoria
- Tachycardia
- Blood pressure effects
- Conjunctival reddening
- Decreased skin temperature
- Decreased intraocular pressure
- Bronchodilatation
- Memory effects
- Altered time perception
- Psychomotor and perceptual impairment
- Paranoia
- Hallucinations, delusions

Pharmacologic effects of chronic marijuana exposure

- Apathy
- Impairment of judgment
- Inhibition of spermatogenesis
- Bronchitis and asthma
- Tolerance

Note: Acute effects are listed in approximate order of increasing dose of THC.

When marijuana is smoked by non-tolerant individuals, physiological and behavioral effects appear rapidly. Huestis and colleagues (1992) found that subjects displayed mean peak heart rate increases (N = 6) of 46.0 ± 18.6 and 55.8 ± 22.2 beats per minute over baseline levels following the smoking of a single 1.75 per cent or 3.55 per cent THC cigarette, respectively. Peak effects occurred at 17.4 ± 4.8 and 13.8 ± 4.2 minutes after initiation of smoking of the low- or high-dose cigarette. Maximum effects were recorded within four to six minutes after the last puff of marijuana smoke.

The euphoria or subject-rated "high" reported from marijuana smoking occurs after the end of smoking. Time lapses of 5 to 20 minutes from the end of smoking have been reported in earlier studies (Cocchetto, Owens et al., 1981; Hollister, Gillespie et al., 1981; Lemberger, Weiss et al., 1972; Lindgren, Ohlsson et al., 1981; Perez-Reyes, Di Guiseppi et al., 1982). However, in a study of the rapid onset of marijuana effects following smoking, Huestis and colleagues (Huestis, Sampson et al., 1992) reported that peak subjective effects appeared concurrently or within minutes of smoking. Three of six subjects reported increases in drug "liking" scores after the first puff, 15 seconds after smoking began. All subjects reported increases after the second puff of the high dose (3.55 per cent THC) cigarette and maximum drug liking was reported at 10.2 minutes (eight puffs).

PERFORMANCE, MEMORY AND COGNITION

The feelings of well-being and euphoria induced by marijuana are accompanied by signs of central nervous system depression along with some stimulatory components (Dewey, 1986). This unique profile of pharmacological effects complicates the overt characterization of marijuana's effects on behavior. Many studies have addressed the issue of whether marijuana exerts detrimental effects on cognitive functions, psychomotor performance and memory, and these topics have been reviewed (Chait & Pierri, 1992; Ferraro, 1980; Murray, 1986). Generally, decrements in information processing, cognition and memory tests have been reported as a result of acute marijuana exposure

(Braff, Silverton et al., 1981; Heishman, Stitzer & Bigelow, 1988; Moskowitz, 1984; Moskowitz, Sharma & McGlothlin, 1972; Schaefer, Gunn & Dubowski, 1977; Solowij, Michie & Fox, 1991; Tinklenberg, Kopell et al., 1972; Wilson, Ellinwood et al., 1994), but some investigators have failed to demonstrate significant effects on some measures (Heishman, Stitzer & Bigelow, 1988; Huestis, Sampson et al., 1992). Effects were usually short-lived and disappeared within four to eight hours; however, Heishman et al. (1990) reported decreased accuracy and increased response time on arithmetic and digit recall tasks up to 24 hours after subjects smoked two and four marijuana cigarettes (2.57 per cent THC). Plasma THC concentrations were also measured in this study (Heishman, Huestis et al., 1990). As shown in Figure 6, THC plasma concentrations parallelled subjective "high" and heart rate and were predictive of digit recall accuracy.

Psychomotor performance decrements have been reported (Bird, Boleyn et al., 1980; Cone, Johnson et al., 1986; Heishman, Huestis et al., 1990; Manno, Kiplinger et al., 1970; 1971), but the effects have been variable and often slight when compared to alcohol-induced impairment. Heishman et al. (1988) compared the effects of three doses of marijuana (0, 1.3, 2.7 per cent THC) to three doses of alcohol (0, 0.6 and 1.2 g/kg) in six male subjects with histories of moderate alcohol and marijuana use. The study was performed in a double-blind randomized cross-over design. The results of that study are illustrated in Figures 7 and 8. Alcohol produced dose-related elevations on subjective measures of drug effect. Impairment was produced by alcohol on circular lights, tracking and digit-symbol substitution (DSST) tasks. In contrast, although marijuana produced elevations on subjective measures, there was minimal effect on performance measures. Marijuana did not significantly impair response accuracy on the DSST, but did produce significant slowing. Unfortunately, blood levels were not measured and it is possible that the doses administered in this study were low compared to those normally used. Also, the performance tasks may not have been suitable for

FIGURE 6.

Temporal relationship between plasma THC concentration and per cent correct trials on digit recall task (top panel), heart rate (middle panel) and subjective rating of drug high (bottom panel) for Subject NU in drug condition 3. Arrows indicate time of administration of one active and one placebo marijuana cigarette in the morning (0900) and afternoon (1300) on day 1.

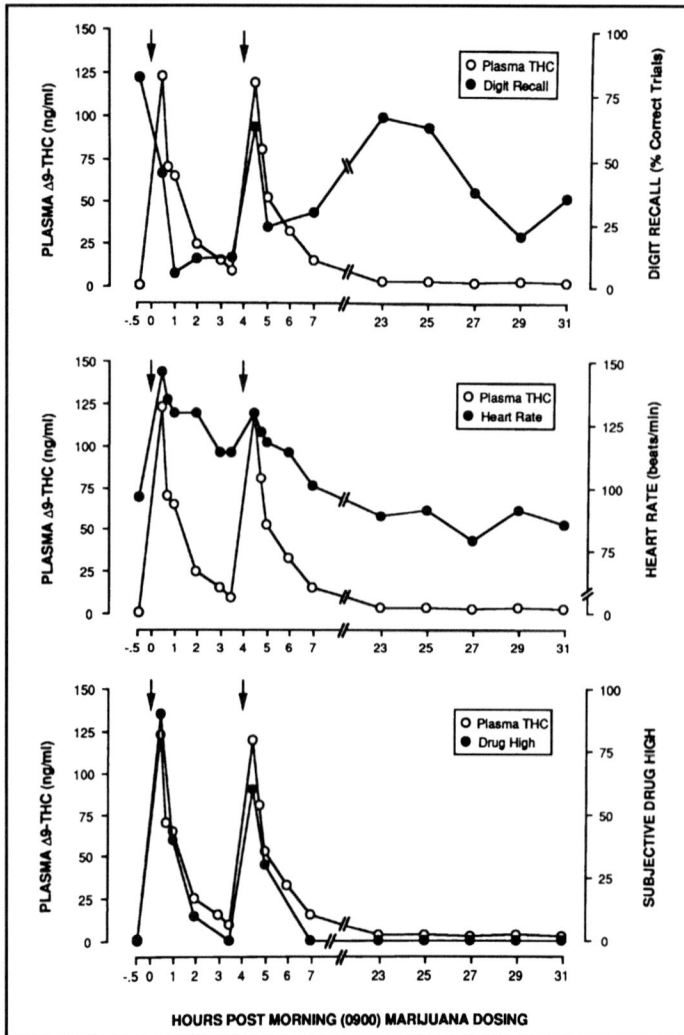

SOURCE.

From "Acute and residual effects of marijuana: Profiles of plasma, THC levels, physiological, subjective, and performance measures," by S.J. Heishman, M. Huestis, J. Henningfield & E. Cone, 1990, *Pharmacology, Biochemistry and Behavior, 37*, pp. 561–565. Reprinted by permission of Pergamon Press.

most clearly demonstrated when complex psychomotor-cognitive tasks are performed.

The combined use of marijuana and alcohol produces performance decrements greater than when either drug is administered alone (Bird, Boleyn et al., 1980; Manno, Kiplinger et al., 1971; Perez-Reyes, Hicks et al., 1988). Neither drug appeared to affect blood concentrations of the other drug when administered in combination (Bird, Boleyn et al., 1980; Perez-Reyes, Hicks et al., 1988). In the study by Perez-Reyes et al., it was concluded that "decrements due to ethanol in performance of skills necessary to drive an automobile were significantly enhanced by marijuana in an additive and perhaps synergistic manner."

MARIJUANA'S EFFECTS ON DRIVING AND FLYING

Driving an automobile is a complex task that requires psychomotor co-ordination, skill, memory, orientation in time and space, concentration and vigilance. Experienced drivers have described city-driving as "a tedious, rote-memory operation occasionally punctuated by moments of sheer terror." The effects of marijuana on driving skills can be variable. Performance decrements become increasingly more evident with higher marijuana doses, in combination with alcohol and with increasing task-situational demand. Moskowitz (1984) provided an elegant description of two attention tasks, vigilance and divided attention, that were useful for laboratory evaluation of drug effects on

optimal assessment of marijuana's effects on performance. Most investigators have concluded that the effects of marijuana are dose-related and

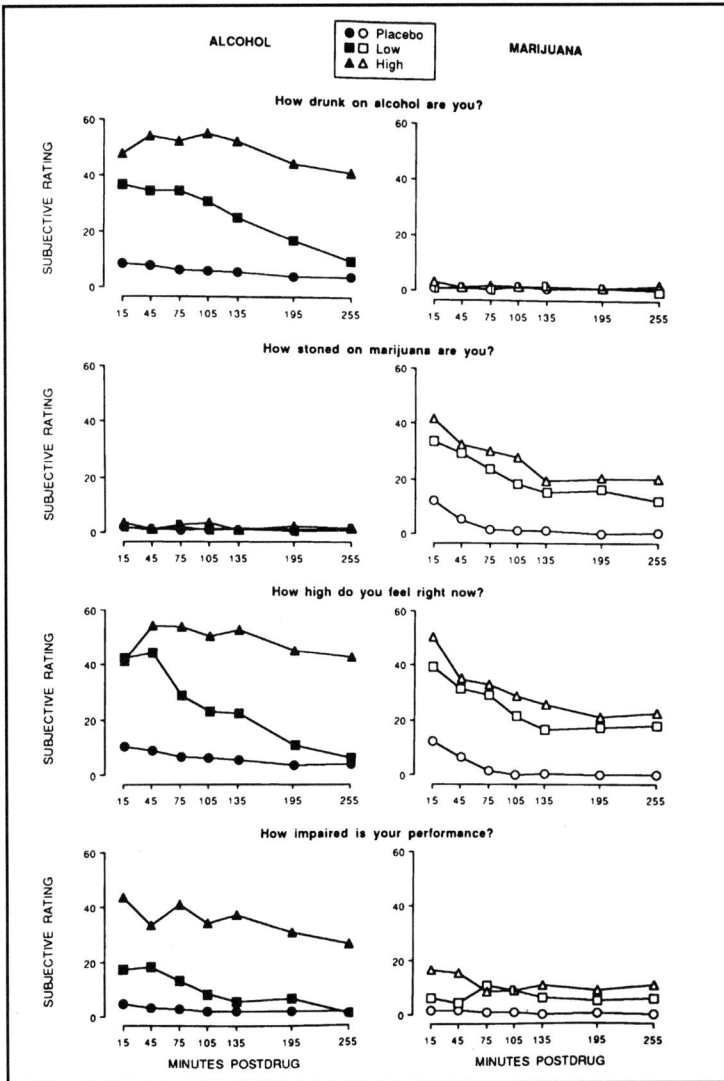

FIGURE 7.

Time course date of four subjective report questions for three doses of oral alcohol (left column) and three doses of smoked marijuana (right column). Alcohol doses were 0, 0.6 and 1.2 g/kg 95 per cent ethanol. Marijuana doses were 16 puffs from cigarettes containing 0, 1.3 and 2.7 per cent THC. Data points are adjusted for predrug baseline values and represent means of six subjects.

SOURCE.

From "Alcohol and marijuana: Comparative dose effect profiles in humans," by S.J. Heishman, M.L. Stitzer & G.E. Bigelow, 1988, *Pharmacology, Biochemistry and Behavior, 31,* pp. 649–655. Reprinted by permission of Pergamon Press.

information overload. Earlier studies indicated that the divided-attention task was sensitive to the presence of ethanol, whereas marijuana impaired vigilance behavior (Moskowitz, Sharma & McGlothlin, 1972).

Other researchers also have reported that marijuana impaired performance in simulated driving tests (Perez-Reyes, Hicks et al., 1988; Rafaelsen, Bech & Rafaelsen, 1973; Smiley, Moskowitz & Ziedman, 1985), closed course tasks (Attwood, Williams et al., 1981; Hansteen, Miller & Lonero, 1976) and driving in real-life situations (Klonoff, 1974). A variety of effects were noted in these studies including reductions in task accuracy, prolongation of reaction time, reduction in lane position control, impaired ability to follow a lead car, increased crashes, increased brake time and start time. However, not all subjects showed impairment. A few subjects demonstrated improved performance with marijuana, possibly as a result of overcompensation for the sedative effects of the drug. In one study of nine male graduate students who participated in an evaluation of the effects of alcohol (0.06 per cent), and marijuana (2 per cent THC), administered separately and in combination, no significant impairment was evident from either alcohol or marijuana administered alone (Sutton, 1983). Significant impairment was recorded from

humans performing tedious, repetitive tasks, but needing to respond appropriately to important cues, as required in industrial work, driving or flying and for emergency situations in which there is combined alcohol and marijuana administration. The author noted that the controlled obstacle course used in the driving trials had few manoeuvres to test perception and attention. Moskowitz (1985) has noted that the perceptual demands of driving are particularly sensitive to the effects of marijuana.

Flying, like driving, is a complex series of tasks requiring a high level of perceptual and motor skills at times of high demand. Janowsky et al. (1976) evaluated the effects of smoked marijuana (2.1 per cent THC, 0.09 mg/kg) on 10 certified airplane pilots in a flight simulator under placebo-controlled conditions. All 10 pilots showed significant impairment of flying performance 30 minutes after smoking. Errors were principally associated with deviations in altitude and heading from the assigned flight path. A non-significant decrease in flying ability also was noted for 6 of the pilots two hours after smoking marijuana. Performance returned to baseline by four hours. The effects of marijuana on short-term memory and sense of time were particularly prominent in this study. The authors noted that 30 minutes after smoking, pilots often forgot where they were in a given flight sequence or had difficulty recounting how long they had been performing a specific manoeuvre, in spite of the presence of a stopwatch and written instructions.

FIGURE 8.

Time course data of four performance measures for three doses of oral alcohol (left column) and three doses of smoked marijuana (right column). Data points are adjusted for predrug baseline values and represent means of six subjects.

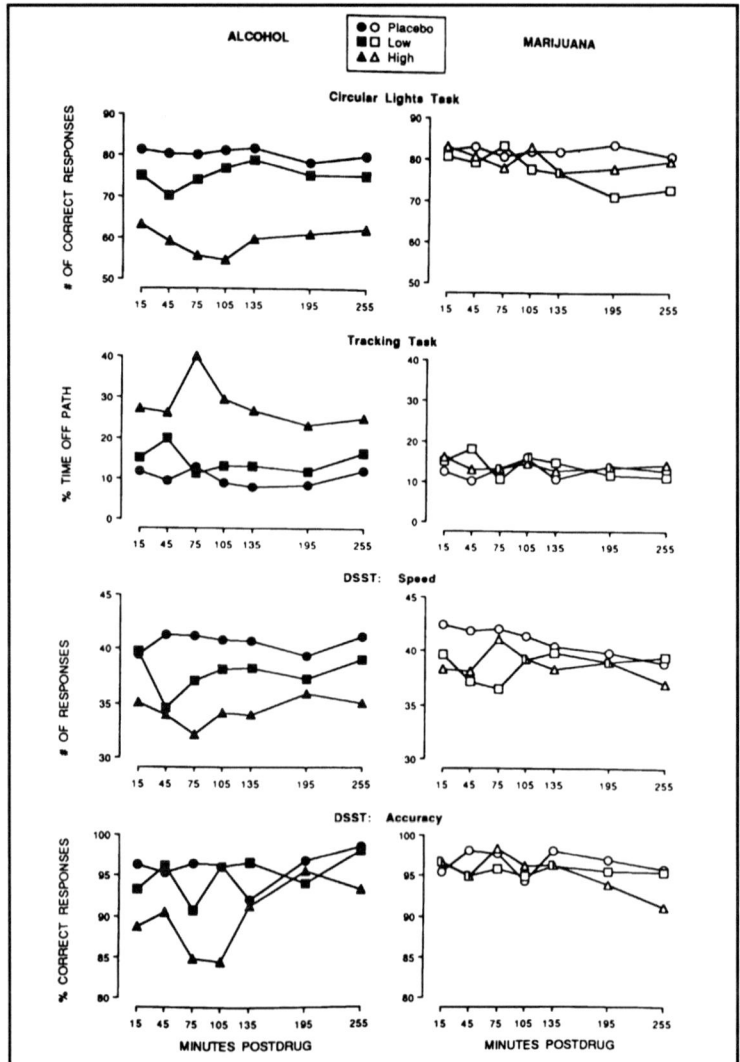

SOURCE.
From "Alcohol and marijuana: Comparative dose effect profiles in humans," by S.J. Heishman, M.L. Stitzer & G.E. Bigelow, 1988, *Pharmacology, Biochemistry and Behavior, 31*, pp. 649–655. Reprinted by permission of Pergamon Press.

Carry-over effects from marijuana have been reported for 10 experienced pilots in a flight simulator task (Yesavage, Leirer et al., 1985). The pilots smoked a marijuana cigarette containing 19 mg of THC and were tested 1, 4 and 24 hours later.

Compared to predrug baseline, significant differences occurred in all variables at 1 and 4 hours. At 24 hours, there were trends toward impairment in all measures and significant changes in several tasks, including a task that measured distance off-centre on landing. Subjective measures indicated that the pilots were unaware of their impairment at 24 hours. Unfortunately, this study did not include a placebo control and has been criticized for this omission. In a subsequent study, impairment was reported in pilots who were in a light aircraft simulator with turbulent flight conditions for 1 and 4 hours following a high-dose marijuana condition (20 mg THC). However, no significant effects were recorded at 24 or 48 hours, or at any time in the study with a lower marijuana dose of 10 mg THC (Leirer, Yesavage & Morrow, 1989). In a more recent report, this group again reported a carry-over effect for marijuana with pilots tested in a flight simulator 24 hours after smoking marijuana (Leirer, Yesavage & Morrow, 1991). Marijuana (20 mg THC) impaired performance at 0.25, 4, 8 and 24 hours. These results were more convincing since the study was conducted under placebo-controlled conditions. Seven of nine pilots showed impairment at 24 hours after smoking and only one reported awareness of the drug effect. Mean serum THC concentrations at test points following the 20-mg THC cigarette were as follows: predrug, < 0.2 ng/mL; 0.25 hours, 4.5 ng/mL; 4 hours, 0.7 ng/mL; 8 hours, 0.3 ng/mL; 24 hours, < 0.2 ng/mL.

Alcohol is generally considered to be the greatest contributor to motor vehicle accidents. However, there is growing awareness of involvement of other drugs as contributors. Evidence for the involvement of cannabis in vehicular and other types of accidents originates from several sources. A number of surveys have documented the presence of cannabinoids in the blood of impaired motorists (Christophersen, Gjerde et al., 1990; Gjerde & Kinn, 1991; McLean, Parsons et al., 1987; Poklis, Maginn & Barr, 1987; Sutton & Praegle, 1992; Zimmerman, Yeager et al., 1983). After alcohol, marijuana and benzodiazepines were the second most commonly detected drugs. In many cases, marijuana was detected in combination with alcohol. In alcohol-negative cases (< 0.05 per cent), THC prevalence ranged from 14.4 per cent (Zimmerman, Yeager et al., 1983) to 56 per cent (Gjerde & Kinn, 1991). Zimmerman et al. (1983) defined positive blood specimens as having THC ≥ 5.5 ng/mL. In that study, THC concentrations of positive specimens obtained from impaired motorists (N = 252) ranged from 5.5 ng/mL to 23 ng/mL. The high prevalence of THC in alcohol-negative cases led to the recommendation that all blood samples with blood alcohol concentration below legal limits be screened for other drugs (Christophersen, Gjerde et al., 1990). The authors have reviewed epidemiological studies of drugs in various subpopulations of drivers along with recent studies on psychomotor performance and drugs in an effort to define the role of drugs of abuse and alcohol in determining disability to drive (Ferrara, Giorgetti & Zancaner, 1994).

Marijuana use has been detected in surveys of truck drivers (Lund, Preusser et al., 1988), drivers in Tasmania (McLean, Parsons et al., 1987), motor vehicle collision victims (Stoduto, Vingilis et al., 1993), homicide victims and vehicular fatalities (Garriott, Di & Rodriguez, 1986; Soderstrom & Carson, 1988), and trauma patients (Soderstrom & Carson, 1988). The frequency of detection of cannabinoids ranged from 6 per cent to 34 per cent. In one study, concentrations of THC in blood (RIA, 2 ng/mL cutoff) ranged from 2 ng/mL to 75 ng/mL (Soderstrom & Carson, 1988). No correlation was found between injury severity and the presence of THC in blood. Of the 1,006 patients that were tested for both marijuana and alcohol, 18.3 per cent were positive for marijuana alone, 16.1 per cent were positive for alcohol and 16.5 per cent had used both drugs. The prevalence of drug use among automobile drivers and passengers in the three groups was approximately equal. There were no significant differences in marijuana use between vehicular and non-vehicular trauma victims, but marijuana use was higher among victims aged 30 years or younger and among men versus women.

Surveys of autopsy specimens from fatally injured drivers also indicate that marijuana and benzodiazepines are most often detected after alcohol. In most studies, marijuana was most often detected in combination with alcohol (Budd, Muto & Wong, 1989; Cimbura, Lucas et al., 1982; Gjerde, Belich & Morland, 1993; Haley, Iwuc et al., 1992; Mason & McBay, 1984; Williams, Peat et al., 1985). Due to alcohol involvement, low concentrations and frequency of detection of THC and other factors, several investigators (Mason & McBay, 1984; Haley, Iwuc et al., 1992) have concluded that the presence of drugs other than alcohol in blood does not prove causality in motor accidents or establish impairment. Cannabinoid concentrations vary widely in autopsy cases of marijuana users involved in fatal crashes. In a study of 162 drivers fatally injured: 38 per cent of the cases had THC in the range 0.2 to 0.9 ng/mL; 22 per cent had a range of 1.0 to 1.9 ng/mL; 26 per cent had a range of 2.0 to 4.9 ng/mL; and 14 per cent had a range of > 5 ng/mL (Williams, Peat et al., 1985). In the same cases, 11-*nor*-9-car-

boxy-THC was found in the following ranges: 30 per cent, < 10 ng/mL; 25 per cent, 10 to 24.9 ng/mL; 24 per cent, 25 to 49.9; and 22 per cent, > 50 ng/mL. However, marijuana was found alone in these cases only 12 per cent of the time. The causal role of drugs in this study was assessed by comparing drivers with and without drugs in terms of their responsibility for the crash. For the 19 drivers in which marijuana was found alone, 53 per cent were assigned responsibility compared with 71 per cent of the drug-free drivers (N = 78) leading the authors to conclude that there was insufficient evidence that marijuana contributes to crashes.

Pharmacokinetic-Pharmacodynamic (PK/PD) Modelling of THC

RELATIONSHIP OF THC TO EFFECTS

Although marijuana contains over 60 cannabinoids, the major active ingredient, $\varnothing$-THC, appears to be primarily responsible for its psychoactive effects. The THC molecule is a neutral, lipophilic substance that readily crosses alveolar membranes when marijuana is smoked resulting in nearly instantaneous appearance in blood. Subjects begin to report behavioral effects after a single puff of marijuana smoke and these effects culminate at a time similar to or somewhat delayed with respect to blood THC concentrations (Huestis, Sampson et al., 1992). The delay between peak blood concentrations and peak drug effects is likely related to delays in penetration of the central nervous system and to subsequent redistribution of THC following rapid uptake by adipose tissues. The delay

FIGURE 9.

Hysteresis relationships between 'Feel Drug Score" versus simultaneously obtained plasma THC concentrations in six male subjects following the smoking of a single 3.55 per cent THC marijuana cigarette

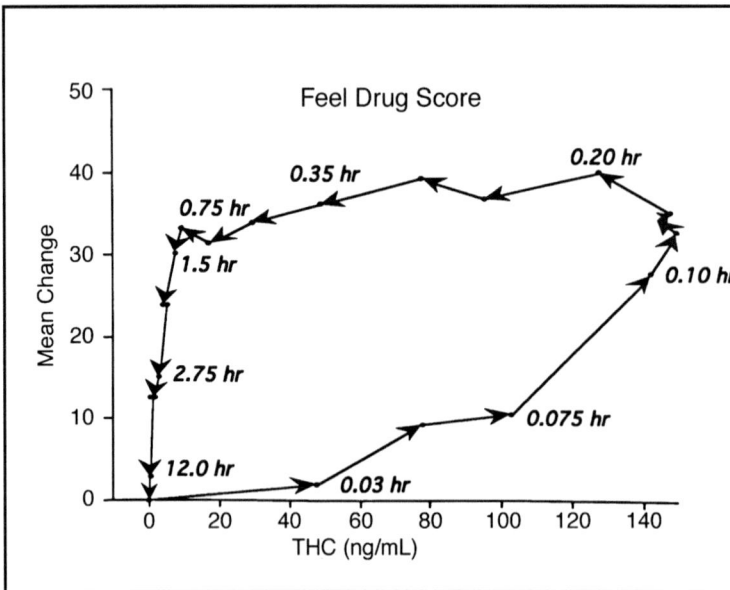

SOURCE.
From "Relating blood concentrations of tetrahydrocannabinol and metabolites to pharmacologic effects and time of marihuana usage," by E.J. Cone & M.A. Huestis, 1993, *Therapeutic Drug Monitoring, 15*, pp. 527–532. Reprinted by permission of Raven Press.

is characterized by counter-clockwise hysteresis between THC blood concentrations and drug (Barnett, Chiang et al., 1982; Barnett, Licko & Thompson, 1985). An example of the hysteresis relationship between "Feel Drug Score" and plasma THC concentrations is illustrated in Figure 9. The data represent mean data from six male subjects following the smoking of a single 3.55 per cent THC marijuana cigarette (Cone & Huestis, 1993). Prior to equilibrium, plasma concentrations increase rapidly while effects develop more slowly. Consequently, at early times after smoking marijuana, plasma concentrations are high while effects are low, whereas at later times, plasma concentrations may be diminishingly low while effects become highly prominent.

PK/PD MODELS

The lack of synchrony between blood THC concentrations and effects immediately after smoking marijuana confounds interpretation of blood THC concentrations. Thus, *ipso facto* concentrations of THC in blood have not been established that imply a person is impaired or under the influence of THC. Nonetheless, it was suggested (Chiang & Barnett, 1984) that once THC distribution is complete and equilibrium is established, the intensity of marijuana's effects become proportional to plasma concentrations. These investigators developed a kinetic and dynamic model linking THC plasma concentrations of marijuana smokers to drug effects (see Figure 10). In this figure, C and V represent THC concentrations and compartment volumes, respectively. A_e represents the amount of THC in the effect compartment (central nervous system) that is linked to the central compartment (blood and highly perfused tissues). The rate constants K_a, K_{12}, K_{21} and K_{10} describe the kinetics of THC in the two-compartment model and K_{1e} and K_{eo} characterize the dynamic effect compartment. K_{1e} represents a non-destructive first-order transfer from the central compartment to the effect compartment (brain) and K_{eo} represents elimination from the effect compartment. In

FIGURE 10.
Kinetic and dynamic model for THC

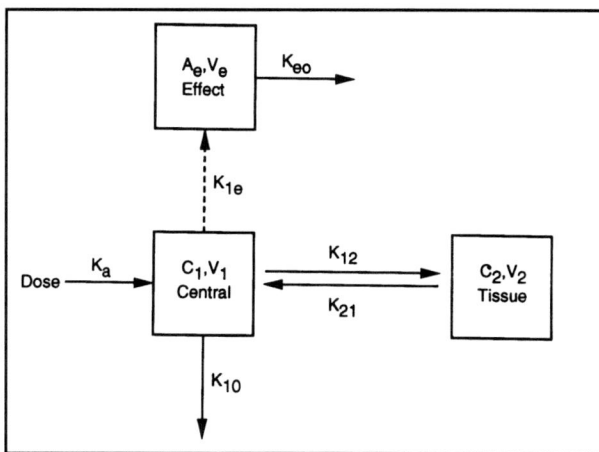

SOURCE.
From "Relating blood concentrations of tetrahydrocannabinol and metabolites to pharmacologic effects and time of marihuana usage," by E.J. Cone & M.A. Huestis, 1993, *Therapeutic Drug Monitoring, 15,* pp. 527–532. Reprinted by permission of Raven Press.

addition, K_{eo} is a constant that defines the temporal relationship between drug effect and drug levels in blood when the system is not at equilibrium. With this model, Chiang and Barnett (1984) related response data to the amount of THC in the effect compartment by means of the Hill equation:

$$E = \frac{(k_{eo}A_e/K_{1e}V_1)^\gamma}{(k_{eo}A_e/K_{1e}V_1)^\gamma + C_{ss}(50)^\gamma}$$

where E is the intensity of subjective measures, $C_{ss}(50)$ is the steady-state THC plasma concentration at 50 per cent of maximum effect, and γ determines the sigmoidicity of the effect/concentration relationship. Application of this equation to the data revealed that K_{eo} varied from 0.03 min^{-1} to 0.04 min^{-1}. This indicates that effect changes occur somewhat slowly during the distribution phase. Sigmoidicity ranged from 1.5 to 2.0 and $C_{ss}(50)$ had a range of 25 to 29 ng/mL. Domino et al. (1984) utilized a similar model and found that plasma THC concentrations at 50 per cent maximal subject high were 7.2 ng/mL and 16.8 ng/mL in light and heavy users. The difference between the groups was suggested to be due to tolerance to the effects of marijuana. Based on their model, they predicted a parallel decline between plasma THC concentrations and drug effect once pseudoequilibrium between blood and brain was established. The estimated time for pseudoequilibrium was 40 minutes for heavy users and 60 minutes in light users. These predictions appear to be borne out in Figure 9 in which a linear relationship was observed between THC plasma concentrations and Feel Drug Scores once equilibrium had been established (0.75 hours) for the six subjects who smoked a single 3.55 per cent THC cigarette.

THC Cutoff Concentrations Indicative of Impairment

The difficulties of defining cutoff concentrations for drugs that impair driving performance were outlined succinctly by a Consensus Development Panel (1985). Only a few attempts have been made at establishing acceptable cutoff concentrations for THC. Table 5 lists some suggested values or ranges based on widely differing sources such as PK/PD modelling theory, controlled-dosing studies and "per se" concentrations. Perhaps the most applicable study addressing this issue was performed by Reeve and colleagues (Reeve, Grant et al., 1983; Reeve, Robertson et al., 1983) who attempted to correlate passing or failing on roadside sobriety tests (RST) with THC plasma concentrations. The goal of the study was to determine a range of plasma

concentrations of THC that could be used as evidence of impairment. A total of 59 subjects (37 male, 22 female) smoked either 1, 2, 3 or 4 marijuana cigarettes (18 mg THC). Unfortunately, no controls were included in the study and conditions were not blind to the smokers. Plasma concentrations of THC and performance measures on the RST were determined prior to smoking and at 5, 30, 90 and 150 minutes after smoking. Only clear signs of impairment on the RST were used. THC concentrations were measured by RIA. Plasma concentrations were greatest at 5 minutes, but impairment was often greater at later times when THC concentrations were declining. The investigators reasoned that it was unlikely that persons apprehended for erratic driving would have completed smoking only 5 minutes earlier; consequently, the 5-minute data were eliminated from further consideration. Evaluation of performance at later times indicated that smokers consistently failed the Romberg test, a component of the RST, when they had a plasma concentration higher than 24 ng/mL. Only three passes on the finger-nose test occurred at THC concentrations > 25 ng/mL and only one pass occurred at concentrations > 22 ng/mL for the standing-on-one-foot test. It was concluded that plasma THC concentrations of 25 to 30 ng/mL, taken at some time after smoking, would be presumptive evidence of impairment. However, a majority of failures (80 per cent) on

---

TABLE 5.

THC Cutoff Concentrations in Blood Indicative of Impairment

Basis for establishing THC cutoff concentration	THC cutoff range	Reference
PK/PD models, THC concentration at 50% maximum effect	25–29 ng/mL plasma	Chiang & Barnett, 1984
PK/PD models, THC concentration at 50% maximum effect	7.2 ng/mL (light users; 16.8 ng/m (heavy users) plasma	Domino, Domino & Domino, 1984
Suggested performance on roadside sobriety test	10 ng/mL plasma 25–30 ng/mL plasma	McBay, 1985 Reeve, Grant et al., 1983
Per se	5 ng/mL plasma	Nelemans, 1985

these tests occurred at THC concentrations of 3 to 20 ng/mL. Consequently, a THC cutoff concentration > 20 ng/mL would miss many seriously impaired drivers.

Predicting Time of Marijuana Usage from THC and Metabolite Concentrations in Blood

Occasionally, forensic toxicologists are requested to estimate the elapsed time since marijuana was used based on measurements of THC and 11-*nor*-9-carboxy-THC in blood samples. This may occur in criminal and accident investigations in which only a single blood specimen was obtained after the incident. The time of marijuana usage may be an extremely important factor in assigning responsibility for criminal behavior, loss of property, injury or loss of life. Various attempts have been made to interpret time of marijuana use based on measurement of concentrations of THC and metabolites in blood (Foltz, McGinnis & Chinn, 1983; Hanson, Buonarti et al., 1983; Law, Mason et al., 1984), but have not been highly accurate or tested thoroughly. Recently, Huestis et al. (1992a) proposed two mathematical models for the estimation of time elapsed since marijuana usage based on THC plasma concentrations (Model I) and 11-*nor*-9-carboxy-THC/THC blood ratios (Model II). These models were derived from data obtained from a controlled marijuana dosing study with six male subjects who smoked a single marijuana

FIGURE 11.

Mathematical models for the prediction of time of marijuana exposure based on cannabinoid plasma concentrations: (a) Model I was derived from linear regression analysis of plasma THC concentrations versus elapsed time after marijuana smoking; (b) Model II was derived from linear regression analysis of plasma THCCOOH/THC ratios versus elapsed time after marijuana smoking. Plasma data were obtained from a controlled clinical study of acute marijuana use analysed by GC/MS. Dotted lines represent 95 per cent confidence intervals.

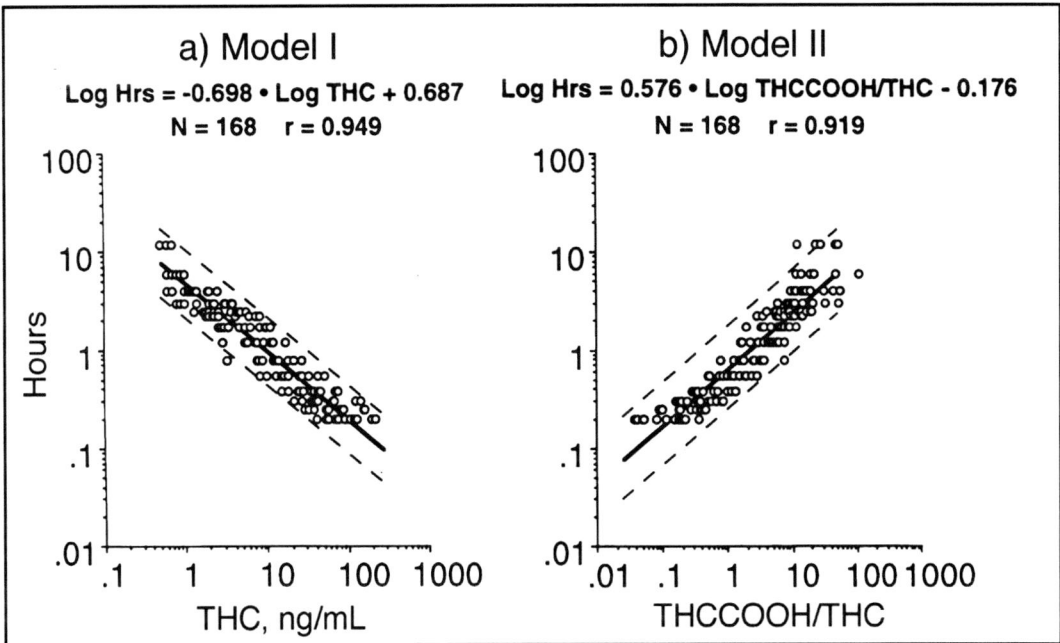

a) Model I

Log Hrs = -0.698 • Log THC + 0.687

N = 168 r = 0.949

b) Model II

Log Hrs = 0.576 • Log THCCOOH/THC - 0.176

N = 168 r = 0.919

SOURCE.

From "Blood cannabinoids: II. Models for the prediction of time of marijuana exposure from plasma concentrations of Δ^9-tetrahydrocannabinol (THC) and 11-*nor*-9-carboxy-Δ^9-tetrahydrocannabinol (THCCOOH)," by M.A. Huestis, J.E. Henningfield & E.J. Cone, 1992, *Journal of Analytical Toxicology, 16,* pp. 283-290. Reprinted by permission of Preston Publications, a division of Preston Industries, Inc.

cigarette containing 1.75 per cent THC and 3.55 per cent THC on two occasions. Equations for estimation of the time of marijuana usage are illustrated together with the clinical data in Figure 11.

Models I and II were validated by testing data from nine separate clinical studies reported in scientific literature in which the time, dose and route of administration of marijuana were known. The populations tested consisted of frequent and infrequent smokers and naive subjects who received THC orally. Generally, Model I accurately predicted the elapsed time after marijuana use for infrequent and frequent smokers, but was less accurate with sample data from oral administration. Model II was generally accurate with all groups, but somewhat less so than Model I with samples from frequent smokers. Model II tended to overestimate the time of usage slightly for samples from frequent smokers, but this was preferable to underestimation for use in forensic investigations. Both models provided 95 per cent confidence intervals for estimates of time of marijuana usage. Because of the nature of the models, the confidence intervals become progressively larger as the time elapsed since marijuana usage increased. Considerable interest has been expressed in the forensic community regarding the usefulness of these models in the interpretation of cannabinoid plasma concentrations.

Conclusion

Marijuana continues to be one of society's most highly abused illicit substances. The psychoactive effects include the production of feelings of euphoria, physiological changes and performance impairment in tests related to driving skills and the operation of complex machinery. There is continued interest in the pharmacokinetics of cannabinoids for several reasons. Detection of 11-*nor*-9-carboxy-THC in urine remains the primary means for determining whether an individual has used marijuana. Sensitive assays have been developed that can routinely detect this metabolite for one week or longer after marijuana exposure. Prevalence studies indicate that marijuana is frequently present in victims of homicide, trauma and traffic accidents. Marijuana is also abused in combination with alcohol. As a consequence, there is a need for understanding the relationship of body fluid concentrations of these drugs to pharmacological effects induced by their presence. Immediately following marijuana smoking, high concentrations of THC are present in blood and are distributed to tissues. During the distribution phase, the physiological and psychic effects of marijuana are on the increase, but may peak at times when blood concentrations of THC are falling. Once equilibrium between brain and blood concentrations is established (approximately 45 minutes after usage), a linear relationship between blood concentrations and pharmacological effects appears. Recently developed mathematical models are useful in the interpretation of the relationship of THC and metabolite concentrations in blood to drug-induced effects and for estimation of time elapsed since marijuana usage.

Some investigators have attempted to establish a range of THC concentrations in blood or other body fluids, similar to that for alcohol, that can be related to behavioral changes, drug influence and impairment. Establishment of cutoff concentrations for THC is greatly complicated by the wide individual variability observed in responses from subjects undergoing performance testing. This variability can be associated with a host of factors related to dose, physiological and pharmacological differences, complexity of performance tasks, situational demand during testing, and drug experience of the subject. Adoption of "per se" cutoff concentrations for THC in blood has been suggested as an alternative approach, similar to the manner in which alcohol limits were established. Although less appealing scientifically, this latter approach would allow adoption of standards for detection and routine monitoring of marijuana usage in circumstances involving increased risks to society.

Toxicity

A major concern with the recreational use of any drug is the adverse consequences that arise. Since the health consequences of cannabis use are discussed extensively in other chapters, only brief mention will be made of some selected findings in laboratory animals as they pertain to the central nervous system. The toxicity of cannabinoids was reviewed in depth in the last WHO report (Rosenkrantz, 1983). A great deal of new information has not emerged since that time to alter our concept of cannabis toxicity. The psychoactive constituents of cannabis are relatively non-toxic agents. As yet, there are not convincing cases of cannabis-induced lethality in humans, and very large doses are required to produce death in laboratory animals.

Recent reviews have emphasized that toxicity or adverse effects of cannabinoids are more likely to arise from repeated exposure to the drug (Compton & Martin, 1995; Scallet, 1991). Scallet (1991) described several reports of memory deficits in rodents that were exposed to THC or cannabis extracts. Additionally, Scallet et al. (1987) observed morphological changes in brain of rats up to seven months after chronic treatment with THC. These changes included axodendritic contact regions that were shortened and broken, enhanced extracellular space and less separation between vesicles/mitochondria and intact membranes. Statistical analysis revealed significantly smaller neurons and significantly decreased synaptic density in the THC-treated rats. These morphological changes were highly dependent on the treatment regimen. The above findings were observed in rats receiving 20 mg/kg (PO) of THC Monday through Thursday and 60 mg/kg on Friday. In a repeat experiment, rats receiving either 10 or 20 mg/kg per day for five days per week failed to exhibit ultrastructural abnormalities, although dendrites were shortened. Slikker et al. (1992) exposed rhesus monkeys to different quantities of daily marijuana smoke for one year and then evaluated them for behavioral, neurochemical and neurohistological changes. They concluded that long-term inhalation of marijuana smoke did not compromise the overall health of the animal although it did serve as a daily stressor. Behavioral changes were described as a decrease in "motivation" to work for food. The chronic marijuana smoke exposure failed to produce any neurochemical or neurohistological changes that could be detected seven months after smoking cessation.

The discovery of the endogenous ligand provides an additional opportunity to examine the toxicity that might arise from cannabinoid exposure. Future studies conducted with anandamide could provide clues to toxic effects that might not be detected with the exogenous substance. Certainly, if pharmacological effects are produced by chronic stimulation of the cannabinoid system, new insights will be gained regarding the functional role of anandamide.

Summary

One of the major goals of cannabinoid research has been to elucidate the mechanisms by which this class of compounds produce their behavioral effects. The long-held notion that these highly lipophilic substances exert psychotomimetic effects by disordering membranes, much like general anaesthetics, has been dispelled. There is now compelling evidence that the psychoactive constituent in cannabis, i.e., $\varnothing$-tetrahydrocannabinol (THC), produces its effects by interacting with specific receptors in the central nervous system. There are several lines of evidence to support this notion.

Structure–activity relationship studies have clearly shown that subtle alterations in the structure of THC dramatically influence its pharmacological potency. Moreover, numerous derivatives have been developed that are considerably more potent than THC, compounds that have proven to be valuable in probing the mechanism of THC action. In addition, several structurally distinct classes of cannabinoids have been developed. One of these compounds (CP-55,940) was used to characterize the binding properties of the cannabinoid receptor in brain. These studies revealed that the brain contains very high quantities of the cannabinoid receptor. Autoradiographic studies have shown a heterogeneous distribution in brain that is conserved throughout a variety of mammalian species, including humans, with most of the sites in the basal ganglia, hippocampus and cerebellum. Binding sites are also abundant in the cerebral cortex and striatum. It is interesting to speculate that these sites correlate with some of the pharmacological effects of cannabis, for example, cognitive impairment (hippocampus and cortex), ataxia (basal ganglia and cerebellum) and low toxicity (lack of receptors in the brainstem).

The receptor has been cloned and is known to be a member of a family of receptors coupled to G-proteins. It appears that this receptor is responsible for most of the centrally mediated effects of THC. There is a high correlation between receptor affinities and pharmacological potencies for THC analogues in several pharmacological paradigms. In addition, no other cannabinoid receptor subtypes have been identified in brain. Although multiple cannabinoid receptors have not been found in the brain, a peripheral receptor has been identified that is structurally different from the brain receptor. This cloned receptor, expressed in macrophages in the marginal zone of the spleen, exhibits 44 per cent homology with the brain receptor reported earlier. The spleen receptor is also a member of G-protein-coupled receptors. Its functional role in the immune system has not been established, but it is well known that cannabinoids are capable of producing immune suppression in several model systems.

There is also strong evidence that activation of central cannabinoid receptors results in inhibition of adenylyl cyclase and inhibition of calcium influx through N-type ion channels, second messenger systems that predominate in brain.

The characterization of cannabinoid receptors led to the discovery of the endogenous ligand, anandamide. This substance was initially isolated from pig brain and is an ethanolamide derivative of arachidonic acid. Brain is capable of both synthesis and metabolism of anandamide. Its pharmacological properties are similar to those of THC, with the exception that it is less potent and has a shorter duration of action. These differences are most likely due to rapid metabolism of anandamide *in vivo*. There are several indications that endogenous cannabinoids other than anandamide may exist. Two other unsaturated fatty acid ethanolamides (homo-γ-linolenylethanolamide and docosatetraenylethanolamide) have been isolated from pig brain that bind to the cannabinoid receptor.

The search for an antagonist eluded investigators until the recent development of SR141716A, which was found to have high affinity (Ki = 2 nM) for the CB_1 cannabinoid receptor but very low affinity for the CB_2 spleen receptor. It effectively antagonized cannabinoid-induced inhibition of adenylyl cyclase and neuronally stimulated smooth muscle contractions. More importantly, orally and intraperitoneally administered SR141716A antagonized cannabinoid-induced hypothermia, catalepsy and antinociception in mice with high potency. It also appears that this antagonist is highly selective for the cannabinoid receptor, because it failed to bind to histamine, dopamine, adrenergic, purinergic, adenosine, opioid, neurotensin, cholecystokinin, benzodiazepine, sigma, tachykinin, serotonin, excitatory or inhibitory amino acid receptors. The discovery of this antagonist completes the basic requirements for a receptor system and provides a valuable tool for establishing the functional role of the cannabinoids in the central nervous system.

Acknowledgments

Portions of this research were supported by the NIDA research grant DA-03672.

References

Abadji, V., Lin, S., Taha, G., Griffin, G., Stevenson, L.A., Pertwee, R.G. & Makriyannis, A. (1994). (R)-methanandamide: A chiral novel anandamide possessing higher potency and metabolic stability. *Journal of Medicinal Chemistry, 37,* 1889–1893.

Adams, I.B., Ryan, W., Singer, M., Thomas, B.F., Compton, D.R., Razdan, R.K. & Martin, B.R. (1995). Evaluation of cannabinoid receptor binding and *in vivo* activities for anandamide analogs. *Journal of Pharmacology and Experimental Therapeutics, 273,* 1172–1181.

Attwood, A., Williams, R., McBurney, L. & Frecker, R. (1981). Cannabis, alcohol and driving: Effects on selected closed-course tasks. *Alcohol, Drugs and Traffic Safety,* 3, 938–953.

Barnett, C., Chiang, C., Perez-Reyes, M. & Owens, S. (1982). Kinetic study of smoking marijuana. *Journal of Pharmacokinetics and Biopharmaceutics, 10,* 495–506.

Barnett, G., Licko, V. & Thompson, T. (1985). Behavioral pharmacokinetics of marijuana. *Psychopharmacology, 85,* 51–56.

Beltramo, M., Stella, N., Calignano, A., Lin, S.Y., Makriyannis, A. & Piomelli, D. (1997). Functional role of high-affinity anandamide transport, as revealed by selective inhibition. *Science, 277,* 1094–1097.

Bidaut-Russell, M., Devane, W.A. & Howlett, A.C. (1990). Cannabinoid receptors and modulation of cyclic AMP accumulation in the rat brain. *Journal of Neurochemistry, 55,* 21–26.

Binder, M., Witteler, F.-J., Schmidt, B. & Franke, I. (1984). Triglyceride/phospholipid partitioning and pharmacokinetics of some natural and semi-synthetic cannabinoids: Further evidence for the involvement of specific receptors in the mediation of the psychotropic effects of D1-THC and D6-THC. In S. Agurell, W.L. Dewey & R.E Willette (Eds.), *The Cannabinoids: Chemical, Pharmacologic and Therapeutic Aspects* (pp. 709–727). New York: Academic Press.

Bird, K.D., Boleyn, T., Chesher, G.B., Jackson, D.M., Starmer, G.A. & Teo, R.K.C. (1980). Intercannabinoid and cannabinoid-ethanol interactions and their effects on human performance. *Psychopharmacology, 71,* 181–188.

Bouaboula, M., Poinot-Chazel, C., Bourrié, B., Canat, X., Calandra, B., Rinaldi-Carmona, M., Le Fur, G. & Casellas, P. (1995). Activation of mitogen-activated protein kinases by stimulation of the central cannabinoid receptor CB1. *Biochemical Journal, 312*, 637–641.

Braff, D., Silverton, L., Saccuzzo, D. & Janowsky, D. (1981). Impaired speed of visual information processing in marijuana intoxication. *American Journal of Psychiatry, 138*, 613–617.

Budd, R.D., Muto, J.J. & Wong, J.K. (1989). Drugs of abuse found in fatally injured drivers in Los Angeles County. *Drug and Alcohol Dependence, 23*, 153–158.

Caulfield, M.P. & Brown, D.A. (1992). Cannabinoid receptor agonists inhibit Ca current in NG108-15 neuroblastoma cells via a pertussis toxin-sensitive mechanism. *British Journal of Pharmacology, 106*, 231–232.

Chait, L.D. & Pierri, J. (1992). Effects of smoked marijuana on human performance: A critical review. In L. Murphy & A. Bartke (Eds.), *Marijuana/Cannabinoids: Neurobiology and Neurophysiology* (pp. 387–423). Boca Raton, FL: CRC Press.

Chaudry, A., Thompson, R.H., Rubin, R.P. & Laychock, S.G. (1988). Relationship between $\varnothing^9$-tetrahydrocannabinol-induced arachidonic acid release and secretagogue-evoked phosphoinositide breakdown and Ca^{2+} mobilization of exocrine pancreas. *Molecular Pharmacology, 34*, 543–548.

Chen, J., Marmur, R., Pulles, A., Paredes, W. & Gardner, E. (1993). Ventral tegmental microinjection of $\varnothing^9$-tetrahydrocannabinol enhances ventral tegmental somatodendritic dopamine levels but not forebrain dopamine levels: Evidence for local neural action by marijuana's psychoactive ingredient. *Brain Research, 621*, 65–70.

Chiang, C.W. & Barnett, G. (1984). Marijuana effect and D9-tetrahydrocannabinol plasma level. *Clinical Pharmacology and Therapeutics, 36*, 234–238.

Christophersen, A., Gjerde, H., Sakshaug, A. & Morland, J. (1990). Screening for drug use among Norwegian drivers suspected of driving under influence of alcohol or drugs. *Forensic Science International, 45*, 5–14.

Cimbura, G., Lucas, D.M., Bennett, R.C., Warren, R.A. & Simpson, H.M. (1982). Incidence and toxicological aspects of drugs detected in 484 fatally injured drivers and pedestrians in Ontario. *Journal of Forensic Sciences, 27*, 855–867.

Cocchetto, D., Owens, S., Perez-Reyes, M., Di Guiseppi, S. & Miller, L. (1981). Relationship between plasma delta-9-tetrahydrocannabinol concentration and pharmacologic effects in man. *Psychopharmacology, 75*, 158–164.

Compton, D.R., Gold, L.H., Ward, S.J., Balster, R.L. & Martin, B.R. (1992). Aminoalkylindole analogs: Cannabimimetic activity of a class of compounds structurally distinct from $\varnothing$-tetrahydrocannabinol. *Journal of Pharmacology and Experimental Therapeutics, 263*, 1118–1126.

Compton, D.R., Johnson, M.R., Melvin, L.S. & Martin, B.R. (1992). Pharmacological profile of a series of bicyclic cannabinoid analogs: Classification as cannabimimetic agents. *Journal of Pharmacology and Experimental Therapeutics, 260*, 201–209.

Compton, D.R. & Martin, B.R. (1995). Marijuana neurotoxicology. In L.W. Chiang & R.S. Dyer (Eds.), *Handbook of Neurotoxicology* (pp. 871–890). New York: Marcel Dekker.

Compton, D.R., Rice, K.C., De Costa, B.R., Razdan, R.K., Melvin, L.S., Johnson, M.R. & Martin, B.R. (1993). Cannabinoid structure–activity relationships: Correlation of receptor binding and in vivo activities. *Journal of Pharmacology and Experimental Therapeutics, 265*, 218–226.

Cone, E.J. & Huestis, M.A. (1993). Relating blood concentrations of tetrahydrocannabinol and metabolites to pharmacologic effects and time of marihuana usage. *Therapeutic Drug Monitoring, 15*, 527–532.

Cone, E.J., Johnson, R.E., Moore, J.D. & Roache, J.D. (1986). Acute effects of smoking marijuana on hormones, subjective effects and performance in male human subjects. *Pharmacology, Biochemistry and Behavior, 24*, 1749–1754.

Cone, E.J., Johnson, R.E., Paul, B.D., Mell, L.D. & Mitchell, J. (1988). Marijuana-laced brownies: Behavioral effects, physiologic effects, and urinalysis in humans following ingestion. *Journal of Analytical Toxicology, 12*, 169–175.

Consensus Development Panel. (1985). Drug concentrations and driving impairment. *Journal of the American Medical Association, 254*, 2618–2621.

Cook, E. (1986). Analytical methodology for delta-9-tetrahydrocannabinol and its metabolites. *Advances in Alcohol and Substance Abuse, 2*, 79–85.

Crawley, J., Corwin, R., Robinson, J., Felder, C., Devane, W. & Axelrod, J. (1993). Anandamide, an endogenous ligand of the cannabinoid receptor, induces hypomotility and hypothermia in vivo in rodents. *Pharmacology, Biochemistry and Behavior, 46*, 967–972.

D'Ambra, T.E., Estep, K.G., Bell, M.R., Eissenstat, M.A., Josef, K.A., Ward, S.J., Haycock, D.A., Baizman, E.R., Casiano, F.M., Beglin, N.C., Chippari, S.M., Grego, J.D., Kullnig, R.K. & Daley, G.T. (1992). Conformationally restrained analogues of pravadoline — Nanomolar potent, enantioselective, (aminoalkyl)indole agonists of the cannabinoid receptor. *Journal of Medicinal Chemistry, 35*, 124–135.

Deutsch, D.G. & Chin, S.A. (1993). Enzymatic synthesis and degradation of anandamide, a cannabinoid receptor agonist. *Biochemical Pharmacology, 46*, 791–796.

Devane, W.A. & Axelrod, J. (1994). Enzymatic synthesis of anandamide, and endogenous ligand for the cannabinoid receptor by brain membranes. *Proceedings of the National Academy of Sciences of the United States of America, 91*, 6698–6701.

Devane, W.A., Breuer, A., Sheskin, T., Järbe, T.U.C., Eisen, M.S. & Mechoulam, R. (1992). A novel probe for the cannabinoid receptor. *Journal of Medicinal Chemistry, 35*, 2065–2069.

Devane, W.A., Dysarz, F.A., III, Johnson, M.R., Melvin, L.S. & Howlett, A.C. (1988). Determination and characterization of a cannabinoid receptor in rat brain. *Molecular Pharmacology, 34*, 605–613.

Devane, W.A., Hanus, L., Breuer, A., Pertwee, R.G., Stevenson, L.A., Griffin, G., Gibson, D., Mandelbaum, A., Etinger, A. & Mechoulam, R. (1992). Isolation and structure of a brain constituent that binds to the cannabinoid receptor. *Science, 258*, 1946–1949.

Dewey, W.L. (1986). Cannabinoid pharmacology. *Pharmacological Reviews, 38*, 151–178.

Domino, L., Domino, S. & Domino, E. (1984). Relation of plasma delta-9-THC concentrations to subjective "high" in marijuana users: A review and reanalysis. In S. Agurell, W.L. Dewey & R.E. Willette (Eds.), *The Cannabinoids: Chemical, Pharmacologic and Therapeutic Aspects* (pp. 245–261). New York: Academic Press.

Edery, H., Grunfeld, Y., Ben-Zvi, Z. & Mechoulam, R. (1971). Structural requirements for cannabinoid activity. *Annals of the New York Academy of Sciences, 191*, 40–53.

Eldridge, J.C. & Landfield, P.W. (1990). Cannabinoid interactions with glucocorticoid receptors in rat hippocampus. *Brain Research, 534*, 135–141.

Eldridge, J.C. & Landfield, P.W. (1992). Cannabinoid-glucocorticoid interactions in the hippocampal region of the brain. In L. Murphy & A. Bartke (Eds.), *Marijuana/Cannabinoids: Neurobiology and Neurophysiology* (pp. 93–117). Boca Raton, FL: CRC Press.

Evans, C.J., Keith, D.E., Morrison, H., Magendzo, K. & Edwards, R.H. (1992). Cloning of a delta opioid receptor by functional expression. *Science, 258*, 1952–1955.

Evans, D., Lake, J.T., Johnson, M.R. & Howlett, A. (1994). Endogenous cannabinoid receptor binding activity released from rat brain slices by depolarization. *Journal of Pharmacology and Experimental Therapeutics, 268*, 1271–1277.

Fan, F., Compton, D.R., Ward, S., Melvin, L., Martin, B.R. (1994). Development of cross-tolerance between D9-THC, CP 55,940 and WIN 55,212. *Journal of Pharmacology and Experimental Therapeutics, 271*, 1383–1390.

Felder, C.C., Briley, E.M., Axelrod, J., Simpson, J.T., Mackie, K. & Devane, W.A. (1993). Anandamide, an endogenous cannabimimetic eicosanoid, binds to the cloned human cannabinoid receptor and stimulates receptor-mediated signal transduction. *Proceedings of the National Academy of Sciences of the United States of America, 90*, 7656–7660.

Felder, C.C., Veluz, J.S., Williams, H.L., Briley, E.M. & Matsuda, L.A. (1992). Cannabinoid agonists stimulate both receptor- and nonreceptor-mediated signal transduction pathways in cells transfected with an expressing cannabinoid receptor clones. *Molecular Pharmacology, 42*, 838–845.

Ferrara, S., Giorgetti, R. & Zancaner, S. (1994). Psychoactive substances and driving: State of the art and methodology. *Alcohol, Drugs and Driving, 10*, 1–55.

Ferraro, D.P. (1980). Acute effects of marijuana on human memory and cognition. In R.C. Petersen (Ed.), *Marijuana Research Findings: 1980* (NIDA Research Monograph No. 31, pp. 98–119). Washington, DC: U.S. Government Printing Office.

Foltz, R.L., McGinnis, K.M. & Chinn, D.M. (1983). Quantitative measurement of $\varnothing$- tetrahydro-cannabinol and two major metabolites in physiological specimens using capillary column gas chromatography negative ion chemical ionization mass spectrometry. *Biomedical Mass Spectrometry, 10*, 316–323.

Fride, E. & Mechoulam, R. (1993). Pharmacological activity of the cannabinoid receptor agonist, anandamide, a brain constituent. *European Journal of Pharmacology, 231*, 313–314.

Gardner, E.L. & Lowinson, J.H. (1991). Marijuana's interaction with brain reward systems — Update 1991. *Pharmacology, Biochemistry and Behavior, 40*, 571–580.

Garriott, J.C., Di, M.V.J. & Rodriguez, R.G. (1986). Detection of cannabinoids in homicide victims and motor vehicle fatalities. *Journal of Forensic Sciences, 31*, 1274–1282.

Gérard, C.M., Mollereau, C., Vassart, G. & Parmentier, M. (1990). Nucleotide sequence of a human cannabinoid receptor cDNA. *Nucleic Acids Research, 18*, 7142.

Gérard, C.M., Mollereau, C., Vassart, G. & Parmentier, M. (1991). Molecular cloning of a human cannabinoid receptor which is also expressed in testis. *Biochemical Journal, 279*, 129–134.

Gjerde, H. (1991). Screening for cannabinoids in blood using emit: Concentrations of delta-9-tetrahydrocannabinol in relation to EMIT results. *Forensic Science International, 50*, 121–124.

Gjerde, H., Belich, K. & Morland, J. (1993). Incidence of alcohol and drugs in fatally injured car drivers in Norway. *Accident Analysis and Prevention, 25*, 479–483.

Gjerde, H. & Kinn, G. (1991). Impairment in drivers due to cannabis in combination with other drugs. *Forensic Science International, 50*, 57–60.

Glass, M., Faull, R. & Dragunow, M. (1993). Loss of cannabinoid receptors in the substantia nigra in Huntington's disease. *Neuroscience, 56*, 523–527.

Gold, L., Balster, R.L., Barrett, R.L., Britt, D.T. & Martin, B.R. (1992). A comparison of the discriminative stimulus properties of $\varnothing$-THC and CP-55,940 in rats and rhesus monkeys. *Journal of Pharmacology and Experimental Therapeutics, 262,* 479–486.

Goldberger, B. & Cone, E. (1994). Confirmatory tests for drugs in the workplace by gas chromatography-mass spectrometry. *Journal of Chromatography, 674,* 73–86.

Haley, N., Iwuc, P., Ogilvie, L. & Carria, L. (1992). Motor vehicle fatalities in Rhode Island (FY1990-1991): A report on driver impairment. *Medicine and Health—Rhode Island, 75,* 397–400.

Hanson, V.W., Buonarati, M.H., Baselt, R.C., Wade, N.A., Yep, C., Biasotti, A.A., Reeve, V.C., Wong, A.S. & Orbanowsky, M.W. (1983). Comparison of ^{3}H- and ^{125}I-radioimmunoassay and gas chromatography/mass spectrometry for the determination of delta 9-tetrahydrocannabinol and cannabinoids in blood and serum. *Journal of Analytical Toxicology, 7,* 96–102.

Hansteen, R.W., Miller, R.D. & Lonero, L. (1976). Effects of cannabis and alcohol on automobile driving and psychomotor tracking. *Annals of the New York Academy of Science, 282,* 240–256.

Hanus, L., Gopher, A., Almog, S. & Mechoulam, R. (1993). Two new unsaturated fatty acid ethanolamides in brain that bind to the cannabinoid receptor. *Journal of Medicinal Chemistry, 36,* 3032–3034.

Hardman, H.F., Domino, E.F. & Seevers, M.H. (1971). General pharmacological actions of some synthetic tetrahydrocannabinol derivatives. *Pharmacological Reviews, 23,* 295–315.

Harris, L.S., Carchman, R.A. & Martin, B.R. (1978). Evidence for the existence of specific cannabinoid binding sites. *Life Sciences, 22,* 1131–1138.

Harris, R.A. & Stokes, J.A. (1982). Cannabinoids inhibit calcium uptake by brain synaptosomes. *Journal of Neuroscience, 2,* 443–447.

Harvey, D.J., Leuschner, J.T.A. & Paton, W.D.M. (1980). Measurement of $\varnothing$-tetrahydrocannabinol in plasma to the low picogram range by gas chromatography-mass spectrometry using metastable ion detection. *Journal of Chromatography, 202,* 83–92.

Hawks, R.L. (Ed.). 1982. The Analysis of Cannabinoids in Biological Fluids (NIDA Research Monograph No. 42). Washington, DC: U.S. Government Printing Office.

Heishman, S.J., Huestis, M.A., Henningfield, J.E. & Cone, E.J. (1990). Acute and residual effects of marijuana: Profiles of plasma THC levels, physiological, subjective, and performance measures. *Pharmacology, Biochemistry and Behavior, 37,* 561–565.

Heishman, S.J., Stitzer, M.L. & Bigelow, G.E. (1988). Alcohol and marijuana: Comparative dose effect profiles in humans. *Pharmacology, Biochemistry and Behavior, 31,* 649-655.

Herkenham, M., Lynn, A.B., De Costa, B.R. & Richfield, E.K. (1991a). Neuronal localization of cannabinoid receptors in the basal ganglia of the rat. *Brain Research, 547,* 267–274.

Herkenham, M., Lynn, A.B., Johnson, M.R., Melvin, L.S., De Costa, B.R. & Rice, K.C. (1991b). Characterization and localization of cannabinoid receptors in rat brain: A quantitative in vitro autoradiographic study. *Journal of Neuroscience, 11,* 563–583.

Herkenham, M., Lynn, A.B., Little, M.D., Johnson, M.R., Melvin, L.S., De Costa, B.R. & Rice, K.C. (1990). Cannabinoid receptor localization in the brain. *Proceedings of the National Academy of Sciences of the United States of America, 87,* 1932–1936.

Hillard, C.J., Edgemond, S., Jarrahian, A. & Campbell, W.B. (1997). Accumulation of N-arachidonoylethanolamine (anandamide) into cerebellar granule cells occurs via facilitated diffusion. *Journal of Neurochemistry, 69,* 631–638.

Hollister, L.E., Gillespie, H.K., Ohlsson, A., Lindgren, J.-E., Wahlen, A. & Agurell, S. (1981). Do plasma concentrations of $\varnothing$-tetrahydrocannabinol reflect the degree of intoxication? *Journal of Clinical Pharmacology, 21,* 171S–177S.

Howlett, A.C. (1985). Cannabinoid inhibition of adenylate cyclase: Biochemistry of the response in neuroblastoma cell membranes. *Molecular Pharmacology, 27,* 429–436.

Howlett, A.C., Bidaut-Russell, M., Devane, W.A., Melvin, L.S., Johnson, M.R. & Herkenham, M. (1990). The cannabinoid receptor: Biochemical, anatomical and behavioral characterization. *Trends in Neuroscience, 13,* 420–423.

Howlett, A.C., Champion, T.M., Wilken, G.H. & Mechoulam, R. (1990). Stereochemical effects of 11-OH-D8-tetrahydrocannabinol-dimethylheptyl to inhibit adenylate cyclase and bind to the cannabinoid receptor. *Neuropharmacology, 29,* 161–165.

Howlett, A.C., Evans, D.M. & Houston, D.B. (1992). The cannabinoid receptor. In L. Murphy & A. Bartke (Eds.), *Marijuana/Cannabinoids: Neurobiology and Neurophysiology* (pp. 35–72). Boca Raton, FL: CRC Press.

Howlett, A.C. & Fleming, R.M. (1984). Cannabinoid inhibition of adenylate cyclase: Pharmacology of the response in neuroblastoma cell membranes. *Molecular Pharmacology, 26,* 532–538.

Howlett, A.C., Johnson, M.R., Melvin, L.S. & Milne, G.M. (1988). Nonclassical cannabinoid analgetics inhibit adenylate cyclase: Development of a cannabinoid receptor model. *Molecular Pharmacology, 33,* 297–302.

Howlett, A.C., Qualy, J.M. & Khachatrian, L.L. (1986). Involvement of Gi in the inhibition of adenylate cyclase by cannabimimetic drugs. *Molecular Pharmacology, 29,* 307–313.

Huestis, M.A., Henningfield, J.E. & Cone, E.J. (1992a). Blood cannabinoids: II. Models for the prediction of time of marijuana exposure from plasma concentrations of $\varnothing$-tetrahydrocannabinol (THC) and 11-*nor*-9-carboxy-$\varnothing$-tetrahydrocannabinol (THCCOOH). *Journal of Analytical Toxicology, 16*, 283–290.

Huestis, M.A., Henningfield, J.E. & Cone, E.J. (1992b). Blood cannabinoids: I. Absorption of THC and formation of 11-OH-THC and THCCOOH during and after smoking marijuana. *Journal of Analytical Toxicology, 16*, 276–282.

Huestis, M.A., Sampson, A.H., Holicky, B.J., Henningfield, J.E. & Cone, E.J. (1992). Characterization of the absorption phase of marijuana smoking. *Clinical Pharmacology and Therapeutics, 52*, 31–41.

Huffman, J.W., Dai, D., Martin, B.R. & Compton, D.R. (1994). Design, synthesis and pharmacology of cannabimimetic indoles. *Bio-organic and Medicinal Chemistry Letters, 4*, 563–566.

Hunt, C.A. & Jones, R.T. (1980). Tolerance and disposition of tetrahydrocannabinol in man. *Journal of Pharmacology and Experimental Therapeutics, 215*, 35–44.

Janowsky, D., Meacham, M., Blaine, J., Schoor, M. & Bozzetti, L. (1976). Marijuana effects on simulated flying ability. *American Journal of Psychiatry, 133*, 384–388.

Jansen, E.M., Haycock, D.A., Ward, S.J. & Seybold, V.S. (1992). Distribution of cannabinoid receptors in rat brain determined with aminoalkylindoles. *Brain Research, 575*, 93–102.

Järbe, T.U.C., Hiltunen, A.J. & Mechoulam, R. (1989). Stereospecificity of the discriminative stimulus functions of the dimethylheptyl homologs of 11-hydroxy-$\varnothing$-tetrahydro-cannabinol in rats and pigeons. *Journal of Pharmacology and Experimental Therapeutics, 250*, 1000–1005.

Johansson, E., Agurell, S., Hollister, L. & Halldin, M. (1988). Prolonged apparent half-life of delta-9-tetrahydrocannabinol in plasma of chronic marijuana users. *Journal of Pharmacy and Pharmacology, 40*, 374–375.

Johansson, E., Ohlsson, A., Lindgren, J.E., Agurell, S., Gillespie, H. & Hollister, L.E. (1987). Single-dose kinetics of deuterium-labelled cannabinol in man after intravenous admin-istration and smoking. *Biomedical and Environmental Mass Spectrometry, 14*, 495–499.

Johnson, M.R. & Melvin, L.S. (1986). The discovery of nonclassical cannabinoid analgetics. In *Cannabinoids as Therapeutic Agents* (pp. 121–144). Boca Raton, FL: CRC Press.

Jones, R.T. (1980). Human effects: An overview. In R.C. Petersen (Ed.), *Marijuana Research Findings: 1980* (National Institute on Drug Abuse Research Monograph No. 31, pp. 54–80) (DHHS Publication No. ADM 80-1001). Washington, DC: U.S. Government Printing Office.

Kaminski, N.E., Abood, M.E., Kessler, F.K., Martin, B.R. & Schatz, A.R. (1992). Identification of a functionally relevant cannabinoid receptor on mouse spleen cells that is involved in cannabinoid-mediated immune modulation. *Molecular Pharmacology, 42*, 736–742.

Kelly, P. & Jones, R.T. (1992). Metabolism of tetrahydrocannabinol in frequent and infrequent marijuana users. *Journal of Analytical Toxicology, 16*, 228–235.

Kemp, P.M., Abukhalaf, I.K., Manno, J.E., Manno, B.R., Alford, D.D., McWilliams, M.E., Nixon, F.E., Fitzgerald, M.J., Reeves, R.R. & Wood, M.J. (1995). Cannabinoids in humans. II: The influence of three methods of hydrolysis on the concentration of THC and two metabolites in urine. *Journal of Analytical Toxicology, 19*, 292–298.

King, D.L., Martel, P.A. & O'Donnell, C.M. (1987). Laboratory detection of cannabinoids. *Clinics in Laboratory Medicine, 7*, 641–653.

Klonoff, H. (1974). Marijuana and driving in real-life situations. *Science, 186*, 317–324.

Koe, B.K., Milne, G.M., Weissman, A., Johnson, M.R. & Melvin, L.S. (1985). Enhancement of brain [3H]flunitrazepam binding and analgesic activity of synthetic cannabimimetics. *European Journal of Pharmacology, 109*, 201–212.

Koe, W.S., Crawford, R.B. & Kaminski, N.E. (1997). Inhibition of protein kinase A and cyclic AMP response element (CRE)-specific transcription factor binding by $\varnothing^9$-tetrahydrocannabinol ($\varnothing^9$-THC). *Biochemical Pharmacology, 53*, 1477–1484.

Koutek, B., Prestwich, G.D., Howlett, A.C., Chin, S.A., Salehani, D., Akhavan, N. & Deutsch, D.G. (1994). Inhibitors of arachidonyl ethanolamide hydrolysis. *Journal of Biological Chemistry, 269*, 22937–22940.

Kruszka, K. & Gross, R. (1994). The ATP-and CoA-independent synthesis of arachidonoylethanolamide. *Journal of Biological Chemistry, 269*, 14345–14348.

Kumbaraci, N.M. & Nastuk, W.L. (1980). Effects of $\varnothing^9$-tetrahydrocannabinol on excitable membranes and neuromuscular transmission. *Molecular Pharmacology, 17*, 344–349.

Landfield, P.W., Cadwallader, L.B. & Vinsant, S. (1988). Quantitative changes in hippocampal structure following long-term exposure to $\varnothing^9$-tetrahydrocannabinol: Possible mediation by glucocorticoid systems. *Brain Research, 443*, 47–62.

Law, B., Mason, P.A., Moffat, A.C., Gleadle, R.I. & King, L.J. (1984). Forensic aspects of the metabolism and excretion of cannabinoids following oral ingestion of cannabis resin. *Journal of Pharmacy and Pharmacology, 36*, 289–294.

Lawrence, D.K. & Gill, E.W. (1975). The effects of $\varnothing^9$-tetrahydrocannabinol and other cannabinoids in spin-labeled liposomes and their relationship to mechanisms of general anesthesia. *Molecular Pharmacology, 11*, 595–602.

Leader, J.P., Koe, B.K. & Weisman, A. (1981). GABA-like actions of levonantradol. *Journal of Clinical Pharmacology, 21*, 2625–2705.

Leirer, V.O., Yesavage, J.A. & Morrow, D.G. (1989). Marijuana, aging and task difficulty effects on pilot performance. *Aviation, Space and Environmental Medicine, 60*, 1145–1152.

Leirer, V.O., Yesavage, J.A. & Morrow, D.G. (1991). Marijuana carry-over effects on aircraft pilot performance. *Aviation, Space and Environmental Medicine, 62*, 221–227.

Lemberger, L., Crabtree, R.E. & Rowe, H.M. (1972). 11-Hydroxy-$\varnothing$-tetrahydrocannabinol: Pharmacology, disposition, and metabolism of a major metabolite of marihuana in man. *Science, 177*, 62–64.

Lemberger, L., Tamarkin, N.R., Axelrod, J. & Kopin, I.J. (1971). $\varnothing$-Tetrahydrocannabinol: Metabolism and disposition in long-term marihuana smokers. *Science, 173*, 72–73.

Lemberger, L., Weiss, J.L., Watanabe, A.M., Galanter, I.M., Wyatt, R.J. & Cardon, P.V. (1972). D9-Tetrahydrocannabinol: Temporal correlation of the psychologic effects and blood levels after various routes of administration. *New England Journal of Medicine, 286*, 685–688.

Lindgren, J., Ohlsson, A., Agurell, S., Hollister, L. & Gillespie, H. (1981). Clinical effects and plasma levels of delta-9-tetrahydrocannabinol in heavy and light users of cannabis. *Psychopharmacology, 74*, 208–212.

Little, P.J., Compton, D.R., Johnson, M.R., Melvin, L.S. & Martin, B.R. (1988). Pharmacology and stereoselectivity of structurally novel cannabinoids in mice. *Journal of Pharmacology and Experimental Therapeutics, 247*, 1046–1051.

Little, P.J., Compton, D.R., Mechoulam, R. & Martin, B.R. (1989). Stereochemical effects of 11-OH-dimethylheptyl-$\varnothing$-tetrahydrocannabinol. *Pharmacology, Biochemistry and Behavior, 32*, 661–666.

Lund, A.K., Preusser, D.F., Blomberg, R.D. & Williams, A.F. (1988). Drug use by tractor-trailer drivers. *Journal of Forensic Sciences, 33*, 648–661.

Lynn, A. & Herkenham, M. (1994). Localization of cannabinoid receptors and nonsaturable high-density cannabinoid binding sites in peripheral tissues of the rat: Implications for receptor-mediated immune modulation by cannabinoids. *Journal of Pharmacology and Experimental Therapeutics, 268*, 1612–1623.

Mackie, K., Devane, W. & Hille, B. (1993). Anandamide, an endogenous cannabinoid, inhibits calcium currents as a partial agonist in N18 neuroblastoma cells. *Molecular Pharmacology, 44*, 498-503.

Mackie, K. & Hille, B. (1992). Cannabinoids inhibit N-type calcium channels in neuroblastoma-glioma cells. *Proceedings of the National Academy of Sciences of the United States of America, 89*, 3825–3829.

Mailleux, P. & Vanderhaeghen, J. (1993a). Dopaminergic regulation of cannabinoid receptor mRNA levels in the rat caudate-putamen: An in situ hybridization study. *Journal of Neurochemistry, 61*, 1705–1712.

Mailleux, P. & Vanderhaeghen, J. (1993b). Glucorticoid regulation of cannabinoid receptor messenger RNA levels in the rat caudate-putamen: An in situ hybridization study. *Neuroscience Letters, 156*, 51–53.

Manno, J., Kiplinger, G., Haine, S., Bennett, I. & Forney, R. (1970). Comparative effects of smoking marijuana or placebo on human motor and mental performance. *Clinical Pharmacology and Therapeutics, 11*, 808–815.

Manno, J., Kiplinger, G., Scholz, N., Forney, R. & Haine, S. (1971). The influence of alcohol and marijuana on motor and mental performance. *Clinical Pharmacology and Therapeutics, 12*, 202–211.

Martin, B.R., Compton, D.R., Thomas, B.F., Prescott, W.R., Little, P.J., Razdan, R.K., Johnson, M.R., Melvin, L.S., Mechoulam, R. & Ward, S.J. (1991). Behavioral, biochemical, and molecular modeling evaluations of cannabinoid analogs. *Pharmacology, Biochemistry and Behavior, 40*, 471–478.

Martin, B.R., Howlett, A.S. & Welch, S.P. (1989). Cannabinoid action in the central nervous system. *Problems of Drug Dependence 1988: Proceedings of the 50th Annual Scientific Meeting* (pp. 275–283). Washington, DC: U.S. Government Printing Office.

Martin, B.R., Welch, S.P. & Abood, M. (1994). Progress toward understanding the cannabinoid receptor and its second messenger systems. In M.W. Anders (Ed.), *Advances in Pharmacology* (pp. 341–397). San Diego, CA: Academic Press.

Mason, A.P. & McBay, A.J. (1984). Ethanol, marijuana, and other drug use in 600 drivers killed in single-vehicle crashes in North Carolina, 1978–1981. *Journal of Forensic Sciences, 29*, 987–1026.

Mason, A.P. & McBay, A.J. (1985). Cannabis: Pharmacology and interpretation of effects. *Journal of Forensic Sciences, 30*, 615–631.

Matsuda, L.A., Lolait, S.J., Brownstein, M.J., Young, A.C. & Bonner, T.I. (1990). Structure of a cannabinoid receptor and functional expression of the cloned cDNA. *Nature, 346*, 561–564.

McBay, A. (1985). Cannabinoid testing: Forensic and analytical aspects. *Laboratory Management, 23*, 36–41.

McBay, A. (1986). Drug concentrations and traffic safety. *Alcohol, Drugs and Driving, 2*, 51–59.

McLean, S., Parsons, R.S., Chesterman, R.B., Dineen, R., Johnson, M.G. & Davies, N.W. (1987). Drugs, alcohol and road accidents in Tasmania. *Medical Journal of Australia*, *147*, 6–11, 1987.

Mechoulam, R., Ben-Shabat, S., Hanus, L., Ligumsky, M., Kaminski, N.E., Schatz, A.R., Gopher, A., Almog, S., Martin, B.R., Compton, D.R., Pertwee, R.G., Griffin, G., Bayewitch, M., Barg, J. & Vogel, Z. (1995). Identification of an endogenous 2-monoglyceride, present in canine gut, that binds to cannabinoid receptors. *Biochemical Pharmacology*, *53*, 1477–1484.

Mechoulam, R., Feigenbaum, J.J., Lander, N., Segal, M., Järbe, T.U.C., Hiltunen, A.J. & Consroe, P. (1988). Enantiomeric cannabinoids: Stereospecificity of psychotropic activity. *Experientia*, *44*, 762–764.

Mechoulam, R., Hanus, L., Ben-Shabat, S., Fride, E. & Weidenfeld, J. (1994). The anandamides, a family of endogenous cannabinoid ligands: Chemical and biological studies. *Neuropsychopharmacology*, *10*, 145S.

Mechoulam, R., Hanus, L. & Martin, B.R. (1994). The search for endogenous ligands of the cannabinoid receptor. *Biochemical Pharmacology*, *48*, 1537–1544.

Melvin, L.S., Johnson, M.R., Harbert, C.A., Milne, G.M. & Weissman, A. (1984). A cannabinoid derived prototypical analgesic. *Journal of Medicinal Chemistry*, *27*, 67–71.

Milne, G.M. & Johnson, M.R. (1981). Levonantradol: A role for central prostanoid mechanisms. *Journal of Clinical Pharmacology*, *21*, 367S–374S.

Moskowitz, H. (1984). Attention tasks as skills performance measures of drug effects. *British Journal of Clinical Pharmacology*, *1*, 51S–61S.

Moskowitz, H. (1985). Marijuana and driving. *Accident Analysis and Prevention*, *17*, 323–345.

Moskowitz, H., Sharma, S. & McGlothlin, W. (1972). Effect of marijuana upon peripheral vision as a function of the information processing demands in central vision. *Perceptual Motor Skills*, *35*, 875–882.

Mountjoy, K.G., Robbins, L.S., Mortrud, M.T. & Cone, R.D. (1992). The cloning of a family of genes that encode the melanocortin receptors. *Science*, *257*, 1248–1251.

Munro, S., Thomas, K.L. & Abu-Shaar, M. (1993). Molecular characterization of a peripheral receptor for cannabinoids. *Nature*, *365*, 61–64.

Murray, J. (1986). Marijuana's effects on human cognitive functions, psychomotor functions, and personality. *Journal of General Psychology*, *113*, 23–55.

Nakahara, Y., Sekine, H. & Cook, C. (1989). Confirmation of cannabis use: II. Determination of tetrahydrocannabinol metabolites in urine and plasma by HPLC with ECD. *Journal of Analytical Toxicology*, *13*, 22–24.

Naor, Z. (1990). Cyclic GMP stimulates inositol phosphate production in cultured pituitary cells: Possible implications to signal transduction. *Biochemical and Biophysical Research Communications, 167*, 982–992.

Navarro, M., Fernandez-Ruiz, J.J., De Miguel, R., Hernandez, M.L., Cebeira, M. & Ramos, J.A. (1993). Motor disturbances induced by an acute dose of $\varnothing$-tetrahydrocannabinol: Possible involvement of nigrostriatal dopaminergic alterations. *Pharmacology, Biochemistry and Behavior, 45*, 291–298.

Nelemans, F. (1985). Medicines and narcotics: The impairment in drivers' ability to drive safely. *Journal of Traffic Medicine, 13*, B5.

Nye, J.S., Seltzman, H.H., Pitt, C.G. & Snyder, S.H. (1984). Labelling of a cannabinoid binding site in brain with a [³H]quarternary ammonium analogue of $\varnothing$-THC. *Marijuana '84: Proceedings of the Oxford Symposium on Cannabis* (pp. 253–262). Oxford, UK: IRL Press.

Nye, J.S., Seltzman, H.H., Pitt, C.G. & Snyder, S.S. (1985). High-affinity cannabinoid binding sites in brain membranes labeled with [³H]-5[1]-trimethylammonium-$\varnothing$-tetrahydrocannabinol. *Journal of Pharmacology and Experimental Therapeutics, 234*, 784–791.

Ohlsson, A., Lindgren, J.-E., Wahlen, A., Agurell, S., Hollister, L.E. & Gillespie, H.K. (1980). Plasma delta-9-tetrahydrocannabinol concentrations and clinical effects after oral and intravenous administration and smoking. *Clinical Pharmacology and Therapeutics, 28*, 409–416.

Ohlsson, A., Lindgren, J.-E., Wahlen, A., Agurell, S., Hollister, L.E. & Gillespie, H.K. (1982). Single dose kinetics of deuterium labelled $\varnothing$-tetrahydrocannabinol in heavy and light cannabis users. *Biomedical Mass Spectrometry, 9*, 6–11.

Okada, M., Urae, A., Mine, K., Shoyama, Y., Iwasaki, K. & Fujiwara, M. (1992). The facilitating and suppressing effects of $\varnothing$-tetrahydrocannabinol on the rise in intrasynaptosomal Ca^{2+} concentration in rats. *Neuroscience Letters, 140*, 55–58.

Onaivi, E.S., Green, M.R. & Martin, B.R. (1990). Pharmacological characterization of cannabinoids in the elevated plus maze. *Journal of Pharmacology and Experimental Therapeutics, 253*, 1002–1009.

Pacheco, M., Childers, S.R., Arnold, R., Casiano, F. & Ward, S.J. (1991). Aminoalkylindoles: Actions on specific G-protein-linked receptors. *Journal of Pharmacology and Experimental Therapeutics, 257*, 170–183.

Pacheco, M., Ward, S. & Childers, S. (1994). Differential requirements of sodium for coupling of cannabinoid receptors to adenylyl cyclase in rat brain membranes. *Journal of Neurochemistry, 62*, 1773–1782.

Paton, W.D.M., Pertwee, R.G. & Temple, D. (1972). The general pharmacology of cannabinoids. In J. Crown & W. Patten (Eds.), *Cannabis and Its Derivatives* (pp. 50–75). London: Oxford University Press.

Perez-Reyes, M. (1985). Pharmacodynamics of certain drugs of abuse. In G. Barnett & C.N. Chiang (Eds.), *Pharmacokinetics and Pharmacodynamics of Psychoactive Drugs: A Research Monograph* (pp. 287–310). Foster City, CA: Biomedical Publications.

Perez-Reyes, M., Di Guiseppi, S., Davis, K.H., Schindler, V.H. & Cook, C.E. (1982). Comparison of effects of marihuana cigarettes of three different potencies. *Clinical Pharmacology and Therapeutics, 31*, 617–624.

Perez-Reyes, M., Hicks, R.E., Bumberry, J., Jeffcoat, A.R. & Cook, C.E. (1988). Interaction between marihuana and ethanol: Effects on psychomotor performance. *Alcoholism: Clinical and Experimental Research, 12*, 268–276.

Perez-Reyes, M., Owens, S. & Di Guiseppi, S. (1981). The clinical pharmacology and dynamics of marijuana cigarette smoking. *Journal of Clinical Pharmacology, 21*, 201S–207S.

Pertwee, R. (1990). The central neuropharmacology of psychotropic cannabinoids. In D.J.K. Balfour (Ed.), *Psychotropic Drugs of Abuse* (p. 355–429). New York: Pergamon Press.

Pertwee, R.G. (1992). In vivo interactions between psychotropic cannabinoids and other drugs involving central and peripheral neurochemical mediators. In L. Murphy & A. Bartke (Eds.), *Marijuana/Cannabinoids: Neurobiology and Neurophysiology* (pp. 165–218). Boca Raton, FL: CRC Press.

Pertwee, R., Stevenson, L. & Griffin, G. (1993). Cross-tolerance between delta-9-tetrahydrocannabinol and the cannabimimetic agents, CP 55,940, WIN 55,212-2 and anandamide. *British Journal of Pharmacology, 110*, 1483–1490.

Pertwee, R.G., Stevenson, L.A., Elrick, D.B., Mechoulam, R. & Corbett, A.D. (1992). Inhibitory effects of certain enantiomeric cannabinoids in the mouse vas deferens and the myenteric plexus preparation of guinea-pig small intestine. *British Journal of Pharmacology, 105*, 980–984.

Poklis, A., Maginn, D. & Barr, J.L. (1987). Drug findings in "Driving Under the Influence of Drugs" cases: A problem of illicit drug use. *Drug and Alcohol Dependence, 20*, 57–62.

Rafaelsen, O.J., Bech, P. & Rafaelsen, L. (1973). Simulated car driving influenced by cannabis and alcohol. *Pharmakopsychiatry, 6*, 71–83.

Razdan, R.K. (1986). Structure–activity relationships in cannabinoids. *Pharmacological Reviews, 38,* 75–149.

Reeve, V.C., Grant, J.D., Robertson, W., Gillespie, H.K. & Hollister, L.E. (1983). Plasma concentrations of delta-9-tetrahydrocannabinol and impaired motor function. *Drug and Alcohol Dependence, 11,* 167–175.

Reeve, V., Robertson, W., Grant, J., Soares, J., Zimmerman, E., Gillespie, H. & Hollister, L. (1983). Hemolyzed blood and serum levels of delta-9-THC: Effects on the performance of roadside sobriety tests. *Journal of Forensic Sciences, 28,* 963–971.

Rinaldi-Carmona, M.R., Barth, F., Héaulme, M., Shire, D., Calandra, B., Congy, C., Martinez, S., Maruani, J., Néliat, G., Caput, D., Ferrara, P., Soubrié, P., Brelière, J.C. & Le Fur, G. (1994). SR 141716A, a potent and selective antagonist of the brain cannabinoid receptor. *FEBS Letters, 350,* 240–244.

Rodríguez de Fonseca, F., Hernandez, M.L., de Miguel, R., Fernández-Ruiz, J.J. & Ramos, J.A. (1992). Early changes in the development of dopaminergic neurotransmission after maternal exposure to cannabinoids. *Pharmacology, Biochemistry and Behavior, 41,* 469–474.

Rosenkrantz, H. (1983). Cannabis, marihuana, and cannabinoid toxicological manifestations in man and animals. In K.O. Fehr & H. Kalant (Eds.), *Cannabis and Health Hazards: Proceedings of an ARF/WHO Scientific Meeting on Adverse Health and Behavioral Consequences of Cannabis Use* (pp. 91–175). Toronto: Addiction Research Foundation.

Roth, S.H. & Williams, P.J. (1979). The non-specific membrane binding properties of $\varnothing$-tetrahydrocannabinol and the effects of various solubilizers. *Journal of Pharmacy and Pharmacology, 31,* 224–230.

Ryan, W.J., Banner, W.K., Wiley, J.L., Martin, B.R. & Razdan, R.K. (1997). Potent anandamide analogs: The effect of changing the length and branching of the end pentyl chain. *Journal of Medicinal Chemistry, 40,* 3617–3625.

Scallet, A.C. (1991). Neurotoxicology of cannabis and THC: A review of chronic exposure studies in animals. *Pharmacology, Biochemistry and Behavior, 40,* 671–676.

Scallet, A.C., Uemura, E., Andrews, A., Ali, S.F., McMillan, D.E., Paule, M.G., Brown, R.M. & Slikker, W., Jr. (1987). Morphometric studies of the rat hippocampus following chronic $\varnothing$-tetrahydrocannabinol (THC). *Brain Research, 436,* 193–198.

Schaefer, C., Gunn, C. & Dubowski, K. (1977). Dose-related heart rate, perceptual, and decisional changes in man following marijuana smoking. *Perceptual Motor Skills, 44,* 3–16.

Seltzman, H.H., Fleming, D.N., Thomas, B.F., Gilliam, A.F., McCallion, D.S., Pertwee, R.G., Compton, D.R. & Martin, B.R. (1997). Synthesis and pharmacological comparison of dimethylheptyl and pentyl analogs of anandamide. *Journal of Medicinal Chemistry, 40,* 3626–3634.

Shivachar, A.C., Martin, B.R. & Ellis, E.F. (1996). Anandamide- and $\varnothing$-tetrahydrocannabinol-evoked arachidonic acid mobilization and blockade by SR 141716A [N-(piperidin-1-yl)-5-(4-chlorophenyl)-1-(2,4-dichlorophenyl)-4-methyl-1H-pyrrazole-3-carboximide hydrochloride]. *Biochemical Pharmacology, 51*, 669–676.

Slikker, W., Jr., Paule, M.G., Ali, S.F., Scallet, A.C. & Bailey, J.R. (1992). Behavioral, neuro-chemical, and neurohistological effects of chronic marijuana smoke exposure in the nonhuman primate. In L. Murphy & A. Bartke (Eds.), *Marijuana/Cannabinoids: Neurobiology and Neurophysiology* (pp. 219–273). Boca Raton, FL: CRC Press.

Smiley, A.M., Moskowitz, H. & Ziedman, K. (1985). *Effects of Drugs on Driving: Driving Simulator Tests of Secobarbital, Diazepam, Marijuana, and Alcohol.* Rockville, MD: U.S. Department of Health and Human Services.

Smith, P.B., Compton, D.R., Welch, S.P., Razdan, R.K., Mechoulam, R. & Martin, B.R. (1994). The pharmacological activity of anandamide, a putative endogenous cannabinoid, in mice. *Journal of Pharmacology and Experimental Therapeutics, 270*, 219–227.

Soderstrom, C. & Carson, S. (1988). Update: Alcohol and other drug use among vehicular crash victims. *Makerere Medical Journal, 37*, 541–545.

Solowij, N., Michie, P.T. & Fox, A.M. (1991). Effects of long-term cannabis use on selective attention: An event-related potential study. *Pharmacology, Biochemistry and Behavior, 40*, 683–688.

Stoduto, G., Vingilis, E., Kapur, B., Sheu, W., McLellan, B. & Liban, C. (1993). Alcohol and drug use among motor vehicle collision victims admitted to a regional trauma unit: Demographic, injury, and crash characteristics. *Accident Analysis and Prevention, 25*, 411–420.

Sugiura, T., Kondo, S., Sukagawa, A., Nakane, S., Shinoda, A., Itoh, K., Yamashita, A. & Waku, K. (1995). 2-Arachidonoylglycerol: A possible endogenous cannabinoid receptor ligand in brain. *Biochemical and Biophysical Research Communications, 215*, 89–97.

Sutton, L. (1983). The effects of alcohol, marijuana and their combination on driving ability. *Journal of Studies on Alcohol, 44*, 438–445.

Sutton, L. & Praegle, I. (1992). The drug impaired driver detection and forensic specimen analysis. *Blutalkohol, 29*, 134–138.

Thomas, B.F., Wei, X. & Martin, B.R. (1992). Characterization and autoradiographic localization of the cannabinoid binding site in rat brain using [^{3}H]11-OH-$\varnothing$-THC-DMH. *Journal of Pharmacology and Experimental Therapeutics, 263*, 1383–1390.

Thompson, L. & Cone, E. (1987). Determination of delta-9-tetrahydrocannabinol in human blood and saliva by high-performance liquid chromatography with amperometric detection. *Journal of Chromatography, 421*, 91–97.

Tinklenberg, J.R., Kopell, B.S., Melges, F.T. & Hollister, L.E. (1972). Marihuana and alcohol: Time production and memory functions. *Archives of General Psychiatry, 27*, 812–815.

Van der Kloot, W. (1994). Anandamide, a naturally-occurring agonist of the cannabinoid receptor, blocks adenylate cyclase at the frog neuromuscular junction. *Brain Research, 649*, 181–184.

Vogel, Z., Barg, J., Levy, R., Saya, D., Heldman, E. & Mechoulam, R. (1993). Anandamide, a brain endogenous compound, interacts specifically with cannabinoid receptors and inhibits adenylate cyclase. *Journal of Neurochemistry, 61*, 352–355.

Wall, M.E., Sadler, B.M., Brine, D., Taylor, H. & Perez-Reyes, M. (1983). Metabolism, disposition, and kinetics of $\varnothing^9$-tetrahydrocannabinol in men and women. *Clinical Pharmacology and Therapeutics, 34*, 352–363.

Ward, S.J., Childers, S.R. & Pacheco, M. (1989). Pravadoline and aminoalkylindole (AAI) analogues: Actions which suggest a receptor interaction. *British Journal of Pharmacology* (Suppl. 98), 831P.

Ward, S.J., Mastriani, D., Casiano, F. & Arnold, R. (1990). Pravadoline: Profile in isolated tissue preparations. *Journal of Pharmacology and Experimental Therapeutics, 255*, 1230–1239.

Weidenfeld, J., Feldman, S. & Mechoulam, R. (1994). Effect of the brain constituent anandamide, a cannabinoid receptor agonist, on the hypotholamo-pituitary-adrenal axis in the rat. *Neuroendocrinology, 59*, 110–112.

Welch, S.P., Thomas, C. & Patrick, G.S. (1995). Modulation of cannabinoid-induced antinociception following intracerebroventricular versus intrathecal administration to mice: Possible mechanisms for interaction with morphine. *Journal of Pharmacology and Experimental Therapeutics, 272*, 310–321.

Westlake, T.M., Howlett, A.C., Ali, S.F., Paule, M.G., Scallet, A.C. & Slikker, W., Jr. (1991). Chronic exposure to delta-9-tetrahydrocannabinol fails to irreversibly alter brain cannabinoid receptors. *Brain Research, 544*, 145–149.

Wickens, A.P. & Pertwee, R.G. (1993). $\varnothing^9$-Tetrahydrocannabinol and anandamide enhance the ability of muscimol to induce catalepsy in the globus pallidus of rats. *European Journal of Pharmacology, 250*, 205–208.

Wiley, J., Balster, R. & Martin, B.R. (1995). Discriminative stimulus effects of anandamide in rats. *European Journal of Pharmacology, 276*, 49–54.

Williams, A.F., Peat, M.A., Crouch, D.J., Wells, J.K. & Finkle, B.S. (1985). Drugs in fatally injured young male drivers. *Public Health Reports, 100* (1), 19–25.

Wilson, W.H., Ellinwood, E.H., Mathew, R.J. & Johnson, K. (1994). Effects of marijuana on performance of a computerized cognitive-neuromotor test battery. *Psychiatry Research, 51*, 115–125.

Yesavage, J.A., Leirer, V.O., Denari, M. & Hollister, L.E. (1985). Carry-over effects of marijuana intoxication on aircraft pilot performance: A preliminary report. *American Journal of Psychiatry, 142*, 1325–1329.

Zimmerman, E.G., Yeager, E.P., Soares, J.R., Hollister, L. & Reeve, V.C. (1983). Measurement of D9- tetrahydrocannabinol (THC) in whole blood samples from impaired motorists. *Journal of Forensic Sciences, 28*, 957–962.

Epidemiology
of Cannabis Use
and Its Consequences

Epidemiology of Cannabis Use and Its Consequences

WAYNE HALL, LLOYD JOHNSTON AND NEIL DONNELLY

This chapter summarizes and critically reviews the epidemiological evidence on patterns of cannabis use and their effects on health and psychological functioning. The chapter is divided into two parts reflecting the comparative independence of the epidemiological literatures on patterns of cannabis use and their health consequences. Smart's remark on reviewing this literature in the early 1980s is still true today: "the epidemiology of cannabis use and the clinical epidemiology of adverse reactions are fields that have grown up separately" (1983, p. 755).

The epidemiological literature on patterns of cannabis use and their health and psychological consequences is largely based on studies conducted in English-speaking countries, most particularly the United States. Countries with a long tradition of heavy cannabis use are not well represented in the research literature. The exceptions are studies of patterns of cannabis use and their consequences in those developing countries studied by American researchers in the 1970s (namely, Costa Rica, Greece, Jamaica), and a small number of studies of the cognitive effects of chronic cannabis use conducted by Egyptian and Indian investigators.

The preponderance of American research on the health effects of cannabis use reflects the emergence over the past several decades of widespread cannabis use among adolescents and young adults in the United States. The novelty of this development raised considerable societal concern that led to the allocation of the resources necessary to undertake large-scale surveys of cannabis use and epidemiological studies of the health and psychological consequences of its use among young adults.

The first section of the chapter describes what can be inferred about patterns of cannabis use from the findings of surveys of the general population, high school students and special populations at high risk of illicit drug use in English-speaking countries. This is preceded by a brief discussion of the validity of self-reported drug use, and its implications for the interpretation of apparent trends in cannabis use over time. We also briefly describe the characteristics of users that predict earlier initiation of cannabis use, and the transition to heavy, chronic cannabis use, the pattern of use that probably poses the most serious threat to the health of users.

The second section summarizes the epidemiological evidence on the health and psychological consequences of cannabis use. For the purpose of this section, epidemiological evidence is taken to include controlled studies that examine and attempt to explain associations between cannabis use and human disease and dysfunctional behavior. Although this definition includes case-control studies, cross-sectional studies, cohort studies and experiments, the emphasis will be on large sample cross-sectional and prospective studies of health outcomes among cannabis users. This has been done to minimize duplication of the material covered in other chapters where case-control and controlled clinical studies of particular health effects are described in detail.

Patterns of Cannabis Use

Methodological Issues in Assessing Cannabis Use

Because cannabis is an illegal drug in most English-speaking countries, data on the patterns of its use in these countries are less readily available than data on the use of legal drugs like alcohol and tobacco. Thus, there are practically no data on the volume of cannabis produced or imported, on wholesale or retail sales, nor are there regular market research surveys as there are for alcohol and tobacco. Information about cannabis use has had to be collected by special purpose surveys of drug use which, because of their expense, have often been conducted intermittently and opportunistically by different groups of researchers, using highly varied sampling and survey methods.

Surveys of illicit drug use face a number of obstacles. Because use of these drugs is illegal there are a number of potential biases that operate to underestimate the prevalence of use. First, illicit drug users are likely to be undersampled in household surveys, and those who are contacted may be reluctant to participate in a survey for fear of the consequences of admitting to an illegal act. Second, even if users agree to participate they may be less inclined to give truthful

responses for the same reason. Third, even if users can be persuaded to give honest answers to questions, it is probable that they will underestimate both the frequency of their use and the quantities that they consume (Bachman & O'Malley, 1981).

These sampling and response biases are well known to drug survey researchers who have developed various methods to minimize them. For example, subjects can be given guarantees of anonymity and confidentiality which encourage honest answers to questions about drug use. Non-existent drugs can be included to catch out those respondents who are exaggerating their drug use (Spooner & Flaherty, 1992). These and other methods minimize but do not eliminate sampling and response biases in surveys of drug use, most of which operate in the direction of underestimating use.

Despite the biases toward underreporting, particularly the frequency of use, the evidence of validity of self-reported drug-use measures in carefully designed studies is quite strong. O'Malley et al. (1983), for example, demonstrated reliability levels comparable to most other psychometric measures, using a three-wave panel analysis of a national sample of high school seniors followed for three to four years beyond high school. They have also shown that although over time there is some later denial of earlier reported lifetime drug use, such denial is quite low for marijuana use (Johnston & O'Malley, 1997). Co-ordinated cross-sectional studies of secondary school students in six Western countries, sponsored by the Council of Europe, have also shown good evidence of reliability and validity (Johnston, Driessen & Kokkevi, 1994).

Further, whatever biases there may be towards underestimation of cannabis use, they are probably fairly constant across time, making their impact on trend estimates of less concern. While it has been hypothesized that an increase in societal disapproval of using a drug may lead to an increasing degree of underreporting, Johnston et al. (1996) argued that this is not necessarily the case. Using cross-time data over two decades, they have shown that reported levels of cannabis use for respondents' unidentified friends, about whom there is presumably much less motivation to conceal use, closely parallel trends in self-reported use. Despite considerable changes in peer norms over that historical interval, Johnston and colleagues concluded that the degree of underreporting remained relatively stable.

The United States

The United States has undertaken the longest series of surveys of illicit drug use. Two major drug survey projects have collected nationwide data on self-reported drug use in the United States for over the last 20 years. The "Monitoring the Future" project, directed by researchers at the University of Michigan Institute for Social Research and sponsored by the National Institute on Drug Abuse, has conducted nationwide surveys of samples of high school seniors, college students and young adults annually since 1975 (Johnston, O'Malley & Bachman, 1996). The National Household Survey on Drug Abuse (sponsored by the U.S. Substance Abuse and Mental Health Services Administration) has conducted surveys of household samples throughout the United States on a regular basis since 1972.

NATIONAL HOUSEHOLD SURVEY ON DRUG ABUSE

The National Household Survey surveyed approximately 9,000 persons, aged 12 years and older, in randomly selected households throughout the United States every two to three years a number of times between 1971 and 1990. After 1990, the surveys were conducted on an annual basis and from 1991 through 1993 had much larger sample sizes, ranging from 26,000 to 33,000 per year. Since 1993,

the sample sizes have been about 18,000 per year (SAMHSA, 1997a).

In 1996, one-third (33 per cent) of the national household sample reported that they had tried cannabis, 9 per cent had used in the past year, and 4 per cent reported that they were current users (see Table 1). Lifetime use was related to age, increasing from 17 per cent among those aged 12 to 17 years to a peak of 51 per cent among those aged 26 to 34 years and declined to 27 per cent among those over the age of 35 years. Clearly, different birth cohorts have had different degrees of experience related to cannabis use, with those finishing adolescence before the mid-1960s having had much less experience than those who grew up in subsequent years. Rates of discontinuation of use were high, with over 90 per cent of the population not having used cannabis in the prior year. Put another way, nearly three-quarters of all people who had tried cannabis were no longer using it. Weekly cannabis use was uncommon and its prevalence was strongly related to gender (9 per cent of men and 6 per cent of women) and to age (with a peak prevalence of 21 per cent among those aged 12 to 17 years who had ever used, or 11 per cent of all 12- to 17-year-olds [see Table 2]).

Trends in the prevalence of cannabis use in the National Household Survey series from 1974 to 1990 are shown in Table 3. These results show that the prevalence of cannabis use increased throughout the 1970s, peaking in 1979, before declining steadily throughout the 1980s to reach

TABLE 1.
Prevalence Rates of Cannabis Use: U.S. Household Survey 1996

	% ever used	% last year	% last month
12–17 yrs	16.8	13.0	7.1
18–25 yrs	44.0	23.8	13.2
26–34 yrs	50.5	11.3	6.3
35+ yrs	27.0	3.8	2.0
Total	32.0	8.6	4.7

SOURCE.
Substance Abuse and Mental Health Services Administration (SAMHSA) (1997b)

TABLE 2.

Per Cent Weekly Use, and Discontinuation Rates Among Those Who Ever Used Cannabis: U.S. Household Survey 1996

	Weekly use	Weekly use as a per cent of ever use	Per cent lifetime users who did not use in past year
Gender			
Females	1.6	5.8	78.2
Males	4.1	11.1	69.2
Total	2.8	8.8	73.1
Age			
12–17	3.6	21.4	22.6
18–25	8.8	20.0	45.9
26–34	4.0	7.9	77.6
35+	1.1	4.1	85.9
Age by gender			
Females			
12–17	2.8	16.4	25.7
18–25	5.2	13.4	53.7
26–34	2.7	5.9	82.0
35+	0.4	1.8	91.3
Males			
12–17	4.3	26.1	20.0
18–25	12.4	25.2	39.4
26–34	5.4	9.8	73.6
35+	1.8	5.5	82.1

SOURCE.
Estimates derived from information contained in SAMHSA (1997b)

TABLE 3.

Trends in Past Month Prevalence of Cannabis: U.S. Household Survey 1974–1996

Age group	1974	1976	1977	1979	1985	1988	1990	1992	1995	1996
12–17	12.0	12.3	16.6	16.3	13.2	8.1	7.1	5.3	10.9	9.0
18–25	25.2	25.0	27.4	38.0	25.3	17.9	15.0	13.1	14.2	15.6
26+	2.0	3.5	3.3							
26–34				20.8	23.1	14.7	10.9	11.4	8.3	8.4
35+				2.8	3.9	2.3	3.1	2.5	2.8	2.9

SOURCES.
National Institute on Drug Abuse (1992) for years 1974–77; Substance Abuse and Mental Health Services Administration (SAMHSA) (1997a) for subsequent years

levels in 1990 that were often lower than those reported in 1974. In the 1990s, however, use among adolescents once again began to rise.

THE MONITORING THE FUTURE PROJECT

In this ongoing series of surveys, estimates of the prevalence of cannabis use are provided among samples of secondary school students, college students and young adults. Each year since 1975 approximately 17,000 high school seniors have been surveyed. The samples of college students and young adults comprised a proportion of those who were originally surveyed as high school seniors (about 14 per cent) and were subsequently followed up every two years. Starting in 1991, national samples of 8th and 10th grade students have also been surveyed annually.

In the 1993 survey, lifetime use increased for each higher age level (see Table 4), but annual use was highest at about age 18 (senior year of high school), before beginning a gradual decline with age (Johnston, O'Malley & Bachman, 1996). Current daily use, defined as use on 20 or more occasions in the 30 days prior to the survey, was also highest at age 18. About 1 in every 20 high school seniors (4.9 per cent) reported current daily use, far fewer than in the peak year of 1978 when nearly 1 in every 9 high school seniors (10.7 per cent) reported such use.

Because of the high prevalence of daily use in the late 1970s, in 1982 the investigators added more questions to the survey of 12th graders on the lifetime prevalence and duration of daily use. In 1982, they found that 20.5 per cent of the 12th graders had smoked cannabis daily for a month or more — a statistic that fell steadily to 8.4 per cent by 1992, before rising again to 12.1 per cent by 1995. Such behavior consistently has been higher among males than females, and much higher among those who did not plan to attend college than among those who did. Of the 1995 seniors who by 12th grade (age 18) had become daily cannabis smokers for at least a month, more than two-thirds had this pattern of heavy use by 10th grade (age 16). In 1993, 3.6 per cent of all American 12th graders surveyed reported that they had smoked cannabis daily for two years or more on a cumulative basis. Earlier in the epidemic it had been feared that a much larger proportion of youth would become long-term, heavy users, but this did not occur because of a dramatic decline in overall use.

Table 5 shows wide fluctuations since 1975 in cannabis use among American adolescents in secondary school. Among 12th graders, lifetime prevalence peaked at 65 per cent in 1980, then fell by nearly half by the early 1990s; annual prevalence peaked at 51 per cent in 1979 and fell by more than three-fifths (to 22 per cent) by 1992. Not only did the initiation rate decline, as evidenced by the fall in lifetime prevalence, but the rate of discontinuation rose considerably (see Table 5, third column). The factors which appear

TABLE 4.
1993 U.S. Monitoring the Future Survey: Cannabis Prevalence

	% ever used	% last year	% last month	% daily
8th grade (12 years)	23.1	18.3	11.3	1.5
10th grade (14 years)	39.8	33.6	20.4	3.5
12th grade (18 years)	44.9	35.8	21.9	4.9
College	45.1	33.1	17.5	2.8
19–28 years	53.4	27.0	15.1	3.3

SOURCE.
Monitoring the Future Study, University of Michigan

TABLE 5.

Trends in Cannabis Use Among Twelfth Graders

	% any lifetime use	% any use in past 12 months	% discontinuation rates among those who had:	
			Used any	Used 10+ times
1975	47	40	15	4
1980	60	49	19	5
1985	54	41	25	8
1990	41	27	34	12
1992	33	22	33	11
1993	45	36	20	8

SOURCE.
Monitoring the Future, The University of Michigan

to explain these large declines in use will be discussed below, but also it should be noted that other drugs, both licit and illicit had quite different cross-time trends in use, suggesting that the changes in cannabis use reflected factors specific to that drug. While most users of other illicit drugs also had used cannabis, trends in the use of other illicit drugs were fairly independent of the cannabis-use trends. (This was possible because cannabis prevalence is generally much higher than the prevalence of other illicit drugs by late adolescence.)

One other point to note in Table 5 is how few of those who had used cannabis 10 or more times, stopped their use by 12th grade. Most of the discontinuation (defined as the population of lifetime users who reported no use in the prior 12 months) has occurred among those who did not yet have a great deal of experience with cannabis.

Following more than a decade of fairly steady decline in cannabis use among American secondary students, the 1992 surveys of 8th graders and 1993 surveys of 8th, 10th and 12th graders showed an abrupt turnaround. Cannabis use began to rise sharply in all three grades. The turnaround was evident in both an increasing initiation rate and a higher rate of continued use (see Table 5).

Johnston and his colleagues have marshalled considerable evidence to suggest that changes in certain attitudes and beliefs about cannabis use have been pivotal in driving down the epidemic levels of use during the late 1970s and more recently in driving it up again. For some years, they have reported a strong negative correlation across time between the prevalence of cannabis use and both the perceived risk of using cannabis and peer disapproval of use (e.g., Johnston, Bachman & O'Malley, 1981; Johnston, O'Malley & Bachman, 1996). Over the interval 1979 to 1992, there was a dramatic increase in perceived risk, a somewhat less dramatic increase in personal disapproval of use, and large decline in use. Additional analyses of quitters and abstainers (Johnston, 1982; 1985a) showed that the two most frequently checked reasons for not using cannabis were concerns about adverse effects on physical and psychological health. These concerns were mentioned with increasing frequency, particularly by quitters from 1976 onward. Johnston concluded:

A logical interpretation of these data is that changes in the beliefs concerning the harmfulness of regular marijuana use led to changes in personal disapproval which, when shared among friends, translated into changes in perceived peer norms. The fact that personal disapproval rose more quickly than perceived peer disapproval . . . helps to substantiate the last link in this sequence. The much more rapid increase in perceived harmfulness than in personal disapproval provides some substantiation for the first. (Johnston, 1985a, pp. 157–158)

Johnston subsequently expanded this theoretical interpretation, according to which perceived risk affects drug use both directly and indirectly (through peer norms), into a more elaborated theory that identified societal forces that are likely to influence perceived risk and social disapproval (Johnston, 1991). This line of work has also shown that the perceived availability of cannabis did not change much over the last 18 years and therefore cannot explain the long period of decline or the more recent increase (e.g., Johnston, O'Malley & Bachman, 1996).

Johnston et al. (1991) report a strong negative correlation between the perceived risks of cannabis use and cannabis prevalence rates over time. In an analysis of the data to 1986, Bachman et al. (1988) found that while lifestyle variables (e.g., truancy, school performance, hours worked, income, religiosity, political beliefs, number of nights out) were strong predictors of cannabis use at any given point in time, changes in these variables could not account for the decrease in prevalence of cannabis use. Rather, the decline in cannabis use rates occurred consistently across the different categories of each of these lifestyle risk factors, suggesting a secular trend of declining use. Thus, the alternative hypothesis that the decline in use occurring in the 1980s was attributable to an increased "conservatism" among young people, did not stand up to empirical test.

Johnston et al. (1996) attributed the recent sharp upturn in the use of cannabis (and some other drugs) to a decline in perceived risk, which preceded the turnaround in use, as well as a decline in social disapproval of use, which occurred concurrently. They hypothesized that these attitudes and beliefs have changed as a result of lower public attention to the drug-use problem in general in recent years; a growth in pro-drug messages in the culture, especially from rock musicians; and to "generational forgetting" — the replacement generation of young people having less opportunity than the preceding generation to learn vicariously about the dangers of drug use from those around them and from those they see in the media.

Canada

A national telephone survey was conducted in Canada in 1989 by Health and Welfare Canada. The sample comprised 11,634 persons aged 15 years and older. Some of the results of this survey have been documented by Williams et al. (1992) in their profile of Canadian drug and alcohol use, but unfortunately they did not provide detailed information on the sampling methodology or questionnaire format. Overall, 23 per cent of the sample reported that they had used cannabis at some time in their lives, with higher rates among males than females across all age groups. Prevalence of use declined with age from a high of 43 per cent among those aged 20 to 24 years to 10 per cent among those aged 45 to 54 years and 2 per cent among those aged 55 to 64 years. Rates of discontinuation were substantial with only 14 per cent of those who had ever used cannabis having done so in the past year.

There have been a number of school surveys conducted in various provinces throughout Canada since the mid-1970s. The most regular of these have been carried out in Ontario biennially since 1977. Adlaf and Smart (1991) reviewed findings across 6 of the 10 provinces where surveys had been conducted intermittently between the early 1970s and the late 1980s. The most consistent trend pattern for cannabis suggested an increase in prevalence through the 1970s, then a sharp decline through the 1980s.

The Ontario data provide the most reliable source for comparing trend patterns with other countries. The Ontario series surveyed students in grades 7, 9, 11 and 13 (corresponding to ages 10 through 19 years old) with sample sizes between 3,000 and 5,000. Age-adjusted prevalence of cannabis use during the previous 12 months has declined from 32 per cent in 1979 to 14 per cent in 1989. Declines were also reported for nine other drug types including tobacco and alcohol. Rates of illicit drug use were lower in Ontario than in the neighboring United States. The size of the decline in rates of annual cannabis use was greater than for other substances. Among cannabis users, frequency of use has also declined over successive samples (Smart & Adlaf, 1989).

Unlike in the United States, Adlaf and Smart (1991) reported that the perceived availability of cannabis among Ontario students declined during the period 1985 to 1989. However, the percentage reporting a high likelihood of apprehension by the authorities for using cannabis had also decreased. More importantly, the Ontario data agreed with the U.S. finding that the perceived health risks of cannabis use have increased over time. Further, as with the U.S. data, the decline in cannabis use could not be explained by a decrease in "deviant" behavior, as none of these measures had decreased, and some had actually increased (Adlaf & Smart, 1991).

Recently, McKenzie, Williams and Single (1997) reported an analysis of trends in cannabis use in Canada between 1989 and 1994. This revealed a decline in the percentage of persons who had used cannabis in the past year between 1989 (5.6 per cent) and 1993 (4.2 per cent), followed by a small increase in use in 1994 (7.4 per cent). Throughout the period, males were consistently more likely to use cannabis than females. In 1994, detailed analyses by age showed that the highest rates of lifetime use and use in the past year were among young adults aged 15 to 24 years.

Australia and New Zealand

Cannabis continues to be the most widely used illicit drug in Australia, with approximately a third of adults reporting that they have ever used the drug in national household surveys of those aged 15 years and older conducted in 1993 (Donnelly & Hall, 1994) and in 1995 (Makkai & McAllister, 1997). Cannabis use was strongly related to gender and age. Men were more likely to have used cannabis than women. Young adults in the 20 to 25 age group had the highest rates of use, and adults over the age of 45 years were much less likely to have used than younger adults, reflecting the initiation of widespread cannabis use among young Australian adults in the early 1970s (Donnelly & Hall, 1994).

Most use was "experimental" in that more than half of those who have ever used cannabis

(three-quarters of women and two-thirds of men) have discontinued their use, or used less than weekly. The proportion of users who become weekly users was 7 per cent of women and 15 per cent of men. Weekly cannabis use (defined as using three or more times in the previous month) was most common among the younger age groups, and highest among those aged 20 to 24 years, declining steeply thereafter (see Donnelly & Hall, 1994).

There appears to have been a small increase in the percentage of Australians who have ever tried cannabis between 1985 and 1995, from 28 per cent in 1985 to 31 per cent in 1995 (Makkai & McAllister, 1997). The increase in lifetime, more recent and regular marijuana use was more marked among adolescents aged 14 to 19 years. Over the decade, in this age group the prevalence of lifetime use increased from 32 per cent to 41 per cent, use in the past year increased from 23 per cent to 31 per cent, and weekly use increased from 6 per cent to 10 per cent.

Standardized surveys of drug use in the general population were not conducted in Australia before 1985 but "omnibus" household surveys conducted throughout the 1970s by market research companies included questions on cannabis use (McAllister, Moore & Makkai, 1991). These show an increase in the prevalence of cannabis use for all age groups between 1973 and 1984. Among 20- to 29-year-olds, for example, the prevalence of ever having used cannabis increased from 23 per cent in 1973 to 39 per cent in 1984. An apparently sharp increase in the prevalence of cannabis use between the 1984 market research survey and the 1985 national household survey probably reflected a change in the degree of anonymity afforded to respondents (Donnelly & Hall, 1994).

In New Zealand, a 1990 telephone survey of over 5,000 persons showed that 43 per cent of adults between the ages of 15 and 45 years of age had used cannabis at some time in their lives, and 12 per cent had used in the previous year (Black & Casswell, 1993). Just over half of all males (52 per cent) and a third of all females (35 per cent) reported that they had ever used cannabis. Use was lowest among those aged 15 to 17 years and increased for older aged groups, and there was a decline in use after age 40.

Europe

Few European countries have undertaken regular series of community or high school surveys of cannabis and other illicit drug use. WHO Regional Office for Europe collected data from 21 countries that had surveyed illicit drug use in the general population (Harkin, Anderson & Goos, 1997). The few that had trend data on the prevalence of cannabis use (e.g., Denmark, France, Switzerland and the United Kingdom) showed increases in the prevalence of cannabis use in the early 1990s (Harkin, Anderson & Goos, 1997). In all cases, the prevalence of current use was substantially less than lifetime use, indicating that cessation of cannabis use was common. Rates of current use were highest among those aged 15 to 24 years.

The Pompidou Group (Johnston, Driessen & Kokkevi, 1994) undertook a study of the feasibility and validity of using school surveys to monitor illicit drug use among high school students in Belgium, France, Greece, Italy, Netherlands, Portugal and Sweden (using a sample from the United States as the comparison). The study showed that it was possible to obtain valid data on illicit drug use. It found that the prevalence rates for almost all illicit drugs were at least two times higher in the U.S. sample (which had prevalence rates that were typical of the United States). In the European samples, marijuana had been used at least once by 10 per cent to 36 per cent of the older student population, and had been used in the past 30 days by between 3 and 14 per cent of the European students, as against 19 per cent of the U.S. students. Marijuana was used on a near daily basis by 1 per cent or less of European samples compared with 3 per cent of the U.S. sample.

In the Netherlands, a large national survey of drug use was undertaken in 1992 of over 10,000 students aged 10 to 18 years (de Zwat, Mensink & Kuipers, 1994). About one-third of males and one-fifth of females had used cannabis at some time in their lives. Data from three national school surveys in 1984, 1988 and 1992 showed large increases in use between 1988 and 1992, particularly among males. This limited data suggests that the prevalence of cannabis use by young people in Europe is probably much lower than that in the United States, Australia and New Zealand, although rates may have increased over the past decade.

Cannabis Use in Other Regions

There is limited survey data on trends in cannabis use in other parts of the world. Occasional surveys have been reported from specific countries but their results have often been reported in ways that make it difficult to compare rates between countries. In many cases, the data only provide crude rates of cannabis use in these countries. Survey methods are poorly reported, and results are often published only in summary form. It is sometimes unclear whether reported rates refer to lifetime use or to more recent cannabis use, and only rarely are data reported on rates of cannabis use in different age groups for men and women. Often only an overall rate of cannabis use is reported for all adults, which understates the extent of cannabis use among young adults who are the heaviest users. With these caveats the following data are briefly reviewed.

AFRICA

There is limited survey data from Egypt and Morocco, two countries with a long tradition of cannabis use (predominantly in the form of hashish). In Egypt, a prevalence estimate of 5 per cent has been cited in the United Nations Drug Control Program's (UNDCP) regional report (1994), but it is uncertain whether this refers to the percentage who have ever used cannabis or to the percentage who have used in the last year. A survey of about 5,000 workers reported that 11.5 per cent had ever used cannabis.

In Morocco, Lamasouri (1993, cited in UNDCP, 1994) reported the results of a survey of drug use among 500 students aged 14 to 26 in

Tangier, one of the regions of Morocco with reputedly a high prevalence of cannabis use. Two-thirds of the sample reported ever having used cannabis: 11.3 per cent were "frequent" users; 18.6 per cent were occasional users; and 8.1 per cent had used only once.

Low rates of ever having used cannabis have been reported in small surveys in Namibia and Nigeria (UNDCP, 1994). A 1991 survey of 600 Namibian school children and their parents reported that 8.2 per cent of parents had ever used cannabis, and 3.3 per cent were daily users. Among the school children, 7.0 per cent had ever used cannabis, 3.7 per cent were occasional users and 0.7 per cent were daily users. In Nigeria a 1991 survey in Lagos State (age range unspecified) reported that 5 per cent of the sample had ever used cannabis.

Two surveys of drug use have been reported among secondary school students in Zimbabwe in 1990 and 1994 (Eide & Acuda, 1995; 1996). In 1990, the prevalence of lifetime use among 12- to 14-year-olds was 5.5 per cent for boys and 1.0 per cent for girls. This increased to 12.7 and 3.2 per cent among 17- to 18-year-old boys and girls respectively. There was suggestive evidence of an increase in the prevalence of use between 1990 and 1994.

Surveys of drug use in the general population and among school children have been reported from a number of regions of South Africa (Rocha-Silva, 1991; Rocha-Silva, de Miranda & Erasmus, 1996). In a 1990 survey of over 3,000 adults aged over 14 years, 13 per cent of males in urban areas reported current use, as against 9 per cent in towns, 22 per cent in squatter camps and 5 per cent in tribal areas (Rocha-Silva, 1991). A survey of African youth in rural and urban areas reported that 5.5 per cent were current cannabis users (Rocha-Silva, de Miranda & Erasmus, 1996).

LATIN AMERICA AND THE CARIBBEAN

Brazil is one of the few Latin American countries to report a series of surveys of cannabis use among high school students. Carlini et al. (1990) reviewed Brazilian survey data, including two large national school based surveys conducted in 1987 (n = 16,151) and 1989 (n = 30,770), and several smaller surveys of street children. The age range of students in the school surveys was not specified; only overall rates were provided. The rate of ever having used cannabis was 2.9 per cent in 1987 and 3.4 per cent in 1989. The highest prevalence levels occurred in Brasilia (5.6 per cent in 1987 and 4.0 per cent in 1989) and Sao Paulo (3.5 per cent in 1987 and 4.7 per cent in 1989). Drug use among street children was much higher: 72 per cent had used cannabis at some point, and 44 per cent in the past year in 1987.

Ospina et al. (1993) reported the findings of a 1992 National Household Survey on Drug Abuse in Colombia. In the household sample of 8,975 adults, 5.3 per cent of respondents reported having used cannabis at least once (10.4 per cent of males and 1.7 per cent of females). Usage was highest among those aged 18 to 24 years, with 1.5 per cent having used during the previous year. Only 0.5 per cent of 12- to 17-year-olds had used during the past 12 months.

The Centros de Integración Juvenil (1992) summarized the findings of a number of surveys conducted in Mexico since the mid-1970s. A National Survey of Addictions was conducted in 1988, which sampled 15,000 respondents aged between 12 and 65 years. It found a lifetime prevalence rate for cannabis use of 3 per cent. Cannabis use was higher among males than females (7.6 per cent versus 2.2 per cent ever used) and more prevalent among younger age groups. The highest rates of use were in the northwest region where 15.4 per cent of respondents aged 12 to 34 years old reported ever having used cannabis, 7.9 per cent having used during the past year, and 4.0 per cent having used during the past month.

The Institute on Alcoholism and Drug Dependency conducted a survey of drug use in Costa Rica in 1988 (cited in UNDCP, 1994). Since no methodological details were provided, it is not clear what the prevalence rate of 9.1 per cent for cannabis referred to. A rate of "ever use" of 17 per cent has been reported in El Salvador, with

3 per cent current users. A 1990 survey of three urban areas in Guatemala of persons aged 12 to 45 years reported a prevalence rate of 7 per cent.

Reported rates of cannabis use in other countries in South America have been low. The UNDCP regional report (1994) quotes an annual prevalence rate of 7.6 per cent and a daily prevalence rate of 4 per cent for Chile, and a lifetime prevalence rate of 4.2 per cent for Ecuador in 1992. A 1988 survey of persons aged 12 years and over in Venezuela found a prevalence of use in the last six months of 5.6 per cent. The prevalence of use in the last 30 days was 3.8 per cent and the prevalence of daily use was 1.2 per cent.

A recent analysis has been published of the prevalence of lifetime cannabis use in a number of Latin American and Caribbean countries, including Bolivia, Colombia, the Dominican Republic, Ecuador, Guatemala, Haiti, Jamaica, Panama, Paraguay and Peru (Jutkowitz & Eu, 1994). This found that the highest lifetime prevalence of use was in Jamaica where 29 per cent of adults had used the drug. The equivalent prevalence rates in the other countries was much lower, ranging between 1.2 per cent in Paraguay and 7.3 per cent in Guatemala (Jutkowitz & Eu, 1994). In all countries except Haiti, males were more likely to report cannabis use than females.

ASIA

India has a long tradition of cannabis use from Vedic times for religious, medical and nutritional purposes, but until recently there has been very little data collected on patterns of cannabis use or on trends in the use of cannabis for its psychoactive effects. This data has only been collected in a small number of regions, which makes it difficult to generalize to the whole population of this large and diverse nation (Channabasavanna, Ray & Kaliaperumal, 1989; Indian Council on Medical Research, 1993; National Institute for Social Defense, 1992). Surveys in three northern Indian states in 1989 and 1991 found a lifetime prevalence rate of 3 per cent and a prevalence of current use of 1 per cent and no evidence of an increase between 1989 and 1991. Rates in southern states were higher, with 7 per cent having used at some time in their lives and 3 per cent current users.

One of the few detailed studies of patterns of cannabis use is that of Machado (1994) who conducted household surveys in three geographic regions of India. The regions were chosen so as to comprise a rural area, an urban slum area and an urban area. All members of selected households aged 10 years and older were interviewed (rural area n = 963; slum area n = 254; city n = 183). There was a poor response rate in the city where many who were approached refused to participate. The percentage of each sample that was reported to have ever used cannabis were: 3.2 per cent in the rural area; 3.2 per cent in the slum area; and 2.7 per cent in the city.

Machado (1994) reported that cannabis use in the rural area was predominantly for religious purposes whereas in the two urban areas its use was mainly recreational. Users also tended to be older in the rural region (over 35 years) reflecting initiation as part of religious ceremonies. Cannabis use was not perceived as a problem behavior in the rural area given the socioreligious context of use, but it was in the urban areas where its use was perceived as a deviant form of behavior.

SUMMARY

This brief review of the limited data on patterns of cannabis use in various regions of the world exemplifies the difficulties in comparing rates when there are variations in methods of sampling, in the questions used to assess cannabis use, and in the ways in which the data have been reported. Despite these difficulties, the data suggest that the prevalence of cannabis use for recreational purposes is higher in the populations of North America, Australia and New Zealand, and some European countries, than it is in many developing countries, including those with a long tradition of cannabis use for religious and other purposes. It would be desirable if this finding could be more rigorously tested by studies that used similar sampling strategies, questionnaire items and methods of statistical analysis and reporting. The publication of the *WHO Guide to Drug Abuse Epidemiology* should facilitate such studies.

Factors Affecting Cannabis Use

AGE

One of the most consistent findings from school-based survey research in English-speaking countries is that the prevalence of both cannabis initiation and heavy cannabis use increases during the teenage years. Community-based research complements this picture, finding that cannabis use remains relatively high during the early twenties, but declines thereafter. Kandel (1984) found in her cohort study that the majority of young adults who experimented with cannabis had done so by age 18. More recently, Johnston and colleagues (1996) have shown that lifetime prevalence continues to grow in the twenties (though active use declines), particularly when corrections are made for those who "forget" their earlier reported use of cannabis. O'Malley et al. (1988) and Bachman et al. (1997) have shown that over multiple class cohorts, annual prevalence increases with age and then decreases over the late twenties, even when period and cohort effects are controlled. The limited data on the prevalence of cannabis use by age from other regions of the world is broadly consistent with the U.S. data.

GENDER

Rates of cannabis use are consistently higher among males than females in English-speaking countries (Adlaf & Smart, 1991; Bachman, Wadsworth et al., 1997; Donnelly & Hall, 1994; Johnston, O'Malley & Bachman, 1996). The same pattern has been generally reported in studies in developing countries (see above). Given this gender difference, prevalence estimates of cannabis use from studies that have not reported rates separately by gender could be misleading. Daily use and chronic daily use are particularly concentrated among males (Johnston, O'Malley & Bachman, 1996).

INCOME

A positive relationship has been found between adolescent's income and income in early adult life and cannabis use. In Australia, in school surveys in Victoria and South Australia, researchers have found an association between the amount of money either earned or received per week and the prevalence of use of a number of different drugs including tobacco, alcohol and cannabis. Similarly, in the United States, Johnston (1981) reported that daily cannabis use correlated with income and hours worked on a paid job.

SOCIOECONOMIC STATUS

The relationship between cannabis use and socioeconomic status (SES) is weak at most. When relative rates of cannabis use are examined across SES groupings, higher rates of cannabis use are sometimes found among lower SES individuals. However, among 12th grade students in the United States, there has been no relationship between level of parents' education and cannabis use for the past two decades, except that the lowest parental education group of the five has slightly lower cannabis use than the others (Johnston, O'Malley & Bachman, 1996). Even that difference may be more explainable in terms of associated differences (e.g., income during adolescence) rather than social class differences.

ETHNICITY

The current state of knowledge about the relationship between various ethnicity indicators and cannabis usage is limited. Ethnic differences in one country may not generalize to others for a number of reasons, including the fact that a given ethnic group may be in the majority in one country, but a minority in another. Further, limitations in sample size often make ethnic comparisons untenable. Even in the very large Monitoring the Future survey, conducted annually in the United States, samples from multiple years must be combined to allow reliable comparison of just three ethnic groups (Bachman, Wallace et al., 1991; Johnston, O'Malley & Bachman, 1996). They show some important differences as a function of ethnicity, with African-American students showing considerably lower rates in all grades than white or Hispanic students. Hispanics, on the other hand, tend to have the highest rates of use in the early grades, before the rates of school drop-out increase.

REASONS FOR USE

One way to get at the question of why young people use cannabis is simply to ask them. In so far as they are aware of the reasons and willing to admit them, some valuable insights may emerge. Examining daily cannabis users, Johnston (1981) gave respondents a checklist of 13 possible reasons for use. Nearly all daily users checked "to feel good or get high" (94 per cent) and "to have a good time with my friends" (79 per cent), the latter showing the importance of cannabis in social ritual. Two-thirds (67 per cent) said they used it to relax, while 45 per cent said they used it to relieve boredom. Daily users were distinguished from lighter users by mentioning more reasons for use, and by more often mentioning reasons having to do with psychological coping: "to get away from my problems" (27 per cent), "because of anger and frustration" (23 per cent), or "to get through the day" (22 per cent).

In a later and more extensive analysis, Johnston and O'Malley (1986) confirmed these general findings, and showed that the profile of reasons given for using cannabis matched the profile of reasons given for drinking alcohol. They also pointed out that a number of important motivations might be missed in the approach they used — in particular, rebellion against parents and their values, as well as symbolic defiance of the larger social order. In the counter-culture era, cannabis use in the United States was associated with holding counter-culture beliefs, in particular an antipathy toward the Vietnam War (Johnston, 1973). These beliefs were uncorrelated with being delinquent, another important correlate of use.

AVAILABILITY

A popular generalization in drug policy analysis is that the availability of a drug affects the prevalence of its use. In general, and all other

things being equal, the more freely available a drug is, the higher will be the prevalence of its use in the population. This generalization has been broadly supported in the case of alcohol consumption, where the larger the number of licensed outlets and the longer the hours of trading, the higher the levels of community alcohol consumption and alcohol-related problems (e.g., Bruun, Edwards et al., 1975; Moore & Gerstein, 1981).

There is very little evidence that would permit a rigorous test of the availability hypothesis in the case of cannabis use. The only indicators of availability of cannabis are self-reported estimates from surveys of how easy respondents believe it would be to obtain cannabis if they wanted to (e.g., Johnston, O'Malley & Bachman, 1996). These reports have typically shown very little change over long periods of time for cannabis (although they have for other drugs). More fine-grained indicators of cannabis use may be needed to detect changes in cannabis use as a result of changes in availability. A separate issue, of course, is whether government attempts to manipulate the supply of an illicit drug are likely to be successful in the face of vigorous market demand. Johnston and his colleagues, as well as other American analysts, have argued that in the main, the supply control efforts of their government have been futile.

Epidemiological Studies of the Health and Psychological Consequences of Cannabis Use

There is a much larger body of epidemiological studies on the health and psychological effects of cannabis than was available when Smart (1983) last reviewed the literature. Nonetheless, it is still uneven in its coverage of specific health effects. It is much more comprehensive in its coverage of the psychological effects, particularly in adolescence, than on health effects more generally. This partly reflects the greater concern about the psychological effects of cannabis use on adolescents and young adults, and partly the greater amenability to the study of psychological consequences by surveys.

Psychological Consequences

ACUTE EFFECTS

The major motive for the widespread recreational use of cannabis is the experience of a subjective "high" — an altered state of consciousness that is characterized by mild euphoria and relaxation, and by perceptual alterations, such as time distortion, and the intensification of experiences, such as eating, listening to music and engaging in sex. Cognitive changes include impaired short-term memory and loosening of associations, which enables users to become lost in reverie and makes it difficult for them to engage in goal-directed mental activity. Motor skills, reaction time and motor co-ordination are also affected (Hall, Solowij & Lemon, 1994; Jaffe, 1985).

Some cannabis users report unpleasant psychological reactions, ranging from anxiety to panic (Smith, 1968; Thomas, 1993; Weil, 1970). These experiences are often reported by naive users who are unfamiliar with the effects of cannabis, and by some patients given THC for therapeutic purposes. More experienced users may report these experiences after the oral ingestion of cannabis when the effects may be more pronounced and of longer duration than usual. These effects can usually be successfully prevented by adequate preparation of users about the type of effects they may experience. If these effects develop they can be managed by reassurance and support (Smith, 1968; Weil, 1970). Psychotic symptoms, such as delusions and hallucinations, are very rare experiences that have been reported to occur at very high doses of THC (Smith, 1968; Thomas, 1993; Weil, 1970).

In terms of the number of persons affected, the most common adverse psychological effects are likely to be anxiety and unpleasant psycho-logical reactions in naive users. These may occur in as many as a third of those who ever use the drug, and their occurrence may be a major explanation for the high rates of discontinuation of its use (Goodstadt, Chan et al., 1986; Smart, 1983). The majority of these experiences are self-limited and rarely lead to help-seeking.

The psychological effects of cannabis use that are of major concern are those that may arise from its chronic use. A special cause for concern, given the widespread use by young adults, has been the psychological effects of daily cannabis use over a period of years from late adolescence into early adulthood. It is to the results of studies prompted by these concerns to which we now turn.

ADOLESCENT DEVELOPMENT

The evidence that initially raised concern about the effects of cannabis use on adolescents were clinical reports of bright adolescents whose heavy use of cannabis preceded marked declines in social relationships and educational performance, leading to high school drop-out and immersion in illicit drug use (e.g., Kolansky & Moore, 1971; Lantner, 1982; Milman, 1982). These reports were of limited value in deciding to what extent cannabis use was a symptom rather than a cause of personality, or other psychiatric, disorders. But they prompted a number of important prospective studies of the consequences of adolescent drug use (e.g. Kandel, 1988; Kaplan, Martin & Robbins, 1982; Newcombe & Bentler, 1988).

Is Cannabis a Gateway Drug?

A major concern about cannabis has been that its use in adolescence may lead to the use of other more dangerous illicit drugs, such as cocaine and heroin (DuPont, 1984; Goode, 1974; Kleiman, 1992). There is now abundant evidence of an association between cannabis and heroin use from cross-sectional studies of adolescent drug use in the United States and elsewhere. In the late 1970s and into the 1990s in the United States there was a strong relationship between degree of involvement with cannabis and the use of other illicit drugs such as heroin and cocaine (Kandel, 1988; Kandel & Davies, 1996).

Kandel (1984), for example, found that the prevalence of other illicit drug use increased with degree of marijuana involvement: 7 per cent of those who had never used marijuana, 33 per cent of those who had used in the past, and 84 per cent of those who were currently daily cannabis users, had used other illicit drugs. Johnston (1981) reported that in a national sample of daily cannabis-using 12th grade students, 59 per cent were daily cigarette smokers and 27 per cent were daily drinkers — much higher than average rates for the age groups — and daily cannabis users used most other illicit drugs at rates five to seven times the average.

A relationship between cannabis and other illicit drug use has also been observed in the small number of longitudinal studies of drug use among American adolescents (e.g., Donovan & Jessor, 1983; Johnston, 1973; Kandel, Davies et al., 1986; Robins, Darvish & Murphy, 1970). These studies identified a predictable sequence of involvement with licit and illicit drugs among American adolescents in which progressively fewer adolescents tried each drug class in the sequence but almost all of those who tried drug types later in the sequence had used all the drugs earlier in the sequence (Kandel, 1988; Kandel & Faust, 1975).

Typically, psychoactive drug use began with the use of alcohol and tobacco which were almost universally used. A smaller group of the regular alcohol and tobacco users also started using cannabis, and the smaller group who became regular cannabis users were more likely to use amphetamines and tranquillizers. Users of these "pills" were more likely to use heroin and cocaine. Generally, the earlier that any particular drug in the sequence was used, and the heavier its use, the more likely users were to move on to the next drug type in the sequence (Kandel, 1988; Kandel, Davies et al., 1986; Kandel & Logan, 1984).

Yamaguchi and Kandel (1984) examined variables that predicted progression to illicit drug use beyond cannabis use. They used statistical methods to see if the relationship between cannabis use and subsequent illicit drug use persisted after controlling for pre-existing adolescent behaviors and attitudes, interpersonal factors, and age of initiation into drug use. Among men, those who initiated marijuana use under the age of 16 were more likely to use other illicit drugs (and this was not explained by their having been at risk for longer because of their early age of onset). Persons who had not used marijuana, had very small probabilities of using other drugs, (0.01 to 0.03 in men, and 0.02 in women). These findings suggest that marijuana is a necessary condition for the initiation of other illicit drugs.

The work of Kandel and colleagues does not imply that a high proportion of those who experiment with marijuana will go on to use heroin. In fact, the majority of cannabis users do not use harder drugs like heroin. Rather, cannabis use is largely a behavior of late adolescence and early adulthood. Its frequency of use peaks in the early twenties when 50 per cent of males and 33 per cent of females reported using, and rapidly declines by age 23, with the assumption of the roles of adulthood, for example, getting married, entering the labor force and becoming a parent, all roles that are incompatible with involvement in illicit drugs and deviant lifestyles (Bachman, Wadsworth et al., 1997; Kandel & Logan, 1984). Most illicit drug use, including marijuana, ceases by age 29, when there are very few new recruits (Chen & Kandel, 1995).

Kandel's work does show that heavy cannabis use greatly increases the chance of using other illicit drugs. But this type of relationship does not necessarily mean that heavy cannabis use "causes" heroin use. A more plausible explanation is that deviant and non-conformist persons with a predilection for the use of intoxicating substances are more likely to be early recruits to cannabis use (Fergusson & Horwood, 1997; Kandel & Davies, 1996). On this hypothesis, the sequence in which drugs are typically used reflects their availability and the societal disapproval of their use (e.g., Donovan & Jessor, 1983). The drugs that are the least available, and the most strongly socially disapproved "hard" drugs, are used last by the most socially deviant members of their age cohort. On this hypothesis, cannabis use and other illicit drug use are common manifestations of adolescent deviance and non-conformity (Kaplan, Martin & Robbins, 1982; Newcombe & Bentler, 1988; Osgood, Johnston et al., 1988).

The selective recruitment hypothesis has been supported by a number of studies that have found substantial correlations between various forms of non-conforming adolescent behavior, such as high school drop-out, early premarital sexual experience and pregnancy, delinquency and alcohol and illicit drug use (Hays & Ellickson, 1996; Jessor & Jessor, 1977; Osgood, Johnston et al., 1988). All such behaviors are correlated with non-conformist and rebellious attitudes and antisocial conduct in childhood (Shedler & Block, 1990) and early adolescence (Fergusson & Horwood, 1997; Jessor & Jessor, 1977; Newcombe & Bentler, 1988).

Recent research also indicates that those who are most likely to use other illicit drugs are more likely to have a history of antisocial behavior (Brook, Cohen et al., 1992; Johnston, 1973; McGee & Feehan, 1993), non-conformity and alienation (Brook, Cohen et al., 1992; Jessor & Jessor, 1978; Shedler & Block, 1990), perform more poorly at school (Bailey, Flewelling & Rachal, 1992; Fergusson & Horwood, 1997; Hawkins, Catalano & Miller, 1992; Johnston, 1973; Kandel & Davies, 1992), and use drugs to deal with personal distress and negative affect (Kaplan & Johnson, 1992; Shedler & Block, 1990). In general, the more of these risk factors that adolescents have, the more likely they are to become intensively involved with cannabis, and to use other illicit drugs (Brook, Cohen et al., 1992; Maddahian, Newcombe & Bentler, 1988; Newcombe, 1992; Scheier & Newcombe, 1991).

One way of testing the selective recruitment hypothesis is to see whether cannabis use continues to predict progression to "harder" illicit drugs after statistically controlling for pre-existing differences in personality and other characteristics between cannabis users and non-users. In several such studies (e.g., Kandel, Davies et al., 1986; O'Donnell & Clayton, 1982; Robins, Darvish & Murphy, 1970) the relationship between cannabis and heroin use has been substantially reduced but not eliminated when pre-existing differences have been statistically controlled for. O'Donnell and Clayton (1982) have interpreted the fact that the relationship persists after statistical adjustment as evidence for a causal connection between cannabis and heroin use.

The credibility of this causal interpretation depends upon whether the most important prior characteristics have been adequately measured and statistically controlled for in these studies. It would be difficult to argue that this has been the case. Kandel et al. (1986), for example, did not measure the users' attitudes and family characteristics at the time of drug initiation, or differential drug availability, while O'Donnell and Clayton (1982) and Robins et al. (1970) retrospectively assessed deviance "prior" to drug use.

If we assume that the association between cannabis and heroin use is in part causal, it remains to be explained how cannabis use "causes" heroin use. Although it may seem plausible that the pharmacological effects of cannabis predisposes heavy users to use other intoxicants, there are non-pharmacological explanations that need to be considered. There is, for example, good evidence that the pattern of progression observed among American adolescents in the 1970s was conditioned by drug availability (Kandel, 1988). In earlier cohorts of U.S. heroin users prior involvement with cannabis was confined to those geographic areas of the United States in which it was readily available (Goode, 1974). Research on African-American adolescents has also found that the use of the more readily available cocaine and heroin preceded the use of the less available hallucinogens and "pills" (Kandel, 1988). Similarly, American soldiers in Vietnam were more likely to use heroin before alcohol because heroin was cheaper and more freely available to soldiers who were below the minimum drinking age of 21 (Robins, 1993).

These historical and geographical variations in sequences of illicit drug use suggest a sociological explanation of the sequence and of the higher rates of progression to heroin use among heavy cannabis users. One of the most popular explanations is that heavy cannabis use increases the chance of using other illicit drugs because it increases contact with other drug users. That is, heavy cannabis use leads to greater involvement in a drug-using subculture, which, in turn, exposes cannabis users to peers who have used other illicit drugs. Such exposure also increases opportunities to use other illicit drugs because of their increased availability within these social networks. Heavy cannabis use therefore puts individuals in a context in which illicit drug use is encouraged and approved (e.g., Goode, 1974).

Although plausible, there is little direct evidence for this hypothesis. Goode (1974) presented data from the late 1960s indicating that the number of friends who used heroin was a stronger predictor of heroin use than was frequency of cannabis use. These observations have been supported by Kandel's (1984) finding that the strongest predictor of continued cannabis use in early adulthood was the number of friends who were cannabis users. Examining daily cannabis users in the early years of the Monitoring the Future study, Johnston (1981) reported that they had heavily drug-using friendship circles, with over 85 per cent saying that most or all of their friends smoked cannabis and that at least a few of their friends used a number of other illicit drugs.

Selective recruitment and socialization in a drug-using subculture are not mutually exclusive possibilities; both processes could independently explain the relationship between regular marijuana use and progression to heroin use (Goode, 1974). As already noted, the selective recruitment hypothesis is supported by the consistent finding of pre-existing differences between those who use marijuana and those who do not (e.g., Fergusson, Lynskey & Horwood, 1996; Maddahian, Newcombe & Bentler, 1988), and the fact that these characteristics are most marked in those who are heavy cannabis users and most likely to use other illicit drugs. Once initiated into cannabis use, heavy users become further distinguished from non-users and ex-users by the number of their social relationships

which involve the use of marijuana, and their involvement in buying and selling illicit drugs.

Educational Performance

Another major concern about adolescent cannabis use has been that it may impair educational performance and increase the chances of students discontinuing their education. Heavy cannabis use in the high school years may impair memory and attention, thereby interfering with learning in and out of the classroom (Baumrind & Moselle, 1985). If use became chronic, persistently impaired learning would produce poorer school performance in high school and increase the chance of a student dropping out of school. If an adolescent's school performance was marginal to begin with, then regular use could increase the risk of high school failure. Because of the importance of high school education to occupational choice, this potential effect could have consequences throughout the affected individual's adult life.

Cross-sectional studies (e.g., Johnston, 1973; Kandel, 1984; Robins, Darvish & Murphy, 1970) have found a positive relationship between degree of involvement with cannabis as an adult and the risk of dropping out of high school. Studies of relationships between performance in college and marijuana smoking have usually failed to find consistent evidence that the performance of cannabis users was more impaired than would be predicted by their performance prior to cannabis use. These studies have been criticized on the grounds that grade point average is an insensitive measure of adverse educational effects among bright high school and college students (Baumrind & Moselle, 1985), and that students whose learning has been most adversely affected by chronic heavy cannabis use would not be found in college samples (Cohen, 1982).

Longitudinal studies of the effect of cannabis use on educational achievement have generally supported the hypothesis (e.g., Friedman, Bransfield & Kreisher, 1994; Kandel, Davies et al., 1986; Newcombe & Bentler, 1988). Kandel et al. (1986), for example, reported a negative relationship between marijuana use in adolescence and years of education completed in early adulthood, but this relationship disappeared once account was taken of the much lower educational aspirations among those who used cannabis. Newcombe and Bentler (1988) found negative correlations between adolescent drug use and high school completion, but there was only a modest negative relationship between drug use and college involvement after controlling for the higher non-conformity and lower academic potential of adolescent cannabis users.

Using the quite different approach of asking users what adverse consequences they ascribe to their use, Johnston (1981) reported that about one-third of 12th grade students who were active daily cannabis users felt that their use hurt their school and/or job performance. One has to evaluate how to interpret such information, but it should probably be recalled that heavy users of other drugs, including alcohol, are probably more likely to deny problems that exist than to exaggerate them.

On the whole then, the available evidence suggests that there may be a modest statistical relationship between cannabis use in adolescence and poor educational performance. The strong relationship observed in cross-sectional studies exaggerates the adverse impact of cannabis use on school performance because adolescents who perform poorly at school, and have lower academic aspirations, are more likely to use cannabis. But even if the relationship is modest, it may be substantively important among those whose educational performance was marginal to begin with, thereby adversely affecting their subsequent life choices, such as their occupation, and choice of marital partner.

Occupational Performance

Among those young adult cannabis users who enter the workforce the continued use of cannabis and other illicit drugs in young adulthood might impair job performance for the same reasons that it has been suspected of impairing school performance. There is some suggestive support for this hypothesis in that cannabis users report higher rates of unemployment than non-users (e.g., Fergusson & Horwood, 1997; Friedman, Granick et al., 1996; Kandel, 1984; Robins, Darvish & Murphy, 1970), but this comparison is confounded by the different educational qualifications of the two groups.

Longitudinal studies have suggested that there is a relationship between adolescent marijuana use and job instability among young adults which is not explained by differences in education and other characteristics that precede cannabis use (e.g., Friedman, Granick et al., 1996; Kandel, Davies et al., 1986). Newcombe and Bentler (1988) examined the relationships between adolescent drug use and income, job instability, job satisfaction, and resort to public assistance in young adulthood, while controlling for differences between users and non-users in social conformity, academic potential and income in adolescence. Their findings supported those of Kandel and colleagues in that adolescent drug users had a larger number of changes of job than nondrug users.

Interpersonal Relationships

There are developmental and empirical reasons for suspecting that cannabis use may adversely affect interpersonal relationships. Heavy adolescent drug use may produce a developmental lag, entrenching adolescent styles of thinking and coping that impair the ability to form adult interpersonal relationships (Baumrind & Moselle, 1985). There are strong positive correlations between drug use and precocious sexual activity resulting in early marriage, which in turn predicts a high rate of relationship failure (Newcombe & Bentler, 1988).

Cross-sectional studies of drug use in young adults have indicated that a high degree of involvement with marijuana predicts a reduced probability of marriage, an increased rate of cohabiting, an increased risk of divorce or terminated *de facto* relationships, and a higher rate of unplanned parenthood and pregnancy termination (Kandel, 1984; Robins, Darvish & Murphy, 1970). Kandel (1984) also found that heavy cannabis users were more likely to have a social network in which friends and the spouse or partner were also cannabis users. These findings have been largely confirmed in analyses of the longitudinal data from this cohort of young adults (Kandel, Davies et al., 1986).

Newcombe and Bentler (1988) found similar relationships between drug use and early marriage in their analysis of the cross-sectional data from their cohort of young adults in Los Angeles. Drug use in adolescence predicted an increased rate of early family formation in late adolescence and of divorce in early adulthood which they interpreted as evidence that "early drug involvement leads to early marriage and having children which then results in divorce" (p. 97).

Johnston (1981), reporting on daily cannabis users among 12th grade students, found that a number felt that their use hurt their relationship with their parents (31 per cent), their teachers (24 per cent), and their partner of the opposite sex (16 per cent). Relatively few felt it hurt their relationships with their friends (10 per cent), perhaps because so many were immersed in friendship networks with other cannabis users.

Mental Health

Since cannabis is a psychoactive drug that affects the user's mood and feelings, its chronic heavy use could possibly adversely affect mental health. This might be a special risk among those whose adjustment prior to their cannabis use was poor, as well as among those who use cannabis to control their negative mood states and emotions. The relationships between cannabis use and the risks of developing dependence upon cannabis or major mental illnesses such as schizophrenia are reviewed below. In this section attention is confined to symptoms of depression and distress.

A number of studies have suggested an association between cannabis use and poor mental health. Kandel's (1984) cross-sectional study found that the more intense the involvement with marijuana, the lower the degree of satisfaction with life, and the greater the likelihood of having consulted a mental health professional and of having been hospitalized for a psychiatric disorder. Longitudinal analyses of this same

cohort found weaker associations between adolescent drug use and these outcomes in early adult life (Kandel, Davies et al., 1986).

The cross-sectional adult data in Newcombe and Bentler's (1988) study showed strong relationships between adolescent drug use and emotional distress, psychoticism and lack of a purpose in life. Emotional distress in adolescence predicted emotional distress in young adulthood, but there were no relationships between adolescent drug use and the experience of emotional distress, depression and lack of a sense of purpose in life in young adulthood. Adolescent drug use predicted psychotic symptoms in young adulthood, and hard drug use in adolescence predicted increased suicidal ideation in young adulthood, after controlling for other drug use and earlier emotional distress.

More recently, Fergusson and Horwood (1997) have shown in a birth cohort of New Zealand youth that early cannabis initiation (before age 16) was associated with poorer mental health, as indicated by higher rates of major depression, anxiety disorders and suicide attempts. These relationships were substantially reduced and no longer statistically significant after adjustment for differences between cannabis and non-cannabis users in pre-existing characteristics that predicted a higher risk of these outcomes.

Delinquency and Crime

Since initiation into illicit drug use and the maintenance of regular illicit drug use are both strongly related to degree of social non-conformity or deviance (e.g., Jessor & Jessor, 1977; Newcombe & Bentler, 1988; Polich, Ellickson et al., 1984) it is reasonable to expect adolescent illicit drug use to predict social non-conformity and various forms of delinquency and crime in young adulthood. Cross-sectional studies of adult drug users indicate that there is a relationship between the extent of marijuana use as an adult and a history of lifetime delinquency (e.g., Kandel, 1984; Robins, Darvish & Murphy, 1970), having been convicted of an offence, and having had a motor vehicle accident while intoxicated (Kandel, 1984).

Johnston et al. (1978) reported a detailed analysis of the relationship between intensity of drug use and delinquency across two waves of interviews of adolescent males. They found in their cross-sectional data that there was a strong relationship between self-reported rates of delinquent activity and degree of involvement with illicit drugs. However, a series of analyses looking at changes in drug use and crime over time indicated that the groups defined by intensity of drug involvement differed strongly in their rate of delinquent acts *before* their drug use. Moreover, the onset of illicit drug use (including cannabis) had little effect on delinquent acts, except possibly among those who used heroin. Those who used only marijuana had no higher rates of interpersonal aggression than those who abstained from all illicit drug use. Finally, rates of delinquent acts declined over time in all drug-use groups at about the same rate. The findings were interpreted as delivering "a substantial, if not mortal, blow" to the hypothesis that "drug use short of addiction somehow causes other kinds of delinquency" (p. 156).

Newcombe and Bentler (1988) reported a positive correlation between drug use and criminal involvement in adolescence, but found more mixed results in the relationship between adolescent drug use and criminal activity in young adulthood. Adolescent drug use predicted *drug* crime involvement in young adulthood, but after controlling for other variables, it was *negatively* correlated with violent crime, and general criminal activities in young adulthood. Newcombe and Bentler argued that these negative correlations indicated that the correlation between different forms of delinquency in adolescence decreased with age, as criminal activities became differentiated into drug-related and non-drug-related offences.

Fergusson and Horwood's (1997) study of a birth cohort of New Zealand youth also examined the association between early cannabis initiation (before age 16) and juvenile property and violent offences. As in the other studies, early cannabis users were much more likely to engage in juvenile offences than their peers.

In this case, however, the association persisted after statistical adjustment for differences in risk factors, although it was substantially reduced.

MOTIVATIONAL EFFECTS IN ADULTS

There have been anecdotal reports that chronic heavy cannabis use impairs motivation and social performance in societies with a long history of use, such as Egypt, the Caribbean and elsewhere (e.g., Brill & Nahas, 1984). In these societies, heavy cannabis use occurs primarily among the poor, impoverished and unemployed. There were clinical reports of a similar syndrome occurring among heavy cannabis users in the early 1970s (e.g., Kolansky & Moore, 1971; Millman & Sbriglio, 1986; Tennant & Groesbeck, 1972), which was described as an "amotivational syndrome" (e.g., McGlothlin & West, 1968; Smith, 1968). All these reports were uncontrolled, and often poorly documented so it was impossible to disentangle the effects of chronic cannabis use from those of poverty and low socioeconomic status, or pre-existing personality and other psychiatric disorders (Edwards, 1976; Institute of Medicine, 1982; Millman & Sbriglio, 1986; Negrete, 1983).

Two major types of investigation have been carried out in an attempt to assess the motivational effects of chronic heavy cannabis use: field studies of chronic heavy cannabis-using adults in societies with a tradition of such use, for example, Costa Rica (Carter, Coggins & Doughty, 1980) and Jamaica (Rubin & Comitas, 1975); and laboratory studies of the effects on the motivation and performance of volunteers who have been administered heavy doses of cannabis over periods of several weeks (e.g., Mendelson, Rossi & Meyer, 1974). There is only limited epidemiological evidence on the prevalence of symptoms of the "amotivational syndrome" among chronic cannabis users in the United States (e.g., Halikas, Weller et al., 1982).

Rubin and Comitas (1975) examined the effects of ganja smoking on the performance of Jamaican farmers who regularly smoked cannabis in the belief that it enhanced their physical energy and work productivity. Four case histories were reported which indicated that the level of physical activity increased immediately after smoking ganja, but not productivity. It seemed to be that after smoking ganja the workers engaged in more intense and concentrated labor but this was done less efficiently. Rubin and Comitas concluded: "In all Jamaican settings observed, the workers are motivated to carry out difficult tasks with no decrease in heavy physical exertion, and their perception of increased output is a significant factor in bolstering their motivation to work" (p. 79).

A study of Costa Rican cannabis smokers produced mixed evidence on the impact of chronic cannabis use on job performance (Carter, Coggins & Doughty, 1980). A comparison of the employment histories of 41 pairs of heavy users (10 marijuana cigarettes per day for 10 or more years) and non-users who had been matched on age, marital status, education, occupation and alcohol and tobacco consumption indicated that non-users were more likely than users: to have attained a stable employment history, to have received promotions and raises, and to be in full-time employment. Users were also more likely to spend all or more than their incomes and to be in debt. Among users, however, the relationship between average daily marijuana consumption and employment was the obverse of what the amotivational hypothesis would predict, that is, those "who had steady jobs or who were self-employed were smoking more than twice as many marijuana cigarettes per day as those with more frequent job changes, or those who were chronically unemployed" (p. 153). This could, of course, reflect differences among users in having the resources necessary to purchase and consume larger amounts of ganja.

Evidence from these field studies has usually been interpreted as failing to demonstrate the existence of the amotivational syndrome (e.g., Dornbush, 1974; Hollister, 1986; Negrete, 1988). There are critics, however, who raise doubts about how convincing such apparently negative evidence is. Cohen (1982), for example, has argued that the chronic users in three field studies have

come from socially marginal groups so that the cognitive and motivational demands of their everyday lives were insufficient to detect any impairment caused by chronic cannabis use. Moreover, the sample sizes of these studies have been too small to exclude the possibility of an effect occurring among a minority of heavy users.

Evidence from prospective studies of long-term cannabis users suggests that any amotivational syndrome is likely to be a relatively rare occurrence, if it exists. Halikas et al. (1982) followed up 100 regular cannabis users six to eight years after initially recruiting them and asked them about the experience of symptoms suggestive of an amotivational syndrome. They found only three individuals who had ever experienced such a cluster of symptoms in the absence of significant symptoms of depression. These individuals were not distinguished from the other smokers who did not experience such symptoms by their heaviness of use. Nor was their experience of these symptoms obviously related to changes in pattern of use; they seemed to come and go independently of continued heavy cannabis use.

In the light of Halikas and colleagues' low estimate of the prevalence of amotivational symptoms among chronic heavy cannabis users it is perhaps unsurprising that the small number of laboratory studies of long-term heavy cannabis use (e.g., Campbell, 1976; Mendelson, Rossi & Meyer, 1974) have failed to provide evidence of impaired motivation (Edwards, 1976). Such studies have also examined heavy use over short periods (e.g., 21 days) by comparison with the life histories of 15 or more years' daily use in heavy cannabis users in the field studies. The subjects have typically been healthy young volunteers with a college education, and tasks that they were asked to perform have been undemanding.

The motivational effects of chronic cannabis use were examined in a recent study of 243 Australian cannabis users who had been at least weekly cannabis users for 19 years (Didcott, Reilly et al., 1997). The findings were as equivocal as the findings of many earlier studies. Supporters of the amotivational syndrome would see evidence for their views in the lifestyles of these 243 long-term cannabis users. They were university-educated people who have made little use of their abilities or education; they were underemployed, or at least, arguably underusing their education and ability, by working part-time; and they spent a substantial part of their time using cannabis and growing it for their personal use. The study participants argued that the way they spent their time reflected the lifestyle choices that they had made. They continued to be actively involved in family and community life, and many played a role in local politics and community affairs. Long-term cannabis use did not prevent some study participants from holding responsible professional or managerial positions. Interviews with partners and others provided an opportunity to assess the motivational effects of long-term cannabis use from the perspective of non-using friends and family. Here too the evidence was equivocal. Some noticed an effect of cannabis use on motivation; others did not, and some reported the opposite effect.

The status of the amotivational syndrome remains contentious in part because of differences in the appraisal of evidence from clinical observations and controlled studies. On the one hand, there are those who find the small number of cases of amotivational syndrome compelling clinical evidence of the marked deterioration in functioning that chronic heavy cannabis use can produce. On the other hand, there are those who are more impressed by the largely unsupportive findings of the small number of field and laboratory studies.

Finally, Johnston's (1981) study of daily cannabis users in a large national sample of 12th grade students, yielded some findings of relevance. Over 40 per cent reported that their cannabis use had caused them to have less energy (the most frequently mentioned on a checklist of 15 potential problems) and a third indicated that it caused them to be less interested in other activities than they were before their use. The fact that all had become daily users, averaging two-and-one-half joints per day, within a few years previous may have allowed them to judge

the changes more accurately than the long-term, chronic users in some of the other studies. On the other hand, we would have thought that their less intense and less prolonged use would have been less likely to have had discernible effects.

CANNABIS DEPENDENCE

During the 1960s and 1970s, the apparent absence of a withdrawal syndrome analogous to that seen in alcohol and opioid dependence led many to believe that cannabis was not a drug of dependence. This changed with the adoption of a more liberal definition of drug dependence by the World Health Organization (Edwards, Arif & Hodgson, 1981). This reduced the emphasis upon tolerance and withdrawal, and placed greater emphasis on symptoms of a compulsion to use, a narrowing of the drug-using repertoire, rapid reinstatement of dependence after abstinence, and the high salience of drug use in the user's life.

Since the middle 1970s, human and animal studies have shown that chronic administration of high doses of THC results in the development of marked tolerance to a wide variety of cannabinoid effects, such as cardiovascular effects, and the subjective high in humans (Compton, Dewey & Martin, 1990; Fehr & Kalant, 1983; Hollister, 1986; Jones, Benowitz & Herning, 1981; Institute of Medicine, 1982). The abrupt cessation of chronic high doses of THC generally produces a mild withdrawal syndrome like that produced by other long-acting sedative drugs (Compton, Dewey & Martin, 1990; Jones & Benowitz, 1976; Jones, Benowitz & Herning, 1981).

Epidemiological Evidence on Cannabis Dependence

The population prevalence of cannabis abuse and dependence in the community was estimated in the Epidemiological Catchment Area (ECA) study (Robins & Regier, 1991). This study involved face-to-face interviews with 20,000 Americans in five catchment areas: Baltimore, Maryland; Los Angeles, California; New Haven, Connecticut; Durham, North Carolina; and St. Louis, Missouri. A standardized and validated

Chapter 3

clinical interview schedule was used to elicit a history of psychiatric symptoms for 40 major psychiatric diagnoses, including drug abuse and dependence, which were used to diagnose the presence or absence of a *DSM-III (Diagnostic and Statistical Manual of Mental Disorders*, third edition) diagnosis (Anthony & Helzer, 1991).

The criteria used to define drug abuse and dependence were derived from the *DSM-III*, which divided symptoms of abuse and dependence into four main groups: (1) tolerance to drug effects; (2) withdrawal symptoms; (3) pathological patterns of use; and (4) impairments in social and occupational functioning due to drug use. Drug abuse required a pattern of pathological use and impaired functioning. In the case of cannabis, a diagnosis of dependence required pathological use, or impaired social functioning, in addition to either signs of tolerance or withdrawal. The problem had to have been present for at least one month although there was no requirement that all criteria had to be met within the same period of time. In reporting the results Anthony and Helzer analyse the prevalence of drug abuse and/or dependence combined for all drug types.

Drug abuse and dependence were diagnosed in 6.2 per cent of the population. Cannabis abuse and/or dependence was the most common type, with 4.4 per cent of the population being so diagnosed. When *DSM-III-R* diagnoses were approximated, 60 per cent of those with a diagnosis of drug dependence and/or abuse met the criteria for dependence. The proportion of current users who were dependent increased with age, from 57 per cent in the 18- to 29-year age group to 82 per cent in the 45- to 64-year age group, reflecting the remission of less severe drug abuse problems with age. Only a minority of those who had a diagnosis of abuse and/or dependence (20 per cent of men and 28 per cent of women) had mentioned their drug problem to a health professional.

There were predictable age and gender differences in the prevalence of drug abuse and/or dependence. Men had a higher prevalence than women (7.7 per cent versus 4.8 per cent).

This was largely because fewer women used cannabis. The prevalence of abuse and/or dependence among persons who had used an illicit drug more than five times was about the same for men and women (21 per cent and 19 per cent). The highest prevalence of drug abuse and/or dependence (13.5 per cent) was in the 18- to 29-year age group (16.0 per cent among men and 10.9 per cent among women), declining steeply thereafter in both sexes.

Similar estimates of the population prevalence of cannabis dependence were produced by a community survey of psychiatric disorder conducted in Christchurch, New Zealand, in 1986 using the same sampling strategy and diagnostic interview as the ECA study (Wells, Bushnell et al., 1992). This survey used the Diagnostic Interview Schedule (DIS) to diagnose a restricted range of *DSM-III* diagnoses in a community sample of 1,498 adults aged 18 to 64 years of age. The prevalence of having used cannabis on five or more occasions was 15.5 per cent, remarkably close to that of the ECA estimate, as was the proportion who met *DSM-III* criteria for marijuana abuse or dependence, namely, 4.7 per cent. The fact that this survey largely replicated the ECA findings for other diagnoses, including alcohol abuse and dependence, enhances confidence in the validity of the ECA study findings.

The National Comorbidity Survey (NCS) also estimated the prevalence of cannabis dependence in a nationally representative sample of the U.S. population. According to the *DSM-III-R* classification, using a modified version of the Composite International Diagnostic Interview (CIDI) schedule. The NCS produced a higher lifetime prevalence of any mental disorder than the ECA (48 per cent versus 32 per cent) but a similar gender difference in pattern of disorders, for example, a male excess for substance use disorders and antisocial personality disorders (ASPD), and a female excess in affective disorders and anxiety disorders.

The NCS estimated that 4 per cent of the U.S. population had met lifetime criteria for cannabis dependence, compared to 24 per cent for tobacco, 14 per cent for alcohol, 3 per cent for cocaine and 0.4 per cent for heroin (Anthony, Warner & Kessler, 1994). Correlates of cannabis dependence in the NCS were very similar to those reported in the ECA (Anthony, Warner & Kessler, 1994).

The Risk and Consequences of Cannabis Dependence

A variety of estimates suggest that the risk of becoming dependent on cannabis is probably more like that for alcohol than nicotine or the opioids. As with all drugs of dependence, persons who use cannabis on a daily basis over periods of weeks to months are at greatest risk of becoming dependent upon it. The ECA data suggested that approximately half of those who used any illicit drug on a daily basis satisfied *DSM-III* criteria for abuse or dependence (Anthony & Helzer, 1991). Kandel and Davies (1992) estimated the risk of dependence among near-daily cannabis users (according to approximated *DSM-III* criteria) at one in three. Johnston (1981) reported that just over half of the active daily cannabis users he identified at the end of high school were still daily users four years later, and two-thirds of the remainder were still current users. O'Malley, Bachman and Johnston (1984) also report some evidence of a cohort effect for daily cannabis use, much as is found for cigarettes, also suggestive of a dependence-producing property.

The risk of developing dependence among less than daily users of cannabis would be substantially less. A crude estimate from the ECA study was that approximately 20 per cent of persons who used any illicit drug more than five times met *DSM-III* criteria for drug abuse and dependence at some time. The specific rate of abuse and dependence for cannabis was 29 per cent. A more conservative estimate which removed cases of abuse (40 per cent) from the overall estimate of cannabis abuse and dependence would be that 17 per cent of those who used cannabis more than five times would meet *DSM-III* criteria for dependence.

Estimates derived from a number of other studies suggest that the ECA estimates of the risk of dependence are reasonable. The percentage of

cases of dependence and abuse among persons who had used cannabis five or more times in the Christchurch epidemiology study (Wells, Bushnell et al., 1992) was 30 per cent, whereas an estimate derived from Newcombe's community survey of young adults was 25 per cent. On Kandel and Davies' (1992) data the estimated rate of abuse and dependence among those who had used cannabis 10 or more times was 39 per cent, the higher rate reflecting the higher number of times of use required to be counted as a cannabis user in Kandel and Davies' study (10 times versus 5 times in ECA). It is reassuring that these estimates are within a limited range (12 per cent to 37 per cent), and that they vary in predictable ways with the ages of the samples and the stringency of the criteria used in defining cannabis use. These estimates are broadly in line with the NCS estimate that 9 per cent of those who had ever used cannabis had met criteria for cannabis dependence during their lifetime (Anthony, Warner & Kessler, 1994).

THE COGNITIVE EFFECTS OF CANNABIS USE

Concerns about the cognitive effects of chronic cannabis use were prompted by clinical reports of mental deterioration in persons who had used cannabis at least weekly for more than one year (Fehr & Kalant, 1983; Kolansky & Moore, 1971). The National Institute on Drug Abuse (NIDA) commissioned three cross-cultural studies of long-term heavy cannabis users in Jamaica, Greece and Costa Rica to assess the effects of chronic cannabis use on cognitive functioning (among other things).

The results of the cross-cultural studies of long-term heavy cannabis users provided at most equivocal evidence of an association between cannabis use and more subtle long-term cognitive impairments (Fehr & Kalant, 1983; Hall, Solowij & Lemon, 1994). Given that cognitive impairments are most likely to be found in subjects with a long history of heavy use, it is reassuring that these studies have found few and typically small differences between heavy cannabis users and controls. It is unlikely that the negative results of these studies can be attributed to an insufficient duration or intensity of cannabis use within the samples studied since the duration of cannabis use ranged between 16.9 to 23 years, and the estimated amount of THC consumed daily ranged from 20 to 90 milligrams daily in Rubin and Comitas's (1975) Jamaican study to 120 to 200 milligrams daily in the Greek sample.

It has been argued that if cannabis use produced cognitive impairment, then these studies should have revealed it (Wert & Raulin, 1986). The force of this argument is weakened by the fact that most of these studies also suffered from methodological difficulties that may have operated against finding a difference. For example, many of these studies were based on small samples of questionable representativeness, with an overrepresentation of illiterate, rural, older and less intelligent or less educated subjects. Moreover, many studies were only capable of detecting gross deficits, and few attempted to examine relationships between neuropsychological test performance and frequency and duration of cannabis use (see chapter 6 in this volume).

Despite these problems, there was suggestive evidence of more subtle cognitive deficits. Slower psychomotor performance, poorer perceptual motor co-ordination, and memory dysfunction were the most consistently reported deficits. In terms of memory function, four studies detected persistent short-term memory and attentional deficits (Page, Fletcher & True, 1988; Soueif, 1976; Varma, Malhotra et al., 1988; Wig & Varma, 1977), while three failed to detect such deficits (Bowman & Pihl, 1973; Mendhiratta, Wig & Verma, 1978; Satz, Fletcher & Sutker, 1976).

A number of epidemiological studies have been conducted on the cognitive performance of American or Canadian cannabis users (e.g., Brill & Christie, 1974; Hochman & Brill, 1973). They have generally failed to find any significant differences between users, non-users or former users in grade point average. These samples have generally been young and well-educated college students with relatively short-term exposure to cannabis by comparison with the long history of use among chronic users in the cross-cultural studies.

A crucial requirement for evaluating the performance of chronic marijuana users is an appropriately matched group of non-using subjects. Although the studies described have made substantial progress in this regard, the possibility remains that some of the impairments were present prior to their cannabis use. Block et al. (1990) reported one of the few studies that matched their user and non-user samples (aged 18 to 42 years) on a test administered in the fourth grade of grammar school to ensure that they were comparable in intellectual functioning before they began using marijuana. The results showed that heavy users performed more poorly than controls on two tests of verbal expression and mathematical skills.

CANNABIS AND SCHIZOPHRENIA

Precipitation

There is good epidemiological evidence of a cross-sectional association between schizophrenia and drug abuse and dependence. In the ECA study (Anthony & Helzer, 1991) there was an increased risk of schizophrenia among men and women with a diagnosis of any form of drug abuse and dependence (relative risks of 6.2 for men and 6.4 for women). Bland, Newman and Orn (1987) also found that the odds of receiving a diagnosis of drug abuse and dependence were 11.9 times higher among persons with schizophrenia in a population survey of the prevalence of psychiatric disorder in Edmonton, Alberta, using the same ECA interview schedule and diagnostic criteria.

Many researchers have inferred that this association indicates that cannabis and other drug use precipitates schizophrenic disorders in persons who may not otherwise have experienced them. In support of this hypothesis are the common findings that drug-abusing schizophrenic patients have an earlier age of onset of psychotic symptoms (with their drug use typically preceding the onset of symptoms), a better premorbid adjustment, fewer negative symptoms (e.g., withdrawal, anhedonia, lethargy), and a better response to treatment and outcome than schizophrenic patients who do not use drugs (Allebeck, Adamsson et al., 1993; Dixon, Haas et al., 1990; Schneier & Siris, 1987).

There are other interpretations of these findings, however (Thomas, 1993; Thornicroft, 1990). The association between cannabis use and an early onset of schizophrenia in persons with a good premorbid personality and outcome may be spurious (e.g., Arndt, Tyrrell et al., 1992). Schizophrenics with a better premorbid personality were simply more likely to be exposed to illicit drug use among peers than those who were withdrawn and socially inept. Because of this exposure they are more likely to use illicit drugs to cope with the symptoms of their psychoses. A related possibility is that cannabis use is a form of self-medication to deal with some of the unpleasant symptoms of schizophrenia, such as depression, anxiety, the negative symptoms of lethargy and anhedonia, and the side effects of the neuroleptic drugs used to treat it (Dixon, Haas et al., 1990).

The most convincing indication that cannabis use may precipitate schizophrenia comes from a prospective study of cannabis use and schizophrenia in Swedish conscripts (Andreasson, Allebeck et al., 1987). These investigators used data from a 15-year prospective study of 50,465 Swedish conscripts to investigate the relationship between self-reported cannabis use at age 18 and the risk of receiving a diagnosis of schizophrenia in the Swedish psychiatric case register over the subsequent 15 years.

Their results showed that the relative risk of receiving a diagnosis of schizophrenia was 2.4 times higher for those who had ever tried cannabis compared to those who had not. There was also a dose-response relationship between the risk of a diagnosis of schizophrenia and the number of times that the conscript had tried cannabis by age 18. The crude relative risk of developing schizophrenia was 1.3 times higher for those who had used cannabis 1 to 10 times, 3.0 times higher for those who had used

cannabis between 10 and 50 times, and 6.0 times higher for those who had used cannabis more than 50 times (compared in each case to those who had not used cannabis).

The relative risk was substantially reduced after statistically controlling for variables that independently predicted an increased risk of developing schizophrenia (having a psychiatric diagnosis at conscription, and having parents who had divorced). Nevertheless, the relationship remained statistically significant and still showed a dose-response relationship. The adjusted risk of a diagnosis of schizophrenia for those who had smoked cannabis from 1 to 10 times was 1.5 times that of those who had never used, and the relative risk for those who had used 10 or more times was 2.3 times that for those who had never used.

Andreasson et al. (1987) and Allebeck (1991) argued that their data showed that cannabis use precipitated schizophrenia in vulnerable individuals. A number of criticisms have been made of this causal interpretation (e.g., Johnson, Smith & Taylor, 1988; Negrete, 1989). First, there was a large temporal gap between self-reported cannabis use at age 18 and the development of schizophrenia over the next 15 years (Johnson, Smith & Taylor, 1988; Negrete, 1989), and there was no information on whether the individuals used cannabis up until the time that schizophrenia was diagnosed. Andreasson et al. (1987) responded that self-reported cannabis use at age 18 was strongly related to the risk of subsequently attracting a diagnosis of drug abuse. This suggests that cannabis use at age 18 was predictive of continued drug use, and the more so the more frequently it had been used by age 18.

A second possibility is that the cases of "schizophrenia" among the heavy cannabis users were acute cannabis-induced toxic psychoses that were mistakenly diagnosed as schizophrenia (Johnson, Smith & Taylor, 1988; Negrete, 1989). Andreasson et al. (1989) responded by citing data on the validity of the schizophrenia diagnoses in 21 conscripts in the case register (8 of whom had used cannabis and 13 of whom had not).

A third possibility is that the relationship between cannabis use and schizophrenia may be a consequence of the use of other illicit psychoactive drugs. Intensity of cannabis use in adolescence predicts the later use of stimulant drugs, such as amphetamine and cocaine (e.g., Kandel, 1988; Kandel & Faust, 1975), which can produce an acute paranoid psychosis (Angrist, 1983; Bell, 1973; Connell, 1959; Gawin & Ellinwood, 1988; Grinspoon & Hedblom, 1975). Since amphetamine was the major illicit drug of abuse in Sweden during the study period (Goldberg, 1968a; 1968b; Inghe, 1969) it may be that intervening amphetamine use produced the apparent correlation between cannabis use and schizophrenia. Andreasson and colleagues' (1989) study reported that only two of their eight schizophrenic cannabis users had also been abusers of amphetamines prior to the diagnosis of their schizophrenia, but with a sample size as small as this the true rate could be anywhere between 0 and 55 per cent.

A fourth criticism is that cannabis use at age 18 may have been a symptom of emerging schizophrenia. Statistical adjustment for a psychiatric diagnosis at conscription substantially reduced the relative risk but there was still a dose-response relationship between cannabis use and the risk of a schizophrenia among those who did not have a psychiatric history.

A fifth criticism relates to the validity of self-reported cannabis use at conscription. Andreasson et al. (1987) argued that any underreporting of cannabis use was most likely to lead to an underestimation of the relationship between cannabis use and the risk of schizophrenia.

When all these criticisms are considered, the Andreasson et al. (1987) study still provides prospective evidence of an association between cannabis use and schizophrenia that is not completely explained by prior psychiatric history. Uncertainty remains about the causal significance of the association, however, because it is unclear to what extent the relationship is a result of drug-induced psychoses being mistaken for schizophrenia, and to what extent it is attributable to amphetamine use rather than cannabis use.

Exacerbation of Schizophrenia

There is reasonable clinical evidence that schizophrenic patients who use cannabis and other drugs experience exacerbations of symptoms (Weil, 1970) and have more frequent psychotic episodes than those who do not (Knudsen & Vilmar, 1984; Perkins, Simpson & Tsuang, 1986; Negrete, Knapp et al., 1986; Turner & Tsuang, 1990). This is reviewed in detail in chapter 7.

SUMMARY OF PSYCHOLOGICAL EFFECTS

The most commonly experienced adverse psychological effects of cannabis use are anxiety and panic among naive users. These are probably of minor concern because they are not life-threatening and their major effect is likely to be to discourage further cannabis use.

Adolescent Use

There is more cause for concern about psychological effects of chronic cannabis use during adolescence and young adulthood. There has been a predictable sequence of initiation into the use of illicit drugs among American adolescents throughout the 1970s and 1980s in which the use of licit drugs preceded experimentation with cannabis, which in turn preceded the use of other drugs such as the hallucinogens, "pills," cocaine and heroin. Generally, the earlier the age of initiation into cannabis use, and the greater the involvement with it, the greater the likelihood of progression to the use of other illicit drugs.

The causal significance of cannabis in the sequence of illicit drug use remains controversial. The hypothesis that the sequence reflects a direct pharmacological effect of cannabis use upon the use of later drugs in the sequence is the least compelling. A more plausible explanation is that it reflects a combination of the selective recruitment into cannabis use of non-conforming and deviant adolescents who have a propensity to use illicit drugs, and the socialization of cannabis users within an illicit drug-using subculture that increases the exposure, opportunity and encouragement to use other illicit drugs.

There has been some support for the hypothesis that heavy adolescent use of cannabis impairs educational performance. Cannabis use appears to increase the risks of failing to complete a high school education and of job instability in young adulthood. The apparent strength of these relationships in cross-sectional studies has been exaggerated because those who are most likely to use cannabis have lower academic aspirations and poorer high school performance than those who do not. Even though more modest than has sometimes been supposed, the adverse effects of cannabis and other drug use upon the educational performance of persons whose performance was marginal to begin with may cascade throughout young adult life, affecting choice of occupation, level of income and quality of life.

There is weaker suggestive evidence that heavy cannabis use has adverse effects upon family formation, mental health and involvement in crime. In the case of each of these outcomes, the apparently strong associations revealed in cross-sectional data are much more modest in longitudinal studies after statistically controlling for associations between cannabis use and other variables that predict these adverse outcomes.

Adult Use

There is a variety of evidence that chronic heavy cannabis use may adversely affect psychological health in adults. The situation is least clear with the motivational effects of chronic cannabis use in adults. Case reports of an amotivational syndrome have not been well supported by epidemiological studies of chronic heavy users, although these studies may have had a limited capacity to detect such a syndrome.

It is clearer that some chronic heavy cannabis users develop a dependence syndrome like that defined in the *DSM-III-R*. There is good experimental evidence that chronic heavy cannabis users can develop tolerance to drug effects, and there is suggestive evidence that some may experience a withdrawal syndrome on the abrupt cessation of cannabis use. There is epidemiological evidence that some heavy cannabis users experience problems in controlling their cannabis use and continue to use the drug despite experiencing adverse personal consequences of use. If the estimates of the community prevalence of drug dependence provided by the Epidemiological Catchment Area study are correct, cannabis dependence is the most common form of dependence on illicit drugs.

The weight of the epidemiological evidence suggests that the long-term use of cannabis does not result in any severe or grossly debilitating impairment of cognitive function. However, there is some experimental evidence (see chapter 6) to suggest that long-term cannabis use may produce more subtle cognitive impairments in specific aspects of memory, attention and the organization and integration of complex information.

There is suggestive evidence that chronic cannabis use may precipitate schizophrenia in vulnerable individuals. There is still some uncertainty about the relationship because in the best study conducted to date (Andreasson, Allebeck et al., 1987) the use of cannabis was not documented at the time of diagnosis, there was a possibility that cannabis use was confounded by amphetamine use, and there remains a question about the ability of the study to reliably distinguish between schizophrenia and acute cannabis or other drug-induced psychoses.

Health Consequences of Cannabis Use

Very few of the major potential health effects of cannabis have been the subject of epidemiological research. These include: an increased risk of accidents when cannabis users drive while intoxicated, and effects of chronic cannabis use on the immune, respiratory and reproductive systems. Other major areas of potential interest such as cardiovascular effects and effects on brain structure have not been investigated by epidemiological methods.

CANNABIS USE AND ACCIDENT RISK

There is no doubt that cannabis adversely affects performance on a number of psychomotor tasks, and that these effects are related to dose, and are larger, more consistent and persistent in difficult tasks involving sustained attention (Chait & Pierri, 1992; see also chapter 5 in this volume). The acute effects on performance of doses of cannabis that are used recreationally are similar to, if smaller than, those of intoxicating doses of alcohol. Alcohol and cannabis differ in their effects on the apparent willingness of intoxicated users to take risks in simulated driving tasks in the laboratory and on-road (Smiley, 1986). Persons intoxicated by cannabis are less likely to engage in risky behavior than are persons intoxicated by alcohol.

While cannabis produces decrements in psychomotor performance in laboratory and controlled settings, it has been difficult to assess the impact of cannabis use on motor vehicle accidents. Surveys (e.g., Dalton, Martz et al., 1975; Klonoff, 1974; Robbe, 1994; Robbe & O'Hanlon, 1993; Thompson, 1975) have found that cannabis users are generally aware that their driving is impaired after using cannabis but the majority had driven, or would still drive, after using cannabis (Klonoff, 1974).

There have been no controlled epidemiological studies to show that cannabis users are at increased risk of being involved in motor vehicle or other accidents. This is in contrast to alcohol use and accidents where case-control studies have shown that persons with blood alcohol levels indicative of intoxication are over-represented among accident victims in comparison to their prevalence in the community (English, Holman et al., 1995). There are retrospective studies of the prevalence of cannabinoids in the blood of motor vehicle and other accident victims (see McBay, 1986 for a review). These studies have found that between 4 and 37 per cent of blood samples contain cannabinoids, typically in combination with blood alcohol levels indicative of intoxication (e.g., Cimbura, Lucas et al., 1982; Mason & McBay, 1984; Williams, Peat et al., 1985). Similar prevalence data on blood cannabinoid levels have been found among Californian motorists tested by the highway patrol because of suspicion of impairment (Zimmerman, Yeager et al., 1983)

and among trauma patients (Soderstrom, Triffilis et al., 1988).

These studies are difficult to evaluate because we do not know whether persons with cannabinoids are overrepresented among accident victims (Terhune, 1986). Although a prevalence of 35 per cent may seem high, this is the prevalence of cannabis use among young males who are at highest risk of motor vehicle and other accidents (Soderstrom, Triffilis et al., 1988). There are also major problems in using cannabinoid blood levels to determine whether a driver or pedestrian was intoxicated with cannabis at the time of an accident. The simple presence of cannabinoids indicates only recent use, not necessarily intoxication at the time of the accident (Consensus Development Panel, 1985). Finally, there are problems of causal attribution since more than 75 per cent of drivers with cannabinoids in their blood also have blood levels indicative of alcohol intoxication (Gieringer, 1988; McBay, 1986).

There is some epidemiological evidence to suggest that cannabis use produces an increase in the risk of accidents. Two surveys of self-reported accidents among adolescent drug users found a relationship between marijuana use and self-reported involvement in accidents, with marijuana smokers having approximately twice the risk of being involved in accidents that non-marijuana smokers do (Hingson, Heeren et al., 1982; Smart & Fejer, 1976).

More direct evidence of an association between cannabis use and accidents is provided by two epidemiological studies of the relationship between cannabis use and mortality (Andreasson & Allebeck, 1990; Sidney, Beck et al., 1997) and health service utilization (Polen, Sidney et al., 1993). Andreasson and Allebeck reported a prospective study of mortality over 15 years among 50,465 Swedish military conscripts. They found an increased risk of premature mortality among men who had smoked cannabis 50 or more times by age 18 (relative risk of 4.6). Violent deaths were the major cause contributing to this excess mortality, with 26 per cent of deaths being motor vehicle and 7 per cent other accidents. The increased risk was no longer statistically significant (relative risk of 1.2 [95 per cent CI: 0.7, 1.9]) after multivariate statistical adjustment for confounding variables such as antisocial behavior, and alcohol and other drug use in adolescence (Andreasson & Allebeck, 1990).

Sidney et al. (1997) reported a 10-year study of mortality in cannabis users among 65,171 Kaiser Permanente Medical Care Program members aged between 15 and 49. In the sample, 38 per cent had never used cannabis, 20 per cent were experimenters who had used less than six times, 20 per cent were former cannabis users, and 22 per cent were current cannabis users. Overall, regular cannabis use had only a small impact on all cause mortality (RR = 1.33). This was wholly explained by an increase in AIDS-related deaths among men in the cohort. This was probably because marijuana use was a marker for male homosexual behavior in this cohort of men from the San Francisco Bay area. It is too early to conclude that marijuana use does not increase mortality from motor vehicle accidents (or indeed for any other causes of death). The average age at follow-up was only 43 years; there was a possibility that deaths were missed among cohort members who left the state, and cigarette smoking and alcohol use, which have been shown to predict premature death in other cohorts (English, Holman et al., 1995), were only modestly associated with premature mortality in this cohort.

Polen et al. (1993) compared health service utilization by non-smokers (N = 450) and daily cannabis-only smokers (N = 450) who were screened at Kaiser Permanente Medical centres between July, 1979, and December, 1985. They reported an increased rate of medical care utilization by cannabis smokers for accidental injury over a one- to two-year follow-up. There was also an interaction between cannabis and alcohol use in that cannabis users who were the heaviest alcohol users showed the highest rates of utilization. This result is difficult to interpret in terms of the risks of motor vehicle accidents because all forms of accidental injury were aggregated.

IMMUNOLOGICAL EFFECTS OF CANNABIS

The animal evidence indicates that cannabinoids produce impairments of the cell-mediated and humoral immune systems, as well as decreased resistance to bacteria and viruses. There is also evidence that the non-cannabinoid components of cannabis smoke can impair the functioning of alveolar macrophages, the first line of the body's defence system. However, the doses required to produce these immunological effects have been very high (see Hall, Solowij & Lemon, 1994). The very limited human experimental evidence is mixed, with a small number of studies suggesting immunosuppressant effects that have not been replicated by others (Munson & Fehr, 1983).

Three field studies of the effects of chronic cannabis use in Costa Rica (Carter, Coggins & Doughty, 1980), Greece (Stefanis, Dornbush & Fink, 1977), and Jamaica (Rubin & Comitas, 1975) failed to demonstrate any evidence of increased susceptibility to infectious diseases among chronic cannabis users. But less than 100 users were studied, far too few to detect a small increase in the incidence of common infectious and bacterial diseases. Large-scale epidemiological studies are needed to exclude the latter possibility.

Given the duration of large-scale cannabis use by young adults in Western societies, some have argued that the absence of an epidemic of infectious disease is arguably sufficient to rule out the hypothesis that cannabis smoking produces major impairments in the immune systems of users comparable to those caused by AIDS (Hollister, 1992). The absence of such epidemics among cannabis users does not, however, exclude the possibility that chronic heavy use may produce minor impairments in immunity, since this would produce small increases in the rate of occurrence of common bacterial and viral illnesses (Munson & Fehr, 1983) that would have escaped the notice of clinical observers. Such an increase could nonetheless be of public health significance because of the increased expenditure on health services and the loss of productivity among the young adults who are the heaviest users of cannabis.

Epidemiological studies of cannabis users whose immune systems have been compromised by AIDS may provide the best ways of detecting any adverse immunological effects of cannabinoids. One such study has been conducted by Kaslow et al. (1989) who examined predictors of progression to AIDS among HIV-positive homosexual men. They conducted a prospective study of progression to AIDS among HIV-positive men in a cohort of 4,954 homosexual and bisexual men. Among the predictor variables studied were licit and illicit drug use, including cannabis use. Illicit drug use predicted an increased risk of infection with HIV, as has been consistently found in studies of risk factors for HIV infection, but neither cannabis use, nor any other psychoactive drug use, predicted an increased rate of progression of the disease to AIDS among men who were HIV-positive. Cannabis use was also unrelated to changes in a limited number of measures of immunological functioning.

RESPIRATORY EFFECTS OF CANNABIS

There is good reason to expect that chronic heavy cannabis smoking may have adverse effects upon the respiratory system (Tashkin, 1993). Cannabis smoke is similar in constitution to tobacco smoke and in fact contains substantially more particulate matter and more of some carcinogens (e.g., benz[a]pyrene) than does tobacco smoke (Institute of Medicine, 1982; Leuchtenberger, 1983). Cigarette smoking is known to cause diseases of the respiratory system, such as bronchitis, emphysema and various forms of cancer affecting the lung, oral cavity, trachea and esophagus (English, Holman et al., 1995).

Despite the reasonableness of this hypothesis, it has been difficult to investigate the contribution of chronic heavy cannabis smoking to diseases of the respiratory system (Huber, Griffith & Langsjoen, 1988; Institute of Medicine, 1982). Most marijuana smokers also smoke tobacco, which makes it difficult to disentangle the effects of cannabis from those of tobacco smoking. The difficulties in quantifying current and lifetime exposure to cannabis because of variations in

quality and potency make it difficult to examine dose-response relationships between cannabis use and the risk of developing various respiratory diseases. There is also likely to be a long latency period between exposure and the development of these diseases, especially in the case of cancers of the aerodigestive tract. This period exceeds the length of time since cannabis smoking became widespread in Western societies. Finally, the number of cases on which research data would be needed is likely to be quite large.

Bronchitis and Airways Obstruction

The most convincing evidence that chronic cannabis use may be a contributory cause of impaired lung function and symptoms of respiratory disease comes from a series of prospective controlled studies that have been conducted by Tashkin and his colleagues since the mid-1970s (see chapter 9). These studies have found that the prevalence of bronchitic symptoms of cough, sputum and wheeze is higher among all types of smokers than among non-smokers, and there was an additive adverse effect of marijuana and cigarette smoking on these symptoms. Tashkin and his colleagues (Fligiel, Beals et al., 1988; Fligiel, Roth et al., 1997; Gong, Fligiel et al., 1987) have also shown that subjects who smoked (whether cannabis, tobacco or both) had more prevalent and severe histopathological abnormalities than non-smokers. Many of these abnormalities were more prevalent in marijuana smokers, and they were most marked in those who smoked both marijuana and tobacco.

Bloom et al. (1987) have reported a cross-sectional epidemiological study that broadly confirmed the findings of Tashkin and his colleagues. Bloom et al. studied the relationship between smoking "non-tobacco" cigarettes and respiratory symptoms and respiratory function in a general population sample. Their study sample was a community sample of 990 individuals aged under 40 years who were being followed as part of a prospective community study of obstructive airways disease. Subjects were asked about symptoms of cough, phlegm, wheeze and shortness of breath, and they were also measured on a number of indicators of respiratory function, including forced expiratory volume and forced vital capacity.

The prevalence of ever having smoked a non-tobacco cigarette was 14 per cent (the same as the prevalence of marijuana smoking in general population surveys), with 9 per cent being current smokers and 5 per cent ex-smokers. The mean frequency of current non-tobacco smoking was seven times per week, and the average duration of use was nine years. Non-tobacco smokers were more likely than non-tobacco non-smokers to have smoked tobacco, and more likely to inhale deeply than tobacco smokers.

Non-tobacco smoking was related to the prevalence of the self-reported respiratory symptoms of cough, phlegm and wheeze, regardless of whether the person smoked tobacco or not. There were also mean differences in forced expiratory volume and forced vital capacity, with those who had never smoked having the best functioning, followed in decreasing order of function by current cigarette smokers, current non-tobacco smokers and current smokers of both tobacco and non-tobacco cigarettes. Non-tobacco smoking alone had a larger effect on all flow indices than tobacco smoking alone, and the effect of both types of smoking was additive.

Most recently, Tashkin et al. (1997) have reported data on rates of decline in respiratory function over eight years among marijuana and tobacco smokers in their cohort (65 per cent of whom were reassessed). They found that tobacco smokers showed the greatest rate of decline in respiratory function. The rate of decline in marijuana-only smokers did not differ from that in non-smokers. This was in contrast to a follow-up study of the Tucson cohort (Sherrill, Krzyzanowski et al., 1991), which found a greater rate of decline in respiratory function among marijuana-only than tobacco smokers, and additive effects of tobacco and marijuana smoking. The studies of Tashkin et al. and Bloom et al. are consistent in showing that chronic cannabis smoking increases the prevalence of bronchitic symptoms, but they disagree in their findings on the rate of decline in respiratory function with cannabis smoking.

Cancers of the Aerodigestive Tract

The work of Fligiel et al. (1988) has indicated that histopathological changes of the type that are believed to be precursors of carcinoma can be observed in the lung tissue of chronic marijuana smokers. These observations have recently received support from case reports of cancers of the upper aerodigestive tract in young adults who have been chronic cannabis smokers. These include series of: 13 cases of advanced head and neck cancer occurring in young adults under 40 years of age, 11 of whom had been daily cannabis smokers (Donald, 1991a; 1991b); 10 cases of upper respiratory tract cancer occurring in adults under the age of 40 years over a four-year period, 7 of whom were probably regular cannabis smokers (Taylor, 1988); and 2 cases of squamous cell carcinoma of the tongue in men aged 37 and 52 years, whose only shared risk factor was a history of long-term daily cannabis use (Caplan & Brigham, 1990).

These case reports provide limited support for the hypothesis that cannabis use is a cause of upper respiratory tract cancers. None of them compare the prevalence of cannabis use in cases with that in a control sample, and cannabis exposure was not assessed in a standardized way or in ignorance of case or control status, all standard controls to minimize bias in case-control studies of cancer etiology. Interpretation is complicated by the fact that many of these patients also smoked tobacco, and were alcohol consumers, both risk factors for cancers of the upper aerodigestive tract, although the average age of onset in smokers and drinkers is over 60 rather than under 40 years (Holman, Armstrong et al., 1988; Vokes, Weichelsbaum et al., 1993). Nonetheless, there is a worrying consistency about these reports that should be addressed by case-control studies that compare the proportions of cannabis smokers among patients with cancers of the upper aerodigestive tract and appropriate controls (Institute of Medicine, 1982).

REPRODUCTIVE EFFECTS

Fetal Development and Birth Defects

Given animal evidence that THC affects female reproductive function, one might expect it to have a potentially adverse effect on the outcome of pregnancy (Bloch, 1983). The possibility of adverse pregnancy outcomes is increased by evidence that THC crosses the placenta in animals (Bloch, 1983) and humans (Blackard & Tennes, 1984). This raises the possibility that THC, and possibly other cannabinoids, are teratogens, i.e., substances that may interfere with the normal development of the fetus *in utero*.

Reproductive Effects

Chronic administration of high doses of THC disrupts male and female reproductive function in animals, reducing the secretion of testosterone, impairing sperm production, motility and viability, and disrupting the ovulatory cycle in females (Bloch, 1983; Institute of Medicine, 1982). It is uncertain whether marijuana smoking has these effects in humans because the limited literature on human males is inconsistent (Mendelson & Mello, 1984) and there is almost no research on human females (Hollister, 1986).

Cannabis use during pregnancy impairs fetal development in animals, reducing birthweight (Abel, 1985; Behnke & Eyler, 1993). Epidemiological studies of the effects of cannabis use on human development have produced more mixed results for a number of reasons. First, adverse reproductive outcomes and the prevalence of heavy cannabis use during pregnancy are relatively rare, so very large samples are required to detect associations between cannabis use and fetal development (Richardson, Day & McGauhey, 1993).

Second, the stigma associated with illicit drug use during pregnancy probably discourages honest reporting, compounding the usual problem of forgetting when women are asked about their drug use during early pregnancy, late in their pregnancy or even after the birth (Day, Wagener & Taylor, 1985; Richardson, Day & McGauhey, 1993). If a substantial proportion of cannabis users are misclassified as non-users, any relationship between cannabis use and adverse outcomes will be attenuated, requiring even larger samples to detect it (Zuckerman, 1985).

Third, even when large samples are studied and associations are found, there are difficulties in interpreting the associations because cannabis users are more likely to use tobacco, alcohol and other illicit drugs during their pregnancy. They also differ from non-users in other ways (e.g., social class, education, nutrition) that predict an increased risk of experiencing an adverse outcome of pregnancy (Fried, 1980; 1982; 1993; Institute of Medicine, 1982; Tennes, Avitable et al., 1985).

It is doubtful whether cannabis smoking during pregnancy produces an increase in the risk of birth defects. There is some animal evidence of such effects although these studies have usually involved very high doses by the oral route (Abel, 1985). In humans, there were early reports of children with features akin to the fetal alcohol syndrome born to women who had smoked cannabis during pregnancy and not used alcohol (e.g., Milman, 1982, p. 42). Subsequent studies have not reported an increased rate of major congenital abnormalities among children born to women who use cannabis (Gibson, Baghurst & Colley, 1983; Hingson, Alpert et al., 1982; Tennes, Avitable et al., 1985; Zuckerman, Frank et al., 1989). The study by Zuckerman et al. provides the most convincing failure to find an increased risk. It included a large sample of women with a substantial prevalence of cannabis use that was verified by urinalysis. There was a low rate of birth abnormalities among the cannabis users, and no suggestion of an increase by comparison with the controls.

There is marginally more evidence that cannabis smoking in pregnancy is associated with reduced birthweight (e.g., Gibson, Baghurst & Colley, 1983; Hatch & Bracken, 1986; Zuckerman, Frank et al., 1989) and length at birth (Tennes, Avitable et al., 1985). This relationship has been found in some of the best controlled studies in which it has persisted after statistically controlling for potential confounding variables (e.g., Hatch & Bracken, 1986;

Zuckerman, Frank et al., 1989). Other studies (e.g., Gibson, Baghust & Colley, 1983; Linn, Schoenbaum et al., 1983; Tennes, Avitable et al., 1985; Witter & Niebyl, 1990) and some recent studies on large samples (Shiono, Klebanoff et al., 1995) have not found any such association. In studies that report the effect, it is small by comparison with the effects of tobacco smoking on birthweight (Behnke & Eyler, 1993; Cornelius, Taylor et al., 1995).

Postnatal Development

Cannabis use by the mother during pregnancy and breast feeding could affect the postnatal development of the child either because of the enduring developmental impairment arising from *in utero* exposure, or because the infant continues to be exposed to cannabinoids via breast milk. There are a small number of animal studies that provide suggestive evidence of such effects (Nahas, 1984; Nahas & Frick, 1987).

The most extensive research evidence in humans comes from the Ottawa Prospective Prenatal Study (OPPS) that studied developmental and behavioral abnormalities in children born to women who reported using cannabis during pregnancy (Fried and colleagues, 1980; 1982; 1983; 1985; 1986; 1989; 1990; 1992; 1993; 1995) (see also chapter 12 in this volume). In this study, mothers were asked about their drug use during pregnancy, and their children were measured on the Brazelton scales after birth, neurologically assessed at one month, and assessed again by standardized scales of ability at 6 and 12 months. The results indicated that there was some developmental delay shortly after birth in the infants' visual system, and there was also an increased rate of tremors and startle among the children of cannabis users.

The behavioral effects discernible after birth had faded by 1 month, and no effects were detectable in performance on standardized ability tests at 6 and 12 months. Effects were subsequently reported at 36- and 48-month follow-ups (Fried & Watkinson, 1990), but these did not persist in a more recent follow-up at 60 and 72 months (Fried, O'Connell &

Watkinson, 1992). These results are suggestive of a developmental impairment occurring among children who had experienced a shorter gestation and prematurity, or they indicate a more subtle effect on cognitive performance analogous to those reported in adult cannabis users (Fried, 1995). The possibility that the tests used in later follow-ups are insufficiently sensitive to the subtle effects of prenatal cannabis exposure seems unlikely since they were able to detect effects of maternal tobacco smoking during pregnancy on behavioral development at 60 and 72 months (Fried et al., 1990; 1992; 1993).

Attempts to replicate the OPPS findings have been mixed. Tennes et al. (1985) conducted a prospective study of the relationship between cannabis use during pregnancy and postnatal development in 756 women, a third of whom reported using cannabis during pregnancy. The children were assessed shortly after birth using the same measurement instruments as Fried (1980), and a subset were followed up and assessed at one year of age. There was no evidence of impaired development of the visual system, and no increased risk of tremor or startle among the children of users. There was also no evidence of any differences at one year. More recently, Richardson et al. (1993) have followed up at age three children born to 655 women who were questioned about their substance use during pregnancy. They found a relationship between the mothers' cannabis use during pregnancy and the children's performances on memory and verbal scales of the Stanford-Binet Intelligence Scale.

Childhood Cancers

Several case-control studies have provided suggestive evidence that cannabis use during pregnancy may have more serious and life-threatening effects on postnatal development. The first of these was a case-control study of acute non-lymphoblastic leukemia (ANLL), a rare form of childhood cancer (Neglia, Buckley & Robinson, 1991; Robinson, Buckley et al., 1989). The study was designed to examine the etiological role of maternal and paternal environmental exposures to petrochemicals, pesticides and radiation. Maternal drug use, including marijuana use, before and during pregnancy, was assessed as a possible confounder to be statistically controlled in any relationships observed between ANLL and environmental exposures.

An unexpected but strong association was observed between maternal cannabis use and ANLL. The mothers of cases were 11 times more likely to have used cannabis before and during their pregnancy than were the mothers of controls. The relationship persisted after statistical adjustment for many other risk factors. Comparisons of cases whose mothers did and did not use cannabis during their pregnancies showed that cases with cannabis exposure were younger, and had a higher frequency of ANLL with cell types of a specific pathological origin than did the cases without such exposure. The authors argued that these differences made it unlikely that the relationship was due to chance.

Reporting bias on the part of the mothers of cases is an alternative explanation of the finding. The reports of cannabis use were obtained retrospectively after diagnosis of the ANLL, so it is possible that the mothers of children who developed ANLL were more likely to report cannabis use than were mothers of controls. The authors investigated this possibility by comparing the rates of cannabis use reported in this study with the rates reported in several earlier case-control studies of other childhood cancers that they had conducted using the same methods. The rate was lower among controls in the ANLL study, but even when the rate of cannabis use among the controls in these other studies was used the odds ratio was still greater than three and statistically significant. Nonetheless, since this was an unexpected finding that emerged from a large number of exploratory analyses conducted in a single study, it should be replicated as a matter of some urgency.

There are two other case-control studies that report an increased risk of rhabdomyosarcoma (Grufferman, Schwartz et al., 1993) and astrocytomas (Kuitjen, Bunin et al., 1992) in children born to women who reported using cannabis during their pregnancies. Neither of these studies

was planned as an investigation of the association between these childhood cancers and maternal cannabis use. In each case, cannabis use was one of a large number of possible confounding variables that were measured and controlled for in the statistical analysis of the relationship between the exposure of principal interest and the childhood cancer. Their replication is nonetheless a research priority.

SUMMARY OF HEALTH EFFECTS

There is no doubt that cannabis adversely affects the performance of a number of psychomotor tasks relevant to driving a motor vehicle. While cannabis produces decrements in performance under laboratory and controlled on-road conditions, it has been difficult, for technical and ethical reasons, to discover whether cannabis intoxication increases the risk of involvement in motor vehicle accidents. There is sufficient consistency and coherence in the evidence from studies of cannabinoid levels among accident victims and a small number of epidemiological studies to argue on the grounds of plausibility that there probably is an increased risk of motor vehicle accidents among persons who drive when intoxicated with cannabis. This increased risk may be largely explained by the combined use of cannabis with intoxicating doses of alcohol. Further research is required to elucidate this issue.

The limited experimental evidence on immune effects in humans is conflicting, with the small number of studies producing adverse effects not being replicated. There has not been any evidence of increased rates of disease among chronic heavy cannabis users analogous to that seen among homosexual men in the early 1980s. Given the duration of large-scale cannabis use by young adults in Western societies, the absence of such epidemics makes it unlikely that cannabis smoking produces major impairments in the immune system.

It is more difficult to exclude the possibility that chronic heavy cannabis use produces minor impairments in immunity. Such effects would produce small increases in the rates of infectious diseases that have public health significance because of the increased expenditure on health services and the loss of productivity among the young adults who are the heaviest users. There is one large prospective study of HIV-positive homosexual men which indicates that continued cannabis use did not increase the risk of progression to AIDS (Kaslow, Blackwelder et al., 1989). The most sensitive assay of any small immunological effects of cannabis may come from studies of the therapeutic usefulness of cannabinoids in immunologically compromised patients, such as those undergoing cancer chemotherapy or those with AIDS.

Chronic heavy cannabis smoking probably causes chronic bronchitis and impairs functioning of the large airways. Given the documented adverse effects of cigarette smoking, it is likely that chronic cannabis use predisposes individuals to develop lung diseases. There is suggestive evidence that chronic cannabis smoking produces histopathological changes in lung tissues that are precursors of lung cancer. Case studies raise a strong suspicion that cannabis may cause cancers of the aerodigestive tract. The conduct of case-control studies of these cancers is a high priority for research that aims to identify the possible adverse health effects of chronic cannabis smoking.

Cannabis use during pregnancy probably impairs fetal development, leading to smaller birthweight. It is unlikely that cannabis use during pregnancy increases the risk of birth defects as a result of exposure of the fetus *in utero*. Prudence suggests that until this issue is resolved, we should err in the conservative direction by recommending that women not use cannabis during pregnancy or when attempting to conceive (Hollister, 1986). There is suggestive evidence that infants exposed *in utero* to cannabis may experience transient behavioral and developmental effects during the first few months after birth. There is also a single study that raises concern about an increased risk of childhood leukemia occurring among the children born to women who used cannabis during their pregnancies.

Conclusions and Implications for Research

The epidemiological literature provides uneven coverage of the possible health and psychological effects of cannabis, and it has primarily been conducted on cannabis users in the United States. The best coverage is of the possible psychological consequences of cannabis use among adolescents and young adults. This research has helped to clarify the role that cannabis use plays in increasing the risk of using other illicit drugs and in impairing educational performance.

There is also reasonable epidemiological evidence for the existence of a cannabis-dependence syndrome. The cognitive consequences of long-term use remain unclear: it is unlikely that cannabis produces gross cognitive impairment of the kind found among heavy alcohol users but it may produce more subtle forms of impairment. There is consistent evidence of an association between schizophrenia and cannabis use from cross-sectional studies and one large prospective study. Its causal significance remains uncertain although again prudence would suggest that persons with schizophrenia or a family history of the disorder should be discouraged from using cannabis.

Epidemiological evidence on more narrowly defined health effects of cannabis use is sparser. The only possible exception is in the case of the reproductive effects of maternal cannabis use where there is reasonably consistent evidence of growth impairment. The evidence of respiratory disease from controlled laboratory studies has received some support from the limited epidemiological studies.

As to research priorities, the occurrence of upper respiratory tract cancers among young adults with a history of regular cannabis use indicates that case-control studies of respiratory cancer and cannabis use are a research priority. Now may be the time to conduct such studies since chronic cannabis smokers who began their use in the early 1970s are now entering the period of risk for such cancers. If carcinoma occurs earlier in heavy cannabis smokers, it may be better to restrict attention to early onset cases (e.g., cases occurring in individuals under 50 years of age). Information on cannabis use should also be obtained prospectively in newly diagnosed cases because of the problems with retrospective assessment of cannabis and other drug use from either clinical records or the relatives of those who have died. Other priorities would be replication of the case-control studies of maternal cannabis use and various childhood cancers, and better-controlled studies of the effects of cannabis in immunologically compromised patients, such as those with AIDS.

There is also one possibility not covered in this chapter that deserves priority for epidemiological study: the possibility that chronic cannabis use has adverse effects on the cardiovascular system. There is evidence from laboratory studies that cannabinoids have pronounced acute effects on cardiovascular functioning (Institute of Medicine, 1982). Although these effects are unlikely to be significant in healthy young adults, clinical studies indicate that cannabis smoking can have adverse effects on patients with pre-existing diseases (Aronow & Cassidy, 1975). The fact that the cohort of cannabis users that initiated use in the early 1970s are now entering a period of maximal risk for cardiovascular disease suggests that it may be timely to consider case-control studies of cannabis use and cardiovascular disease.

An overarching priority for all epidemiological research on cannabis use is greater attention to patterns of use and problems in developing countries. Apart from informing governments in these countries about the scale of cannabis use and problems, such work will also enable us to discover which of the findings of American research, especially those on its psychological effects, may be historically and culturally specific. More effective use could also be made of the fact that some cultures have a long history of traditional use, including very heavy use among some subpopulations. It remains true that these populations are the ones most likely to show any adverse health and psychological effects of chronic heavy use, a fact that prompted the National Institute on Drug Abuse to fund research in these countries in the 1970s. A high priority would be to repeat this type of research with more focused inquiries, using more sophisticated research designs and methods of measurement than were available to researchers in the 1970s.

References

Abel, E.L. (1985). Effects of prenatal exposure to cannabinoids. In T.M. Pinkert (Ed.), *Current Research on the Consequences of Maternal Drug Abuse* (NIDA Research Monograph No. 59, pp. 20–35)(DHHS Publication No. 85-1400). Washington, DC: U.S. Government Printing Office.

Adlaf, E.M. & Smart, R.G. (1991). Drug use among adolescent students in Canada and Ontario: The past, present and future. *The Journal of Drug Issues, 21,* 59–72.

Allebeck, P. (1991). Cannabis and schizophrenia: Is there a causal association? In G.G. Nahas & C. Latour (Eds.), *Physiopathology of Illicit Drugs: Cannabis, Cocaine, Opiates.* Oxford: Pergamon Press.

Allebeck, P., Adamsson, C., Engstrom, A. & Rydberg, U. (1993). Cannabis and schizophrenia: A longitudinal study of cases treated in Stockholm county. *Acta Psychiatrica Scandinavica, 88,* 21–24.

Andreasson, S. & Allebeck, P. (1990). Cannabis and mortality among young men: A longitudinal study of Swedish conscripts. *Scandinavian Journal of Social Medicine, 18,* 9–15.

Andreasson, S., Allebeck, P., Engstrom, A. & Rydberg, U. (1987). Cannabis and schizophrenia: A longitudinal study of Swedish conscripts. *Lancet, 2,* 1483–1486.

Andreasson, S., Allebeck, P. & Rydberg, U. (1989). Schizophrenia in users and nonusers of cannabis. *Acta Psychiatrica Scandinavica, 79,* 505–510.

Angrist, B. (1983). Psychoses induced by central nervous system stimulants and related drugs. In I. Creese (Ed.), *Stimulants: Neurochemical, Behavioral and Clinical Perspectives* (pp. 1–30). New York: Raven Press.

Anthony, J.C. & Helzer, J.E. (1991). Syndromes of drug abuse and dependence. In L.N. Robins & D.A. Regier (Eds.), *Psychiatric Disorders in America* (pp. 116–154). New York: Free Press.

Anthony, J.C., Warner, L.A. & Kessler, R.C. (1994). Comparative epidemiology of dependence on tobacco, alcohol, controlled substances and inhalants: Basic findings from the National Comorbidity Study. *Clinical and Experimental Psychopharmacology, 2,* 244–268.

Arndt, S., Tyrrell, G., Flaum, M. & Andreasen, N.C. (1992). Comorbidity of substance abuse and schizophrenia: The role of premorbid adjustment. *Psychological Medicine, 22,* 379–388.

Aronow, W.S. & Cassidy, J. (1975). Effect of smoking marihuana and a high-nicotine cigarette on angina pectoris. *Clinical Pharmacology and Therapeutics, 17,* 549–554.

Bachman, J.G., Johnston, L.D., O'Malley, P.M. & Humphrey, R.H. (1988). Explaining the recent decline in marijuana use: Differentiating the effects of perceived risks, disapproval, and general lifestyle factors. *Journal of Health and Social Behavior, 29*, 92–112.

Bachman, J.G. & O'Malley, P.M. (1981). When four months equal a year: Inconsistencies in students' reports of drug use. *Public Opinion Quarterly, 45*, 536–548.

Bachman, J.G., Wadsworth, K.N., O'Malley, P.M., Johnston, L.D. & Schulenberg, J.E. (Eds.). (1997). *Smoking, Drinking and Drug Use in Young Adulthood*. Mahwah, NJ: Erlbaum.

Bachman, J.G., Wallace, J.M., Jr., O'Malley, P.M., Johnston, L.D., Kurth, C.L. & Neighbors, H.W. (1991). Racial/ethnic differences in smoking, drinking, and illicit drug use among American high school seniors, 1976–1989. *American Journal of Public Health, 81*, 372–377.

Bailey, S.L., Flewelling, R.L. & Rachal, J.V. (1992). The characterization of inconsistencies in self-reports of alcohol and marijuana use in a longitudinal study of adolescents. *Journal of Studies on Alcohol, 53*, 636–647.

Baumrind, D. & Moselle, K.A. (1985). A developmental perspective on adolescent drug abuse. *Advances in Alcohol and Substance Abuse, 5*, 41–67.

Behnke, M. & Eyler, F.D. (1993). The consequences of prenatal substance use for the developing fetus, newborn and young child. *International Journal of the Addictions, 28*, 1341–1391.

Bell, D. (1973). The experimental reproduction of amphetamine psychosis. *Archives of General Psychiatry, 29*, 35–40.

Black, S. & Casswell, S. (1993). *Drugs in New Zealand — A survey 1990. Alcohol and Public Health Research Unit*, University of Auckland.

Blackard, C. & Tennes, K. (1984). Human placental transfer of cannabinoids. *New England Journal of Medicine, 311*, 797.

Bland, R.C., Newman, S.C. & Orn, H. (1987). Schizophrenia: Lifetime co-morbidity in a community sample. *Acta Psychiatrica Scandinavica, 75*, 383–391.

Bloch, E. (1983). Effects of marijuana and cannabinoids on reproduction, endocrine function, development and chromosomes. In K.O. Fehr & H. Kalant (Eds.), *Cannabis and Health Hazards* (pp. 355–432). Toronto: Addiction Research Foundation.

Block, R.I., Farnham, S., Braverman, K., Noyes, R., Jr. & Ghoneim, M.M. (1990). Long-term marijuana use and subsequent effects on learning and cognitive functions related to school achievement: Preliminary study. In J.W. Spencer & J.J. Boren (Eds.), *Residual Effects of Abused Drugs on Behavior* (NIDA Research Monograph No. 101, pp. 96–111). Rockville, MD: U.S. Department of Health and Human Services.

Bloom, J.W., Kaltenborn, W.T., Paoletti, P., Camilli, A. & Lebowitz, M.D. (1987). Respiratory effects of non-tobacco cigarettes. *British Medical Journal, 295*, 1516–1518.

Bowman, M. & Pihl, R.O. (1973). Cannabis: Psychological effects of chronic heavy use. A controlled study of intellectual functioning in chronic users of high potency cannabis. *Psychopharmacologia* (Berl.), *29*, 159–170.

Brill, H. & Nahas, G.G. (1984). Cannabis intoxication and mental illness. In G.G. Nahas (Ed.), *Marihuana in Science and Medicine* (pp. 263–306). New York: Raven Press.

Brill, N.Q. & Christie, R.L. (1974). Marihuana use and psychosocial adaptation: Follow-up study of a collegiate population. *Archives of General Psychiatry, 31*, 713–719.

Brook, J.S., Cohen, P., Whiteman, M. & Gordon, A.S. (1992). Psychosocial risk factors in the transition from moderate to heavy use or abuse of drugs. In M. Glantz & R. Pickens (Eds.), *Vulnerability to Drug Abuse* (pp. 359–388). Washington, DC: American Psychological Association.

Bruun, K., Edwards, G., Lumio, M., Makela, K., Pan, L., Popham, R.E., Room, R., Schmidt, W., Skog, O.J., Sulkunen, P. & Osterberg, E. (1975). *Alcohol Control Policies in Public Health Perspective* (Vol. 25). Helsinki: Finnish Foundation for Alcohol Studies.

Campbell, I. (1976). The amotivational syndrome and cannabis use with emphasis on the Canadian Scene. *Annals of the New York Academy of Sciences, 282*, 33–36.

Caplan, G.A. & Brigham, B.A. (1990). Marijuana smoking and carcinoma of the tongue. Is there an association? *Cancer, 66*, 1005–1006.

Carlini, E.A., Carlini-Cotrim, B. & Nappo, S.A. (1990). Illicit use of psychotropic drugs in Brazilian cities: 1987–1989. In *CEWG Proceedings of Epidemiological Trends in Drug Abuse* (DHHS Publication No. 90-1724, pp. II4–II15). Washington, DC: U.S. Government Printing Office.

Carter, W.E., Coggins, W. & Doughty, P.L. (1980). *Cannabis in Costa Rica: A Study of Chronic Marihuana Use*. Philadelphia: Institute for the Study of Human Issues.

Centros de Integración Juvenil, A.C. (1992). *Epidemiology of Drug Abuse in Mexico: A Comparative Overview of the United States of America*. Mexico City: Centro de Integracion Juvenil.

Chait, L.D. & Pierri, J. (1992). Effects of smoked marijuana on human performance: A critical review. In L. Murphy & A. Bartke (Eds.), *Marijuana/Cannabinoids: Neurobiology and Neurophysiology* (pp. 387–423). Boca Raton, FL: CRC Press.

Channabasavanna, S.M., Ray, Y. & Kaliaperumal, V.G. (1989). *Patterns and problems on non-alcoholic drug dependence in Karnataka*. Government of Bangalore.

Chen, K. & Kandel, D.B. (1995). The natural history of drug use from adolescence to the mid-thirties in a general population sample. *American Journal of Public Health*, 85, 41–47.

Cimbura, G., Lucas, D.M., Bennet, R.C., Warren, R.A. & Simpson, H.M. (1982). Incidence and toxicological aspects of drugs detected in 484 fatally injured drivers and pedestrians in Ontario. *Journal of Forensic Science*, 27, 855–867.

Cohen, S. (1982). Cannabis effects upon adolescent motivation. In *Marijuana and Youth: Clinical Observations on Motivation and Learning* (pp. 2–9). Rockville, MD: National Institute on Drug Abuse.

Compton, D.R., Dewey, W.L. & Martin, B.R. (1990). Cannabis dependence and tolerance production. *Advances in Alcohol and Substance Abuse*, 9, 128–147.

Connell, P.H. (1959). *Amphetamine Psychosis* (Maudlsey Monograph No. 5, Institute of Psychiatry). London: Oxford University Press.

Consensus Development Panel. (1985). Drug concentrations and driving impairment. *Journal of the American Medical Association*, 254, 2618–2621.

Cornelius, M.D., Taylor, P.M., Geva, D. & Day, N.L. (1995). Prenatal tobacco and marijuana use among adolescents: Effects on offspring, gestational age, growth and morphology. *Pediatrics*, 95, 738–743.

Dalton, W.S., Martz, R., Lemberger, L., Rodda, B.E. & Forney, R.B. (1975). Effects of marijuana combined with secobarbitol. *Clinical Pharmacology and Therapeutics*, 14, 298–304.

Day, N.L., Wagener, D.K. & Taylor, P.M. (1985). Measurement of substance use during pregnancy: Methodologic issues. In T.M. Pinkert (Ed.), *Current Research on the Consequences of Maternal Drug Abuse* (NIDA Research Monograph No. 59)(DHHS Publication No. 85-1400). Washington, DC: U.S. Government Printing Office.

de Zwat, W.M., Mensink, C. & Kuipers, S.B.M. (1994). *Key Data: Smoking, Drinking, Drug Use and Gambling Among Pupils Aged 10 Years and Older — The 3rd Sentinal Station Survey with Regard to High Risk Substances.* Utrecht: Netherlands Institute on Alcohol and Drugs.

Didcott, P., Reilly, D., Swift, W. & Hall, W. (1997). *Long Term Cannabis Users on the New South Wales North Coast* (National Drug and Alcohol Research Centre Monograph No. 30). Sydney: National Drug and Alcohol Research Centre.

Dixon, L., Haas, G., Wedien, P.J., Sweeney, J. & Frances, A.J. (1990). Acute effects of drug abuse in schizophrenic patients: Clinical observations and patients' self-reports. *Schizophrenia Bulletin*, 16, 69–79.

Donald, P.J. (1991a). Marijuana and upper aerodigestive tract malignancy in young patients. In G. Nahas & C. Latour (Eds.), *Physiopathology of Illicit Drugs: Cannabis, Cocaine, Opiates* (pp. 39–54). Oxford: Pergamon Press.

Donald, P.J. (1991b). Advanced malignancy in the young marijuana smoker. In H. Freidman, S. Specter, & T.W. Klein (Eds.), *Drugs of Abuse, Immunity, and Immunodeficiency* (pp. 33–36). London: Plenum Press.

Donnelly, N. & Hall, W. (1994). *Patterns of Cannabis Use in Australia*. Review prepared for the Australian National Task Force on Cannabis.

Donovan, J.E. & Jessor, R. (1983). Problem drinking and the dimension of involvement with drugs: A Guttman Scalogram analysis of adolescent drug use. *American Journal of Public Health*, *73*, 543–552.

Dornbush, R.L. (1974). The long-term effects of cannabis use. In L.L. Miller (Ed.), *Marijuana: Effects on Behavior* (pp. 221–231). New York: Academic Press.

DuPont, R. (1984). *Getting Tough on Gateway Drugs*. Washington, DC: American Psychiatric Press.

Edwards, G. (1976). Cannabis and the psychiatric position. In J.D.P. Graham (Ed.), *Cannabis and Health* (pp. 321–342). London: Academic Press.

Edwards, G., Arif, A. & Hodgson, R. (1981). Nomenclature and classification of drug- and alcohol-related problems: A WHO memorandum. *Bulletin of the World Health Organization*, *59* (2), 225–242.

Eide, A.H. & Acuda, S.W. (1995). Drug use among secondary school students in Zimbabwe. *Addiction*, *90*, 1517–1527.

Eide, A.H. & Acuda, S.W. (1996). Adolescents' drug use in Zimbabwe: Comparing two recent studies. *Central African Journal of Medicine*, *42*, 128–135.

English, D., Holman, C.J.D., Milne, E., Winter, M.G., Hulse, G.K., Codde, J.P., Corti, B., Dawes, V., de Klerk, N., Knuiman, M.W., Kurinczuk, J.J., Lewin, G.F. & Ryan, G.A. (1995). *The Quantification of Drug-Caused Morbidity and Mortality in Australia*. Canberra: Commonwealth Department of Human Services and Health.

Fehr, K.O. & Kalant, H. (Eds.). (1983). *Cannabis and Health Hazards*. Toronto: Addiction Research Foundation.

Fergusson, D. & Horwood, J.L. (1997). Early onset cannabis use and psychosocial development in young adults. *Addiction*, *92*, 279–296.

Fergusson, D., Lynskey, M. & Horwood, J.L. (1996). The short-term consequences of early adolescent cannabis use. *Journal of Abnormal Child Psychology*, *24*, 499–512.

Fligiel, S.E.G., Beals, T.F., Venkat, H., Stuth, S., Gong, H. & Tashkin, D.P. (1988). Pulmonary pathology in marijuana smokers. In G. Chesher, P. Consroe & R. Musty (Eds.), *Marijuana: An International Research Report* (National Campaign Against Drug Abuse Monograph No. 7, pp. 43–48). Canberra: Australian Government Publishing Service.

Fligiel, S.E.G., Roth, M.D., Kleerup, E.C., Barsky, S.H., Simmons, M.S. & Tashkin, D.P. (1997). Tracheobronchial histopathology in habitual smokers of cocaine, marijuana and/or tobacco. *Chest*, *112*, 319–326.

Fried, P.A. (1980). Marijuana use by pregnant women: Neurobehavioral effects in neonates. *Drug and Alcohol Dependence*, *6*, 415–424.

Fried, P.A. (1982). Marijuana use by pregnant women and effects on offspring: An update. *Neurobehavioral Toxicology and Teratology*, *4*, 451–454.

Fried, P.A. (1985). Postnatal consequences of maternal marijuana use. In T.M. Pinkert (Ed.), *Current Research on the Consequences of Maternal Drug Abuse* (NIDA Research Monograph No. 59, pp. 61–72) (DHHS Publication No. 85-1400). Washington, DC: U.S. Government Printing Office.

Fried, P.A. (1986). Marijuana and human pregnancy. In I. Chasnoff (Ed.), *Drug Use in Pregnancy: Mother and Child*. Lancaster: MTP Press.

Fried, P.A. (1989). Postnatal consequences of maternal marijuana use in humans. *Annals of the New York Academy of Sciences*, *562*, 123–132.

Fried, P.A. (1993). Prenatal exposure to tobacco and marijuana: Effects during pregnancy, infancy, and early childhood. *Clinical Obstetrics and Gynecology*, *36*, 319–337.

Fried, P.A. (1995). The Ottawa Prenatal Prospective Study (OPPS): Methodological issues and findings — It's easy to throw the baby out with the bath water. *Life Sciences*, *56*, 2159–2168.

Fried, P.A., Buckingham, M. & Von Kulmiz, P. (1983). Marijuana use during pregnancy and perinatal risk factors. *American Journal of Obstetrics and Gynecology*, *146*, 992–994.

Fried, P.A., O'Connell, C.M. & Watkinson, B. (1992). 60- and 72-month follow-up of children prenatally exposed to marijuana, cigarettes, and alcohol: Cognitive and language assessment. *Journal of Developmental and Behavioral Pediatrics*, *13*, 383–391.

Fried, P.A. & Watkinson, B. (1990). 36- and 48-month neurobehavioral follow-up of children prenatally exposed to marijuana, cigarettes, and alcohol. *Journal of Developmental and Behavioral Pediatrics*, *11*, 49–58.

Friedman, A.S., Bransfield, S. & Kreisher, C. (1994). Early teenage substance use on later educational/vocational status. *American Journal of Addiction*, *3*, 326–335.

Friedman, A.S., Granick, S., Bransfield, S., Kreisher, C. & Schwartz, A. (1996). The consequences of drug use/abuse for vocational career: A longitudinal study of a male urban African-American sample. *American Journal of Drug and Alcohol Abuse*, *22*, 57–73.

Gawin, F.H. & Ellinwood, E.H. (1988). Cocaine and other stimulants: Actions, abuse and treatment. *New England Journal of Medicine*, *318*, 1173–1182.

Gieringer, D.H. (1988). Marijuana, driving and accident safety. *Journal of Psychoactive Drugs, 20,* 93–101.

Gibson, G.T., Baghurst, P.A. & Colley, D.P. (1983). Maternal alcohol, tobacco and cannabis consumption and the outcome of pregnancy. *Australian and New Zealand Journal of Obstetrics and Gynaecology, 23,* 15–19.

Goldberg, L. (1968a). Drug abuse in Sweden. Part I. *Bulletin on Narcotics, 20* (1), 1–31.

Goldberg, L. (1968b). Drug abuse in Sweden. Part II. *Bulletin on Narcotics, 20* (2), 9–36.

Gong, H., Jr., Fligiel, S., Tashkin, D.P. & Barbers, R.G. (1987). Tracheobronchial changes in habitual, heavy smokers of marijuana with and without tobacco. *American Review of Respiratory Disease, 136,* 142–149.

Goode, E. (1974). Marijuana use and the progression to dangerous drugs. In L.L. Miller (Ed.), *Marijuana: Effects on Human Behavior* (pp. 303–336). New York: Academic Press.

Goodstadt, M. , Chan, G.C., Sheppard, M.A. & Cleve, J.C. (1986). Factors associated with cannabis nonuse and cessation of use: Between and within survey replications of findings. *Addictive Behaviors, 11,* 275–286.

Grinspoon, L. & Hedblom, P. (1975). *The Speed Culture: Amphetamine Abuse in America.* Cambridge, MA: Harvard University Press.

Grufferman, S., Schwartz, A.G., Ruymann, F.B. & Mauer, H.M. (1993). Parent's use of cocaine and marijuana and increased risk of rhabdomyosarcoma in their children. *Cancer, Causes and Control, 4,* 217–224.

Halikas, J.A., Weller, R.A., Morse, C. & Shapiro, T. (1982). Incidence and characteristics of amotivational syndrome, including associated findings, among chronic marijuana users. In *Marijuana and Youth: Clinical Observations on Motivation and Learning* (pp.11–26). Rockville, MD: National Institute on Drug Abuse.

Hall, W., Solowij, N. & Lemon, J. (1994). *The Health and Psychological Consequences of Cannabis Use* (National Drug Strategy Monograph No. 25). Canberra: Australian Government Publication Services.

Harkin, A.M., Anderson, P. & Goos, P. (1997). *Smoking, Drinking and Drug Taking in the European Region.* Copenhagen: WHO Regional Office for Europe.

Hatch, E.E. & Bracken, M.B. (1986). Effect of marijuana use in pregnancy on fetal growth. *American Journal of Epidemiology, 124,* 986–993.

Hawkins, J.D., Catalano, R.F. & Miller, J.Y. (1992). Risk and protective factors for alcohol and other drug problems in adolescence and early adulthood: Implications for substance abuse prevention. *Psychological Bulletin, 112,* 64–105.

Hays, R.D. & Ellickson, P.L. (1996). Associations between drug use and deviant behavior in teenagers. *Addictive Behaviors, 21*, 291–302.

Hingson, R., Alpert, J., Day, N., Dooling, E., Kayne, H., Morelock, S., Oppenheimer, E. & Zuckerman, B. (1982). Effects of maternal drinking and marijuana use on fetal growth and development. *Pediatrics, 70*, 539–546.

Hingson, R., Heeren, T., Mangione, T., Morelock, S. & Mucatel, M. (1982). Teenage driving after using marijuana or drinking and traffic accident involvement. *Journal of Safety Research, 13*, 33–37.

Hochman, J.S. & Brill, N.Q. (1973). Chronic marijuana use and psychosocial adaptation. *American Journal of Psychiatry, 130*, 132–140.

Hollister, L.E. (1986). Health aspects of cannabis. *Pharmacological Reviews, 38*, 1–20.

Hollister, L.E. (1992). Marijuana and immunity. *Journal of Psychoactive Drugs, 24*, 159–164.

Holman, C.D., Armstrong, B.K., Arias, L.N., Martin, C.A., Hatton, W.M., Hayward, L.D., Salmon, M.A., Shean, R.E. & Waddell, V.P. (1988). *The Quantification of Drug-Caused Morbidity and Mortality in Australia.* Canberra: Commonwealth Department of Community Services and Health.

Huber, G.L., Griffith, D.E. & Langsjoen, P.M. (1988). The effects of marihuana on the respiratory and cardiovascular systems. In G. Chesher, P. Consroe & R. Musty (Eds.), *Marijuana: An International Research Report* (National Campaign Against Drug Abuse Monograph No. 7, pp. 1–18). Canberra: Australian Government Publishing Service.

Indian Council of Medical Research. (1993). *Report on Drug Abuse.* New Delhi.

Inghe, G. (1969). The present state of abuse and addiction to stimulant drugs in Sweden. In F. Sjoqvist & M. Tottie (Eds.), *Abuse of Central Stimulants* (pp. 187–214). New York: Raven Press.

Institute of Medicine. (1982). *Marijuana and Health.* Washington, DC: National Academy Press.

Jaffe, J.H. (1985). Drug addiction and drug abuse. In A.G. Gilman, L.S. Goodman & F. Murad (Eds.), *The Pharmacological Basis of Therapeutics* (7th ed., pp. 532–581). New York: Macmillan.

Jessor, R. & Jessor, S.L. (1977). *Problem Behavior and Psychosocial Development: A Longitudinal Study of Youth.* New York: Academic Press.

Jessor, R. & Jessor, S.L. (1978). Theory testing in longitudinal research on marihuana use. In D.B. Kandel (Ed.), *Longitudinal Research on Drug Use: Empirical Findings and Methodological Issues* (pp. 41–70). New York: John Wiley.

Johnson, B.A., Smith, B.L. & Taylor, P. (1988). Cannabis and schizophrenia. *Lancet, 1*, 592–593.

Johnston, L.D. (1973). *Drugs and American Youth*. Ann Arbor, MI: Institute for Social Research.

Johnston, L.D. (1981). Frequent marijuana use: Correlates, possible effects, and reasons for using and quitting. In R. deSilva, R. Dupont & G. Russell (Eds.), *Treating the Marijuana Dependent Person* (pp. 8–14). New York: American Council on Marijuana.

Johnston, L.D. (1982). A review and analysis of recent changes in marijuana use by American young people. In *Marijuana: The National Impact on Education* (pp. 8–13). New York: American Council on Marijuana.

Johnston, L.D. (1985a). The etiology and prevention of substance use: What can we learn from recent historical changes? In C.L. Jones & R.J. Battjes (Eds.), *Etiology of Drug Abuse: Implications for Prevention* (NIDA Research Monograph No. 56, pp. 155–177). Washington, DC: U.S. Government Printing Office.

Johnston, L.D. (1985b). Techniques for reducing measurement error in surveys of drug use. In L.N. Robins (Ed.), *Studying Drug Abuse* (pp. 117–136). New Brunswick, NJ: Rutgers University Press.

Johnston, L.D. (1991). Toward a theory of drug epidemics. In R. L. Donohew, H. Sypher & W. Bukoski (Eds.), *Persuasive Communication and Drug Abuse Prevention* (pp. 93–132). Mahwah, NJ: Erlbaum.

Johnston, L.D., Bachman, J.G. & O'Malley, P.M. (1981). *Highlights from Student Drug Use in America, 1975–1981*. (DHHS Publication No. ADM 82-1208). Rockville, MD: National Institute on Drug Abuse.

Johnston, L.D., Driessen, F. & Kokkevi, A. (1994). *Surveying Student Drug Misuse: A Six-Country Pilot Study*. Strasbourg, France: Cooperation Group to Combat Drug Abuse and Illicit Trafficking in Drugs (Pompidou Group), Council of Europe.

Johnston, L.D. & O'Malley, P.M. (1986). Why do the nation's students use drugs and alcohol: Self-reported reasons from nine national surveys. *Journal of Drug Issues, 16*, 29–66.

Johnston, L.D. & O'Malley, P.M. (1997). The recanting of earlier reported drug use by young adults. In L. Harrison (Ed.), *The Validity of Self-reported Drug Use: Improving the Accuracy of Survey Estimates* (NIDA Research Monograph No. 167, pp. 59–79). Rockville, MD: National Institute on Drug Abuse.

Johnston, L.D., O'Malley, P.M. & Bachman, J.G. (1991). *Drug Use Among American high School Seniors, College students and Young Adults, 1975–1990* (Vols. 1–2). Rockville, MD: National Institute on Drug Abuse.

Johnston, L.D., O'Malley, P.M. & Bachman, J.G. (1994). *National Survey Results on Drug Use from the Monitoring the Future Study, 1975–1993. Vol 1. Secondary School Students* (NIH Publication No. 94-3809); *Vol 2. College Students and Young Adults* (NIH Publication No. 94-3810). Rockville, MD: National Institute on Drug Abuse.

Johnston, L.D., O'Malley, P.M. & Bachman, J.G. (1996). *National Survey Results on Drug Use from the Monitoring the Future Study, 1975–1995. Vol. 1. Secondary School Students* (NIH Publication No. 96-4139); *Vol. 2. College Students and Young Adults* (NIH Publication No. 98-4140). Rockville, MD: National Institute on Drug Abuse.

Johnston, L.D., O'Malley, P.M. & Eveland, L.K. (1978). Drugs and delinquency: A search for causal connections. In D.B. Kandel (Ed.), *Longitudinal Research on Drug Use: Empirical Findings and Methodological Issues* (pp. 137–159). New York: John Wiley.

Jones, R.T. & Benowitz, N. (1976). The 30-day trip — Clinical studies of cannabis tolerance and dependence. In M.C. Braude & S. Szara (Eds.), *Pharmacology of Marijuana* (Vol. 2, pp. 627-642). New York: Academic Press.

Jones, R.T., Benowitz, N. & Herning, R.I. (1981). The clinical relevance of cannabis tolerance and dependence. *Journal of Clinical Pharmacology*, *21*, 143S–152S.

Jutkowitz, J.M. & Eu, H. (1994). Drug prevalence in Latin American and Caribbean countries: A cross-national analysis. *Drug Education, Prevention and Policy*, *1*, 199–252.

Kandel, D.B. (1984). Marijuana users in young adulthood. *Archives of General Psychiatry*, *41*, 200–209.

Kandel, D.B. (1988). Issues of sequencing of adolescent drug use and other problem behaviors. *Drugs and Society*, *3*, 55–76.

Kandel, D.B. & Davies, M. (1992). Progression to regular marijuana involvement: Phenomenology and risk factors for near daily use. In M. Glantz & R. Pickens (Eds.), *Vulnerability to Drug Abuse* (pp. 211–253). Washington, DC: American Psychological Association.

Kandel, D.B. & Davies, M. (1996). High school students who use crack and other drugs. *Archives of General Psychiatry*, *53*, 71–80.

Kandel, D.B., Davies, M., Karus, D. & Yamaguchi, K. (1986). The consequences in young adulthood of adolescent drug involvement. *Archives of General Psychiatry*, *43*, 746–754.

Kandel, D. & Faust, R. (1975). Sequence and stages in patterns of adolescent drug use. *Archives of General Psychiatry*, *32*, 923–932.

Kandel, D.B. & Logan, J.A. (1984). Patterns of drug use from adolescence to young adulthood: I. Periods of risk for initiation, continued use and discontinuation. *American Journal of Public Health*, *74*, 660–666.

Kaplan, H.B. & Johnson, R.J. (1992). Relationships between circumstances surrounding initial drug use and escalation of drug use: Moderating effects of gender and early adolescent experiences. In M. Glantz & R. Pickens (Eds.), *Vulnerability to Drug Abuse* (pp. 299–358). Washington, DC: American Psychological Association.

Kaplan, H.B., Martin, S. & Robbins, C. (1982). Pathways to adolescent drug use: Self-derogation, peer influence, weakening of social controls, and early substance use. *Journal of Health and Social Behavior, 25*, 270–289.

Kaslow, R.A., Blackwelder, W.C., Ostrow, D.G., Yerg, D., Palenick, J., Coulson, A.H. & Valdiserri, R.O. (1989). No evidence for a role of alcohol or other psychoactive drugs in accelerating immunodeficiency in HIV-1-positive individuals: A report from the Multicenter AIDS Cohort Study. *Journal of the American Medical Association, 261*, 3424–3429.

Kleiman, M.A.R. (1992). *Against Excess: Drug Policy for Results.* New York: Basic Books.

Klonoff, H. (1974). Effects of marijuana on driving in a restricted area and on city streets: Driving performance and physiological changes. In L. Miller (Ed.), *Marijuana: Effects on Human Behavior* (pp. 1–23). New York: Academic Press.

Knudsen, P. & Vilmar, T. (1984). Cannabis and neuroleptic agents in schizophrenia. *Acta Psychiatrica Scandinavica, 69*, 162–174.

Kolansky, H. & Moore, R.T. (1971). Effects of marihuana on adolescents and young adults. *Journal of the American Medical Association, 216*, 486–492.

Kuitjen, R.R., Bunin, G.R., Nass, C.C. & Meadows, A.T. (1992). Parental occupation and childhod astrocytoma. *Cancer Research, 52*, 782–786.

Lantner, I.L. (1982). Marijuana abuse by children and teenagers: A pediatrician's view. In *Marijuana and Youth: Clinical Observations on Motivation and Learning* (pp. 84–91). Rockville, MD: National Institute on Drug Abuse.

Leuchtenberger, C. (1983). Effects of marihuana (cannabis) smoke on cellular biochemistry of *in vitro* test systems. In K.O. Fehr & H. Kalant (Eds.), *Cannabis and Health Hazards* (pp. 127-223). Toronto: Addiction Research Foundation.

Linn, S., Schoenbaum, S.C., Monson, R.R., Rosner, R., Stubblefield, P.C. & Ryan, K.J. (1983). The association of marijuana use with outcome of pregnancy. *American Journal of Public Health, 73*, 1161–1164.

Machado, T. (1994). *Culture and Drug Abuse in Asian Settings: Research for Action.* Bangalore: St. John's Medical College.

Maddahian, E., Newcombe, M.D. & Bentler, P.M. (1988). Risk factors for substance use: Ethnic differences among adolescents. *Journal of Substance Abuse, 1*, 11–23.

Makkai, T. & McAllister, I. (1997). *Marijuana in Australia: Patterns and Attitudes* (National Drug Strategy Monograph No. 31). Canberra: Commonwealth of Australia.

Mason, A.P. & McBay, A.J. (1984). Ethanol, marijuana and other drug use in 600 drivers killed in single-vehicle crashes in North Carolina, 1978–1981. *Journal of Forensic Science, 29*, 987–1026.

McAllister, I., Moore, R. & Makkai, T. (1991). *Drugs in Australian Society: Patterns, Attitudes & Policies*. Melbourne: Longman Cheshire.

McBay, A.J. (1986). Drug concentrations and traffic safety. *Alcohol, Drugs and Driving, 2*, 51–59.

McGee, R.O. & Feehan, M. (1993). Cannabis use among New Zealand adolescents. *New Zealand Medical Journal, 106*, 345.

McGlothlin, W.H. & West, L.J. (1968). The marijuana problem: An overview. *American Journal of Psychiatry, 125*, 370–378.

McKenzie, D., Williams, B. & Single, E. (1997). *Canadian Profile: Alcohol, Tobacco and Other Drugs*. Toronto: Canadian Centre for Substance Abuse and Addiction Research Foundation.

Mendelson, J.H. & Mello, N.K. (1984). Effects of marijuana on neuroendocrine hormones in human males and females. In M.C. Braude & J.P. Ludford (Eds.), *Marijuana Effects on the Endocrine and Reproductive Systems* (pp. 97–114). Rockville, MD: National Institute on Drug Abuse.

Mendelson, J.H., Rossi, A.M. & Meyer, R.E. (Eds.). (1974). *The Use of Marihuana: A Psychological and Physiological Inquiry*. New York: Plenum Press.

Mendhiratta, S.S., Wig, N.N. & Verma, S.K. (1978). Some psychological correlates of long-term heavy cannabis users. *British Journal of Psychiatry, 132*, 482–486.

Millman, R.B. & Sbriglio, R. (1986). Patterns of use and psychopathology in chronic marijuana users. *Psychiatric Clinics of North America, 9*, 533–545.

Milman, D.H. (1982). Psychological effects of cannabis in adolescence. In *Marijuana and Youth: Clinical Observations on Motivation and Learning* (pp. 27–37). Rockville, MD: National Institute on Drug Abuse.

Moore, M.H. & Gerstein, D.K. (Eds.). (1981). *Alcohol and Public Policy: Beyond the Shadow of Prohibition.*. Washington, DC: National Academy Press.

Munson, A.E. & Fehr, K.O. (1983). Immunological effects of cannabis. In K.O. Fehr & H. Kalant (Eds.), Cannabis and health hazards. *Proceedings of an ARF/WHO Scientific Meeting on Adverse Health and Behavioral Consequences of Cannabis Use* (pp. 257–354). Toronto: Addiction Research Foundation.

Nahas, G.G. (1984). Toxicology and pharmacology. In G.G. Nahas (Ed.), *Marihuana in Science and Medicine* (pp. 109–246). New York: Raven Press.

Nahas, G.G. & Frick, H.C. (1987). Developmental effects of cannabis. *Neurotoxicology, 7*, 381–395.

National Institute on Drug Abuse. (1992). *National Household Survey on Drug Abuse: Population Estimates 1991 — Revised November 20, 1992*. Rockville, MD: U.S. Department of Health and Human Services.

National Institute for Social Defense. (1992). *Drug Abuse: Summaries of Research Studies*. New Delhi: Ministry of Welfare, Government of India.

Neglia, J.P., Buckley, J.D. & Robinson, L.L. (1991). Maternal marijuana use and leukemia in offspring. In G. Nahas & C. Latour (Eds.), *Physiopathology of Illicit Drugs: Cannabis, Cocaine, Opiates* (pp. 119–126). Oxford: Pergamon Press.

Negrete, J.C. (1983). Psychiatric aspects of cannabis use. In K.O. Fehr & H. Kalant (Eds.), *Cannabis and Health Hazards* (pp. 577–616). Toronto: Addiction Research Foundation.

Negrete, J.C. (1988). What's happened to the cannabis debate? *British Journal of Addiction, 83*, 359–372.

Negrete, J.C. (1989). Cannabis and schizophrenia. *British Journal of Addiction, 84*, 349–351.

Negrete, J.C., Knapp, W.P., Douglas, D. & Smith, W.B. (1986). Cannabis affects the severity of schizophrenic symptoms: Results of a clinical survey. *Psychological Medicine, 16*, 515–520.

Newcombe, M.D. (1992). Understanding the multidimensional nature of drug use and abuse: The role of consumption, risk factors and protective factors. In M. Glantz & R. Pickens (Eds.), *Vulnerability to Drug Abuse* (pp. 255-297). Washington, DC: American Psychological Association.

Newcombe, M.D. & Bentler, P. (1988). *Consequences of Adolescent Drug Use: Impact on the Lives of Young Adults*. Newbury Park, CA: Sage.

O'Donnell, J.A. & Clayton, R.R. (1982). The stepping stone hypothesis — Marijuana, heroin and causality. *Chemical Dependencies, 4*, 229–241.

O'Malley, P.M., Bachman, J.G. & Johnston, L.D. (1983). Reliability and consistency of self-reports of drug use. *International Journal of the Addictions, 18*, 805–824.

O'Malley, P.M., Bachman, J.G. & Johnston, L.D. (1984). Period, age, and cohort effects on substance use among American youth. *American Journal of Public Health, 74*, 682–688.

O'Malley, P.M., Bachman, J.G. & Johnston, L.D. (1988). Period, age, and cohort effects on substance use among young Americans: A decade of change, 1976–1986. *American Journal of Public Health, 78*, 1315–1321.

Osgood, D.W., Johnston, L.D., O'Malley, P.M. & Bachman, J.G. (1988). The generality of deviance in late adolescence and early adulthood. *American Sociological Review, 53*, 81–93.

Ospina, E.G., Ramirez, L.F.D. & Garcia, J.R. (1993). National Household Survey on Drug Abuse, Colombia: Highlights 1992. In *United Nations Drug Control Program, Regional Report on Drug* Use. Vienna: United Nations Drug Control Program.

Page, J.B., Fletcher, J. & True, W.R. (1988). Psychosociocultural perspectives on chronic cannabis use: The Costa Rican follow-up. *Journal of Psychoactive Drugs, 20*, 57–65.

Perkins, K.A., Simpson, J.C. & Tsuang, M.T. (1986). Ten-year follow-up of drug abusers with acute or chronic psychosis. *Hospital and Community Psychiatry, 37*, 481–484.

Polen, M.R., Sidney, S., Tekawa, I.S., Sadler, M. & Friedman, G.D. (1993). Health care use by frequent marijuana smokers who do not smoke tobacco. *Western Journal of Medicine, 158*, 596–601.

Polich, J.M., Ellickson, P.L., Reuter, P. & Kahan, J.P. (1984). *Strategies for Controlling Adolescent Drug Use.* Santa Monica, CA: The Rand Corporation.

Richardson, G.A., Day, N.L. & McGauhey, P.J. (1993). The impact of prenatal marijuana and cocaine use on the infant and child. *Clinical Obstetrics and Gynecology, 36*, 302–318.

Robbe, H.W.J. (1994). *Influence of Marijuana on Driving.* Maastricht: Institute for Human Psychopharmacology, University of Limberg.

Robbe, H.W.J. & O'Hanlon, J.F. (1993). *Marijuana's Effect on Actual Driving: Final Report.* (DOT HS 808 078). Washington, D.C.: U.S. Department of Transportation.

Robins, L. (1993). Vietnam veterans' rapid recovery from heroin addiction: A fluke or normal expectation? *Addiction, 88*, 1041–1054.

Robins, L., Darvish, H.S. & Murphy, G.E. (1970). The long-term outcome for adolescent drug users: A follow-up study of 76 users and 146 nonusers. In J. Zubin & A.M. Freedman (Eds.), *The Psychopathology of Adolescence.* (pp. 159–178). New York: Grune and Stratton.

Robins, L.N. & Regier, D.A. (Eds.). (1991). *Psychiatric Disorders in America.* New York: Free Press.

Robinson, L.I., Buckley, J.D., Daigle, A.E., Wells, R., Benjamin, D., Arthur, D.C. & Hammond, G.D. (1989). Maternal drug use and the risk of childhood nonlymphoblastic leukemia among offspring: An epidemiologic investigation implicating marijuana. *Cancer, 63,* 1904–1911.

Rocha-Silva, L. (1991). *Alcohol and Other Drug Use by Residents of Major Districts in the Self-Governing States of South Africa.* Pretoria: Human Sciences Research Council.

Rocha-Silva, L., de Miranda, S. & Erasmus, R. (1996). *Alcohol, Tobacco and Other Drug Use Among Black Youth.* Pretoria: Human Sciences Research Council.

Rubin, V. & Comitas, L. (1975). *Ganja in Jamaica: A Medical Anthropological Study of Chronic Marihuana Use.* The Hague: Mouton.

Satz, P., Fletcher, J.M. & Sutker, L.S. (1976). Neuropsychologic, intellectual and personality correlates of chronic marijuana use in native Costa Ricans. *Annals of the New York Academy of Sciences, 282,* 266–306.

Scheier, L.M. & Newcombe, M.D. (1991). Psychosocial predictors of drug use initiation and escalation: An expansion of the multiple risk factors hypothesis using longitudinal data. *Contemporary Drug Problems, 18,* 31–73.

Schneier, F.R. & Siris, S.G. (1987). A review of psychoactive substance use and abuse in schizophrenia: Patterns of drug choice. *Journal of Nervous and Mental Disorders, 175,* 641–652.

Shedler, J. & Block, J. (1990). Adolescent drug use and psychological health. *American Psychologist, 45,* 612–630.

Sherrill, D.L., Krzyzanowski, M., Bloom, J.W. & Lebowitz, M.D. (1991). Respiratory effects of non-tobacco cigarettes: A longitudinal study in general population. *International Journal of Epidemiology, 20,* 132–137.

Shiono, P.H., Klebanoff, M.A., Nugent, R.P., Cotch, M.F., Wilkins, D.G., Rollins, D.E., Covey, J.C. & Behrman, R.E. (1995). The impact of cocaine and marijuana use on low birth weight and preterm birth: A multicenter study. *American Journal of Obstetrics and Gynecology, 172,* 19–27.

Sidney, S., Beck, J.E., Tekawa, I.S., Quesenberry, C.P. & Friedman, G.D. (1997). Marijuana use and mortality. *American Journal of Public Health, 87,* 585–590.

Smart, R.G. (1983). The epidemiology of cannabis use and its health consequences in Western countries. In K.O. Fehr & H. Kalant (Eds.), *Cannabis and Health Hazards* (pp.723–761). Toronto: Addiction Research Foundation.

Smart, R.G. & Adlaf, E. (1989). Student cannabis use and enforcement activity in Canada: 1977–1987. *Drug and Alcohol Dependence, 24,* 67–74.

Smart, R.G. & Fejer, D. (1976). Drug use and driving risk among high school students. *Accident Analysis and Prevention, 8*, 33–38.

Smiley, A. (1986). Marijuana: On-road and driving simulator studies. *Alcohol, Drugs and Driving, 2*, 121–134.

Smith, D.E. (1968). Acute and chronic toxicity of marijuana. *Journal of Psychedelic Drugs, 2*, 37–47.

Soderstrom, C.A., Triffilis, A.L., Shankar, B.S., Clark, W.E. & Cowley, R.A. (1988). Marijuana and alcohol use among 1023 trauma patients. *Archives of Surgery, 123*, 733–737.

Soueif, M.I. (1976). Differential association between chronic cannabis use and brain function deficits. *Annals of the New York Academy of Sciences, 282*, 323–343.

Spooner, C. & Flaherty, B. (1992). *Comparison of Data Collection Methodologies for the Study of Young Illicit Drug Users* (Report Series No. 92-2). Sydney: Drug and Alcohol Directorate, N.S.W. Health Department.

Stefanis, C., Dornbush, R. & Fink, M. (Eds.). (1977). *Hashish: Studies of Long-Term Use.* New York: Raven Press.

Substance Abuse and Mental Health Services Administration (SAMHSA). (1993). *National Household Survey on Drug Abuse: Main Findings 1991* (DHHS Publication No. SMA 93-1980). Rockville, MD: U.S. Department of Health and Human Services; National Institute on Drug Abuse.

Substance Abuse and Mental Health Services Administration (SAMHSA). (1992). *Population Estimates 1991* (DHHS Publication No. ADM 92-1887). Rockville, MD: National Institute on Drug Abuse.

Substance Abuse and Mental Health Services Administration (SAMHSA). (1997a). *Preliminary Results from the 1996 National Household Survey on Drug Abuse* (DHHS Publication No. SMA 97-3149). Washington, DC: Government Printing Office.

Substance Abuse and Mental Health Services Administration (SAMHSA). (1997b). *National Household Survey on Drug Abuse: Population Estimates 1996* (DHHS Publication No. SMA 97-3137). Washington, DC: Government Printing Office.

Tashkin, D.P. (1993). Is frequent marijuana smoking harmful to health? *Western Journal of Medicine, 158*, 635–637.

Tashkin, D.P., Simmons, M.S., Sherrill, D.L. & Coulson, A.H. (1997). Heavy habitual marijuana smoking does not cause an accelerated decline in FEV1 with age: A longitudinal study. *American Journal of Respiratory and Critical Care Medicine, 155*, 141–148.

Taylor, F.M. (1988). Marijuana as a potential respiratory tract carcinogen: A retrospective analysis of a community hospital population. *Southern Medical Journal, 81*, 1213–1216.

Tennant, F.S. & Groesbeck, C.J. (1972). Psychiatric effects of hashish. *Archives of General Psychiatry, 27,* 133–136.

Tennes, K., Avitable, N., Blackard, C., Boyles, C., Hassoun, B., Holmes, L. & Kreye, M. (1985). Marihuana: Prenatal and postnatal exposure in the human. In T.M. Pinkert (Ed.), *Current Research on the Consequences of Maternal Drug Abuse* (NIDA Research Monograph No. 59, pp. 48–60) (DHHS Publication No. 85-1400). Washington, DC: U.S. Government Printing Office.

Terhune, K.W. (1986). Problems and methods in studying drug crash effects. *Alcohol, Drugs and Driving, 2,* 1–13.

Thomas, H. (1993). Psychiatric symptoms in cannabis users. *British Journal of Psychiatry, 163,* 141–149.

Thompson, P. (1975). "Stoned" driving is unpleasant, say marijuana smokers. *The Journal (Addiction Research Foundation), 4,* 13.

Thornicroft, G. (1990). Cannabis and psychosis: Is there epidemiological evidence for association. *British Journal of Psychiatry, 157,* 25–33.

Turner, W.M. & Tsuang, M.T. (1990). Impact of substance abuse on the course and outcome of schizophrenia. *Schizophrenia Bulletin, 16,* 87–95.

United Nations Drug Control Program. (1994). *Regional Report on Drug Use.* Vienna: United Nations Drug Control Program.

Varma, V.J., Malhotra, A.K., Dang, R., Das, K. & Nehra, R. (1988). Cannabis and cognitive functions: A prospective study. *Drug and Alcohol Dependence, 21,* 147–152.

Vokes, E.E., Weichelsbaum, R.R., Lippman, S.M. & Hong, W.K. (1993). Head and neck cancer. *New England Journal of Medicine, 328,* 183–194.

Weil, A. (1970). Adverse reactions to marihuana. *New England Journal of Medicine, 282,* 997–1000.

Weller, M.P.I., Ang, P.C., Latimer-Sayer, D.T. & Zachary, A. (1988). Drug abuse and mental illness. *Lancet, 1,* 977.

Wells, J.E., Bushnell, J.A., Joyce, P.R., Oakley-Browne, M.A. & Hornblow, A.R. (1992). Problems with alcohol, drugs and gambling in Christchurch, New Zealand. In M. Abbot & K. Evans (Eds.), *Alcohol and Drug Dependence and Disorders of Impulse Control.* (pp. 3–13). Auckland: Alcohol Liquor Advisory Council.

Wert, R.C. & Raulin, M.L. (1986). The chronic cerebral effects of cannabis use: II. Psychological findings and conclusions. *The International Journal of the Addictions, 21,* 629–642.

Wig, N.N. & Varma, V.K. (1977). Patterns of long-term heavy cannabis use in North India and its effects on cognitive functions: A preliminary report. *Drug and Alcohol Dependence*, *2*, 211–219.

Williams, A.F., Peat, M.A., Crouch, D.J., Wells, J.K. & Finkle, B.S. (1985). Drugs in fatally injured young male drivers. *Public Health Reports*, *100* (1), 19–25.

Williams, B., Chang, K. & Van Truong, M. (1992). *Canadian Profile: Alcohol & Other drugs 1992*. Toronto: Addiction Research Foundation.

Witter, F.R. & Niebyl, J.R. (1990). Marijuana use in pregnancy and pregnancy outcome. *American Journal of Perinatology*, *7*, 36–38.

Yamaguchi, K. & Kandel, D.B. (1984). Patterns of drug use from adolescence to adulthood: III. Predictors of progression. *American Journal of Public Health*, *74*, 673–681.

Zimmerman, E.G., Yeager, E.P., Soares, J.R., Hollister, L. & Reeve, V.C. (1983). Measurement of $\emptyset^9$-tetrahydrocannabinol (THC) in whole blood samples from impaired motorists. *Journal of Forensic Sciences*, *28*, 957–962.

Zuckerman, B. (1985). Developmental consequences of maternal drug use during pregnancy. In T.M. Pinkert (Ed.), *Current Research on the Consequences of Maternal Drug Abuse* (NIDA Research Monograph No. 59, pp. 36–47) (DHHS Publication No. 85-1400). Washington, DC: U.S. Government Printing Office.

Zuckerman, B., Frank, D., Hingson, R., Amaro, H., Levenson, S., Kayne, H., Parker, S., Vinci, R., Aboagye, K., Fried, L., Cabral, H., Timperi, R. & Bauchner, H. (1989). Effects of maternal marijuana and cocaine use on fetal growth. *New England Journal of Medicine*, *320*, 762–768.

Acute Effects of Cannabis on Human Behavior and Central Nervous System Functions

Acute Effects of Cannabis on Human Behavior and Central Nervous System Functions

PATRICK M. BEARDSLEY AND THOMAS H. KELLY

The acute administration of cannabis, and individually its chief behaviorally active constituent $\varnothing^9$-tetrahydrocannabinol (THC), is able to produce a variety of effects on behavior and central nervous system (CNS) function. Klonoff (1983) has reviewed experimental reports published prior to 1981, providing an overview of the effects of cannabis on perception, affect, memory and psychomotor performance. What follows is an updated (post-1980) review of these effects. Explicitly excluded from this chapter, but reviewed elsewhere in this volume (see chapter 5), are studies directly examining the effects of cannabis on driving and flying. Included in this chapter, but which was not included in the previous Klonoff overview, is a discussion of the effects of cannabis on social behavior and the reinforcing effects of cannabis as explicated under experimental control.

This chapter is divided into six sections: (1) effects of cannabis on memory; (2) effects of cannabis on appetite; (3) effects of cannabis on temporal processing; (4) effects of cannabis on psychomotor performance; (5) reinforcing effects of marijuana; and (6) cannabis and social behavior. Each section is followed by a brief summary that identifies general findings and future research needs.

Effects of Cannabis on Memory

Disruption of memory has been cited as the single, most consistently reported behavioral effect of cannabis (Miller, 1984). Experimental tests of memory are varied but often can be categorized into tests directed at what has historically been referred to as "short-term" and "long-term" memory. Short-term memory functions involve recollections following up to several seconds from initial exposure of the to-be-learned material. One example of a test used to address short-term memory function is the digit span task. In this task, subjects are presented a progressively longer series of digits and are asked to reproduce them. Long-term memory is considered a permanent memory store with a qualitatively longer duration and larger capacity than short-term memory. Tests of long-term memory often entail either free recall or recognition tests. In free recall tests, subjects are presented material, for example, a list of words, and subsequently are asked to reproduce what was presented without an experimenter-imposed structure on the order, or other limitation on how the subject responds. The subject can make errors of omission, omitting previously presented material, or of commission, by including material not actually presented (intrusions). In recognition tests, subjects are presented material, and during testing are presented items that may or may not have been initially presented. The subject's task is to correctly identify (recognize) what items were or were not originally presented.

Testing the effects of cannabis on memory functioning can involve the administration of cannabis at any of several time points. Cannabis can be administered either during learning or during recall, or both. Cannabis can also be administered between the learning and recall components in order to address the possibility of affecting future, drug-free recall of already-learned material.

Studies prior to 1980 have observed that cannabis can impair memory under some conditions but not others, but have not found conditions in which cannabis facilitates memory. For instance, material learned under a cannabis state and later recalled either under a drug-free or a cannabis state is detrimentally affected relative to learning under a non-drugged state (for review, see Ferraro, 1980). Material learned in a drug-free state, however, and later recalled or recognized under a cannabis state is often little affected. Studies published after 1980 have typically confirmed this generalization and have further examined the conditions in which cannabis can affect learning and memory.

One procedure that has been used by researchers to evaluate cannabis effects on short-term memory is the digit span task as described above. The effects observed on the digit span task by smoking marijuana have been inconsistent, and have not regularly been related to either dose or to whether the task required forward or backward recall. Smoking a single 12- or 21-mg THC-containing cigarette impaired digit recall in 12 marijuana-experienced men, in that the number of correct spans and the longest correct span before an error was made was reduced relative to smoking a placebo cigarette (Heishman, Stitzer & Yingling, 1989). Only the lower dose (12 mg), however, significantly reduced these

measures during forward recall, and only the higher dose produced these impairments during reverse recall. There were systematic dose-dependent effects on heart rate, although the doses produced similar subjective report effects on "drug high" and "impaired performance" on the visual analogue scales. No effects were observed, however, in a digit recognition task in which up to 16 controlled puffs on marijuana cigarettes containing 3.55 per cent THC had been consumed (Heishman, Arasteh & Stitzer, 1997). In this task, a set of five to seven digits were presented for two seconds, and following a two-second delay, a test digit was presented and the subjects were required to indicate whether or not it was a member of the initial set. Smoking marijuana did not affect the number of correct responses or the latency to respond.

Chait, Evans and colleagues (1988) also found that marijuana reduced the number of digits correctly recalled in a forward recall digit span task. In their study, they used a cumulative dosing procedure in which marijuana-experienced subjects progressively completed two, two, and four puffs of a cigarette containing about 12 mg of THC.

Unlike the above studies, other reports have shown a lack of effect on the digit span task. In one study, subjects did not show impairments on either the forward or the reverse recall of digit sequences after smoking a 10.7-mg THC-containing cigarette when tested in a memory battery that included a digit span task (Hooker & Jones, 1987). From these results, the authors concluded that cannabis did not impair immediate "attention." There were many differences among these studies that could account for the reported differences in effect, including the type of digit span task employed and the method used to smoke (the topography of smoking was controlled in the studies by Heishman et al. and by Chait et al., but subjects smoked freely in the Hooker & Jones study). This inconsistency of finding cannabis-induced impairments on performance in the digit span task are reflective of the inconsistency also reported in studies published prior to 1981. Both impairments (for example, Galanter, Weingartner et al., 1973) and lack of impairment (for example, Casswell & Marks, 1973) had also been reported.

In several studies involving tests of longer-term memory, cannabis administration slowed retrieval of information, but the degree of impairment was not necessarily correlated with the degree to which memory was required. Block and Wittenborn (1986) examined the effects of smoking marijuana on the ability of 24 marijuana-experienced men (median 2.5 cigarettes per week during the preceding six months) to quickly identify whether two, tachistoscopically presented letters had the same name (for example, "AA," "aa" or "aA"). An assumption was that less memory retrieval is required on same-case (i.e., "AA") than on mere same-name (i.e., "aA") trials, and if marijuana specifically affected retrieval, the reaction times during same-name trials would be increased. Smoking a 10-mg THC-containing marijuana cigarette significantly slowed reaction times during all types of trials equally, suggesting that the drug did not differentially affect retrieval requiring a greater memory dependency.

In other studies, Block and Wittenborn (1984a) investigated whether marijuana produced more uncommon associations and greater vivid imagery during recall, and also whether these affected the degree of memory retrieval. In one study, 36 subjects with marijuana histories were tachistoscopically shown a category word (for example, FRUIT) and subsequently were required to identify whether a noun (for example, APPLE) belonged to it or not. Also manipulated was the degree of familiarity of the nouns (APPLE is a more common example of fruit than is TANGERINE) to determine whether marijuana promoted uncommon associations. Non-drugged subjects typically responded faster to common associations relative to uncommon associations. If marijuana increases the probability of uncommon associations, the authors reasoned that this would result in equalized reaction times during common and uncommon trials. Smoking a 10-mg THC-containing marijuana cigarette did not affect error rates relative to placebo control in this study (Experiment 1, Block & Wittenborn, 1984a). Marijuana did slow reaction times during all types of trials relative to placebo. The differential, however, between common and uncommon trials was similar between drug and placebo conditions, suggesting that uncommon associations were not promoted by marijuana.

In a subsequent experiment, other subjects were required to identify whether two nouns belonged to the same category (for example, APPLE PEACH or APPLE APPLE) or different categories (for example, APPLE BLUEBIRD) and the degree of familiarity of the nouns was again manipulated (Experiment 2, Block & Wittenborn, 1984a). In this experiment, marijuana produced a "marginally significant" increase in errors on "different" trials but in no other contrasts were the differences between drug and placebo conditions significant. The results of this experiment were consistent with the others, leading the authors to conclude that marijuana did not differentially impair semantic-memory retrieval.

Block and Wittenborn further investigated the potential interaction between smoking marijuana and the generation of unusual associations on memory. In these studies, subjects were presented with a category name followed by a letter (for example, WEAPON–G), and they had to name an instance of that category beginning with that letter (for example, GUN) (Experiment 2, Block & Wittenborn, 1985). Each letter-category combination had a "target" instance. The target was the instance most frequently produced with the specified letter by non-drugged subjects. Trials with "common targets" involved letters beginning category instances that were commonly given as examples when no alphabetical restrictions applied. Common targets were mixed with "uncommon targets," which began instances infrequently given. Non-drugged subjects showed a marked facilitation in their speed of responding to, and in the number of examples produced for, common letter-category combinations. The results indicated that, relative to placebo, smoking a 10-mg THC-containing cigarette reduced the advantage that common trials had relative to uncommon trials, both in terms of per cent of targets obtained and in response rate, but not in terms of reaction time. These results were consistent with those from their earlier study (Block & Wittenborn, 1984a) in which they found that marijuana did not differentially reduce the reaction-time advantage on common versus uncommon trials and suggested to them that associative processes were not altered. Contrary to this earlier report, however, there was evidence that uncommon associations were being promoted by marijuana. In a subsequent study, Block and colleagues (1992) found further evidence that uncommon associations could be produced by smoking marijuana during free and constrained association tests.

Block and Wittenborn (1984b) also investigated whether visual imagery could be more effectively used to facilitate paired-associate learning while under marijuana's effects. Subjects were divided into equal groups who either smoked a placebo or a 10-mg THC-containing cigarette and were given paired-associate learning with high-imagery nouns. In each group, half the subjects were instructed to use visual imagery during learning and half were not instructed in any specific learning technique. The instructions to use visual imagery were expected to enhance learning and memory under both placebo and marijuana conditions. The authors reasoned, however, that if marijuana enhanced visual imagery, then the subjects who smoked marijuana and were also told to use visual imagery should show greater improvement than the placebo group told to use visual imagery.

The results showed that marijuana did not impair recall relative to smoking placebo (Block & Wittenborn, 1984b). Instructions to use visual imagery during paired-associate learning enhanced recall under both placebo and marijuana conditions equally, relative to comparable no-instruction conditions. These results suggested that marijuana did not enhance visual imagery relative to placebo conditions. In addition, when the "vividness" of the images used to form the paired associations was independently rated following the recall tests, marijuana was found to decrease the vividness scores significantly. The surprising result that marijuana did not impair recall may have been dose-limited. In subsequent studies in which subjects smoked cigarettes containing a greater THC yield (19 per cent), marijuana produced clear impairments on paired-associate recall, recall of prose material and on the immediate and delayed recall of word lists (Block, Farinpour & Braverman, 1992). The results of this series of experiments by Block and colleagues, indicate that marijuana can impair recall and does not enhance unusual associations or the vividness of imagery in a way that facilitates memory or learning.

Other studies have also found that smoking marijuana can reduce the recall of words from presented word lists (Block, Farinpour & Braverman, 1992; Wetzel, Janowsky & Clopton, 1982; Zacny & de Wit, 1989b). Chait et al. (1985) reported that smoking 1-g marijuana cigarettes containing 2.9 per cent THC significantly reduced the number of words recalled immediately following their presentation in word lists, relative to smoking placebo cigarettes. These researchers also found that marijuana increased the amount of time to complete a playing-card sorting task and impaired subjects' perception of time intervals. When these subjects were subsequently tested in the morning following smoking to determine whether there were "hangover" effects of marijuana, only the perception of time was impaired. Taking 4, 8 and 16 puffs of marijuana cigarettes containing 3.55 per cent THC produced dose-related decreases in the number of correctly recalled concrete nouns from lists of 20 words in length (Heishman, Arasteh & Stitzer, 1997). Impairments in recall were observed following each of the three times a single list was presented during a trial.

In one particularly provocative study, Perez-Reyes et al. (1991) addressed the ability of indomethacin, a prostaglandin synthesis inhibitor, to block several of the effects of THC, including its ability to impair recall of words during a free recall task. In their study, subjects smoked six pipe bowls of marijuana containing 2.57 per cent THC separated by one-minute intervals. Before smoking, and then at 30, 60 and 120 minutes after smoking marijuana, the subjects were tested in a free recall task in which they were presented 24 words on a computer screen and were given five minutes to type out as many of these words as they could remember. A time-estimation and a time-production task were also administered at these intervals. At other intervals following smoking, heart rate, subjective ratings of "high," plasma THC and plasma prostaglandin concentration were calculated. The subjects were either pretreated with placebo or with indomethacin prior to smoking marijuana.

As predicted, smoking marijuana (THC) elevated heart rate, subjective ratings of "high" and the subjective time rate determined in the time-estimation and production tasks (Perez-Reyes, Burstein et al., 1991). Indomethacin pretreatment significantly blocked each of these THC-induced effects. This antagonism was particularly dramatic on the THC-induced disruptions of time estimation and production. Plasma THC levels were not affected by indomethacin pretreatment, indicating that the ability to antagonize THC's effects was not due to modulation of its pharmacokinetics. THC also impaired the recall of words during the free recall tasks. Unlike indomethacin's ability to antagonize these other THC effects, however, it failed to block THC-induced impairments significantly during the free recall tasks. These results suggested to the authors that prostaglandins may mediate THC's effects on time estimation and production but not on its impairments of recent memory. Smoking marijuana has also been reported to reduce the recall of words from word lists in other studies and in the absence of effects on remote (long-term) memory (Wetzel, Janowsky & Clopton, 1982; Zacny & de Wit, 1989a).

Cannabis has also been found to affect short story recall. Marijuana-experienced subjects recalled fewer main elements from short stories after they smoked a 10.7-mg THC-containing cigarette, relative to placebo, under delayed free recall conditions (Hooker & Jones, 1987). This impairment on delayed, free recall of short stories was characterized by both omissions and intrusions of recently acquired information. The performance of these same subjects was not impaired when memory was evaluated under less demanding conditions, including tests for short story retention during immediate recall, the learning and later recall of word and paired-associate lists, as well as during the controlled retrieval of words guided by linguistic association (production of instances of words beginning with a specified letter). These results were similar to those found under similar dosing conditions by Block and Wittenborn (1984b) in that paired-associate recall was not adversely affected. They were unlike results found when tests were conducted with cigarettes containing a greater THC content (19 per cent) in which both immediate and delayed recall of text, paired-associate learning and learning of word lists were adversely affected (Block, Farinpour & Braverman, 1992). In examining these studies, it seems possible that increasing the THC dosage or increasing the demands of the memory task may reveal similar impairments on learning and memory produced by marijuana not observable under less demanding conditions.

Cannabis may have effects on learning new behavior, performing previously learned behavior, or both. A useful paradigm that addresses a drug's potential to affect acquisition of new behavior versus performance of previously learned behavior is the repeated acquisition procedure (Boren & Devine, 1968). This procedure typically has two components. During one component a subject learns, *de novo*, a new task, such as a particular sequence of response keys that must be pressed to produce a reward. This "acquisition" component alternates within a test session with a "performance" component during which the subject completes a previously learned sequence of response-key presses, and its correct completion also results in reward. The repeated acquisition procedure has been used to disentangle the effects on acquisition versus performance by a variety of drugs using both human and non-human subjects (Higgins, Bickel et al., 1987;

McMillan, 1988; Schulze, McMillan et al., 1988; Thompson, 1973).

Using this procedure, Kamien and colleagues (1994) examined the effects of placebo, 10-mg and 20-mg THC-containing capsules on acquiring new sequences and performing previously learned sequences of numeric keypad presses reinforced with monetary reward. They found that both doses of THC significantly increased the peak percentage of errors during acquisition components but not during performance components, relative to pre-drug levels. The effect of THC dose on percentage errors did not show a significant dose-by-component interaction, however, indicating that behavior was not necessarily more sensitive during acquisition than behavior during performance. The authors observed that their results were in contrast to repeated acquisition studies involving non-human subjects that demonstrated a lack of significant effects by THC on repeated-acquisition performance (McMillan, 1988; Schulze, McMillan et al., 1988; Thompson & Winsauer, 1985). As well, the results were in contrast to repeated acquisition studies using human subjects with other drugs that had demonstrated selective effects on acquisition but not performance (Bickel, Higgins et al., 1991; Higgins, Bickel et al., 1987; Thompson & Moerschbaecher, 1979).

SUMMARY

Although several studies before and after 1981 have documented that cannabis can affect memory, the effects are typically modest, at least in comparison to effects reported with other behaviorally active drugs. Free recall, in which to-be-learned items and their recall occur with cannabis present, is often impaired, and the major impairment is often reflected by intrusions of novel items. Also, the few studies evaluating the recall of prose material have generally reported deleterious effects induced by cannabis. Effects of cannabis on recall in the digit span, recognition and paired-associate tasks have, however, been inconsistent. Typically, once something is learned, recall is little impaired by cannabis if cannabis is present only during recall. Although the effects of cannabis on memory appear to be modest, an initial "modest" acute detriment in learning could cascade into a retarding, developmental handicap in an adolescent user who progresses to chronic abuse.

Many questions have been left unanswered by studies that have examined cannabis' effects on memory. The answers to these questions could prove critical to understanding the ramifications cannabis use may have for human learning and memory. For example, it is unclear to what degree the level of difficulty of the memory task determines the magnitude of the effect imposed by cannabis. Few studies have made attempts to manipulate this variable parametrically across cannabis-dosing conditions. It is also unclear how the consequences of performance could modulate the effects of cannabis on performance. Could increases in monetary reward for maximal recall produce corresponding decreases in detriments imposed by cannabis? Earlier reviews have suggested that the consequences of performance can, indeed, modulate the effects of cannabis (e.g., Ferraro, 1980) but it seems that this variable has been largely ignored in recent years. Also, how strong is the correspondence between the magnitude of a subject's perceived detriment, and the actual detriment imposed by cannabis on memory? The answer to this latter question would have obvious relevance in placing cannabis-imposed impairments of learning and memory in their proper perspective.

Effects of Cannabis on Appetite

Since A.D. 300, cannabis has been reported to stimulate food intake (for example, as reported by R.N. Chopra and G.S. Chopra cited in Mattes, Engelman et al., 1994). In addition to numerous, anecdotal accounts that have indicated that cannabis increases food consumption, there have been controlled, laboratory studies demonstrating this effect. Although the ability of cannabis to induce food intake appears well established under some experimental conditions, cannabis' ability to induce reliable, subjective ratings of hunger has been more variable.

Prior to the 1980s, there had been a few controlled studies that had reported that acute administrations of cannabis or THC itself could induce food intake (e.g., Abel, 1971; Hollister, 1971). Subsequent to these early studies, researchers have continued to identify conditions under which cannabis is able to increase food intake. Foltin and colleagues (1986; 1988; Kelly, Foltin et al., 1990) have conducted studies on the effects of smoking marijuana on food intake while subjects were housed in a controlled, residential setting. In these studies, adult male subjects lived in a residential laboratory equipped with private and social rooms for the duration of the study. All contact with the experimenters was made through a networked computer system. Subjects spent the initial part of their day engaged in structured work activities in their private rooms and, during another part of the day, they had access to the social rooms where they could interact with other subjects. Food availability was carefully controlled, and food consumption, including the type of food consumed and whether it was consumed as a snack item or as a meal, was continuously monitored. At various times, subjects smoked either marijuana or placebo cigarettes under a uniform smoking procedure. In some studies, psychomotor assessment tests were also given.

In an initial study by Foltin and colleagues (1986), three subjects smoked either a placebo cigarette or a cigarette containing 1.84 per cent (w/w) THC in their private rooms twice a day and in the social area once a day. Six additional subjects were tested under similar conditions except the number of opportunities to smoke in the social area was increased to twice a day. The results indicated that the average caloric intake for eight of the nine subjects was significantly greater when active marijuana cigarettes were smoked than when placebo cigarettes were smoked. Further analysis of the data indicated that the increases in food intake were attributable to increases in eating occasions and were confined to the social-access periods and to the consumption of "snacks." The authors speculated that the interactive social effects may have played a part in the food consumption increases observed.

In the initial study described above by Foltin and colleagues (1986), marijuana smoking occurred more often later in the day than in the morning, and increases in food intake during the evenings may have been in part controlled by the time of the day or by the cumulative dose obtained. In a follow-up study (Foltin, Fischman & Byrne, 1988), marijuana smoking occurred at equal intervals throughout the day to specifically control for these potential effects. In this study, subjects smoked placebo or active cigarettes (either 1.3 or 2.3 per cent w/w THC depending on subject) twice a day in their private rooms and twice a day in the social areas. Smoking active cigarettes increased food intake during both the private and social periods. The greatest rate of change in caloric intake occurred during the social periods in most subjects. Smoking marijuana cigarettes nearly doubled the number of snack occasions during both the private and social periods without affecting the number of meal occasions, and the increases in caloric intake were mainly attributable to increases in consumption of sweet, solid snacks. The authors concluded that it was most likely a dose effect, rather than a social effect that restricted the increases of food consumption to the social periods of their original study (Foltin, Brady & Fischman, 1986).

Single, acute administrations of THC often do not affect appetite and multiple dosing is required. Mattes et al. (1994) examined the effects of single doses of THC administered through oral and sublingual routes (15 mg for males; 10 mg for females) and through inhalation (2.57 per cent THC-containing cigarettes), and found no change in caloric intake relative to placebo. When THC was administered at 2.5 mg b.i.d. for three days via rectal suppository however, mean daily caloric intake significantly increased relative to all acute dosing conditions except inhalation. Mean daily energy intake was not comparably increased however, when an identical dose of THC was given via oral capsule under a similar, chronic dosing regimen.

Although there have been several studies reporting that cannabis increases the intake of food, there have been fewer and less consistent reports that have documented that "appetite," the individual's self-report of the current level of hunger, is similarly increased. Unfortunately, it is difficult to determine whether there is truly a dissociation between cannabis-increased consumption of food and levels of self-reported hunger ratings because few studies have explicitly assessed both variables.

In most reports evaluating appetite, researchers have employed visual analogue scales (VAS) as the method for assessing appetite following cannabis use. In a typical VAS test for hunger, the subject is presented with a 100-millimetre horizontal drawn line labelled "hungry," with one end of the line indicated "not at all" and the opposite end indicated "extremely." The subject is then required to mark along the line the level of hunger felt at the moment. Testing subjects following cannabis (or specifically THC) administration with VASs for hunger has resulted in reports of either no change (Chait, Evans et al., 1988; Chait, Fischman & Schuster, 1985; Zacny & Chait, 1989; 1991; Zacny & de Wit, 1989b; 1991) or in some cases, increases (Chait, Corwin & Johanson, 1988; Chait & Perry, 1994a; Chait & Zacny, 1992) in self-reports of hunger.

In one study involving 14 experienced marijuana users (Chait, Fischman & Schuster, 1985), smoking 2.9 per cent THC-containing cigarettes significantly increased VAS ratings of "high" but not "hungry" relative to smoking placebo. In two other studies that explicitly examined the effects of manipulating breath hold duration between 0 and 20 seconds on marijuana's effects, smoking neither 1.3 per cent nor 2.3 per cent THC-containing cigarettes affected VAS ratings of "hungry" (Zacny & Chait, 1989; 1991). In these studies, ratings of "high" were significantly increased although their level was not systematically related to breath hold duration (Zacny & Chait, 1989; 1991). Chait and colleagues established a discrimination between smoking a 2.7 and a 0 per cent THC-containing

cigarette maintained by monetary reward in 11 marijuana-experienced smokers (Chait, Evans et al., 1988). When tested with 0, 0.9, 1.4 and 2.7 per cent THC-containing cigarettes following training, subjects' ratings of "high" and their level of drug-appropriate responding increased dose-dependently with increases in the concentration of THC within the cigarette smoked; VAS ratings of "hungry" were not significantly affected.

Not all studies have found a lack of effect of cannabis use on appetite. When cumulative doses of THC were varied by manipulating the number of puffs of a 1.4 per cent THC-containing cigarette, both VAS ratings of "hungry" and of "high" linearly increased with dose (Chait, Corwin & Johanson, 1988). Similarly, ratings of "hungry" and "high" significantly increased after smoking either 2.3 per cent or 3.6 per cent THC-containing cigarettes in a study that examined the self-administration (reinforcing) effects of cannabis (Chait & Zacny, 1992). In this same study, ratings of "high" and "hungry" also were increased following the self-administration of THC-containing capsules (Marinol™ 2.5-, 5- or 10-mg pulvules), although the increased VAS levels for "hungry" did not quite reach levels great enough for statistical significance. Chait and Perry (1994a) reported that smoking a 3.6 per cent THC-containing cigarette, compared to consuming a 10 per cent ethanol drink (0.6 g/kg for males; 0.5 g/kg for females), increased ratings of "hungry" in their study. The effects of marijuana on the VAS levels of "hungry" and "high" followed different time courses in this study as peak self-reports of hunger emerged more than one hour following peak "high" ratings. Observing the delayed effects of marijuana on hunger, these authors speculated that perhaps one reason why researchers have inconsistently reported increases in hunger ratings may be attributable to differences in the times following marijuana administration (Chait & Perry, 1994a).

The studies above addressed whether cannabis use could affect the level of hunger in human subjects. In several studies involving laboratory animals, "hunger," i.e., food deprivation, has been shown to directly affect drug self-administration (for review, see Carroll & Meisch, 1984), possibly by increasing the level of the subjective effects of drugs. Two studies have directly assessed whether food deprivation can affect the subjective and other effects of marijuana in human subjects (Zacny & de Wit, 1989b; 1991). In these studies, subjects were tested during experimental sessions either preceded by 24 hours of normal caloric intake or preceded by 24 hours in which they could not consume any food or beverage containing more than 10 calories. Subjects either smoked a 1.3 per cent THC-containing cigarette according to a controlled puffing procedure (Zacny & de Wit, 1989b) or could smoke freely from 0.8 or 3.6 per cent THC-containing cigarettes during 30-minute self-administration sessions (Zacny & de Wit, 1991). Subjective effects were assessed periodically using questionnaires including a VAS for hunger. As expected, fasting increased the levels of self-reported hunger, relative to the fed conditions. Smoking marijuana, however, did not increase these self-reported levels of hunger during either feeding condition. Fasting did not systematically affect the levels of self-administered marijuana (Zacny & de Wit, 1991), nor did it systematically affect the levels of subjective effects following marijuana administration (Zacny & de Wit, 1989b; 1991).

SUMMARY

Cannabis appears to increase the consumption of food consistently. When a variety of foods are available, those most readily identified as snack foods seemed to be selectively targeted for consumption. Cannabis' effects on appetite, i.e., the individual's self-report of current level of hunger, however, are less consistently shared across studies. Whether there is a true dissociation of cannabis' effects on appetite and on actual food consumption is not known. Conducting future studies concurrently examining these two variables in within-subject study designs would likely be the most direct approach for addressing this issue. Certainly the resolution of this issue between appetite and actual food consumption, as well as the further

clarification as to what foods get targeted for consumption, would have implications for the use of cannabis products as appetite enhancers for medically compromised individuals.

Effects of Cannabis on Temporal Processing

With considerable consistency, researchers prior to the 1980s have reported that cannabis can alter temporal processing (for reviews, see Chait & Pierri, 1992; Klonoff, 1983). Experimentally, temporal processing has been addressed using three methods: temporal estimation, production and reproduction. Temporal estimation requires a subject to estimate verbally (in seconds, minutes, etc.) the time interval between two events produced by the experimenter. In temporal production, the subject is required to initiate two events separated by an interval whose duration is intended to match a specified duration indicated by the experimenter. In temporal reproduction, the experimenter initiates two events separated by an interval. The subject is then required first to estimate the duration of this interval and then to reproduce it.

Generally, these earlier reports have indicated that the perception of time occurring between events is accelerated during cannabis intoxication, where estimates of durations intervening experimenter-generated events are overestimated during time-estimation tasks (e.g., Cappell & Pliner, 1973; Jones & Stone, 1970), while subject-generated intervals of time intended to match temporal targets are underproduced during production tasks (e.g., Carlini, Karniol et al., 1974; Vachon, Sulkowski & Rich, 1974). Cannabis effects in temporal-reproduction tasks have not been well studied. In one study involving a time-reproduction task, marijuana use failed to affect performance significantly (Dornbush, Fink & Freedman, 1971).

More recent studies have also reported that acute cannabis use can affect temporal processing. Hicks et al. (1984) required four male marijuana users to depress foot pedals for durations the subjects thought were equivalent to 5, 10, 20, 30 or 45 seconds. The subjects were tested in this temporal-production task before smoking, and at 30, 60 and 120 minutes after smoking a placebo or a 1.29 or 4.61 per cent THC-containing cigarette. The subjects were explicitly instructed not to count or to otherwise "mark time" during these tasks. In addition, in order to test whether any effects of marijuana could be attributed to THC acting as a cholinergic antagonist, the subjects were intravenously administered either saline or 0.2 mg atropine sulfate following the termination of smoking a placebo marijuana. The results indicated that the subjects underproduced durations relative to target durations following the smoking of either concentration of the THC-containing cigarettes relative to placebo marijuana + saline or to the placebo marijuana + atropine conditions. Atropine did not affect time production relative to saline infusion conditions suggesting that it was unlikely that the THC-induced disruption of temporal production was due to anticholinergic effects of THC.

In another study testing for possible THC-cholinergic involvement mediating temporal impairments, atropine administered intravenously (0.04 mg/kg), alone or in combination with the beta-adrenergic antagonist propranolol (0.2 mg/kg), did not significantly influence levels of time-production impairment induced by intravenous THC (30.0 to 44.8 µg/kg) in four experienced male marijuana users (Bachman, Benowitz et al., 1979). Because the levels of temporal underproduction were not further increased by atropine, these results are consistent with the hypothesis that the effects of THC on time production are not mediated via anticholinergic effects. However, as Hicks and colleagues (1984) have cautioned, THC-induced time-production impairments may have been at ceiling levels in the Bachman study (1979) to preclude the possibility of observing further impairment induced by atropine. Bachman and colleagues also observed that pretreatment with atropine or the atropine + propranolol combination prevented the occurrence of THC-induced heart rate elevations. THC, nevertheless, significantly increased ratings of "high" despite these pharmacological pretreatments indicating a dissociation between the cardiovascular and subjective high effects.

Because cannabis can impair memory functions (see above), Hicks et al. (1984) tested whether the underproductions of durations they observed in their first study were attributable to the disintegration of the memory for a duration after it had passed. In this study, three male and three female experienced marijuana users smoked either placebo or 1.0 per cent THC-containing cigarettes. A block of time-production trials was administered to the subjects before smoking and at 15, 45 and 80 minutes after smoking. During these trials, the subjects were required to count silently to 120 at a subjective one-second rate and to say "30," "60" and "120" as they were reached. The experimenter recorded the actual clock duration at each of these reported time points. It was predicted that counting would eliminate the possibility that memory loss could mediate underproductions of time. Despite the fact that subjects counted during the time-production trials, smoking the THC-containing cigarettes nevertheless resulted in underproductions of intervals. These results led the authors to conclude that the THC-induced impairments of time production were evident as time passed, and not solely in the memory for a duration after it had passed.

Other recent studies have examined the effects of cannabis on temporal processing. Chait and colleagues (Chait, 1990; Chait, Fischman & Schuster, 1985) examined the effects of smoking marijuana on performance in time-production tasks in experienced marijuana users. In one study, 14 male experienced marijuana smokers took five standardized puffs from each of two cigarettes containing either placebo or 2.9 per cent THC and were given a test battery that included a time-production task 20 minutes before smoking the first cigarette, 25 minutes after the first cigarette, 20 minutes before the second cigarette and 25 minutes after the second cigarette. In addition, the subjects were tested 30 minutes after awakening the next morning to determine if there were "hangover" effects attributable to the previous evening's marijuana use. For the time-production task, the subjects were instructed to produce a 10-second time interval by saying "start" and then "stop" when they believed 10 seconds had elapsed. Following this "10-second test," the subjects were required to take another test at a longer interval of 30 seconds. Marijuana, but not placebo, significantly shortened produced intervals relative to real time during the 30-second tests. Time production was not altered by marijuana during the 10-second tests. Contrary to these acute marijuana effects for underproducing time intervals, when tested the next morning following smoking, time intervals were significantly longer during both the 10-second and the 30-second tests following marijuana but not placebo smoking.

The "morning after" effect by marijuana of lengthening produced intervals, relative to placebo (Chait, Fischman & Schuster, 1985), was not replicated, however, in a subsequent study Chait (1990). In this latter study, 12 regular marijuana smokers either received 40 standardized puffs of placebo or a 2.1 per cent THC-containing cigarette distributed during the late afternoon and evening hours of a weekend (Friday evening–Sunday evening). The subjects were given a battery of tests including a time-production test each morning following an evening of smoking. During time-production tests, subjects were to indicate "30," "60" or "120" when they believed that 30, 60 and 120 seconds had elapsed since an experimenter-initiated signal. Subject-produced intervals were longer than targeted intervals during the mornings following both placebo and marijuana smoking. The subject-produced intervals were significantly shorter during the morning following marijuana, relative to placebo smoking, however, which was an effect opposite to that seen during the earlier study (Chait, Fischman & Schuster, 1985). The author suggested that additional studies, preferably including multiple methods of evaluating human time perception, were required before the determinants of this discrepancy could be isolated.

Perez-Reyes et al. (1991) examined the ability of indomethacin, a prostaglandin synthesis inhibitor, to block several of the disruptive effects of smoking marijuana including those on time estimation and production (see above discussions of cannabis effects on memory for additional details). In their study, subjects smoked six pipe bowls of marijuana containing 2.57 per cent THC separated by 1-minute intervals. At 30 minutes prior to smoking and at 30, 60 and 120 minutes following smoking, the subjects were given time-estimation and time-production tasks. In the time-estimation task, a computer determined a time interval and the subject was required to estimate its duration. In the time-production task, the computer stated a verbal standard in time units and the subject attempted to delimit the interval. The results showed that indomethacin abolished the profound effect of THC on time estimation and production, as well as attenuated the subjective "high" and heart rate accelerating effects of THC, but failed to affect the decremental effects of THC on word recall. The authors concluded that it was likely that the prostaglandins were involved in the mediation of the distortion of time perception induced by THC and probably did so via the ventral striatum.

SUMMARY

Cannabis appears to accelerate the internal "clock" relative to real time in that when subjects are asked to produce a given interval, they underproduce the target interval, and when asked to estimate the interval occurring between two experimenter-delimited events, they overestimate it. The neurochemical events mediating the disruptive effects of cannabis on time sense appear at least in part to be under the control of prostaglandins, and to operate via mechanisms different from those mediating the disruptive effects of cannabis on memory functions. Future research will further clarify the conditions under which cannabis impairs temporal processing and also the potential dissociation of cannabis' effects on temporal information processing from its effects on the processing of other information.

Effects of Cannabis on Psychomotor Performance

Tasks used to evaluate the acute effects of cannabis on human psychomotor performance have typically required subjects to respond on manipulanda as rapidly and as accurately as possible in response to presented environmental cues. Differences in latency to respond and in accuracy while responding when cannabis-exposed, relative to when placebo-exposed, are used to infer cannabis' effects on psychomotor performance. This section reviews published studies of the effects of cannabis on psychomotor performance. Although the effects of cannabis on driving or flying, either under simulated or "real-life" conditions, could be included in a review of cannabis' effects on psychomotor performance, these effects are reviewed by Smiley (see chapter 5 in this volume) and are not included here.

Burns and Moskowitz (1981) examined the effects of marijuana, alone and in combination with alcohol, on tracking and divided-attention task performance. Two separate tracking tasks, in which subjects were required to adjust a response manipulandum in order to move the location of stimuli displayed on a computer monitor, were presented during test sessions, as was a divided-attention task consisting of a tracking and a vigilance component. The tracking component, similar to the individual tracking tasks, was presented in the centre of a visual field, and the vigilance component, in which subjects were required to identify the number "2" when it appeared among 24 continually changing numbers, was presented in the periphery of the visual field. Twelve male volunteers (22 to 33 years of age), who reported using marijuana more than 10 times but fewer than 2 times per week, consumed a placebo-alcohol beverage and smoked one marijuana cigarette during test sessions. All subjects received marijuana cigarettes containing 0 and 200 µg/kg of THC with placebo alcohol prior to a single session, and cigarettes were smoked 30 minutes prior to sessions using a steady, 30-second rhythm of inhale-hold-exhale until the entire cigarette was consumed (smoke exposure varied across subjects). Performance on all psychomotor tasks was significantly impaired following active marijuana administration.

Ashton et al. (1981) investigated the effects of THC added to herbal cigarettes on a number of measures including signalled reaction-time, EEG, skin conductance, heart rate and mood. During the signalled reaction-time task, subjects pressed a button to identify the onset of an auditory tone presented after a variable period (2 to 4 seconds) following the offset of a distinct auditory warning cue. The effects of 2.5 and 10 mg of THC were investigated in 20 unpaid adults who were experienced occasional marijuana users (reported use of one marijuana cigarette per week or less). These subjects were asked to smoke the marijuana cigarettes using a paced-smoking procedure, including a puff and an 8-second breath hold, with 30 seconds separating successive puffs (no external cues were provided) until the entire cigarette was smoked (total number of puffs varied across subjects). Each dose was tested in half of the subjects on a single session. During sessions, the reaction-time task was completed before drug administration and intermittently for 65 minutes after administration. THC slowed reaction times, but the effects were not statistically significant. Significant changes in heart rate and subjective report of "high" were found under these same conditions.

Reeve et al. (1983) investigated the effects of marijuana on field-sobriety test performance. Specific components that were sensitive to the effects of marijuana included the Romberg, finger-to-nose, heel-to-toe, one-foot balance, finger-count and hand-pat tests. The male and female subjects (between 20 and 52 years of age) included 19 who reported using marijuana between once per week and once per month, 25 who reported using between once per week and once per day, and 15 who reported using once per day or more. Subjects were asked to smoke standard-strength marijuana cigarettes (containing 18 mg or 2.38 per cent THC) to what they considered a reasonable "high" (smoking parameters, including number of puffs, puff duration, breath hold durations and number of cigarettes varied across subjects). Five minutes after smoking, a police officer explained and demonstrated the field-sobriety task, and subjects were immediately required to perform the task. The field-sobriety task was repeated intermittently for 150 minutes. All but one subject "failed" at least one component of the test up to 30 minutes after smoking, and 60 per cent continued to fail at least one component 2.5 hours after smoking. Impaired performance was most consistent across tasks at blood THC concentrations between 25 and 30 ng/mL. Unfortunately, details of performance evaluation were not included, and because all subjects smoked active marijuana, it seems unlikely that evaluators did not know the dose conditions.

Zaki and Ibraheim (1983) examined the effects of marijuana on handwriting. Two adult male marijuana users (32 and 45 years old) provided handwriting samples before, immediately following and one hour after smoking four marijuana cigarettes of unknown potency. Handwriting after marijuana smoking was increased in size, with some altered letter forms and baseline deviations. Evaluation criteria for handwriting analysis were not provided, but the described changes were readily apparent in the samples of handwriting that were provided by the authors.

A study of the effects of smoked marijuana on performance of a circular-lights task, in addition to those on a variety of other measures including subjective reports of drug effect, THC, cortisol and prolactin plasma levels, was conducted by Cone et al. (1986). During the circular-lights task, 16 buttons and associated lights were displayed in a circle. At the start of the task, one random light was illuminated. When subjects pressed the associated button, the light was turned off and a new randomly determined light was immediately illuminated. Subjects pressed as many buttons as possible in a one-minute interval. The effects of smoked marijuana were investigated in four male adults (22 to 54 years of age), each of whom had been exposed to THC during a previous research protocol. Subjects

participated in three sessions on three consecutive days; two marijuana cigarettes were smoked in an *ad libitum* manner, one 45 minutes and one 15 minutes prior to beginning the circular-lights task. None, one or both cigarettes contained THC (2.8 per cent). Each dose condition was presented prior to a single session in a mixed order. Performance on the circular-lights task was impaired during sessions preceded by smoking two active cigarettes. Impairment was maximal 15 minutes after smoking the second cigarette, and had returned to baseline level (i.e., to the two-placebo-cigarette level) by the end of the session (i.e., 3.15 hours after the second cigarette was smoked). Similar effects were observed on subjective reports of drug effects, although these measures were more sensitive to the effects of marijuana (i.e., significant effects were also observed on subjective reports during sessions preceded by only one active cigarette).

Perez-Reyes et al. (1988) examined the acute effects of smoked marijuana, alone and in combination with ethanol, on divided-attention performance, subjective report of drug effect, heart rate, ECG and plasma THC level. During the divided-attention task, subjects responded on keys or foot pedals to indicate when a centrally displayed two-digit number was above 57 or below 53, or when single digits displayed in the periphery changed from either 4 or 5 to 3 or 7 (i.e., multiple vigilance tasks). Six adult male marijuana users (22 to 29 years of age), who reported using 0.5 to 9 marijuana cigarettes per month, received placebo ethanol doses and either placebo or active marijuana (2.4 per cent THC). Subjects smoked marijuana cigarettes in their preferred manner (smoking parameters, including number of puffs, puff duration, breath hold durations and interpuff intervals varied across subjects), and each dose combination (i.e., placebo ethanol–placebo marijuana, placebo ethanol–active marijuana) was tested in a single session. During each session, the divided-attention task was completed before and repeatedly throughout a six-hour interval following drug administration. Prior to the study, subjects were trained on the task until session-to-session performance did not show systematic increases or decreases, and during the study subjects received financial bonuses when performance was within ranges established during training. Active marijuana decreased response accuracy in four subjects and increased response latency in five subjects; however, response accuracy increased and response latency decreased following active marijuana smoking by one subject.

Heishman et al. (1988) have also investigated the effects of marijuana on multiple dimensions of human behavior. This group investigated the effects of marijuana and alcohol, administered separately, on computerized psychomotor tasks (circular-lights, digit-symbol substitution and tracking tasks), on heart rate, on carbon monoxide (CO) levels (to assess marijuana smoke exposure) and on subjective reports of drug effects. During the digit-symbol substitution task (DSST), subjects matched the locations of asterisks in a three-row by three-column pattern of dashes and asterisks displayed on a computer monitor by pressing keys on an attached three-row by three-column keypad that corresponded with the positions of the asterisks. Rates of correct and incorrect patterns (i.e., trials) in a 90-second interval were recorded. During the tracking task, subjects were required to make manual adjustments on a paddle controller to changes in stimuli presented on a computer monitor. The effects of 0, 1.3 and 2.7 per cent THC were investigated in six males (average age = 26.2 ± 5.3 years) who were experienced marijuana users (reported 10 occasions of marijuana use per month, with an average of 2.5 cigarettes per occasion). Prior to marijuana sessions, subjects smoked two marijuana cigarettes using a paced-smoking procedure consisting of eight puffs per cigarette (*ad libitum* duration) with a 10-second breath hold and a 40-second interpuff interval. Each subject received all three doses on separate days. Three subjects were tested with alcohol before being tested with marijuana, and three were tested with marijuana prior to being tested with alcohol. All doses were presented in random order. Tasks and other measures were collected before and intermittently for 255 minutes after marijuana smoking. Subjects were paid for study participation, but any additional programmed consequences for task performance were not reported. Active marijuana decreased the number of DSST trials completed, but no other changes in psychomotor performance were reported. The effects of both active doses were significantly different from placebo over approximately 105 minutes, but the effects of the two active doses were not different from each other. These same doses increased ratings of drug effect and increased heart rate. Another interesting finding in this study was that CO levels decreased as a function of THC concentration in the marijuana, suggesting that smoking compensation may have occurred during cigarette administration.

A second analysis of the effects of marijuana on human behavior, under conditions in which smoking characteristics were carefully monitored, was conducted by Heishman and colleagues (Heishman, Stitzer & Yingling, 1989). This study investigated the effects of marijuana on psychomotor performance (digit-symbol substitution and divided-attention tasks), heart rate, CO and subjective reports of drug effect. The divided-attention task consisted of a tracking task (Heishman, Stitzer & Bigelow, 1988) presented in the upper half of a computer monitor, and a vigilance task, in which subjects were required to press a key to identify a digit displayed in the centre of a rectangle in the lower half of the computer monitor when it appeared in any of the four corners of the rectangle. Four numbers were continuously displayed in the corners of the rectangle and these numbers changed throughout the two-minute task. The DSST was also presented for two minutes. The effects of 0, 1.3 and 2.7 per cent THC were investigated in 12 males (23 to 43 years old) who were occasional marijuana users (10 subjects reported using marijuana an average of 7.8 times per month with 2.1 cigarettes smoked per occasion). Prior to experimental sessions, subjects took eight puffs from a marijuana cigarette. Subjects had been trained to puff immediately after exhaling smoke from the previous puff, but additional restrictions on smoking parameters were not imposed. Several puff characteristics, including puff duration, volume and air flow rates during smoke inhalation were monitored. Each subject received three doses presented in a counterbalanced order. Tasks and other measures were collected before and intermittently for 65 minutes after marijuana smoking. Subjects were paid for study participation, but other consequences for task performance were not reported. Prior to the study, subjects practised tasks until stable performances were obtained. The 2.7 per cent THC marijuana cigarette decreased the number of correct DSST trials completed on all testing occasions (for the entire 65 minutes). Effects on performance of the divided-attention task were not observed. Dose-related increases in heart rate occurred, and both doses produced similar increases in verbal ratings of drug effect. Differences in puff duration and volume, as well as inhalation volume, occurred across THC concentrations, again suggesting that compensation may have occurred during marijuana administration.

A third study of the effects of marijuana on human behavior by this group, under conditions in which marijuana smoke exposure was manipulated in a systematic manner, was reported by Azorlosa and colleagues (1992). This study included most of the dependent measures used in the previous study, including the DSST (1.5 minutes) and the divided-attention task (2 minutes). In addition, blood levels of THC were determined. The effects of 4, 10 or 25 puffs taken from marijuana cigarettes containing 1.75 or 3.55 per cent THC were investigated in seven males (19 to 28 years old) who were regular marijuana users (2 to 14 occasions per week). Non-smoking control sessions were also conducted. Prior to the study, subjects were trained to smoke marijuana by taking 10-second, 60-millilitre puff volumes. Puffs were administered every 60 seconds. Smoking characteristics were recorded by computer, and auditory signals indicated when required capacities and durations were achieved. Several puff characteristics, including puff duration and volume, and air flow rates during smoke inhalation, were monitored. Each subject

received each of the dose conditions in a counterbalanced order. Tasks, blood samples and other measures were collected before and intermittently for 45 minutes after marijuana smoking. Decreases in the number of trials completed and in the correct number of DSST trials were observed as a function of both THC concentration and the number of puffs. Response latency on the vigilance component of the divided-attention task also increased when subjects took 25 puffs of the 3.55 per cent THC cigarettes. Effects were observed throughout the 45-minute testing interval. Heart rate and plasma THC levels increased, and changes in the verbal ratings of drug effect occurred when either the THC concentration or the number of puffs was increased. CO levels, however, increased as a function of number of puffs but not THC concentration. These results indicate that the smoking controls used in the present study were effective for maintaining standard smoke exposure across THC concentration and puff manipulations.

A fourth study by this group of investigators provided additional evaluation of the effects of smoke exposure on the same measures reported in the previous study (Azorlosa, Greenwald & Stitzer, 1995). In this study, number of puffs, inhalation volume and interpuff interval were held constant, while puff volume (30, 60 and 90 mL) and breath hold durations (0, 10 and 20 seconds) were manipulated in separate studies to determine the effects of systematic changes in smoke exposure (from marijuana containing 1.75 or 3.55 per cent THC). Significant effects were not observed during any experimental condition on psychomotor performance in this study. Plasma THC levels were elevated in response to both increased puff volume and breath hold duration. In contrast, CO levels and verbal ratings of drug effects were elevated only in response to increased puff volume. These studies demonstrate that both THC content and marijuana smoke exposure are critical determinants of the biological and behavioral effects of marijuana smoking, and that differential sensitivity to THC is obtained among biological and behavioral measures of drug effect.

A fifth study by this group has been recently reported (Heishman, Arasteh & Stitzer, 1997) in which the separate effects of alcohol and marijuana were again compared, but under conditions in which puffing and inhalation parameters of marijuana smokers were carefully controlled. Five male subjects (between 18 and 26 years old), who reported smoking one to six marijuana cigarettes per week, completed seven three- to four-hour sessions, separated by one week intervals. Prior to the study, subjects were trained to smoke marijuana using standardized puff and inhalation parameters. Audio signals cued the maintenance of standard puff volume, inhalation volume, lung exposure duration and interpuff interval. During four separate sessions, the effects of 0, 4, 8 and 16 puffs on marijuana cigarettes containing 3.55 per cent THC were evaluated on simple reaction time and on DSST performance, and also on other memory, time-estimation and time-reproduction tasks (see above). Heart rate, THC blood levels and subjective reports of drug effects were also obtained. THC blood levels, heart rate, subjective reports of drug effect and DSST performance were all significantly altered as a function of THC exposure, but not in an orderly puff-dependent manner. The authors noted that the THC blood levels produced by the 8 and 16 puff conditions were not significantly different. There were no effects on the reaction-time task, nor on the time-estimation and time-reproduction tasks.

Pickworth and colleagues (1997) compared the acute behavioral effects of several drugs, including marijuana, on card-sorting tasks, DSST and circular-lights performance, among other measures, in eight males (between 27 and 42 years old) who reported recent use of marijuana. Task training was provided prior to the study until performance was stable. Subjects took eight standardized puffs on marijuana cigarettes containing either 1.3 per cent or 3.9 per cent THC, using the procedures described by Heishman et al. (1988) and completed the performance tasks 30, 105, 180 and 300 minutes after smoking. Each dose was tested on a separate day. Results were compared to those obtained on two days in which no drug was administered. No effects of marijuana were obtained on any measure of performance, although subjective reports of marijuana strength were increased at both THC concentrations. In addition, task performance was altered by other drugs (e.g., ethanol, 1.0 g/kg; pentobarbital, 450 mg).

Kelly and colleagues (1993) had conducted a similar study of the acute behavioral effects of several drugs, including marijuana, on multiple measures of cognitive task performance. In contrast to the Pickworth et al. (1997) study, however, the acute behavioral effects of marijuana (five standardized puffs, each consisting of a 5-second inhalation, 10-second breath hold and 45-second exhale/rest cues by signal lights on cigarettes containing 0, 2.0 and 3.5 per cent THC) were equal to or greater than those of ethanol (0.6 g/kg), amphetamine (10 mg/70 kg) and diazepam (10 mg/70 kg).

Heishman and colleagues (1996) examined the acute effects of marijuana on a number of different measures of human psychomotor performance that are used as part of the drug evaluation and classification (DEC) assessment. Variables that were most predictive of marijuana consumption during the DEC assessment included several measures of the field-sobriety task, including the Romberg balance task, the walk-and-turn task and the finger-to-nose task, which are associated with psychomotor performance. Heart rate and dynamic pupil reactivity were also associated with marijuana use.

Chait and colleagues investigated the effects of cumulative doses of marijuana on multiple measures, including divided-attention task performance (Chait, Corwin & Johanson, 1988). During the divided-attention task, subjects pressed keys as quickly as possible to identify a "0" appearing in a continuous string of random numbers while counting the number of times that the number "5" was displayed. The effects of cumulative numbers of puffs from 0 per cent and 1.4 per cent THC marijuana cigarettes were investigated in five males and three females (18 to 25 years old) who were experienced marijuana users (1 to 24 occasions of marijuana use per month). Subjects participated in four 3.5-hour sessions scheduled once per week. Subjects took four puffs from marijuana cigarettes (0 per cent or 1.4 per cent) on four separate occasions during a session; each four-puff occasion was separated from the next by 20 minutes. On each smoking occasion, puffs were taken once every 60 seconds, and subjects were instructed to inhale for 5 seconds and to hold the smoke in the lungs for 10 seconds before exhaling at each puff. The cumulative number of puffs taken from the active marijuana at each of the four smoking occasions was 0, 2, 4 and 8 puffs, respectively. Divided-attention task performance was measured in five 5-minute intervals during each session. The task was completed prior to marijuana smoking and during the four 20-minute intervals following marijuana smoking. Subjects were paid for study participation, but other programmed consequences for task performance were not reported. Prior to the study, subjects attended a practice session during which the divided-attention task was performed. No change occurred in "0" stimulus identifications or reaction times as a function of marijuana smoking, but increased "0" responses were observed following displays of the number "5" after eight cumulative active marijuana puffs. Puff-dependent increases in other measures, such as heart rate and subjective report of drug effect were observed, indicating that these measures were affected by lower doses of THC than was divided-attention performance.

Marks and MacAvoy (1989) examined the acute effects of smoked marijuana, alone and in combination with ethanol, on divided-attention performance. During their divided-attention task, subjects responded when a centrally displayed flashing light stopped flashing or when peripherally displayed lights flashed (i.e., multiple vigilance task). Twelve college students (six were experienced marijuana users of 1.5 to 6 marijuana cigarettes per week — three were female; six were non-users — three were female) received placebo ethanol doses and marijuana cigarettes containing 0, 2.6 or 5.2 mg of THC. Subjects were asked to smoke the marijuana

cigarettes using a paced-smoking procedure, including a "deep" inhalation of smoke and a 20-second breath hold, with 20 seconds separating successive puffs in the absence of external smoking cues. Puffing continued until the entire cigarette was smoked (total number of puffs varied across subjects). Each dose combination (i.e., placebo ethanol and 0 mg THC; placebo ethanol and 2.6 mg THC; placebo ethanol and 5.2 mg THC) was tested in a single session. During each session, the divided-attention task was repeatedly administered from 0.5 to 1.3 hours after drug administration. Prior to the study, subjects were trained on the task until errorless performance was obtained over a 5-minute interval. Subjects were paid for participation independent of task performance. Feedback lights did indicate, however, correct vigilance responses and missed signals (i.e., signals that were not followed by responses). During the study, active marijuana decreased accuracy (increased missed signals), although significant effects were limited to 0 versus 5.2 mg-dose conditions. Response latency was unaffected. More peripheral signals were missed by non-users than users (i.e., greater potency of marijuana effects in non-users).

In the above study by Marks and MacAvoy (1989), the combination of alcohol consumption followed by marijuana smoking resulted in performance impairment that was similar to the effects of either drug alone when administered in isolation (i.e., minimal interaction). In the alcohol/marijuana combination study by Perez-Reyes et al. (1988), the combination of alcohol consumption followed by marijuana smoking resulted in performance impairment that was often equal to the sum of the effects of each of the drugs when administered in isolation. In the earlier alcohol/marijuana combination study by Burns and Moskowitz (1981), alcohol consumption was also followed by marijuana smoking. Performance impairment on some tasks (e.g., tracking and divided-attention tasks) was greater than that observed following the administration of marijuana or alcohol alone; however, the degree of impairment was less than the sum of the effects of each of the drugs when administered in isolation. Performance impairment on other tasks, however, was no different from, and in some cases, less than that observed when alcohol or marijuana were administered alone. A subsequent report by Perez-Reyes and Cook (1993) indicated that the combined effects of marijuana smoking followed by alcohol consumption resulted in performance impairment that was not different from the effects of marijuana smoking or alcohol consumption in isolation. Lukas et al. (1992) also reported that marijuana smoking prior to alcohol consumption resulted in decreased blood alcohol level. Clearly, the interactive effects of these two drugs on performance is complex and may be related to the task and/or to the order in which the drugs are administered.

In a series of studies, Foltin and colleagues (1989b; 1990a; 1990b) examined the motivational effects of marijuana. Using time-based measures of behavioral probability, the subjects' access to high-probability work and recreational activities was contingent on their performance while participating in low-probability activities. Work activities included the DSST, as well as disk-sorting, word-sorting and vigilance tasks. Twenty-four adult males (19 to 35 years old), who reported smoking between 1 and 12 marijuana cigarettes per week, participated in residential studies lasting 15 to 18 consecutive days. Across studies, marijuana cigarettes (0, 1.3, 1.8 or 2.7 per cent THC) were smoked at different times each day, and dose conditions were maintained over two- to six-day intervals. All cigarettes were smoked using a paced-smoking procedure consisting of five 5-second puffs with a 10-second breath hold and a 45-second inter-puff interval. Subjects were paid for participation but not contingently for quality of task performance. Subjects received training on all tasks prior to the start of each study. Consistent marijuana effects on work-task performance were not observed across these studies, although selective disruption of DSST performance was reported for some individuals (Kelly, Foltin et al., 1990). Contrary, however, to the "amotivational

hypothesis," increases in the amount of time that subjects engaged in low-probability work behaviors were observed following active marijuana administration. In addition, marijuana's effects on the amount of time that subjects engaged in high- and low-probability activities were different for work and recreational activities, indicating that the behavioral effects of marijuana are dependent on the context in which the effects are determined. These data indicate clearly that the amotivational hypothesis is inadequate to account for the diversity of behavioral effects observed following marijuana administration. The maintenance of high levels of behavior following marijuana use (e.g., Mello & Mendelson, 1985), and increases in responding following marijuana administration (Dougherty, Cherek & Roache, 1994), have also been reported.

In their studies of the effects of marijuana on memory, Block and colleagues (1992) had also investigated the acute effects of marijuana on critical flicker fusion performance and discriminant reaction time. The critical flicker fusion task required subjects to differentiate two visual stimuli, one presented continuously and one flickering. The flickering rate was manipulated, and the minimum value at which subjects could differentiate the two stimuli with complete accuracy was determined. In the discriminant reaction-time task, single digits were repeatedly presented on a computer screen for 0.1 seconds, and subjects were required to press a button whenever a "4" appeared. The interstimulus interval, initially set at 0.4 seconds, was varied until the minimum duration at which subjects could respond with accuracy was established. Adult subjects (18 to 42 years of age), who reported being experienced marijuana users, smoked placebo and active marijuana (2.57 per cent THC) according to a paced-smoking procedure consisting of either 7- or 15-second puff/breath hold intervals (puff durations were determined by subjects, combined puff/breath hold durations were timed). Signalled puff/breath hold intervals occurred every 35 seconds until an entire marijuana cigarette was smoked (total number of puffs also varied across subjects). Each subject smoked placebo and active cigarettes under double-blind conditions and were randomly assigned to either the 7- or the 15-second puff/breath hold interval group (N = 24/group). Each subject was tested twice at each dose level. Subjects were not trained on the tasks prior to study participation. They were paid for participation but not contingently for quality of task performance. Active marijuana decreased thresholds for flicker discrimination and slowed discriminant reaction times. The effects of active marijuana were unaffected by puff/breath hold intervals.

Foltin et al. (1993) examined the effects of marijuana on psychomotor performance, alone and in combination with cocaine. A 5-minute test battery used in this study included brief, simple and choice reaction-time components and a 1-minute DSST component, presented sequentially. The battery was completed prior to drug administration, and again 15 minutes after smoking marijuana. Marijuana cigarettes (0, 1.3 or 1.84, and 2.7 per cent THC) were smoked using a paced-smoking procedure consisting of five 5-second puffs with a 10-second breath hold and a 45-second interpuff interval. Cocaine (0, 16 and 32 mg) was administered intravenously 13 minutes after marijuana smoking. Seven males (21 to 45 years old), who reported regular use of marijuana (1 to 7 occasions per week) in combination with intravenous cocaine, participated in daily sessions (Monday through Friday) and received all possible drug combinations prior to one session. Marijuana, alone or in combination with cocaine, did not affect psychomotor performance. In contrast, clear dose-related changes in verbal ratings of marijuana effect were observed.

Kelly and colleagues have also examined the effects of marijuana on multiple measures of human performance on a variety of computer-generated tasks, including the DSST and a differential-reinforcement of low-rate (DRL) schedule of point presentation (Kelly, Foltin & Fischman, 1993).

During the DRL task, button presses that were separated in time from the start of the task or from a preceding press by 45 seconds increased a counter. The effects of 0, 2.0 and 3.5 per cent THC were investigated in six males (24 to 29 years old) who were experienced marijuana users (reported 2 to 30 occasions of marijuana use per month). Prior to sessions, subjects smoked marijuana cigarettes using a paced-smoking procedure consisting of five 5-second puffs with a 10-second breath hold and a 45-second interpuff interval. Smoking durations were cued by stimulus lights. In addition, subjects received puff and breath hold duration feedback following each puff. If a puff duration exceeded 3 seconds or breath hold duration exceeded 7 seconds, corresponding stimulus lights were illuminated. If both feedback cues were presented following a puff, subjects received a 50-cent bonus. Each subject received three doses prior to three sessions, which occurred once per day on 10 consecutive weekdays. Task measures were collected during a 3-hour session that began 15 minutes after marijuana smoking. Intermittently throughout the 3-hour session, subjects participated on the DSST and DRL tasks for 3-minute intervals. Subjects were paid for study participation and for completing tasks in a specified order during the 3-hour session. Monetary contingencies were not placed on task performance, although subjects were required to complete a minimum number of trials during each 3-minute task in order to avoid a mild punishment. The punishment was rarely presented during the study. Prior to the study, subjects received extensive task training until stable patterns of responding were observed. Errors increased when active marijuana was administered, although no differences were observed as a function of THC content. Correct trial rate, however, decreased as a function of THC content. Changes in DRL task performance did not occur as a function of marijuana administration. Despite the use of monetary contingencies designed to maintain stable marijuana smoking patterns, increases in puff duration were observed when the low dose was administered, and decreases in puff duration were observed when the high dose was administered. The level of THC content did not produce differences in breath hold duration.

Wilson et al. (1994) examined the effects of marijuana on tracking, standing steadiness, DSST, choice reaction time and vigilance performance. During the tracking task, subjects operated a steering wheel to keep a line segment, which moved horizontally, in a random manner centred on a computer monitor. During the standing-steadiness task, subjects were instructed to stand still (1) with eyes open but fixed on an object, and (2) with eyes closed. Strain gauges attached to the platform on which subjects were standing were used to automate the measurement of movement. During the choice reaction-time task, subjects pressed keys on a keypad that matched numbers displayed on a monitor. During the vigilance task, subjects pressed a key when an even number followed an odd number, or when an odd number followed an even number, in a series of numbers presented on a monitor. The effects of marijuana cigarettes containing 0, 1.75 and 3.5 per cent THC were investigated in 10 males (19 to 40 years old) who were using marijuana "occasionally" prior to the study. Subjects participated in three four-hour sessions, scheduled no more frequently than once per week. Subjects smoked each marijuana cigarette under double-blind conditions during one session in an *ad libitum* manner (i.e., no control over smoke exposure was attempted). Performance testing, which lasted approximately 15 minutes, occurred prior to marijuana smoking and at 30, 90 and 150 minutes after smoking. Blood samples were collected at 0, 10, 30, 50, 70, 90, 110, 130, 150 and 170 minutes after smoking. Subjects were paid for study participation, but other programmed consequences for task performance were not reported. Prior to the study, subjects received task training until less than 10 per cent variance on performance dimensions was observed during repeated testing. Changes in standing-steadiness or vigilance performance did not occur following marijuana smoking. Tracking performance was differentially affected by active and placebo marijuana smoking, as indicated by a time x dose interaction; however, follow-up testing failed to identify significant dose-related differences at any

specific test time. Dose-related differences in choice reaction time and DSST performance occurred and were statistically significant between smoking marijuana containing 0 and 3.55 per cent THC at the 30-minute post-smoking test for choice reaction time and at all three postsmoking tests (i.e., 30, 90 and 150 minutes) for DSST performance. Peak blood THC levels occurred 10 minutes after smoking, although differences did not occur as a function of THC content of the marijuana cigarette.

Most studies of the acute effects of smoked marijuana on human psychomotor performance report either the absence of an effect of marijuana on performance or decremental effects on performance. Numerous factors, including the performance task itself, the THC content of the smoked marijuana and the extent of exposure to marijuana smoke, influence the performance effects of smoked marijuana. In addition, factors other than smoking topography also influence the bioavailability of THC in marijuana smoke (Perez-Reyes, 1990). In sum, the weight of evidence clearly indicates that decremental effects of smoked marijuana on measures of human psychomotor performance are reliably obtained under conditions in which adequate exposure to THC-containing marijuana smoke is established through experimental manipulations. However, the parameters that determine adequate exposure are not yet well understood (e.g., interactions between THC content, smoke exposure, performance task and testing conditions).

The effects of orally administered THC have also been examined. Kamien and colleagues examined the effects of oral doses of THC on DSST performance (Kamien, Bickel et al., 1994), in addition to the repeated acquisition and performance of response sequences, as described earlier. The effects of 0, 10 and 20 mg of THC were investigated in three female and five male adults (19 to 33 years of age), most of whom had reported using marijuana on more than 40 occasions throughout their lifetimes. Doses were administered in mixed order prior to one, two or three sessions (subjects participated for differing numbers of sessions), and sessions occurred no more frequently than once every three days. Performance measures were collected before and after drug administration, as well as at 30-minute intervals for 5 hours after drug administration. Subjects were paid for study participation and for performance on the repeated-acquisition task, but other monetary contingencies were not placed on DSST performance. THC decreased the number of DSST trials completed, but had no effect on accuracy.

Chesher et al. (1990) also investigated the effects of orally administered THC on multiple measures of psychomotor performance, including standing steadiness, pursuit rotor tracking (a tracking task in which the tracking stimulus rotates on a horizontal plane in a clockwise direction at a fixed rate), and both simple and complex reaction times. The effects of 0, 5, 10, 15 and 20 mg/70 kg THC were investigated in 23 female and 57 male adults (18 to 34 years of age), all of whom had previous experience with cannabis use. Subjects participated in a single session and were randomly assigned to one of the five dose conditions. Performance measures were collected before and 80, 140, 200 and 260 minutes after drug administration. Subjects consumed a light breakfast and participated in "a practice run on all of the tests" prior to the pre-drug test. Standing steadiness and pursuit-rotor tracking performance were impaired on all tests up to and including the 200-minute test. Simple visual reaction time was increased only at the 200-minute test, and simple auditory reaction time was increased only at the 140 minute test. Complex reaction time was unaffected, but response accuracy on one complex reaction-time task was disrupted at the 80- and 140-minute tests. Dose effects on individual tasks were not analysed, but clear dose-related impairments were observed on performance measures averaged across these tasks. The results of these last two studies also indicate that similar to smoked marijuana, orally administered THC produces decremental effects on some measures of human psychomotor performance.

Two studies by Chait and colleagues have also investigated the next-day or residual effects of marijuana administration on psychomotor performance (Chait, Fischman & Schuster, 1985; Chait, 1990). The first study examined marijuana effects on eye-hand co-ordination and DSST performance (Chait, Fischman & Schuster, 1985). The eye-hand co-ordination task consisted of two 40-card sorts, one into four 10-card stacks and the other into four stacks based on suit. The effects of marijuana cigarettes containing 0 and 2.9 per cent THC were investigated in 14 males (21 to 35 years old) who had used marijuana on at least 10 occasions during their lifetime. Marijuana use during the month prior to the study ranged from 0 to 50 cigarettes per week. Subjects participated in two or three sessions, occurring between 8:00 p.m. and approximately 8:00 a.m. the following morning, scheduled no more frequently than once per week. Subjects smoked two marijuana cigarettes 90 minutes apart under blind conditions. On two sessions, both cigarettes were either placebo or active. Subjects participating in a third session received one placebo cigarette and one active cigarette on the third session. Order of dose exposure was varied among subjects. Cigarettes were smoked using a paced-smoking procedure consisting of five 5-second puffs with a 10-second breath hold and a 45-second interpuff interval. Performance testing, which lasted 15 to 20 minutes, occurred prior to marijuana smoking, 25 minutes after the first cigarette, 20 minutes prior to the second cigarette, 25 minutes after the second cigarette and 30 minutes after awakening the following morning. Subjects were paid for study participation, but other programmed consequences for task performance were unreported. Subjects familiarized themselves with the tasks prior to the first session. Card-sorting times were increased immediately after active marijuana was smoked, but residual effects were not observed on this measure the following morning. DSST performance was not altered by marijuana smoking at any time during the study.

The second study of the residual effects of marijuana examined multiple dimensions of psychomotor performance, including simple and choice reaction time, visual divided-attention and DSST performance (Chait, 1990). During the simple reaction-time task, subjects were instructed to press a key as quickly as possible whenever an asterisk appeared on the centre of a monitor. During the choice reaction-time task, subjects pressed one key if a digit presented on the monitor was even, and another key if the digit was odd. During separate versions of this task, the location of the stimuli was either (1) always in the centre of the monitor, or (2) at random locations on the monitor. The visual divided-attention task was identical to that used by Chait as described above (Chait, Corwin & Johanson, 1988). The effects of marijuana cigarettes containing 0 and 2.1 per cent THC were investigated in nine males and three females (18 to 26 years old) who reported using marijuana between one and three times per week. Subjects participated in two weekend sessions (Friday evening through Monday morning), separated by two weeks. Each weekend, subjects smoked marijuana during two-hour smoking intervals scheduled at 9:00 p.m. on Friday, Saturday and Sunday evenings, and at 3:00 p.m. on Saturday and Sunday afternoons. During each smoking interval, subjects received four puffs at both the beginning of each two-hour interval and one hour into the smoking interval (eight total puffs per interval). Puffs consisted of five 5-second inhalations and 10-second breath holds with 45-second interpuff intervals separating successive puffs. During each weekend session, all puffs were from either active or placebo marijuana cigarettes, with order of dose exposure varied among subjects. Performance testing occurred on Saturday, Sunday and Monday mornings between 8:00 and 9:00 a.m. Subjects were wakened at 7:30 a.m. Prior to the study, subjects practised the tasks during a weeknight practice session and prior to the Friday smoking interval on the first weekend session. Reaction time to the "0" stimulus was increased after smoking active marijuana the previous day, but no other dimension of divided-attention performance nor any of the other psychomotor tasks was affected by previous-day marijuana smoking.

Heishman et al. (1990) also evaluated the residual or next-day effects of acute marijuana in three males (between 27 and 29 years old) who reported using an average of 4.7 cigarettes per month. Subjects completed four two-day blocks. On day 1, subjects took eight standardized puffs using the procedures described by Heishman et al. (1988) on zero, one or two marijuana cigarettes containing 2.57 per cent THC at 9:00 a.m. and 1:00 p.m. Performance tasks, including the circular-lights task and four computerized cognitive tasks selected from the Performance Assessment Battery (PAB), were completed before the 9:00 a.m. dose, and at 9:30 a.m., 10:00 a.m., 11:00 a.m., 12:30 p.m., 1:30 p.m., 2:00 p.m. and 4:00 p.m. On day 2, performance tasks were again completed at 8:00 a.m., 10:00 a.m., 12:00 p.m., 2:00 p.m. and 4:00 p.m. THC blood levels, heart rate and subjective report measures were also collected. Subjects received task training prior to the study until performance was stable. Psychomotor performance on the circular-lights task was disrupted immediately after smoking on day 1, but no residual or next-day effects were observed on day 2. Similar effects were observed with heart rate and subjective reports of drug effect, and THC blood levels had also dropped to low levels by day 2. In contrast, cognitive and memory task performance on two of the PAB tasks was disrupted on both days 1 and 2, although the magnitude of effect on the morning of day 2 was less than that observed on day 1. These results suggested that the residual effects of marijuana may differ across tasks.

Kelly et al. (1997) further evaluated the residual or next-day effects of marijuana self-administered by subjects in a residential laboratory. Six males (23 to 33 years old), who reported using marijuana between two and eight times per week, were provided free access to marijuana cigarettes over 14 consecutive days. The concentration of THC in the cigarettes available on a given day remained constant but was systematically manipulated across days between 0, 2.0 and 3.5 per cent. Subjects smoked between two and eight marijuana cigarettes each day between 10:00 a.m. and 3:30 p.m. and between 5:00 p.m. and 10:30 p.m. They were wakened each morning at 9:00 a.m. and completed a number-recall task and received a scan measuring pupil reactivity to a brief light flash between 9:10 a.m. and 9:30 a.m. No changes in number-recall performance or in pupil reactivity were observed as a function of marijuana smoking or THC content, however, the resting diameter of the pupils was decreased as a function of THC content.

Additional studies have evaluated the residual or next-day effects of marijuana use on more global measures of psychomotor performance, such as operating an airplane. These topics will be considered elsewhere (see chapter 5). However, in summary, the results indicate that smoked marijuana may produce residual effects on some measures of next-day psychomotor performance and on other physiological indices, but that these effects are clearly of a smaller magnitude than those obtained immediately following smoke exposure. Additional research on this issue is clearly warranted. In the 15 years following Klonoff's review (1983), several advances have been made in the experimental analysis of the effects of cannabis on human psychomotor performance. Psychomotor performance tasks are now administered under more controlled conditions, objective measures of task performance are being used more consistently, the relationship between marijuana smoke exposure and THC absorption is more clearly understood, the behavioral effects of oral THC dose administration and next-day or residual effects of marijuana smoking are being more carefully examined, and the dose-dependent relationship between THC administration and performance impairment is becoming more clearly defined. Future studies will benefit from even greater considerations of dose administration conditions because of the multiple factors now known to influence actual THC exposure following smoking marijuana.

SUMMARY

Mechanisms of cannabis' effects on psychomotor performance remain obscure. Differential sensitivity of performance on different tasks has been reported in many studies, and many of the factors that influence cannabis' effects on psychomotor performance remain unknown. Greater attention to factors influencing psychomotor task performance, including performance training prior to studies, consequences of performance (e.g., payment conditions, response feedback), and task performance parameters, is clearly needed. Investigations of THC dose-response effects across systematic manipulations of task performance parameters would be extremely helpful in understanding how cannabis affects performance. Greater attention to subject conditions, such as age, sex and prior drug use including prior use of cannabis, would enhance experimental precision. Finally, while recent studies have begun to investigate the duration of cannabis' effects on psychomotor performance more carefully, additional studies in this area are needed to characterize more fully the time course of these effects and its implication for day-to-day functioning.

Reinforcing Effects of Marijuana

Two direct methods and one indirect method have been used to investigate the reinforcing effects of marijuana in experimental settings. The first direct method, called drug self-administration, involves the measurement of amount and/or pattern of drug intake as a function of dose when subjects are given free access to a drug. The second direct method, called drug choice or preference, involves measurement of subject choice when given access to different drugs or different doses of the same drug. Results from studies using these two approaches will be reviewed below. The indirect approach to measurement of the reinforcing effects of drugs involves comparing the interoceptive effects produced by a drug with those produced by drugs with known reinforcing efficacy. Or it can measure those interoceptive effects that have been previously shown to be correlated with the reinforcing effects of drugs. Each of these approaches has both advantages and disadvantages (e.g., de Wit & Griffiths,

1991), and the simultaneous use of two or more of these methods in the same experimental setting provides greater precision than is possible with the use of any single method by itself. A majority of studies of marijuana effects on human behavior have included measures of the interoceptive effects of marijuana. In general, results clearly indicate that the interoceptive effects produced by marijuana are associated primarily with the THC content of the marijuana, and that the profile of interoceptive effects produced by THC are consistent with those engendered by other drugs that function as reinforcers. As such, these data clearly support the observation that the reinforcing effects of marijuana are associated with THC content. These data will not be reviewed as an independent topic in this section, but will be discussed when the results are relevant to considerations of marijuana effects on other measures of behavior.

A number of marijuana intake studies were conducted under free access conditions prior to 1981. These studies demonstrated that experienced marijuana users would self-administer marijuana cigarettes under controlled conditions, but most of the studies did not control for the concentration of THC available in the marijuana.

Mello and Mendelson (1985) investigated marijuana self-administration by female subjects. Twenty-one women (21 to 36 years old), who reported using marijuana for 1 to 15 years, lived on a hospital research ward for 35 consecutive days. Marijuana cigarettes (1.83 per cent THC) were available on days 8 to 28. While on the ward, subjects could earn points, exchangeable for money or marijuana cigarettes when available, by completing response requirements on a hand-held button. Points could be earned and marijuana cigarettes could be smoked at any time. Within a single day, marijuana use was lowest between 4:00 and 8:00 a.m. Use increased throughout the day, reaching a peak between 4:00 p.m. and midnight. Across the 21-day marijuana-availability interval, three different patterns of marijuana smoking were observed. Heavy users averaged between 4 and 12 marijuana cigarettes per day, and marijuana use by this group increased across

the 21 days of marijuana availability. Moderate users averaged between 1 and 4 marijuana cigarettes per day, and light users averaged between 0 and 2 marijuana cigarettes per day. Rates of marijuana smoking by both moderate and low users remained constant across the 21 days of marijuana availability. Increases in marijuana use were also observed at premenstruum in women reporting greater premenstrual dysphoria.

Foltin et al. (1989a) examined marijuana self-administration in three males (32 to 34 years old) who remained in a residential facility for 12 consecutive days. Standardized schedules were in effect for the duration of the study. Subjects remained socially isolated while participating in a variety of work tasks every day from 9:45 a.m. until approximately 3:45 p.m. Between 4:00 p.m. and bedtime (11:45 p.m.), subjects could engage in a variety of recreational activities, such as reading, listening to or playing music, playing board and video games, and working on craft activities, either alone in their private areas, or in a common social-access area. Subjects were required to remain in their private areas sleeping or resting in bed between 11:45 p.m. and 9:00 a.m. Up to five marijuana cigarettes (1.84 per cent THC) were available between 9:45 a.m. and 10:00 p.m. on days 2, 3, 6, 7, 10 and 11. Cigarettes were smoked using a paced-smoking procedure cued by stimulus lights consisting of five 5-second puffs with 10-second breath hold and 45-second interpuff intervals. Subjects smoked all five available cigarettes on most days at regularly spaced intervals throughout the day. The authors noted that the third cigarette of the day was typically smoked after the social-access period began. As in the Mello and Mendelson study (1985), smoking rates were highest between 4:00 p.m. and midnight.

Chait (1989) examined marijuana self-administration in eight males and two females (19 to 33 years old) who reported using marijuana from one to six times per week. Subjects participated in 15 30-minute self-administration sessions twice per week. During the sessions, marijuana (0.5, 1.7 or 2.1 per cent THC) was available *ad libitum*, and subjects smoked in their preferred manner (i.e., no restrictions were imposed on number of puffs, puff durations or breath hold durations). Each THC concentration was tested during five sessions. Differences in marijuana smoking were not observed as a function of THC content, although changes in heart rate and reports of the interoceptive effects of the drug were related to THC concentration.

Kelly and colleagues (1994b) also examined marijuana self-administration in six adult males (27 to 34 years of age) reporting between 4 and 30 occasions of marijuana use per month. Subjects remained in a residential facility for 12 consecutive days. Each day was divided into two 6.5-hour work and social-access periods beginning at 10:00 a.m. and 4:30 p.m. The order of work and social-access periods changed during the study. During the work period, subjects remained socially isolated in their private work areas while participating in a variety of work tasks, and during the social-access period subjects could engage in a variety of recreational activities, such as reading, listening to or playing music, viewing videotaped movies, playing board and video games and working on craft activities, alone in their private areas or in a common social-access area. Up to eight marijuana cigarettes (0 or 2.3 per cent THC) could be smoked between 10:00 a.m. and 3:30 p.m. and between 4:30 p.m. and 10:00 p.m. Active marijuana cigarettes were available on days 4 to 6 and 9 to 11, with placebo cigarettes available on all other days except day 1. Cigarettes were smoked using a paced-smoking procedure cued by stimulus lights consisting of three 5-second puffs with 10-second breath hold and 45-second interpuff intervals. As had been reported in earlier studies, no differences in the number of marijuana cigarettes smoked were observed as a function of THC content, although ratings of interoceptive effects were related to THC content. Three subjects smoked greater numbers of both placebo and active marijuana cigarettes during the social-access periods, regardless of whether they occurred at 10:00 a.m. or at 4:30 p.m. The other three subjects smoked more placebo and active marijuana cigarettes during the 10:00 a.m. period, regardless of whether that period was a work period or a social-access period. These results indicate that marijuana use is not always increased in the late afternoon and evenings, as had been previously reported. No differences in subjective reports of drug effects were observed as a function of the order of work and social-access periods.

Zacny and de Wit (also see above) examined the effects of acute food deprivation on marijuana self-administration (Zacny & de Wit, 1991). Four males and one female (21 to 30 years old) who reported using marijuana from 1 to 3 times per week, participated in six 30-minute self-administration sessions beginning at 8:00 p.m., each separated by a minimum of 48 hours. During the experimental sessions, marijuana (0, 0.8 or 3.6 per cent THC) was available *ad libitum*, and subjects smoked in their preferred manner (i.e., there were no restrictions on the number of puffs, or on puff and breath hold duration). One hour prior to the 30-minute self-administration sessions, subjects took four puffs on marijuana cigarettes containing the THC concentration that would be available during the session, using a uniform-puffing procedure. Prior to three sessions, subjects were instructed to fast for 24 hours, and prior to the other three sessions, subjects were instructed to eat a minimum of two meals in the preceding 24-hour period, including a dinner meal between 5:00 p.m. and 7:00 p.m. Each THC concentration was tested once during a fast condition and once during an eating condition. Seven days separated successive fasting days. Clear changes in urinary ketones and bilirubin, and modest changes in blood glucose levels were observed across the fasting and eating conditions. As in previous studies, THC-related differences in marijuana smoking did not occur, regardless of feeding conditions, although differences in heart rate and reports of the interoceptive effects of the drug were observed across THC conditions. Fasting conditions did not produce differential effects on heart rate or on the subjective reports of THC effects.

Chait and Perry (1994b) examined the effects of alcohol pretreatment on marijuana self-administration. Fifteen males and 5 females (21 to 34 years old), who reported smoking between 0.4 and 5 marijuana cigarettes per week and drinking between 1.5 and 17.3 alcohol beverages per week, participated in six one-hour self-administration sessions beginning at 8:00 p.m. Sessions were scheduled once per week. Subjects finished an alcohol beverage (0, 0.3 or 0.6 g/kg, roughly equivalent to 0, 1.5 or 3 commercial cocktails) 30 minutes prior to the marijuana self-administration session. Each dose was presented prior to two sessions. Marijuana (3.6 per cent THC) was available *ad libitum*, and subjects smoked in their preferred manner during the self-administration sessions. No effects of alcohol on marijuana smoking, or on marijuana's heart rate and subjective effects were observed.

These studies demonstrate that humans will smoke marijuana under controlled laboratory conditions. However, these studies generally observed that the level of cannabis self-administration was not systematically related to THC concentration.

Other clinical laboratory studies have examined the selection of marijuana as a choice among several different options as a function of THC content. The first study using a choice procedure investigated the reinforcing effects of marijuana, oral THC and nabilone, a synthetic cannabinoid (Mendelson & Mello, 1984). Twenty-four males (22 to 30 years old), who reported smoking between one marijuana cigarette per month and three cigarettes per day, participated in five experimental sessions, Monday through Friday from 6:00 p.m. until 7:00 a.m. On the first four days, subjects swallowed two capsules and smoked a marijuana cigarette. Placebo capsules and marijuana were presented on one day. On the other three days, a single active dose of either marijuana (1.83 per cent THC), oral THC (17.5 mg) or nabilone (2 mg) was administered under double-blind, double-dummy conditions. On the fifth day, subjects pressed a button 3,600 times in order to choose between the four doses presented on the previous four days. Choice was not mandatory. Eighteen of 24 subjects chose marijuana, 2 chose oral THC and 3 made no choice. These data indicate a clear preference for active marijuana over oral THC, nabilone and placebo marijuana.

Chait and Zacny (1992) examined choice between active and placebo smoked marijuana, and between active and placebo oral doses of THC. Seven males and three females (18 to 31 years old), who reported using marijuana from one to three times per week, participated in the marijuana-choice portion of the study. Eight males and three females (18 to 27 years old), who reported using marijuana from one to six times per week, completed the oral THC dose-choice portion of the study. Sessions were scheduled on Monday, Wednesday and Friday over two weeks. On Monday and Wednesday, subjects received placebo and active doses of the drug (four fixed-volume puffs of marijuana smoke or oral THC doses) under blind conditions in random order. On Friday, subjects chose between the drug conditions (i.e., placebo or active) administered on Monday and Wednesday. After a condition was chosen, subjects could also choose the amount of drug they wished to take (one to eight puffs of marijuana; half, one or two times the dose of oral THC). The amount of active drug administered on sampling days was adjusted individually for each subject in order to standardize the subjective and heart-rate effects that were produced by sample doses. Dose adjustments were based on effects obtained during practice sessions conducted prior to the study. Subjects in the marijuana-choice portion of the study chose active marijuana on all choice occasions, with a mean of 5.7 puffs selected during the first choice session and 6.5 puffs selected on the second choice session (range: 2 to 8 puffs). Ten of 11 subjects in the oral THC dose-choice portion of the study chose active oral THC doses on both choice days. Placebo was chosen on both sessions by the other subject. The maximum dose (twice the sample dose) was chosen on both occasions by 8 of 10 active dose choosers.

In contrast to previous studies in which subjects were allowed to choose between placebo and active marijuana, Chait and Burke also examined choice between marijuana containing varying concentrations of THC (Chait & Burke, 1994). Nine males and three females (19 to 29 years old), who reported using marijuana from 1 to 16 times per month, participated in three experimental sessions per week, separated by 48 hours for two weeks. During the first two sessions of each week, subjects smoked low (0.63 per cent THC) or high (1.95 per cent THC) doses of marijuana under blind conditions in random order using a paced-smoking procedure consisting of four 5-second puffs with a 10-second breath hold and a 45-second interpuff interval. The staff provided verbal cues to control smoking parameters. On the third session, subjects chose between the marijuana sampled on the previous two sessions. After marijuana was chosen, subjects smoked cigarettes, one-at-a-time, in an *ad libitum* manner, for 60 minutes. All subjects chose the high THC dose on the first choice occasion, and nine also chose the high dose on the second session. Subjects smoked an average of 3.5 cigarettes during the choice session (range: 0 to 8). One subject never smoked a cigarette during choice sessions, and a second subject smoked 0 cigarettes during the second choice session. All other subjects smoked at least one cigarette on every choice session. These data suggest preference for high versus low THC concentrations in marijuana cigarettes by experienced marijuana users.

Kelly and colleagues (1994a; 1997) also examined choice between placebo and active marijuana, as well as choice between different doses of active marijuana. Six males (23 to 33 years old), who reported using marijuana from two to eight times per week, participated in a 14-day residential study. Four three-day blocks of choice tests were presented on days 2 to 13. During the first two days of each three-day choice block, subjects sampled marijuana containing varying amounts of THC (0 versus 3.5 per cent THC or 2.0 versus 3.5 per cent THC). On the third choice day, subjects chose between the samples smoked on the previous two days. During the first two blocks, marijuana samples contained either high (3.5 per cent) or zero (0 per cent) THC content, while during the second two blocks marijuana samples contained high or low (2.0 per cent) THC content. Samples were presented in mixed order. Separate choices were available during the 6.5-hour work period (beginning at 10:00 a.m.) and social-access period (beginning at 5:00 p.m.). Subjects were required to smoke a minimum of one cigarette during each period between 10:00 a.m. and 1:00 p.m. and also between 5:00 p.m. and 8:00 p.m., and could smoke as many as they wanted between 5:00 p.m. and 10:30 p.m. up to a maximum of eight cigarettes per day. All cigarettes were smoked using a paced-smoking procedure consisting of three 5-second puffs with 10-second breath hold and 45-second interpuff intervals. Smoking durations were cued by stimulus lights. With this design, both dose choice and number of cigarettes smoked were measured as a function of THC content. As in previous self-administration studies, minimal differences in the number of marijuana cigarettes smoked per day were observed as a function of THC content, providing little evidence for a role of THC in the reinforcing effects of marijuana. In contrast, the choice data provided clear indications of the reinforcing effects of THC. Subjects chose the high dose over placebo on 11 of 12 occasions during the work period and on all 12 occasions during the social-access period. The high dose was chosen over the low dose on 9 of 12 occasions during the work period and on 10 of 12 occasions during the social-access periods. Subject dose choice, but not number of cigarettes smoked, provided clear evidence for the reinforcing effects of THC content; these data highlight the importance of the use of multiple measures for investigating the reinforcing effects of marijuana.

SUMMARY

Although a variety of measures have been used to assess the reinforcing effects of marijuana, the evidence consistently indicates that THC can function as a reinforcer under laboratory conditions. Verbal reports of drug effects are consistent with those engendered by drugs that function as reinforcers, and studies of dose choice have clearly established that preference for marijuana is determined by THC content. Some evidence for contextual influences on the reinforcing effects of marijuana has also been reported. Additional studies of factors that influence the reinforcing effects of marijuana, particularly by social conditions, will be important for a more comprehensive understanding of the reinforcing effects of marijuana.

Cannabis and Social Behavior

Drugs alter social behavior and social contexts alter the behavioral effects of drugs (Stitzer, Griffiths et al., 1981b). Under experimental conditions, dose-related changes in a variety of social behaviors, including verbal, co-operative and aggressive behaviors have been reported. Similarly, experimental investigations have demonstrated that social context alters the behavioral effects of drugs. It is clear that a thorough review of cannabis and social behavior must consider both cannabis-induced changes in social behavior, as well as changes in the behavioral effects of cannabis as a function of social context.

A series of studies of the effects of drugs on human verbal behavior under both isolated and social conditions have been conducted by Stitzer and colleagues. Most drugs of abuse, including amphetamine, ethanol, secobarbital and hydromorphone increase human verbal behavior (e.g., Higgins & Stitzer, 1988; Stitzer, Griffiths et al., 1981a; Stitzer, Griffiths & Liebson, 1978; Stitzer, McCaul et al., 1984). It has been suggested that the reinforcing effects of drugs may be influenced by such changes in verbal behavior (e.g., Stitzer, Griffiths et al., 1981b). Higgins and Stitzer (1986) examined the effects of marijuana on verbal responding by one member of a social dyad. Male and female occasional marijuana users (more than one smoking occasion per month) smoked marijuana (0, 1.01, 1.84 and 2.84 per cent THC) using a paced-smoking procedure consisting of 10 puffs (*ad libitum* duration) with a 7-second breath hold and a 30-second interpuff interval. Smoking durations were cued by stimulus lights. Both members of a dyad smoked marijuana cigarettes, but only the subject (determined arbitrarily) received active

doses. Sixty-minute experimental sessions began 2 minutes after smoke administration. Experimental sessions occurred three times per week, and each subject received each dose prior to one session. Both members of the dyad wore voice microphones during sessions, allowing for automated measurement of speaking duration. Prior to the study, dyads participated in daily practice sessions until stable rates of verbal responding were observed across sessions. Subjects were paid for participation, but no other experimentally programmed consequences for verbal responding were reported. Dose-related decreases in speaking duration were observed. These same doses produced increases in heart rate and verbal ratings of "high." In addition, under similar conditions, other drugs with abuse liability, including amphetamine, ethanol, secobarbital and hydromorphone, have produced increases in human verbal behavior.

Heishman and Stitzer (1989) extended the analysis of effects of marijuana on human verbal behavior by determining whether marijuana influenced the reinforcing efficacy of verbal interaction. Male marijuana users (78 per cent reported using marijuana on more than one occasion per month and averaged 2.6 occasions of use per week) smoked marijuana (0 and 2.7 per cent THC) using a paced-smoking procedure consisting of eight puffs (*ad libitum* duration) with 10-second breath hold and 40-second interpuff intervals. Subjects participated in six sessions, each consisting of four 30-minute trials. Trials occurred in isolated rooms and consisted of 10 discrete choices. Each choice determined whether or not headphones, which allowed verbal interaction with another person located in a different room, would be operative for the next 3 minutes. Only the subject smoked marijuana cigarettes, and the other person was instructed to be ready to talk when subjects chose the talk option. Choice behavior and speaking duration were monitored. After the first session, subjects were instructed to divide their choices evenly between the headphone-on and headphone-off conditions, but feedback on their distribution of choices was provided only during session 2.

Two placebo cigarettes were smoked prior to all trials on sessions 3 to 6. On one session, two active marijuana cigarettes were smoked prior to the third trial, and on two sessions, one active marijuana cigarette was smoked prior to both the second and third trials. Dyads did not practise prior to the study, and subjects were paid for participation, but other experimentally programmed consequences for headphone choice or speaking duration were not reported. Modest decreases in speaking durations and headphone-on choices were observed, but these changes were not statistically significant. These same doses produced increases in verbal ratings of "high," "liking," and in "drug effect." In summary, these results suggest that at pharmacologically active doses, marijuana produces minimal change in subject preference for engaging in verbal interaction.

The effects of marijuana on social behavior and verbal interaction have also been investigated by Fischman and colleagues in residential studies examining the effects of marijuana on multiple dimensions of human behavior, including food intake, tobacco cigarette smoking, allocation of time to available activities, and task performance rate and accuracy (for an overview see, Kelly, Foltin et al., 1990). In these studies, groups of three male subjects were exposed to standardized daily schedules for the duration of a study (typically 10 to 18 days). Subjects remained socially isolated while participating in a variety of work tasks every day from 9:00 a.m. until approximately 5:00 p.m. Between 5:00 p.m. and bedtime (12:00 a.m.), subjects could engage in a variety of recreational activities alone in their private areas or in a common social-access area. During the social-access period, trained monitors recorded the amount of time spent in social areas in the presence of other subjects (social interaction), as well as the amount of time subjects spent speaking to each other (verbal interaction). Subjects were required to remain in their private areas sleeping or resting in bed between 12:00 a.m. and 9:00 a.m.

Using the general conditions of the residential studies described above, Foltin and colleagues (Foltin, Fischman et al., 1989a) investigated the effects of marijuana on social and verbal interaction in four groups of subjects (22 to 38 years old) who were occasional marijuana users (two cigarettes per week to three cigarettes per day). Four identical marijuana cigarettes (0 or 1.84 per cent) were smoked per day, using a paced-smoking procedure consisting of five 5-second puffs with 10-second breath hold and 45-second interpuff intervals. Smoking durations were cued by stimulus lights. All subjects received the same potency of marijuana cigarettes (0 or 1.84 per cent THC) each day. Cigarettes were smoked immediately prior to both the work and social-access periods, and two additional cigarettes were smoked during the social-access period at 7:25 p.m. and 10:00 p.m. Every subject smoked both placebo and active cigarettes in two- or three-consecutive-day intervals. Subjects were paid for participation, but experimentally programmed consequences for verbal responding were not imposed while these data were obtained. Marijuana effects were dependent on the baseline level of verbal interaction. Marijuana increased verbal interaction in three groups that had high baseline levels of verbal interaction, but had no effect on verbal interaction in a fourth group that had low baseline levels of verbal interaction.

In the previous study, few social activities were available that did not require verbal interaction as a requirement of participation. Under these conditions, subjects were speaking for most of the time that they were engaged in social interaction. Foltin and Fischman (1988) extended the analysis of marijuana effects on social and verbal interaction by providing a wider variety of social activities during social-access periods, and by including options that did not require verbal interaction (e.g., watching videotaped movies). In this study, social behavior and verbal interaction did not co-vary in the manner observed in the previous study. The THC concentration in the smoked marijuana was also increased in this study (0 or 2.7 per cent THC, although 1.3 per cent THC was smoked by one subject who reported untoward effects from smoking the more potent cigarettes). Two groups (19 to 30 years old) of three occasional marijuana users (two cigarettes per week to three cigarettes per day) smoked four identical marijuana cigarettes per day using the paced-smoking procedure described in the previous study. As in the previous study, group members smoked the same potency of marijuana cigarettes every day, and placebo and active cigarettes were smoked in alternating three-consecutive-day intervals. Cigarettes were smoked immediately before and halfway through both the work and social-access periods. Subjects were paid for participation, but experimentally programmed consequences for verbal responding were not imposed while the data were collected. In both groups, regardless of baseline levels of verbal interaction, marijuana decreased verbal interaction but had no effect on the amount of time subjects spent under social conditions. When subjects smoked active marijuana, they spent equal amounts of time with each other, but they spoke less frequently. It remains unclear whether this outcome was related to the higher potency of the marijuana cigarettes used in this study, or to the separation of social and verbal interaction afforded by the wider range of social activities.

Rachlinski examined interpersonal space between subjects in the previous study as a function of smoked marijuana (Rachlinski, Foltin & Fischman, 1989). Interpersonal space was operationally defined as the physical distance between subjects who were interacting socially and was measured from the locations of subjects when they were interacting socially. Marijuana-induced decreases in verbal interaction reported in the previous study were associated with increased interpersonal distances indicating that subjects kept greater distances between themselves when socially interacting following active marijuana administration.

In a recent study, Kelly and colleagues (1994b) described marijuana's effects on social and verbal behavior when the drug was self-administered. When subjects self-administered active marijuana, social behavior was not changed, but verbal interaction was decreased. When placebo marijuana was self-administered, changes in social or verbal behavior were not observed.

Myerscough and Taylor (1985) investigated the effects of marijuana on human aggressive behavior. Thirty male subjects participated in experimental sessions consisting of 33 competitive signalled reaction-time trials. The competitor was an experimental confederate. Prior to each trial, subjects selected a shock intensity to be delivered to the other participant. High-intensity shocks were selected on every trial throughout each session by experimental confederates. After the trial, the participant (i.e., subject or experimental confederate) with the slower reaction time received the shock selected by the other participant. Feedback lights were illuminated after each trial to indicate the intensity of shock selected by the experimental confederate. The shock intensities selected by subjects were used as indicators of aggressive behavior. Subjects were randomly assigned to low-, moderate- or high-dose groups, and 50 minutes prior to an experimental session consumed beverages containing 0.10, 0.25 or 0.40 g/kg of THC, respectively. Subjects were paid for participation, but experimentally programmed consequences for shock-intensity choices were not imposed. Practice was not provided to subjects prior to the first session. Shock-intensity selections were inversely related to THC dose. This result is similar to that obtained in an earlier study using similar dosing conditions and experimental procedures (Taylor, Vardaris et al., 1976). The same paradigm has been used extensively for the investigation of the effects of alcohol on human aggressive behavior. In contrast, dose-related increases in shock-intensity selections have been reported following alcohol administration in a number of studies using a similar paradigm (e.g., Taylor & Gammon, 1976; Taylor, Schmutte et al., 1979).

Cherek and colleagues (1993), using a free-operant paradigm, also examined the effects of marijuana on human aggressive behavior. Eight male subjects (19 to 39 years old), who reported using marijuana between one and four times per month, participated in six, 25-minute sessions per day over an eight-hour day. During sessions, subject lever responses were maintained by the accumulation of points that could be exchanged for money, escape from point subtractions or ostensibly subtracting points from another participant depicted as participating in the study at another location. Responding to deliver an aversive stimulus (point subtraction) to another individual served as aggressive behavior. A computer was programmed to simulate the other participant; periodically during sessions, points were subtracted from the subject, and these point subtractions were attributed to the other participant. One marijuana cigarette (0, 1.75, 2.57 or 3.55 per cent THC) was smoked 15 minutes before the second session according to a paced-smoking procedure. Cigarette smoking consisted of 10 3-second puffs, with 10-second breath holds and 17-second inter-puff intervals. Each subject smoked every dose on two experimental days, with 72 hours separating successive active dose days. Marijuana increased aggressive responding and decreased responding maintained by point presentations. No drug effects were observed on escape responding. The 2.7 per cent THC and 3.57 per cent THC doses affected behavior for 0.5 and 2 hours after drug administration, respectively.

Clear differences in route of THC administration and experimental procedures were observed between these two experimental studies of the effects of THC on human aggressive behavior. Additional studies will be required to understand the relationship between THC, environmental context and human aggressive behavior.

The effects of marijuana on human co-operative behavior was examined in a series of three studies, two residential and one outpatient (Kelly, Foltin & Fischman, 1992). During daily work and social-access periods, subjects had access to time-based high- and low-probability activities, including the DSST. Access to high-probability activities was contingent on the availability of points that could be acquired while participating in low-probability activities. While participating in low-probability activities, each subject could choose to distribute points equally among all three group members (co-operative behavior) or to keep earned points for himself

(non-co-operative behavior). Three groups of adult male subjects (21 to 38 years of age), who reported regular use of marijuana (0.5 to 35 occasions per week), participated. Social-access and work periods were 3 or 6.5 hours in duration. Marijuana cigarettes (0 or 2.28 per cent THC) were smoked prior to each period, and a second cigarette was smoked halfway through the 6.5-hour periods. Cigarettes were smoked using a paced-smoking procedure consisting of five 5-second puffs with 10-second breath hold and 45-second interpuff intervals. Each subject smoked placebo and active marijuana cigarettes before and/or during all work and social periods occurring during two- or five-day intervals. Daily schedules and conditions associated with engaging in co-operative behavior varied across studies, and subjects were trained on all aspects of the study prior to the first day. Marijuana disrupted DSST performance and increased verbal-reports of drug effect, but had no effect on time spent engaging in co-operative and non-co-operative behavior.

SUMMARY

Although relatively few studies have been conducted, changes in a variety of social behaviors, including verbal and aggressive behaviors, have been reported following cannabis use, and the behavioral effects of cannabis can be influenced by social context. Given the potential importance of the influence of social factors on the reinforcing and other behavioral effects of cannabis, additional studies manipulating social variables in the study of the behavioral effects of cannabis are of central importance.

Conclusion

The previous review of acute cannabis effects on psychological functioning by Klonoff (1983) had identified effects which have also been observed in more recent (post-1980) experimental studies. Recent studies have continued to document cannabis' effects on memory and learning, food consumption, perception of time and psychomotor performance. These recent studies have additionally extended the examination of cannabis' effects by using more controlled environments, including those in which subjects are chronically housed in social settings, and by including a greater range of effects, including cannabis' discriminative stimulus and reinforcing effects. Where cannabis has been shown to have effects on memory and learning, the perception of time and psychomotor performance, almost invariably these effects have been construed to be detrimental. Considering that the experimental behaviors studied are likely correlates of components of more complex, integrated real-life behaviors, cannabis use should be viewed as potentially disruptive of education, work performance, and a variety of behaviors involving complex psychomotor control.

Although experimental studies have identified many effects of cannabis administration, it is difficult to predict how and to what degree these effects could disrupt real-life functioning, especially in naive users. One complicating factor is that most experimental studies that have examined the acute effects of cannabis have used experienced cannabis users as subjects. The drug histories of these subjects are often difficult to document accurately. Previous experience with cannabis can possibly attenuate its acute effects through a variety of tolerance mechanisms, or might even result in an exaggerated response, relative to a naive user, through accumulated toxicity. Neither tolerance nor sensitization to cannabis is easily identifiable unless reliable histories are obtained and cannabis-naive users are concurrently evaluated. Although the use of cannabis-naive subjects is experimentally desirable, for ethical reasons it may often be impermissible.

Secondly, although THC dose has been shown to be a determinant of the magnitude of effect, it is often difficult to ascertain what the actual dose is in these experimental studies and subsequently to extrapolate this dose to real-life usage. For instance, although the concentration of THC and the weight of cigarettes smoked is usually provided in studies involving smoked cannabis, the actual amount of THC delivered can be variable due to variability in smoking topography. Studies controlling the volume of smoke inhaled, breath hold duration, and those which assay plasma THC levels are the clearest to evaluate dose-response relationships.

Thirdly, a variety of non-pharmacological factors can modulate the effects of cannabis and these factors are often uncontrolled, unreported or non-standardized across experimental studies. The subject's personality and attitude toward cannabis, experience with tasks that have commonalties with the experimental tasks, variations in the physical environment and the consequences (e.g., payment) for completing the experimental tasks correctly are variable from study to study.

Although substantial research on the psychomotor and cognitive effects of cannabis has resulted in a greater awareness of the functional effects of cannabis consumption, the mechanisms through which these functional effects are produced remain largely obscure. Additional research on the mechanisms through which marijuana alters behavior is necessary. Fewer studies have investigated the reinforcing effects of marijuana. Additional research on the factors influencing marijuana use, including age, environmental and historical factors, and the relationship between behavioral and subjective effects of the drug and its reinforcing effects is also needed. Finally, minimal research on the effects of marijuana on complex human behavior, such as social behavior, has been reported. Such studies will have important implications for our understanding of the etiology of marijuana abuse, and will provide valuable insights into the development of efficacious treatment and prevention approaches.

In the past six years, rapid advancements have been occurring in our understanding of the neurobiological basis of the effects of cannabinoids. Cannabinoid receptors in the central nervous system have been identified, and research into the anatomical and functional significance of these receptors is advancing at a rapid pace. In addition, endogenous ligands that interact with these receptors have also been identified. These recent developments offer many exciting possibilities for future research. Our current understanding of the behavioral effects of these cannabinoid receptors and of the naturally occurring ligands is very limited. Research in this area has important implications for our basic understanding of behavior, as well as for more applied issues, including our understanding of the biology of marijuana abuse and our ability to develop more selective and efficacious medicines for the treatment of a variety of behavioral conditions, including appetite disorders, nausea, movement disorders and chronic pain.

In order to address the issues associated with the functional effects of endogenous cannabinoid receptors more effectively, and to investigate issues associated with the acute behavioral effects of endogenous cannabinoid ligands and/or new medications that are derived from these substances more effectively, future research should incorporate the methodological advances that have been developed from research on the acute effects of marijuana over the past two decades. In addition, efforts to establish measurement standards (e.g., inclusion of standardized measures, such as heart rate or digit-symbol substitution performances, see Chait & Pierri, 1992; Foltin & Evans, 1993), and increased attention to environmental and historical influences on the behavioral effects of these substances, should be encouraged. Finally, greater attention to pharmacological issues in the behavioral effects of cannabinoids should be forthcoming, as our understanding of the biological bases for cannabinoid mechanisms of action become better understood.

References

Abel, E.L. (1971). Effects of marijuana on the solution of anagrams, memory, and appetite. *Nature, 231*, 260–261.

Ashton, H., Golding, J., Marsh, V.R., Millman, J.E. & Thompson, J.W. (1981). The seed and the soil: Effect of dosage, personality and starting state on the response to delta 9-tetrahydrocannabinol in man. *British Journal of Clinical Pharmacology, 12*, 705–720.

Azorlosa, J.L., Greenwald, M.K. & Stitzer, M.L. (1995). Marijuana smoking: Effects of varying puff volume and breath hold duration. *Journal of Pharmacology and Experimental Therapeutics, 272*, 560–569.

Azorlosa, J.L., Heishman, S.J., Stitzer, M.L. & Mahaffey, J.M. (1992). Marijuana smoking: Effect of varying delta-9-tetrahydrocannabinol content and number of puffs. *Journal of Pharmacology and Experimental Therapeutics, 261*, 114–122.

Bachman, J.A., Benowitz, N.L., Herning, R.I. & Jones, R.T. (1979). Dissociation of autonomic and cognitive effects of THC in man. *Psychopharmacology, 61*, 171–175.

Bickel, W.K., Higgins, S.T. & Hughes, J.R. (1991). The effects of diazepam and triazolam on repeated acquisition and performance of response sequences with an observing response. *Journal of the Experimental Analysis of Behaviour, 56*, 217–237.

Block, R., Farinpour, R. & Braverman, K. (1992). Acute effects of marijuana on cognition: Relationships to chronic effects and smoking techniques. *Pharmacology, Biochemistry and Behaviour, 43*, 907–917.

Block, R.I. & Wittenborn, J.R. (1984a). Marijuana effects on semantic memory: Verification of common and uncommon category members. *Psychological Reports, 55*, 503–512.

Block, R.I. & Wittenborn, J.R. (1984b). Marijuana effects on visual imagery in a paired-associate task. *Perceptual and Motor Skills, 58*, 759–766.

Block, R.I. & Wittenborn, J.R. (1985). Marijuana effects on associative processes. *Psychopharmacology, 85*, 426–430.

Block, R.I. & Wittenborn, J.R. (1986). Marijuana effects on the speed of memory retrieval in the letter-matching task. *International Journal of Addictions, 21*, 281–285.

Boren, J.J. & Devine, D.D. (1968). The repeated acquisition of behavioural chains. *Journal of the Experimental Analysis of Behaviour, 11*, 651–660.

Burns, M. & Moskowitz, H. (1981). Alcohol, marijuana and skills performance. *Alcohol, Drugs and Traffic Safety, 3*, 954–968.

Cappell, H.D. & Pliner, P.L. (1973). Volitional control of marijuana intoxication: A study of the ability to "come down" on command. *Journal of Abnormal Psychology, 1*, 428–434.

Carlini, E.A., Karniol, I.G., Renault, P.F. & Schuster, C.R. (1974). Effects of marihuana in laboratory animals and in man. *British Journal of Pharmacology, 50*, 299–309.

Carroll, M.E. & Meisch, R.A. (1984). Increased drug-reinforced behavior due to food deprivation. In T. Thompson & P.B. Dews (Eds.), *Advances in Behavioral Pharmacology* (Vol. 4) (pp. 47–88). New York: Academic Press.

Casswell, S. & Marks, D.F. (1973). Cannabis and temporal disintegration in experienced and naive subjects. *Science, 179*, 803–805.

Chait, L.D. (1989). Δ^9-tetrahydrocannabinol content and human marijuana self-administration. *Psychopharmacology, 98*, 51–55.

Chait, L.D. (1990). Subjective and behavioral effects of marijuana the morning after smoking. *Psychopharmacology, 100*, 328–333.

Chait, L.D. & Burke, K.A. (1994). Preference for high- versus low-potency marijuana. *Pharmacology, Biochemistry and Behavior, 49*, 643–647.

Chait, L.D., Corwin, R.L. & Johanson, C.E. (1988). A cumulative dosing procedure for administering marijuana smoke to humans. *Pharmacology, Biochemistry and Behavior, 29*, 553–557.

Chait, L.D., Evans, S.M., Grant, K.A., Kamien, J.B., Johanson, C.E. & Schuster, C.R. (1988). Discriminative stimulus and subjective effects of smoked marijuana in humans. *Psychopharmacology, 94*, 206–212.

Chait, L.D., Fischman, M.W. & Schuster, C.R. (1985). "Hangover" effects the morning after marijuana smoking. *Drug and Alcohol Dependence, 15*, 229–238.

Chait, L.D. & Perry, J.L. (1994a). Acute and residual effects of alcohol and marijuana, alone and in combination, on mood and performance. *Psychopharmacology, 115*, 340–349.

Chait, L.D. & Perry, J.L. (1994b). Effects of alcohol pretreatment on human marijuana self-administration. *Psychopharmacology, 113*, 346–350.

Chait, L.D. & Pierri, J. (1992). Effects of smoked marijuana on human performance: A critical review. In L. Murphy & A. Bartke (Eds.), *Marijuana/Cannabinoids: Neurobiology and Neurophysiology*, pp. 387–423. Boca Raton, FL: CRC Press.

Chait, L.D. & Zacny, J.P. (1992). Reinforcing and subjective effects of oral delta 9-THC and smoked marijuana in humans. *Psychopharmacology, 107*, 255–262.

Cherek, D.R., Roache, J.D., Egli, M., Davis, C., Spiga, R. & Cowan, K. (1993). Acute effects of marijuana smoking on aggressive, escape and point-maintained responding of male drug users. *Psychopharmacology, 111,* 163–168.

Chesher, G.B., Bird, K.D., Jackson, D.M., Perrignon, A. & Starmer, G.A. (1990). The effects of orally administered delta 9-tetrahydrocannabinol in man on mood and performance measures: A dose-response study. *Pharmacology, Biochemistry and Behavior, 35,* 861–864.

Cone, E.J., Johnson, R.E., Moore, J.D. & Roache, J.D. (1986). Acute effects of smoking marijuana on hormones, subjective effects and performance in male human subjects. *Pharmacology, Biochemistry and Behavior, 24,* 1749–1754.

de Wit, H. & Griffiths, R.R. (1991). Testing the abuse liability of anxiolytic and hypnotic drugs in humans. *Drug and Alcohol Dependence, 28,* 83–111.

Dornbush, R.L., Fink, M. & Freedman, A.M. (1971). Marijuana, memory, and perception. *American Journal of Psychiatry, 128,* 194–197.

Dougherty, D.M., Cherek, D.R. & Roache, J.D. (1994). The effects of smoked marijuana on progressive-interval schedule performance in humans. *Journal of the Experimental Analysis of Behavior, 62,* 73–87.

Ferraro, D.P. (1980). Acute effects of marijuana on human memory and cognition. In R.C. Petersen (Ed.), *Marijuana Research Findings: 1980* (NIDA Research Monograph No. 31, pp. 98–119). Washington, DC: U.S. Government Printing Office.

Foltin, R.W., Brady, J.V. & Fischman, M.W. (1986). Behavioral analysis of marijuana effects on food intake in humans. *Pharmacology, Biochemistry and Behavior, 25,* 577–582.

Foltin, R.W. & Evans, S.M. (1993). Performance effects of drugs of abuse: A methodological survey. *Human Psychopharmacology, 8,* 9–19.

Foltin, R.W. & Fischman, M.W. (1988). Effects of smoked marijuana on human social behavior in small groups. *Pharmacology, Biochemistry and Behavior, 30,* 539–541.

Foltin, R.W., Fischman, M.W., Brady, J.V., Bernstein, D.J., Capriotti, R.M., Nellis, M.J. & Kelly, T.H. (1990a). Motivational effects of smoked marijuana: Behavioral contingencies and low-probability activities. *Journal of the Experimental Analysis of Behavior, 53,* 5–19.

Foltin, R.W., Fischman, M.W., Brady, J.V., Bernstein, D.J., Nellis, M.J. & Kelly, T.H. (1990b). Marijuana and behavioral contingencies. *Drug Development Research, 20,* 67–80.

Foltin, R.W., Fischman, M.W., Brady, J.V., Capriotti, R.M. & Emurian, C.S. (1989a). The regularity of smoked marijuana self-administration. *Pharmacology, Biochemistry and Behavior, 32,* 483–486.

Foltin, R.W., Fischman, M.W., Brady, J.V., Kelly, T.H., Bernstein, D.J. & Nellis, M.J. (1989b). Motivational effects of smoked marijuana: Behavioral contingencies and high-probability recreational activities. *Pharmacology, Biochemistry and Behavior, 34*, 871–877.

Foltin, R.W., Fischman, M.W. & Byrne, M.F. (1988). Effects of smoked marijuana on food intake and body weight of humans living in a residential laboratory. *Appetite, 11*, 1–14.

Foltin, R.W., Fischman, M.W., Pippen, P.A. & Kelly, T.H. (1993). Behavioral effects of cocaine alone and in combination with ethanol or marijuana in humans. *Drug and Alcohol Dependence, 32*, 93–106.

Galanter, M., Weingartner, H., Vaughan, T.B., Roth, W.T. & Wyatt, R.J. (1973). $\emptyset$-Transtetrahydrocannabinol and natural marihuana. *Archives of General Psychiatry, 28*, 278–281.

Heishman, S.J., Arasteh, K. & Stitzer, M.L. (1997). Comparative effects of alcohol and marijuana on mood, memory, and performance. *Pharmacology, Biochemistry and Behavior, 58*, 93–101.

Heishman, S.J., Huestis, M.A., Henningfield, J.E. & Cone, E.J. (1990). Acute and residual effects of marijuana: Profiles of plasma THC levels, physiological, subjective and performance measures. *Pharmacology, Biochemistry and Behavior, 37*, 561–565.

Heishman, S.J., Singleton, E.G. & Crouch, D.J. (1996). Laboratory validation study of drug evaluation and classification program: Ethanol, cocaine, and marijuana. *Journal of Analytical Toxicology, 20*, 468–483.

Heishman, S.J. & Stitzer, M.L. (1989). Effect of d-amphetamine, secobarbital, and marijuana on choice behavior: Social versus nonsocial options. *Psychopharmacology, 99*, 156–162.

Heishman, S.J., Stitzer, M.L. & Bigelow, G.E. (1988). Alcohol and marijuana: Comparative dose effect profiles in humans. *Pharmacology, Biochemistry and Behavior, 31*, 649–655.

Heishman, S.J., Stitzer, M.L. & Yingling, J.E. (1989). Effects of tetrahydrocannabinol content on marijuana smoking behavior, subjective reports, and performance. *Pharmacology, Biochemistry and Behavior, 34*, 173–179.

Hicks, R.E., Gualtieri, C.T., Mayo, J.P., Jr. & Perez-Reyes, M. (1984). Cannabis, atropine, and temporal information processing. *Neuropsychobiology, 12*, 229–237.

Higgins, S.T., Bickel, W.K., O'Leary, D.K. & Yingling, J. (1987). Acute effects of ethanol and diazepam on the acquisition and performance of response sequences in humans. *Journal of Pharmacology and Experimental Therapeutics, 243*, 1–8.

Higgins, S.T. & Stitzer, M.L. (1986). Acute marijuana effects on social conversation. *Psychopharmacology, 89*, 234–238.

Higgins, S.T. & Stitzer, M.L. (1988). Time allocation in a concurrent schedule of social interaction and monetary reinforcement: Effects of d-amphetamine. *Pharmacology, Biochemistry and Behavior, 31*, 227–231.

Hollister, L.E. (1971). Hunger and appetite after single doses of marijuana, alcohol, and dextroamphetamine. *Clinical Pharmacology and Therapeutics, 12*, 44–49.

Hooker, W.D. & Jones, R.T. (1987). Increased susceptibility to memory intrusions and the Stroop interference effect during acute marijuana intoxication. *Psychopharmacology, 91*, 20–24.

Jones, R.T. & Stone, G.C. (1970). Psychological studies of marijuana and alcohol in man. *Psychopharmacologia, 18*, 108–117.

Kamien, J., Bickel, W., Higgins, S. & Hughes, J. (1994). Effects of $\varnothing^9$-tetrahydrocannabinol on repeated acquisition and performance of response sequences and on self-reports in humans. *Behavioural Pharmacology, 5*, 71–78.

Kelly, T.H., Foltin, R.W., Emurian, C.S. & Fischman, M.W. (1990). Multidimensional behavioral effects of marijuana. *Progress in Neuro-Psychopharmacology and Biological Psychiatry, 14*, 885–902.

Kelly, T.H., Foltin, R.W., Emurian, C.S. & Fischman, M.W. (1993). Performance-based testing for drugs of abuse: Dose and time profiles of marijuana, amphetamine, alcohol and diazepam. *Journal of Analytical Toxicology, 17*, 264–272.

Kelly, T.H., Foltin, R.W., Emurian, C.S. & Fischman, M.W. (1994a). Effects of $\varnothing^9$-THC on marijuana smoking, dose choice, and verbal report of drug liking. *Journal of the Experimental Analysis of Behavior, 61*, 203–211.

Kelly, T.H., Foltin, R.W., Emurian, C.S. & Fischman, M.W. (1997). Are choice and self-administration of marijuana related to $\varnothing^9$-THC content? *Experimental and Clinical Psychopharmacology, 5*, 74–82.

Kelly, T.H., Foltin, R.W. & Fischman, M.W. (1992). The influence of social context and absence of marijuana effects on human cooperative behavior. *The Psychological Record, 42*, 479–504.

Kelly, T.H., Foltin, R.W. & Fischman, M.W. (1993). Effects of smoked marijuana on heart rate, drug ratings and task performance by humans. *Behavioral Pharmacology, 4*, 167–178.

Kelly, T.H., Foltin, R.W., Mayr, M.T. & Fischman, M.W. (1994b). Effects of $\varnothing^9$-tetrahydro-cannabinol and social context on marijuana self-administration by humans. *Pharmacology, Biochemistry and Behavior, 49*, 763–768.

Klonoff, H. (1983). Acute psychological effects of marihuana in man, including acute cognitive, psychomotor, and perceptual effects on driving. In K.O. Fehr & H. Kalant (Eds.), *Cannabis and Health Hazards* (pp. 433–474). Toronto: Addiction Research Foundation.

Lukas, S.E., Benedikt, R., Mendelson, J.H., Kouri, E., Sholar, M. & Amass, L. (1992). Marihuana attenuates the rise in plasma ethanol levels in human subjects. *Neuropsychopharmacology, 7,* 77–81.

Marks, D.F. & MacAvoy, M.G. (1989). Divided attention performance in cannabis users and non-users following alcohol and cannabis separately and in combination. *Psychopharmacology, 99,* 397–401.

Mattes, R.D., Engelman, K., Shaw, L.M. & ElSohly, M.A. (1994). Cannabinoids and appetite stimulation. *Pharmacology, Biochemistry and Behavior, 49,* 187–195.

McMillan, D.E. (1988). Failure of acute and chronic administration of $\varnothing$-tetrahydrocannabinol to affect the repeated acquisition of serial position responses in pigeons. Pavlovian *Journal of Biological Sciences, 23,* 57–66.

Mello, N.K. & Mendelson, J.H. (1985). Operant acquisition of marihuana by women. *Journal of Pharmacology and Experimental Therapeutics, 235,* 162–171.

Mendelson, J.H. & Mello, N.K. (1984). Reinforcing properties of oral $\varnothing$-tetrahydrocannabinol, smoked marijuana, and nabilone: Influence of previous marijuana use. *Psychopharmacology, 83,* 351–356.

Miller, L. (1984). Marijuana: Acute effects on human memory. In S. Agurell, W.L. Dewey & R.E. Willette (Eds.), *The Cannabinoids: Chemical, Pharmacologic and Therapeutic Aspects* (pp. 21–46). New York: Academic Press.

Myerscough, R. & Taylor, S. (1985). The effects of marijuana on human physical aggression. *Journal of Personality and Social Psychology, 49,* 1541–1546.

Perez-Reyes, M. (1990). Marijuana smoking: Factors that influence the bioavailability of tetrahydrocannabinol. In C.N. Chiang & R.L. Hawks (Eds.), *Research Findings on Smoking of Abused Substances* (NIDA Research Monograph No. 99, pp. 42–62). Rockville, MD: National Institute on Drug Abuse.

Perez-Reyes, M., Burstein, S.H., White, W.R., McDonald, S.A. & Hicks, R.E. (1991). Antagonism of marihuana effects by indomethacin in humans. *Life Sciences, 48,* 507–515.

Perez-Reyes, M. & Cook, C.E. (1993). On the marihuana attenuation of the rise of ethanol levels in human subjects. *Neuropsychopharmacology, 9,* 247–248.

Perez-Reyes, M., Hicks, R.E., Bumberry, J., Jeffcoat, A.R. & Cook, C.E. (1988). Interaction between marihuana and ethanol: Effects on psychomotor performance. *Alcoholism: Clinical and Experimental Research, 12,* 268–276.

Pickworth, W.B., Rohrer, M.S. & Fant, R.V. (1997). Effects of abused drugs on psychomotor performance. *Experimental and Clinical Psychopharmacology, 5,* 235–241.

Rachlinski, J.J., Foltin, R.W. & Fischman, M.W. (1989). The effects of smoked marijuana on interpersonal distances in small groups. *Drug and Alcohol Dependence, 24*, 183–186.

Reeve, V.C., Grant, J.D., Robertson, W., Gillespie, H.K. & Hollister, L.E. (1983). Plasma concentrations of delta-9-tetrahydrocannabinol and impaired motor function. *Drug and Alcohol Dependence, 11*, 167–175.

Schulze, G.E., McMillan, D.E., Bailey, J.R., Scallet, A., Ali, S.F., Slikker, W. & Paule, M.G. (1988). Acute effects of Ø-tetrahydrocannabinol in rhesus monkeys as measured by performance in a battery of complex operant tests. *Journal of Pharmacology and Experimental Therapeutics, 245*, 178–186.

Stitzer, M.L., Griffiths, R.R., Bigelow, G.E. & Liebson, I.A. (1981a). Human social conversation: Effects of ethanol, secobarbital and chlorpromazine. *Pharmacology, Biochemistry and Behavior, 14*, 353–360.

Stitzer, M.L., Griffiths, R.R., Bigelow, G.E. & Liebson, I.A. (1981b). Social stimulus factors in drug effects in human subjects. In T. Thompson & C.E. Johanson (Eds.), *Behavioral Pharmacology of Human Drug Dependence* (NIDA Research Monograph No. 37, pp. 130–154). Washington, DC: U.S. Government Printing Office.

Stitzer, M.L., Griffiths, R.R. & Liebson, I.A. (1978). Effects of d-amphetamine on speaking in isolated humans. *Pharmacology, Biochemistry and Behavior, 9*, 57–63.

Stitzer, M.L., McCaul, M.E., Bigleow, G.E. & Liebson, I.A. (1984). Hydromorphone effects on human conversational speech. *Psychopharmacology, 84*, 402–404.

Taylor, S.P. & Gammon, C.B. (1976). Aggressive behavior of intoxicated subjects: The effect of third-party intervention. *Journal of Studies on Alcohol, 37*, 917–930.

Taylor, S.P., Schmutte, G.T., Leonard, K.E. & Cranston, J.W. (1979). The effects of alcohol and extreme provocation on the use of a highly noxious electric shock. *Motivation and Emotion, 3*, 73–81.

Taylor, S.P., Vardaris, R.M., Rawtich, A.B., Gammon, C.B., Cranston, J.W. & Lubetkin, A.I. (1976). The effects of alcohol and delta-9-tetrahydrocannabinol on human physical aggression. *Aggressive Behavior, 2*, 153–161.

Thompson, D.M. (1973). Repeated acquisition as a behavioral baseline for studying drug effects. *Journal of Pharmacology and Experimental Therapeutics, 184*, 506–514.

Thompson, D.M. & Moerschbaecher, J.M. (1979). Drug effects on repeated acquisition. *Advances in Behavioral Pharmacology, 2*, 229–259.

Thompson, D.M. & Winsauer, P.J. (1985). Ø-tetrahydrocannabinol potentiates the disruptive effects of phencyclidine on repeated acquisition in monkeys. *Pharmacology, Biochemistry and Behavior, 23*, 1051–1057.

Vachon, L., Sulkowski, A. & Rich, E. (1974). Marihuana effects on learning, attention and time estimation. *Psychopharmacologia, 39*, 1–11.

Wetzel, C.D., Janowsky, D.S. & Clopton, P.L. (1982). Remote memory during marijuana intoxication. *Psychopharmacology, 76*, 278–281.

Wilson, W.H., Ellinwood, E.H., Mathew, R.J. & Johnson, K. (1994). Effects of marijuana on performance of a computerized cognitive-neuromotor test battery. *Psychiatry Research, 51*, 115–125.

Zacny, J.P. & Chait, L.D. (1989). Breathhold duration and response to marijuana smoke. *Pharmacology, Biochemistry and Behavior, 33*, 481–484.

Zacny, J.P. & Chait, L.D. (1991). Response to marijuana as a function of potency and breathhold duration. *Psychopharmacology, 103*, 223–226.

Zacny, J.P. & de Wit, H. (1989a). Effects of food deprivation on subjective responses to d-amphetamine and marijuana in humans. In L.S. Harris (Ed.), *Problems of Drug Dependence 1989* (NIDA Research Monograph No. 95, pp. 490–491). Washington, DC: U.S. Government Printing Office.

Zacny, J.P. & de Wit, H. (1989b). Effects of food deprivation on responses to marijuana in humans. *Behavioral Pharmacology, 1*, 177–185.

Zacny, J.P. & de Wit, H. (1991). Effects of food deprivation on subjective effects and self-administration of marijuana in humans. *Psychological Reports, 68*, 1263–1274.

Zaki, N.N. & Ibraheim, M.A. (1983). Effect of alcohol and Cannabis sativa consumption on handwriting. *Neurobehavioral Toxicology and Teratology, 5*, 225–227.

Marijuana: On-Road and Driving-Simulator Studies

Marijuana: On-Road and Driving-Simulator Studies

ALISON SMILEY

Given that cannabis is an illegal substance, its use is fairly widespread. A 1994 Canadian study by Health Canada surveyed 12,155 persons aged 15 and over. A total of 23.1 per cent said they had ever used cannabis; 7.4 per cent reported its use within the last year. Rates of past-year use were twice as high among males as among females. Current users were much more likely to be young than to be middle-aged or older (Health Canada, 1995). Similar patterns have been found in numerous other countries (WHO, 1997).

Since cannabis is widely used and because it is used mainly by young people, who are less experienced drivers, there has been great concern about its impact on traffic safety. Surveys of users show that most of them have driven after using cannabis and that the most frequent users are those most likely to drive after using cannabis (Johnson & White, 1989). Epidemiological studies have examined levels of THC ($\varnothing$-tetrahydrocannabinol, the active ingredient in cannabis) and levels of alcohol in body fluids of persons involved in traffic accidents. Such studies have shown that cannabis is present in the blood, indicating use within the last few hours, in 7 to 10 per cent of samples (Simpson, 1986; Terhune, Ippolito et al., 1992). One study, using only young male fatalities in California,

found a rate of 37 per cent (Williams, Peat et al., 1985). Thus, there is concern about the accident risk associated with cannabis use.

A complicating factor in the interpretation of these epidemiological data is that approximately 80 per cent of the time, when cannabis is present, alcohol is also present (Simpson, 1986). It is well known that alcohol increases accident risk. The combining of cannabis with alcohol makes it difficult to determine, from epidemiological studies alone, how much contribution cannabis makes to accident risk.

A second complication in data interpretation is that young, socially risk-taking males are overrepresented in accident fatalities. This is the same group who are overrepresented among cannabis users. Therefore, there will be an overrepresentation of cannabis users in accident fatalities whether or not the cannabis actually affects driving.

The complications of interpreting epidemiological studies with respect to cannabis mean that performance studies that look at driving-behavior changes associated with cannabis are particularly important. Performance studies can help determine whether there is merely an association between cannabis use and accident risk or a causal link. Such studies have been carried out by examining the effect of cannabis on laboratory tasks that measure driving-related skills, as well as in driving simulators and actual vehicles. Much work has been done using laboratory tasks (see Moskowitz, 1985 and chapter 4 in this volume for reviews).

This chapter considers only those studies of driving carried out in simulators or on the road. Many of these examine alcohol, as well as marijuana, effects. This is because a great deal is known about alcohol's effects on behavior and on accident risk. Therefore, it is valuable to make comparisons between the effects of marijuana and those of alcohol.

Test Methods

Before starting the chapter, a few words are in order on test methods generally used for a drug and driving study. Subjects are typically recruited from persons who have been licensed for at least three years and who are regular users of cannabis. Giving cannabis to a non-user is ethically unacceptable and also would produce non-representative results of its effects on behavior (just as the effects of alcohol on a non-drinker would result in effects not typical of regular users). Subjects are asked to remain drug-free throughout the experimental period, with the exception of the drug and/or alcohol treatment administered by the experimenter.

Drug treatments are given in a double-blind fashion whereby the person who administers the treatment does not know whether it is an active dose or a placebo. This avoids inadvertently influencing the recipient about his or her behavior by giving clues about what effects to expect from the treatment.

Placebo marijuana is produced by extracting THC from the marijuana leaves. The resulting substance looks and smells like marijuana but has no psychoactive effect.

The marijuana (active or placebo) is usually smoked according to a strict schedule in which the time inhaling, holding the smoke and exhaling are regulated to control the amount of THC taken

in by each subject (and to match the behavior in placebo-exposed subjects). However, because some of the material burns and is not inhaled, it is impossible to be precise about the dose actually received by the subject. Only the dose presented to the subject can be strictly quantified. (See chapter 4 in this volume, as well as Perez-Reyes, 1990 for further discussion of the relationship between received and presented doses when marijuana is smoked.)

Alcohol placebos are usually produced by floating a teaspoon of vodka on top of orange juice. The subject can detect the alcohol odor but the effect of this dose on behavior is essentially a placebo effect only. Unlike the case with marijuana, the alcohol dose received by the subject can be very accurately measured using a breathalyzer or blood sample.

Subjects may be tested for each treatment condition (a within-subjects design) or subjects may be tested on one treatment condition each, with different groups of subjects being compared (a between-groups design). Within-subjects comparisons are better if relatively few treatments are being examined. Because the same group of subjects is used for each treatment condition, one can be more certain that any differences found are due to the different treatments and are not due to differences between subjects. If there are a lot of treatments, a between-groups design must be used to avoid, for example, prolonged experiments and learning effects.

Prior to treatment, subjects are trained using a car or simulator so that they understand the driving tasks to be carried out. During on-road studies, subjects are accompanied by an experimenter who usually has access to the means to stop the vehicle in case of erratic behavior by the subject.

Testing of driving skills may be done using either cars on the road or simulators of varying degrees of sophistication. It is important to realize that both types of studies involve simulations of real driving. Although on-the-road studies would seem to replicate real driving more faithfully, subjects are almost always trained to drive in a particular way, for example, keeping right in the middle of the lane, or are asked to perform tasks not normally part of driving, for example, slalom courses. If subjects are not instructed about the driving tasks, there is a lot of variability in behavior and it is difficult to detect differences between treatment conditions.

In summary, simulator and on-the-road studies have different drawbacks and different advantages. Though they lack realism, simulators have the advantage of allowing dangerous situations to occur, involving both driving situations and the interaction of a drug. To date, simulators used in drug studies have lacked fidelity either in car dynamics or in the visual scene. As we will see, both of these aspects affect results. Both types of study are needed to understand the effects of marijuana on driving.

There are always some inconsistencies in results in a review such as this. Often these can be explained by examining how the research was done: the procedures, number of subjects, type of subjects, doses and so on. Therefore the results of the studies described below are discussed in relation to the methods used. Some of the studies used a very large number of performance measures. In these cases, only those measures which showed significant effects are discussed in detail.

Simulator Studies

The earliest simulator study was by Crancer et al. (1969) who used a simple simulator to compare the treatments of 22 mg of THC (equivalent to 314 mcg THC/kg for a 70-kg subject), alcohol targeted to produce 0.10 per cent blood alcohol content (BAC), and no treatment, on 36 subjects. Although the subjects did use a steering wheel, turn signals, the brake and accelerator, none of these affected the filmed presentation. The use of the accelerator merely changed the speedometer reading.

A 23-minute simulator drive was performed at 1/2 an hour, 2 1/2 hours and 4 hours after the beginning of treatment. The subject was required to maintain the speedometer reading within a particular range depending on whether the film was showing urban streets or highways. The drivers also made appropriate responses when the film required a particular manoeuvre.

Alcohol significantly increased accelerator, brake, signal, speedometer and total errors but only the speedometer measure showed increased errors under marijuana. This increase suggests that the principal effect of marijuana was to reduce the time that subjects spent monitoring the speedometer. Alcohol affected performance up to and including four hours after the beginning of treatment, whereas marijuana affected the first simulator run only.

The lack of marijuana effects may have been due in part to the doses being much smaller than were originally thought. Rafaelsen et al. (1973) reported that other workers who examined the same batch of marijuana suggested the subjects received doses of 3 to 8 mg rather than 22 mg THC.

Rafaelsen et al. (1973), like Crancer and his colleagues, used a driver trainer simulator to examine ingested doses of THC of 8, 12 and 16 mg. (An ingested dose has been estimated to be about 2/3 as effective as the same dose presented by smoking; see Moskowitz, 1973.) An alcohol treatment chosen to produce 0.10 per cent BAC was also tested. The driver trainer was modified to include red and green stop and start lights on the windshield. A rotating drum projected a painted landscape onto the windshield. Both accelerator movement and steering movement produced corresponding changes in the movement of the landscape and thus the apparent movement of the car.

Eight subjects were tested 1.75 hours after cannabis ingestion and 1.25 hours after alcohol ingestion. The simulated drive lasted 10 minutes during which measures of brake time, start time (in response to the red and green lights), number of gear changes and mean speed were collected. The red lights, indicating subjects should stop, came on randomly during the run and stayed on for 10 seconds.

The higher cannabis doses and the alcohol dose significantly increased brake time and start time. One of the subjects on the 12-mg-THC dose passed 8 out of 10 red lights without activating the brake pedal at all. The 16-mg-THC dose also increased start time. The number of gear changes significantly increased with alcohol and tended to decrease, but not significantly so, with cannabis. Neither drug affected mean speed. The authors note that in terms of their behavioral measures, alcohol and cannabis were more similar than different. They also took subjective measures, however, asking subjects for estimates of time and distance. For those measures, cannabis had much more pronounced effects than alcohol.

Two simulator studies carried out in the early 1970s examined the effects of marijuana on risk-taking behavior. Dott (1972) used a continuous belt simulator with model cars. Subjects were required to pass the car in front in the presence of an oncoming car. For some passes, subjects were also signalled that the passing manoeuvre would require a rapid response. Twelve subjects were examined under four treatments: no treatment, and smoked doses of 0, 11.25 and 22.5 mg THC. Under marijuana treatment, subjects more frequently aborted passing manoeuvres when the signal to do so was given. Marijuana increased decision time before passing but in non-emergency situations only. Decision time in emergency situations was not affected. No differences were found between the placebo and the no-treatment conditions.

Ellingstad et al. (1973) also examined risk taking under marijuana and alcohol treatment. There were 6 treatment groups of 16 subjects each: 11.25 and 22.25 mg THC, alcohol doses producing 0.05 per cent and 0.10 per cent BAC and 2 placebo groups of marijuana and non-marijuana users. Subjects saw a filmed presentation of an overtaking manoeuvre, performed in the minimum time necessary. Then they saw a series of film clips showing an oncoming car. Subjects indicated the last point at which a pass could safely be initiated. No actual passes were made.

Subjects on marijuana treatment estimated more time would be required for passing than

subjects on placebo. In addition, they less frequently indicated they would perform an unsafe passing manoeuvre compared to subjects on other treatments. Ellingstad et al. suggest that the reluctance to pass may not be related to a change in risk taking but rather is due to an impairment in time estimation. This would make sense if time available was always underestimated. However, a number of studies have examined time estimation and found impairments in both directions after marijuana treatment (Delong & Levy, 1974).

Moskowitz, Hulbert & McGlothlin (1976) used a full car cab simulator with a filmed presentation to examine the effects of four marijuana treatments: 0, 50, 100 and 200 mcg THC/kg. (For a 70-kg subject, these treatments would be equivalent to 0, 3.5, 7.0 and 14.0 mg THC.) Twenty-three subjects participated, each receiving all four treatments. The subject was required to manipulate the steering wheel in order to follow the contours of the road. Brake and accelerator movements affected the speed of the filmed presentation. In addition to driving, subjects performed a visual-choice reaction-time subsidiary task, requiring an average of 2.5 responses per minute. The drive lasted between 45 and 70 minutes depending on the speed chosen by the drivers.

None of the tracking or car control measures was significantly affected by marijuana. However there were significant increases in initially incorrect responses and reaction time in the subsidiary task.

Moskowitz and his colleagues (1976) carried out a second study using a placebo, 200-mcg/kg dose of THC, and an alcohol dose targeted for 0.075 per cent BAC. Eye movement measures were recorded while subjects drove in the simulator. There was no effect of marijuana on visual search pattern, that is, on the length and the number of fixations. In contrast, alcohol at 0.075 per cent had strong effects, increasing dwell time and reducing the number of glances (Moskowitz, Ziedman & Sharma, 1976).

The results of these early simulator studies showed no significant effects of marijuana on car control. However marijuana did increase decision time, time to start and stop (Rafaelsen, Christup & Bech, 1973) and estimated time needed to overtake (Dott, 1972). Marijuana also impaired monitoring a speedometer display. Risk-taking behavior was reduced after marijuana treatment (Dott, 1972; Ellingstad, McFarling & Struckman, 1973). As will be seen in the simulator studies, the lack of effects on car control found in these earlier studies may have been due to the unrealistic car dynamics in all the simulators.

Smiley et al. (1981) described the first study in which an interactive simulator with accurate car dynamics was used to test marijuana effects. Subjects sat in a cut-down car cab and viewed a life-sized, simplified road scene. Steering, accelerator and brake movements all made appropriate changes in the scene viewed by the driver. In addition to various driving tasks, a visual-choice reaction-time subsidiary task was included to simulate the normal requirement to monitor the visual scene. Subjects saw red and green lights to their left and right sides, which were cancelled using foot pedals.

Three groups of subjects were tested in a mixed between-groups (alcohol), within-subjects (marijuana) design. Each subject received one of the three alcohol treatments: alcohol targeted to produce BAC percentages of 0.0 (15 subjects), 0.05 (15 subjects) or 0.08 (10 subjects), along with each of the three marijuana treatments: 0, 100 and 200 mcg/kg THC. Fifteen minutes after the end of marijuana smoking, subjects drove a 45-minute simulator run.

In contrast to earlier studies, this study did show significant effects of marijuana on car control variables: variability of velocity and lateral position both increased while following curves and while controlling the car in wind gusts. There was increased variability of headway and lateral position while following cars. With the exceptions of increased lane position variability in curves and increased headway variability while following a car, the car control changes were significant at the high dose level only.

In addition to these effects on car control, marijuana was also associated with perceptual changes found in the earlier simulator studies. The

number of correct turnoffs taken decreased (significant for both doses) and reaction time to the subsidiary task increased (significant for the high dose only). Also, in the emergency decision-making task, subjects on the high dose of marijuana crashed into the obstacle on the road significantly more often. Risk taking was reduced under marijuana, as shown by the trend towards increased headways in one of the car following tasks.

In contrast to the within-subjects comparisons used to test the effect of marijuana, alcohol's effects were determined with less-sensitive, between-groups comparisons. Not surprisingly, significant effects were few, and were limited to increased lane position variability.

Subjective measures were taken in an attempt to determine how the administered marijuana treatments compared with the subject's normal use. All subjects were regular users of marijuana (weekly at least). Subjects rated both active marijuana treatments as substantially higher than the doses they normally used. They also estimated they would have smoked the doses over a longer time period than was used in the experiments.

Stein et al. (1983) used a car simulator similar in all important aspects to the one used by Smiley et al. (1981). Again, the visual presentation was sparse but the dynamics were accurate and the simulation was completely interactive. The study used a within-subjects design with 12 male subjects being given each of six treatments. Two levels of alcohol (0 and 0.10 per cent BAC) were tested in combination with three levels of marijuana: 0, 100 and 200 mcg/kg THC (equivalent to 0, 7 and 14 mg THC for a 70-kg subject). Thirty minutes after smoking, subjects completed a 15-minute simulator run.

As in the study by Smiley et al. (1981), subjects performed a variety of tasks. In addition, overall scenario performance was measured in terms of number of speeding tickets (32 "radar" checks were made) and number of crashes (hitting obstacles, exceeding road edges by a full car width).

In terms of overall measures, alcohol was associated with significantly increased accidents and traffic tickets. On individual task measures, alcohol was associated with increased lane deviations, speed variability, response time to signs and errors in sign recognition. In contrast, marijuana was associated with few changes: mean speed dropped, and two measures of steering control style changed significantly.

Stein and his colleagues had subjects rate the "high" obtained with the various alcohol and marijuana treatments. Ratings and comments indicated that both treatments were typical of the subjects' prior experiences. Subjects were not able to clearly differentiate between the low and high doses of marijuana.

The results from these last two simulator studies, where realistic car dynamics were used, suggest that marijuana does affect car control. Most effects were found at the higher, 200-mcg/kg THC dose level. As had been seen in earlier simulator studies, marijuana was associated with delayed response time and more conservative behavior (lower speed, longer headway).

Given the similarity of doses used, and of the equipment used, it is interesting that far fewer effects due to marijuana were found by Stein et al. (1983) than by Smiley et al. (1981). There are two possible reasons for this. The former study tested behavior over a 15-minute period compared to a 45-minute period in the latter study. Also the subsidiary task used by Stein and his colleagues was not a random task. It involved making a number of responses to traffic signs. However the locations of the signs were known to the subject. This was not the case with the subsidiary task used by Smiley and her colleagues. In this task, the signals were randomly presented. And for this task, marijuana was associated with significant impairment.

On-Road Studies

On-road studies of marijuana include both closed-course and city- or highway-traffic studies. Klonoff (1974) carried out a study in which subjects drove both on a closed course and in city traffic. Sixty-four subjects participated (43 males and 21 females) in the closed-course study, and

38 of these were tested on city streets as well. The closed-course study was a between-groups design with three groups of subjects. Treatments were placebo and marijuana containing 4.9 or 8.4 mg THC, which was smoked.

Subjects completed eight types of manoeuvres in the closed-course task. For six of these manoeuvres, the measurement of performance was the number of cones struck. In addition, there was an emergency braking task where braking distance was measured and a risk assessment task, where a subject had to decide whether or not a gap was wide enough for the car to pass through.

Subjects performed 20 trials in blocks of five. The first three blocks were considered learning trials. The second and third block of trials were used to establish an expected score, by means of regression analysis, for the fourth block. Treatments were administered, with the car parked, between blocks three and four. The actual performance on block four was then compared with the expected value, calculated from the regression analysis. Thus, group differences and learning effects were taken into account. A confidence interval was calculated for each expected score. If the actual score did not fall within this interval, this was considered to indicate a significant change. Of the eight tasks, performance was different from that expected for two tasks on the low dose (tunnel and curve) and for five tasks on the high dose (slalom, tunnel 1, tunnel 2, funnel and risk assessment).

In the city street portion of the study, each subject received a placebo in one session, and an active dose in the other session. Half the subjects received an active dose first (either 4.9 or 8.4 mg THC). The treatments were administered one week apart.

After 10 minutes of familiarization with the car, subjects were administered the treatment and they then proceeded to drive in city traffic for approximately 45 minutes. Subjects were told to drive as if they were attempting to pass a driving exam and were scored by a driver examiner. Eleven behavioral components were selected from a standard driving test. These ranged from behavior that appears to be directly related to driving performance, for example, speed and regard for traffic signals, to behaviors that are rather difficult to interpret, for example, co-operation, irritability and posture. Scores on each component were normalized for statistical treatment. Change in either direction from normal was considered impairment. In these terms, the higher marijuana dose was associated with significant impairment while the lower dose was not. In particular there were lower scores on judgment and concentration.

It should be noted that there are a number of serious problems with this method of measuring driver behavior, that is, the use of driver licensing exams. Jones (1978) discusses at length the drawbacks of using such exams, a major one being the lack of correlation between what is measured on the driving test and what is relevant to good driving performance. One could certainly question whether measures of posture and irritability are relevant here. Another problem discussed by Jones is the lack of definition of many measures and the requirement that examiners assess many measures at once. For example, "turning" is a combination of monitoring other traffic, appropriate positioning in the lane and appropriate speed. It is difficult to assess these all at once reliably. Yet driver examiners are called upon to do this. In addition to the use of inappropriate and unreliable measures, this study can also be criticized for assuming that any change from normal indicates impairment. If this must be assumed, then we really do not know what "good" driving performance is.

Hansteen et al. (1976) performed a closed-course study for the Canadian LeDain Commission Inquiry into the Non-Medical Use of Drugs. Sixteen subjects (4 females and 12 males) were each given four treatments: placebo, marijuana containing 21 mcg and 88 mcg/kg THC and alcohol targeted to produce a BAC of 0.07 per cent. Two sets of trials were performed, one immediately after smoking and the other three hours later.

Six, six-minute laps were completed, each involving driving through a 1.8-kilometre course that included both slow forward and backward manoeuvres, and higher speed (40 kmh) straight and curved sections marked out with poles and cones. Subjects were instructed to drive the course as quickly as possible but without hitting cones.

Both the alcohol and the higher dose of marijuana were found to result in poorer car handling performance with significantly more cones being hit under these conditions. Under the higher marijuana dose, driving speed was reduced compared to placebo. The difference was small but consistent. In the second trial, three hours after treatment, differences among conditions were slight.

Thirteen of the 16 subjects who participated had experienced driving after using marijuana or drinking. Seven had driven feeling as "high" as after the high dose of marijuana, 11 felt as "high" as after the alcohol dose, suggesting the high marijuana dose was relatively higher in terms of social use than the alcohol dose.

Casswell (1977) examined marijuana and alcohol effects on driving in a closed-course test. Compared to the two earlier closed-course studies, this study sampled tasks more typical of normal driving. These included overtaking, driving on straight roads, a hairpin bend, driving through narrow gaps, response to road signs and response to traffic signals. In addition, subjects performed a subsidiary task requiring response to auditory signals to simulate the demands for monitoring the environment. This is important in closed-course studies, where, for safety reasons, other traffic and pedestrians are usually non-existent. It is also important to assess changes in the driver's ability to monitor the environment. Any increase in inattention due to drug effects is serious. A sizeable number of accidents are associated with inattention (Treat, Tumbas et al., 1977).

During each of three sessions, the 13 male subjects received alcohol and marijuana treatments twice and drove for 35 minutes after each treatment. In session 1, subjects were tested after alcohol at 0.10 per cent BAC, and again after receiving 6.25 mg THC. In session 2, subjects drove after placebo alcohol and placebo marijuana, and again after receiving 6.25 mg THC. In session 3, subjects drove after receiving alcohol at 0.05 per cent BAC and 3.12 mg THC, and again after a repeat of this alcohol and marijuana treatment.

After alcohol treatment, and after combined alcohol and marijuana treatments, fine steering wheel reversals decreased from the placebo level. This change was associated with poorer tracking performance, as indicated by increased variability of lateral position (obtained from visual recording). Mean speed on the straight and around the hairpin bend increased after these treatments (significantly so for the alcohol alone and the combined low doses of alcohol and marijuana). Mean speed through the narrow gap increased significantly after the alcohol alone treatment only. Marijuana alone was not associated with any changes in lateral positioning measures or steering measures. Mean speed dropped significantly, however, both on the straight portions of the course and on the hairpin bend.

Reaction times to auditory signals showed significant increases following marijuana alone or after combination doses where alcohol was at the high dose level. Responses following alcohol alone or the low combination dose were slowed but not significantly so.

All subjects regularly drove after marijuana and alcohol use. They rated the marijuana as a higher dose relative to their past use than was the alcohol dose. Also, after marijuana alone, or after marijuana in combination with the higher level of alcohol, subjects were significantly less prepared to drive than after other treatments. Ratings of willingness to drive following the combination of low-dose marijuana and low-dose alcohol or alcohol alone were not significantly different from placebo.

The author suggested that drivers under the influence of marijuana appeared to compensate for what they perceived as adverse effects on driving ability by driving more slowly and thus reducing the rate of information processing required. Casswell does point out, however, that the increase in subsidiary task reaction time was similar in size to that measured after eight hours of continuous driving in an earlier study and could presumably increase the probability of crashes occurring. Alcohol effects differed in that speeds increased and control effort decreased, resulting in poorer tracking performance.

Attwood et al. (1981) performed a closed-course study, similar to Casswell's study in the use of normal driving tasks, but with doses of marijuana approximately double those used by Casswell. The study used a within-subjects design with eight male subjects being given each of four treatments: (1) double placebo; (2) placebo marijuana, alcohol producing 0.08 per cent BAC; (3) marijuana containing 200 mcg/kg THC, placebo alcohol; and (4) marijuana containing 100 mcg/kg THC, alcohol producing 0.04 per cent BAC.

The driving tasks were: velocity maintenance at 60 kmh and at 80 kmh along a 2-kilometre runway, following a lead car that was varying in speed, making a smooth stop on the occasion of a green light in the car changing to red, and overtaking in the face of an oncoming car. Though the experiment was performed on a closed course with little to distract the subjects, no subsidiary task was used to help simulate the usual demands on the subject to monitor the roadway environment for other traffic.

Many measures were taken during these tasks, of speed, lateral position, acceleration and headway. However, the number of significant comparisons was small, no more than would be expected by chance. Discriminant analysis, however, showed that the various treatment groups could be distinguished from one another. One must conclude that differences were not very robust, if it was possible to find them only using such methods. Possible explanations for the lack of findings are the low number of subjects (eight) and the lack of a subsidiary task which increases the need for the subject to divide attention between monitoring and car control.

Peck et al. (1986) examined the effects of alcohol and marijuana on closed-course driving. A between-groups design was used with 21 subjects in each of four treatment groups. Two levels of alcohol (0 and 0.08 per cent BAC) were tested in combination with two levels of marijuana, 0 and 19 mg (equivalent to 270 mcg/kg THC).

Each subject performed a training run, a baseline run and then, following treatment, four additional runs, the last one of which was four hours after treatment. Each run took approximately 12 minutes.

Including the various ratings, field-sobriety tests and observer measures of car control, 72 measures were made. Marijuana treatment was associated with a significant underestimation of speed with the speedometer covered and lower estimates of the speed at which the driver expected to be able to traverse the slalom course. An interesting measure obtained in this study was the rating of impairment by a California Highway Patrol Officer who followed each subject through the course. The percentage of drivers the officer would have stopped to check for impairment was recorded. Subjects on placebo would have been stopped about 15 per cent of the time, subjects on marijuana about 32 per cent of the time, subjects on alcohol about 50 per cent of the time, and subjects on the combined dose about 60 per cent of the time. (These percentages are much higher than would be anticipated in real life — the officer knew beforehand that some of the subjects would be impaired by alcohol and marijuana. Thus, he had a high expectation of seeing impaired drivers.)

Two objective measures showed significant effects associated with marijuana treatment. Subjects touched fewer cones in the slalom course (they drove more slowly) and when asked to drive a particular speed with the speedometer covered, drove faster than that speed. Both the subjective and objective measures affected by marijuana were also significantly affected by the alcohol treatment and by the combined alcohol and marijuana treatment. The direction of impairment was the same except that more rather than fewer cones were touched in the slalom. At four hours after the initial treatment, only the combination dose of alcohol and marijuana was associated with significant effects on performance.

Smiley et al. (1986) examined the effects of marijuana alone, and combined with alcohol, on driving an instrumented car in a closed-course study. The alcohol and marijuana treatments were administered to groups of subjects over a three-hour period in a partylike atmosphere in the evening. The aim of the experimenters was to test marijuana and alcohol effects in as realistic a setting as possible. Both extended consumption and fatigue at the end of the day may exacerbate effects of marijuana and alcohol use.

Three levels of marijuana, (0, 100 and 200 mcg/kg THC) were tested in combination with two levels of alcohol (0 and 0.05 per cent BAC). In addition, alcohol alone targeted for 0.08 per cent BAC was tested. The study was a between-groups design comparing 7 groups of 9 subjects. Subjects were males (21 to 30 years of age), who were moderate users of marijuana and alcohol. After training, evening and morning-after baseline runs were recorded. A few days later, subjects returned for a treatment run in the evening and a morning-after run.

Twenty-two measures of performance were recorded by the instrumented car during a number of driving tasks that were selected as being representative of normal driving and included situations found to be associated with alcohol- and drug-involved collisions. Throughout the run, subjects also performed a secondary task requiring visual monitoring.

Compared to placebo, the high dose of marijuana significantly increased headway (by a mean of 6 metres) in a car-following task. Standard deviation of headway was also highest for the high dose of marijuana. Alcohol at the 0.05 per cent BAC level was associated with significantly higher velocity on a section of road where subjects had some leeway in choosing their speed and, in particular, higher velocity on curved sections of that roadway. Number of subsidiary task detections decreased at the 0.05 per cent BAC but increased at the 0.08 per cent BAC level. Unfortunately, lane-tracking data were unavailable and it is not possible to say whether subjects at the 0.08 per cent BAC level were paying more attention to the subsidiary task than to the tracking task, resulting in this unexpected better performance.

Subjects were asked to rate the marijuana doses they received subjectively in comparison with their normal self-administered doses. On average, they reported themselves as being less "stoned" on the lower dose but more "stoned" on the high dose compared to their normal usage. Subjects used marijuana at least once every two weeks and at most, once daily.

The most ambitious testing of marijuana effects on actual driving to date is a study which was sponsored by the U.S. National Highway Traffic Safety Administration and carried out in the Netherlands (Robbe & O'Hanlon, 1993). This study involved both public highway and city driving using doses normally used by the subjects involved.

An initial pilot study was run to determine the doses to be used in the main study by having subjects smoke marijuana until they reached the desired "high." All 24 subjects (12 male, 12 female) were current users of marijuana and admitted having driven within one hour after smoking marijuana during the previous year. The only restriction on the smoking was that subjects had to smoke continuously and for a period not exceeding 15 minutes. Doses consumed varied from 11 to 35 mg THC. For males, the mean dose was 22.3 mg and for females, 19.4 mg (or 324 and 293 mcg/kg THC). The highest dose used in the main study was then selected based on these results and was 300 mcg/kg bodyweight. The subjects who participated in the pilot study also took part in the main study.

Selecting a dose level by using levels selected by subjects is to be commended. We know a great deal about how much alcohol drinkers consume. We know very little about typical doses of marijuana users. Thus the pilot study makes a valuable contribution to this knowledge.

The second phase of the study involved driving in an instrumented vehicle at night on a divided highway closed to other traffic. One objective of this study was to determine the safety of carrying out subsequent studies on the open road. Four treatments of 0, 100, 200 and 300 mcg/kg were administered on separate occasions in a counterbalanced order to the same 24 subjects who had participated in the previous pilot study. Subjects were asked to maintain a steady speed of 90 kmh and to maintain a constant lane position over a distance of 22 kilometres. The test began 40 minutes after initiation of smoking and was repeated one hour later. Subjects were accompanied by a driving instructor.

The authors report that "all subjects were willing and able to finish the driving tests without great difficulty." All three marijuana doses were found to increase lane position variability. Effects persisted at the same level in the second test, although subjective "high" had declined. Given the demonstrated safety of the situation, the second study was conducted on a public highway, with 16 new subjects participating. The speed and lane maintenance task was repeated as in the first study, except that subjects were asked to maintain a speed of 95 kmh and pass slower vehicles when it was safe to do so over a 64-kilometre route. In addition, subjects carried out a car-following task, requiring them to maintain a constant headway behind a car whose speed was varying. This task was performed on a 16-kilometre segment of highway. In order to be absolutely sure of the safety of the situation, subjects drove first at the 100-mcg/kg THC dose, followed by the 200-mcg, and then the 300-mcg. In each case, a placebo run was carried out in half the subjects before the active dose run and half after. Results for each dose level were compared to the related placebo run.

In the public highway study, significant increases in lane position were found at the 200- and 300-mcg doses. Speed decreased after the marijuana treatments, in comparison with placebo, but effects were significant for the 200-mcg dose only. Standard deviations of speed and steering movements were unaffected by the treatments. With respect to the lead car-following task, significant and dose-related increases in headway were found after each of the three active doses. The lowest dose of marijuana, which was the first active dose experienced by the subjects, showed the largest effect.

Since O'Hanlon and his colleagues have carried out many studies of drug effects using the same highway driving tasks and headway variability, there exists the potential for comparing marijuana effects with those of other drugs, where equivalent behavior was examined. The one concern that might be raised about the methods used in these studies is that no measure is taken of monitoring ability while subjects are driving. Without such a measure we do not know whether subjects' abilities to respond to an unexpected event are affected.

The third study involved driving a 17.5-kilometre route on city streets. Here, the low dose of marijuana (100 mcg/kg THC) was compared with a low dose of alcohol (0.04 per cent BAC). Driving performance was assessed on one trial by a driving instructor according to a standard licensing test. In this test, the instructor made the rating on a number of items at the end of the test. In a second trial, a test adopted from Jones (1978) was used. In this case the observer attends to only one event and measure at a time and makes the rating immediately after the task is performed.

Only the first type of observer rating showed significant effects. Observer ratings showed that marijuana at 100 mcg/kg THC did not impair performance, although subjects rated their driving as being impaired. In contrast, observer ratings showed that alcohol at 0.04 per cent BAC impaired performance, but subjects did not perceive themselves as being impaired.

Discussion

The simulator and on-road studies reviewed have examined a wide range of tasks and dose levels of both marijuana and alcohol. The measures of driving performance can be categorized as follows: lane position control, speed control, risk-taking behavior, response to subsidiary tasks and other perceptual tasks. From these studies, the effects of alcohol and marijuana appear to show consistently different patterns.

Lane Position Control

The effects of marijuana on lane position control were variable (see Table 1). There were two studies that used simulators with accurate car dynamics. In one, 200 mcg/kg THC was associated with significantly poorer lane position variability in all four tasks in which it was measured; the 100-mcg/kg THC dose was associated with impairment on only the most sensitive of those

---

TABLE 1.

Marijuana and Alcohol Effects on Lane Control and Mean Speed

| Marijuana | | Alcohol | | |
Lane control	Speed	Lane control	Speed	Reference
				Simulator
*	–	*	–	Smiley, Moskowitz & Zeidman, 1981
–	*(–)	*	–	Stein, Allen et al., 1983
				On-Road
*	–	n/a	n/a	Klonoff, 1974
*	*(–)	*	–	Hansteen, Miller & Lonero, 1976
–	*(–)	*	*(+)	Casswell, 1977
				Attwood, Williams et al., 1977
–	–	*	–	Peck, Biasotti et al., 1986
n/a	–	n/a	*(+)	Smiley, Noy & Tostowaryk, 1986
*	–	n/a	n/a	Robbe & O'Hanlon, 1993 (1)
*	–	n/a	n/a	Robbe & O'Hanlon, 1993 (2)

Note: * significant at least at $p < 0.05$.
Dashes indicate variable not significant; all lane position changes with the exception of Peck, Biasotti et al. were in a negative direction; (–), (+) indicate direction of speed change; n/a indicates variable not measured.

tasks, curve following (Smiley, Moskowitz & Zeidman, 1981).

In contrast, the exact same doses did not produce significant impairment of lane position control in the Stein et al. (1983) study. This may be because there was a significant reduction in speed under marijuana treatment in the second study that may have allowed those subjects to maintain lane position control at the placebo level. In addition the subsidiary task used by Stein et al. (1983), in contrast to that used by Smiley et al. (1981), did not create a true divided-attention situation since the position of occurrence of the task was known.

Both studies were in agreement in finding significant effects of alcohol on lane position control. With respect to comparisons of the degree of effect of marijuana and alcohol, the Stein et al. (1983) study should be used. Here all subjects received all treatment conditions. Therefore, within-subjects comparisons are made. In contrast, Smiley et al. (1981) used a mixed design study, appropriate for comparing effects of various levels of marijuana and for looking at alcohol-marijuana interactions, but not designed for making direct comparisons of alcohol alone and marijuana alone effects.

In some on-road studies, lane position control was measured in terms of cones hit (Hansteen, Miller & Lonero, 1976; Klonoff, 1974; Peck, Biasotti et al., 1986). In the Klonoff and Hansteen et al. studies, marijuana was found to increase the number of cones hit significantly; in the Peck et al. study, the number of cones hit declined. The Hansteen and the Peck studies measured alcohol effects and found a significant increase in cones hit.

A number of on-road studies required lane position control more typical of normal driving. Casswell (1977) found impairment in lane control at 0.10 per cent BAC but not for marijuana doses equivalent to 90 mcg/kg THC. Attwood et al. (1981) found that neither the alcohol nor the marijuana treatment increased lane position variability. Casswell used a subsidiary task to divide attention; Attwood and his colleagues did not. In two studies of highway driving involving more

subjects than Attwood et al. (16 and 24 versus 8) and a more precise measurement of lane tracking than Casswell, Robbe and O'Hanlon (1993) found significant increases in lane position variability for marijuana doses of 100, 200 and 300 mcg/kg THC.

Speed Control

In four out of eight studies when speed was measured, marijuana was associated with a decrease in speed (see Table 1). This is despite the fact that in all of these studies, subjects were requested to maintain a particular speed. Where marijuana and alcohol were compared, alcohol more consistently impaired lane position control than did marijuana. This is likely related to the tendency for alcohol to be associated with speed increases, making lane position control more difficult.

Risk-taking Behavior

Changes in speed are a manifestation of the differences in risk-taking behavior that are associated with alcohol and marijuana treatment. Two simulator studies (Dott, 1972; Ellingstad, McFarling & Struckman, 1973), found subjects on marijuana treatment were less likely to engage in overtaking manoeuvres. The second study showed that alcohol was associated with the opposite effect.

Smiley et al. (1981; 1986) found that headway increased in a car-following task, both in a simulator and on the road, also indicating less risky behavior under marijuana treatment. In the study of public highway driving, Robbe and O'Hanlon (1993) found significant increases in headway, but the size of the effect diminished with each run.

In a study of urban driving behavior, observer ratings showed that marijuana at 100 mcg/kg THC did not impair performance, although subjects rated their driving as being impaired. In contrast, observer ratings showed that alcohol at 0.04 per cent BAC impaired performance, but subjects did not perceive themselves as being impaired.

In summary, in terms of car control measures, marijuana appears to induce more conservative behavior, that is lower speeds, in order to offset the effects of feeling impaired. In contrast, alcohol appeared to induce higher speeds, that is, more risky behavior.

Emergency Decision Making

The ability to make decisions in an emergency was tested in four studies. Dott (1972) found marijuana increased decision time for passing but not when it had been indicated subjects must respond quickly. Rafaelsen et al. (1973) found a dose equivalent to approximately 150 mcg/kg smoked THC and a 0.10 per cent BAC dose were associated with significantly increased time for braking when a green light in the car suddenly changed to red. Smiley et al. (1981) found subjects on the 200-mcg/kg THC dose crashed into an obstacle which suddenly appeared in the road more frequently than when on placebo.

In an on-road study, Smiley et al. (1986) examined the response to a task in which subjects approached an array of vertical tubes. The tubes dropped suddenly, either blocking the subject's path entirely or allowing him to go to the left or the right. Neither the marijuana nor the alcohol treatment had any effect on this task.

In summary, it appears that when subjects on marijuana treatment are given some warning when they must respond (as in Dott, 1972) or know where they will have to respond (as in Smiley, Noy & Tostowaryk, 1986), they can gather their resources and make the correct response. However, when a response is called for unexpectedly (as in Rafaelsen, Christup & Bech, 1973; Smiley, Moskowitz & Zeidman, 1981), behavior is impaired.

TABLE 2.

Marijuana and Alcohol Effects on Subsidiary Task Performance

Marijuana	Alcohol	
		Simulator
*	*	Crancer, Dille et al., 1969
*	n/a	Moskowitz, Hulbert & McGlothlin, 1976
*	–	Smiley, Moskowitz & Zeidman, 1981
–	*	Stein, Allen et al., 1983
		On-Road
*	–	Casswell, 1977
–	*[1]	Smiley, Noy & Tostowaryk, 1986

Note: [1] Significant increase for BAC of 0.05% (n = 27); significant decrease for BAC of 0.08% (n = 9).
* Significant impairment at least at $p < 0.05$.

Subsidiary Task Performance

As noted earlier, drug effects on subsidiary task measures are important because they indicate how well the driver is likely to monitor other traffic and whether the risk of an accident due to inattention is increased. Table 2 shows a summary of results from studies using subsidiary tasks.

For two simulator studies (Moskowitz, Hulbert & McGlothlin, 1976; Smiley, Moskowitz & Zeidman, 1981), the subsidiary task was a visual-choice reaction-time task using red and green lights. Stein et al. (1983) used a sign detection task where 16 signs were randomly presented at four locations during the tracking tasks. In a simulator study, Crancer et al. (1969) required subjects to monitor a speedometer continuously. In on-road studies, Casswell (1977) used an auditory reaction-time task and Smiley et al. (1986) used a visual recognition choice reaction-time task where subjects had to distinguish, from a hood-monitored display, the profiles of cars pointing across the road or away from the car.

In two simulator studies, marijuana was associated with a significant dose-related increase in mean reaction time (Moskowitz, Hulbert & McGlothlin, 1976; Smiley, Moskowitz & Zeidman, 1981) and in the number of initially incorrect responses (Smiley, Moskowitz & Zeidman, 1981). In contrast, Stein et al. (1983)

found no effect of marijuana on a subsidiary sign detection task. One reason for this may have been that subjects knew when the signs would appear (though not which one) and were able to prepare themselves to respond. Crancer et al. (1969) found marijuana to be associated with poorer monitoring of a speedometer.

In one on-road study, mean reaction time to the subsidiary task increased on the marijuana treatment by a similar amount to that found to occur after eight hours driving (Casswell, 1977). In a second on-road study (Smiley, Noy & Tostowaryk, 1986), marijuana did not have a significant effect on the subsidiary task. In this study, the 0.05 per cent BAC treatment but not the 0.08 per cent BAC treatment was associated with decreased number of detections.

In summary, four out of six studies showed marijuana impairment of subsidiary monitoring tasks.

Extended Effects

Five studies, one simulator and four on-road studies, looked at extended effects of marijuana and alcohol. The results are summarized in Table 3. The only one of these five studies that showed

any effects of marijuana on driving performance after the initial test was the study by Robbe and O'Hanlon (1993) showing effects of the run one hour after treatment to be as strong as the effects found immediately after treatment. This study used the highest dose, 300 mcg/kg, of any of the studies reported in this review. Three of the studies showed alcohol-alone effects on driving for extended time periods (four hours: Crancer, Dille et al., 1969; three hours: Hansteen, Miller & Lonero, 1976; eight hours: Smiley, Noy & Tostowaryk, 1986). One of the two studies that looked at alcohol and marijuana combination effects found significant effects four hours after treatment (Peck, Biasotti et al., 1986). Smiley et al. (1986) found significantly slower speed after the high dose of alcohol (0.08 BAC) the morning after consumption (eight hours later).

Subjective Measures of Treatment Doses

In a number of studies, subjects were asked to rate the treatment doses (Casswell, 1977; Hansteen, Miller & Lonero, 1976; Smiley, Moskowitz & Zeidman, 1981; Smiley, Noy & Tostowaryk, 1986; Stein, Allen et al., 1983). The Hansteen et

TABLE 3.
Extended Effects of Alcohol and Marijuana

Hours after treatment	Marijuana/Alcohol (highest doses tested)	Treatment effects	Reference
4	314 mcg/kg	–	Crancer, Dille et al., 1969
	0.10% BAC	*	
3	88 mcg/kg	–	Hansteen, Miller & Lonero, 1976
	0.07% BAC	*	
4	270 mcg/kg	–	Peck, Biasotti et al., 1986
	0.10% BAC	–	
	270 mcg + 0.10%	*	
1	300 mcg /kg	*	Robbe & O'Hanlon, 1993
8	200 mcg /kg	–	Smiley, Noy & Tostowaryk, 1986
	0.08% BAC	*	
	200 mcg + 0.05%	–	

*significant impairment at $p < 0.05$ or better

al. and the Casswell studies found the dose levels used (approximately 90 mcg/kg bodyweight) were higher than subjects' normal use. Stein et al. (1983) found 100 and 200 mcg/kg to be typical of normal use. Smiley et al. (1981; 1986) using the same dose levels, found subjects on average rated the higher dose as making them more "stoned" than they were used to. Subjects in all these studies were regular marijuana users. These subjective ratings indicate the treatment doses in the earlier studies were, if anything, slightly higher than what subjects normally used.

Only one study, the most recent, has looked at self-selected dose levels. Mean dose consumed was 308 mcg/kg THC, higher than those used in earlier studies (Robbe & O'Hanlon, 1993).

Marijuana versus Alcohol Comparisons

Six simulator and six on-road studies included alcohol treatments and allowed comparisons to be made between driving performance changes due to marijuana and those due to alcohol. With respect to lane position control, impairment was found both for marijuana and for alcohol. Where speed was significantly affected by treatment, it decreased for marijuana but increased for alcohol. Both substances impaired response time to subsidiary tasks. Besides reductions in mean speed, there were other indications of reduced risk taking for subjects on marijuana treatments — increased headways when following other cars and fewer unsafe passes. One study of visual search patterns showed no change after marijuana treatment, but increased dwell time and decreased numbers of eye movements on alcohol treatment.

Studies by O'Hanlon and his colleagues, carried out with large subject groups (16 or more) allowed comparisons of a number of marijuana (Robbe & O'Hanlon, 1993) and alcohol (Louwerens, Gloerich et al., 1985; 1987) levels examined in different studies using the same methodology. For lane control, impairment associated with marijuana at 100 mcg/kg THC was equivalent to a BAC level of 0.03 to 0.05 per cent; at 200 mcg/kg THC, approximately 0.06 per

cent; and at 300 mcg/kg THC, 0.05 to 0.07 per cent. Two caveats must be kept in mind. First, ability to control lane position is associated with speed, which in turn tends to decrease after marijuana treatment and to increase after alcohol treatment. Second, these results only relate to lane control. The equivalence is different for other tasks. For example, Moskowitz et al. (1976) found that a 200-mcg/kg dose of THC showed no effect on visual search patterns in simulated driving. In contrast, alcohol at 0.075 per cent had strong effects, increasing dwell time and reducing the number of glances. In an urban driving study, marijuana at 100 mcg/kg THC was not associated with observable driving impairment, whereas alcohol at 0.04 per cent was (Robbe & O'Hanlon, 1993). In a study on a closed track, Casswell (1977) found marijuana equivalent to about 90 mcg/kg THC significantly increased reaction time to an auditory detection task performed while driving, whereas alcohol at levels up to 0.10 per cent BAC had no significant effects.

Extended effects were found for marijuana alone, for alcohol alone and for combined alcohol and marijuana treatments. The effects of alcohol persisted longer than those of marijuana, the latter being found for one hour after treatment only after the highest dose tested in any study. The subjective measures of treatment doses suggest that the marijuana treatments used have been relatively higher than the alcohol treatments used. In light of this, and in light of the comparisons between treatment effects, it would appear that, while both marijuana and alcohol individually impair driver performance, marijuana leads to decreased risk taking while alcohol has the opposite effect. The combination of alcohol and marijuana is more impairing than either substance taken alone.

Conclusion

In conclusion, marijuana impairs driving behavior. However, this impairment is mitigated in that subjects under marijuana treatment appear to perceive that they are indeed impaired. Where they can compensate, they do, for example by not overtaking, by slowing down and by focusing their attention when they know a response will be required. Such compensation is not possible, however, where events are unexpected or where continuous attention is required. Effects on driving behavior are present up to an hour after smoking but do not continue for extended periods.

With respect to comparisons between alcohol and marijuana effects, these substances tend to differ in their effects. In contrast to the compensatory behavior exhibited by subjects under marijuana treatment, subjects who have received alcohol tend to drive in a more risky manner. Both substances impair performance; however, the more cautious behavior of subjects who have received marijuana decreases the impact of the drug on performance, whereas the opposite holds true for alcohol.

Acknowledgments

This article is an updated and revised version of an article that was published by the same author in 1986 in *Alcohol, Drugs and Driving, Abstracts and Reviews,* published by the Alcohol Information Service, Neuropsychiatric Institute, University of California, Los Angeles.

References

Attwood, D., Williams, R., McBurney, L. & Frecker, R. (1981). Cannabis, alcohol and driving: Effects on selected closed course tasks. *Alcohol, Drugs, and Traffic Safety, 3,* 938–953.

Casswell, S. (1977). Cannabis and alcohol: Effects on closed course driving behaviour. In I. Johnson (Ed.), *Seventh International Conference on Alcohol, Drugs, and Traffic Safety, Melbourne, Australia* (pp. 238–246).

Crancer, A.J., Dille, J.M., Delay, J.C., Wallace, J.E. & Haken, M. (1969). Comparison of the effects of marijuana and alcohol on simulated driving performance. *Science, 164,* 851–854.

Delong, F.L. & Levy, B.I. (1974). A model of attention describing the cognitive effects of marijuana. In L.L. Miller, (Ed.), *Marijuana, Effects on Human Behaviour* (pp. 103–117). New York: Academic Press.

Dott, A.B. (1972). *Effect of marijuana on risk acceptance in a simulated passing task* (Public Health Service Report ICRL-RR-71-3, DHEW Publication No. HSM-72-10010). Washington, DC: U.S. Government Printing Office.

Ellingstad, V.S., McFarling, L.H. & Struckman, D.L. (1973). *Alcohol, marijuana and risk taking.* Vermillion, SD: South Dakota University, Vermillion Human Factors Laboratory.

Hansteen, R.W., Miller, R.D. & Lonero, L. (1976). Effects of cannabis and alcohol on automobile driving and psychomotor tracking. *Annals of the New York Academy of Science, 282,* 240–256.

Health Canada, (1995). *Canada's Alcohol and Other Drug Survey.* Ottawa: Ministry of Supply and Services, Canada.

Johnson, V. & White, H.R. (1989). An investigation of factors related to intoxicated driving behaviors among youth. *Journal of Studies on Alcohol, 50,* 320–330.

Jones, M.H. (1978). *Safe Performance Curriculum* (Final Report No. DOT-HS-461). Los Angeles: University of Southern California, Performance Measures.

Klonoff. H. (1974). Marijuana and driving in real-life situations. *Science, 186*, 317–324.

Louwerens, J.W., Gloerich, A.B.M., De Vries, G., Brookhuis, K.A. & O'Hanlon, J.F. (1985). *De Invloed van Verschillende Bloedalcoholspiegels op Objectief Meetbare Aspekten van Feitelijk Rijgedrag* (Technical Report No. VK 85-03). University of Groningen, Traffic Research Centre. In H.W.J. Robbe & J.F. O'Hanlon (Eds.), *Marijuana and Actual Driving Performance* (National Highway Traffic Safety Administration Final Report No. DOT-HS-808078, November, 1993). U.S. Department of Transportation.

Louwerens, J.W., Gloerich, A.B.M., De Vries, G., Brookhuis, K.A. & O'Hanlon, J.F. (1987). The relationship between drivers' blood alcohol concentration (BAC) and actual driving performance during high speed travel. In P.C. Noordzij (Ed.), *Proceedings of the 10th International Conference on Alcohol, Drugs, and Traffic Safety* (pp. 183–186). Amsterdam: Elsevier.

Moskowitz, H. (1973, September). A marijuana dose response study of performance in a driving simulator. Paper presented at the First International Conference on Driver Behaviour in Zurich, Switzerland.

Moskowitz, H. (1985). Marijuana and driving. *Accident Analysis and Prevention, 17*, 323–345.

Moskowitz, H., Hulbert, S. & McGlothlin, W. (1976). Marijuana: Effects on simulated driving performance. *Accident Analysis and Prevention, 8*, 45–50.

Moskowitz, H., Ziedman, K. & Sharma, S. (1976). Visual search behavior while viewing driving scenes under the influence of alcohol and marijuana. *Human Factors, 18*, 417–432.

Peck, R.C., Biasotti, A., Boland, P.N., Mallory, C. & Reeve, V. (1986). The effects of marijuana and alcohol on actual driving performance. *Alcohol, Drugs and Driving: Abstracts and Reviews, 2* (3–4), 135–154.

Perez-Reyes, M. (1990). Marijuana smoking: Factors that influence the bioavailability of tetrahydrocannabinol. In C.N. Chiang & R.L. Hawks (Eds.), *Research Findings on Smoking of Abused Substances* (NIDA Research Monograph No. 99, pp. 42–62). Rockville, MD: National Institute on Drug Abuse.

Rafaelsen, L., Christup, H. & Bech, P. (1973). Effects of cannabis and alcohol on psychological tests. *Nature, 242*, 117–118.

Robbe, H.W.J. & O'Hanlon, J.F. (1993). *Marijuana and Actual Driving Performance* (National Highway Traffic Safety Administration Final Report No. DOT-HS-808078). U.S. Department of Transportation.

Simpson, H.M. (1986). Epidemiology of road accidents involving marijuana. *Alcohol, Drugs and Driving: Abstracts and Reviews, 2* (3–4), 15–30.

Smiley, A.M., Moskowitz, H. & Zeidman, K. (1981). Driving simulator studies of marijuana alone and in combination with alcohol. *Proceedings of the 25th Conference of the American Association for Automotive Medicine* (pp. 107–116).

Smiley, A.M., Noy, Y.I. & Tostowaryk, W. (1986). The effects of marijuana, alone and in combination with alcohol, on driving an instrumented car. *Proceedings of the 10th International Conference on Alcohol, Drugs, and Traffic Safety, Amsterdam* (pp. 203–206).

Stein, A.C., Allen, R.W., Cook, M.L. & Karl, R.L. (1983). *A Simulator Study of the Combined Effects of Alcohol and Marijuana on Driving Behaviour* (National Highway Traffic Safety Administration Report No. DOT-HS-806405). Hawthorne, CA: Systems Technology Inc.

Terhune, K.W., Ippolito, C.A., Hendricks, D.L., Michalovic, J.G., Bogema, S.C., Santinga, P., Blomberg, R. & Preusser, D.F. (1992). *Incidence and Role of Drugs in Fatally Injured Drivers* (National Highway Traffic Safety Administration Final Report No. DOT-HS-808065).

Treat, J.R., Tumbas, N.S., McDonald, S.T., Shinar, D., Hume, R.D., Mayer, R.E., Stansfin, R.L. & Castellen, N.J. (1977). *Tri-level Study of the Causes of Traffic Accidents* (Report No. DOT-HS-034-3-535-77, TAC). Indiana.

Williams, A.F., Peat, M.A., Crouch, D.J., Wells, J.K. & Finkle, B.S. (1985). Drugs in fatally injured young male drivers. *Public Health Reports, 100* (1), 19–25.

World Health Organization (WHO). (1997). *Cannabis: A Health Perspective and Research Agenda.* Geneva: World Health Organization.

CHAPTER 6

Long-term Effects of Cannabis on the Central Nervous System

Long-term Effects of Cannabis on the Central Nervous System

NADIA SOLOWIJ

I. BRAIN FUNCTION AND NEUROTOXICITY

A major concern about the recreational use of cannabis has been whether it may lead to functional or structural neurotoxicity, or "brain damage" in ordinary language. Fehr and Kalant (1983a, p. 27a) defined neurotoxicity as functional aberrations qualitatively distinct from the characteristic usual pattern of reversible acute and chronic effects, and that may be caused by identified or identifiable neuronal damage. On this definition an enduring impairment of cognitive functioning could be interpreted as a manifestation of neurotoxicity if neuronal damage was also demonstrated. But cognitive deficits may be the end result of secondary changes associated with drug use, as opposed to a direct toxic effect on neurons. A thorough review of the cognitive literature in relation to long-term cannabis use is presented in section II, "Cognitive Functioning." This first section of the chapter will concentrate on direct investigations of neurological function and toxicity arising from exposure to cannabinoids.

A number of terms that have been used interchangeably throughout the literature require

definition and clarification at the outset. Terms frequently used to describe the toxicity of a drug are *acute, subacute* and *chronic*. These terms strictly apply to the duration of the treatment given to experimental animals in a toxicity study. When applied to human research, they refer to the effects that may follow the acute, subacute or chronic use of the drug.

Acute effects often refer to those effects produced by a single dose of a drug and this includes the effects sought after by the user, as well as the short-lived unwanted side effects that are usually associated with higher doses. The duration of the acute effects depends essentially on the dose and the route of administration, but may also depend on the specific drug effect measured and on whether the user is experienced or naive. Subacute effects are those which result from repeated administration over several days; each dose itself does not necessarily produce a detrimental effect, but cumulatively may result in an adverse response.

Chronic effects refer to the consequences of repeated administration of a drug over a prolonged period. Chronic (long-term) effects, while not necessarily permanent, persist beyond the phase of elimination of cannabinoids from the body, and hence are not attributable to a direct (acute) action of cannabinoids. They can be either a result of neuroadaptive mechanisms (such as have been described in the opioid literature; see Cox, 1990), or the result of drug-induced neurotoxicity. In the former case, the effects are self-limiting if no further drug is taken but may be expressed as a "withdrawal" syndrome. In the latter case, the neurotoxicity may be functional or structural, and reversible or irreversible.

This chapter begins with an examination of the evidence for functional neurotoxicity from animal behavioral studies. Neurochemical, electrophysiological and brain substrate investigations of functionality follow, and the chapter concludes with the findings of more invasive examinations of brain structure and morphology in animals, and of less invasive techniques for imaging the human brain.

Animal Behavioral Studies

Animal research provides the ultimate degree of control over extraneous variables; it is possible to eliminate factors known to influence research findings in humans, such as nutritional status, age, sex, previous drug history and concurrent drug use. The results, however, are often difficult to extrapolate to humans because of between-species differences in brain and behavior and in drug dose, patterns of use, routes of administration and methods of assessment. It is beyond the scope of this chapter to cover the vast animal literature, particularly since most animal studies have involved acute administration only. It should be noted, however, that recent studies of that nature are helping to elucidate the actions of cannabinoids in the brain, which will in turn enable a more thorough understanding of its long-term effects (e.g., Hampson, Byrd et al., 1996; Heyser, Hampson & Deadwyler, 1993; Lichtman & Martin, 1996; Sim, Hampson et al., 1996; Terranova, Storme et al., 1996).

Animal research into the effects of cannabis on brain function has typically involved administration of known quantities of cannabinoids to animals for an extended period of time and then examined performance on various tasks assessing brain function, before using histological and morphometric methods to study the brains of the exposed animals. In general, the results of studies with primates produce results that most closely resemble the likely effects in humans; the monkey is physiologically similar to humans, while rats, for example, metabolize drugs in a different way, and monkeys are able to perform complex behavioral tasks. Nevertheless, every animal species examined to date, including the fruit fly, has been found to have cannabinoid receptors in the brain. In animal models, non-targeted staring into space following administration of cannabinoids is suggestive of psychoactivity comparable to that in humans. The most characteristic responses to cannabinoids in animals are mild behavioral aberrations following small doses, and signs of gross neurotoxicity manifested by tremors and convulsions following excessively large doses. Where small doses are given for a prolonged period of time, behavioral evidence of neurotoxicity has emerged (Rosenkrantz, 1983). Chronic exposure produces lethargy, sedation and depression in many species, and/or aggressive irritability in monkeys.

A clear manifestation of neurotoxicity in rats, which has been called the "popcorn reaction" (Luthra, Rosenkrantz & Braude, 1976), is a pattern of sudden vertical jumping in rats exposed to cannabinoids for five weeks or longer. It is also seen in young animals exposed to cannabinoids *in utero* and then given a small-dose challenge at 30 days of age. Several studies of prenatal exposure indicate that the offspring of cannabis-treated animals show small delays in various stages of postnatal development, such as eye opening, various reflexes and open field exploration, although after several weeks or months their development is indistinguishable from normal (e.g., Fried & Charlebois, 1979). This means that either the developmental delay was not chronic, the remaining damage is too subtle to be detected by available measures, or the "plasticity of nervous system organisation in the newborn permitted adequate compensation for the loss of function of any damaged cells" (Fehr & Kalant, 1983a, p. 29).

Behavioral tests in rodents have included conventional and radial-arm maze learning, operant behavior involving time discriminations, open field exploration and two-way shuttle box avoidance learning. Correct performance on these tests is dependent on spatial orientation or on response inhibition, both of which are believed to depend heavily on intact hippocampal functioning and the involvement of prefrontal cortex. Nakamura et al. (1991) used an eight-arm radial maze to measure the effects of acute and chronic THC administration on working memory in the rat. In the investigation of chronic effects, rats were tested 18 hours after each drug administration of 5 mg/kg THC 6 days per week for 90 days. There was gradual deterioration of performance, measured by the number of errors, in delayed memory conditions, but this impairment was reversible only after 30 days of discontinuation of the drug. Some studies have found decreased learning ability on such tasks several months after long-term treatment with cannabinoids (see Fehr & Kalant, 1983b). For example, Stiglick and Kalant (1982a; 1982b) reported altered learning behavior in rats one to six months after a three-month oral-dosing regimen of marijuana extract or $\varnothing$-tetrahydrocannabinol (THC). Both they and Nakamura et al. (1991) claimed that the deficits observed in their studies were reminiscent of behavioral changes seen after damage to the hippocampus. Long-lasting impairment of learning ability and hippocampal dysfunction suggests that long-lasting damage may result from exposure to cannabis. However, some studies have been carried out too soon after the final drug administration to exclude the possibility that the observed effects may still be acute or subacute effects, or may be due to the continued action of accumulated cannabinoids.

Memory function in rats and monkeys has often been assessed by delayed matching-to-sample tasks. A study with rats (Heyser, Hampson & Deadwyler, 1993) found that an acute THC-induced disruption of performance on such a task was similar to that produced by damage to the hippocampus, and was associated with a specific decrease in hippocampal cell discharge only during the encoding phase of the task. The effects were completely reversible within 24 hours of dosing, but this does not rule out the possibility of a neurotoxic effect following repeated or prolonged administration. Continuing studies from this group have shown that THC-induced impairments on a delayed-non-match-to-sample task were the same as those resulting from complete removal of the hippocampus, and further, that these effects were completely blocked by co-administration of the cannabinoid antagonist SR141716A, thus confirming that the disruption in memory processes occurs via cannabinoid receptor-mediated effects on hippocampal neural activity (Hampson, Byrd et al., 1996).

Deadwyler, Heyser and Hampson (1995) showed that initially severe disruption of performance on a delayed-match-to-sample task following administration of 10 mg/kg THC, was completely eliminated after 30 to 35 days of continuous exposure to the drug, thus reflecting tolerance. Withdrawal from the drug temporarily impaired performance, but this resolved within 2 days and no further effects on performance were apparent up to 15 drug-free days later. The authors discussed these results in terms of their consistency with recovery from a hippocampal deficit, and postulated a receptor-coupled biochemical mechanism (this was supported by a study reported by Sim, Hampson et al., 1996; see below). These results should not be taken to imply that there would be no long-term deleterious effects developing gradually over a period of much longer exposure to the drug, and it must be remembered that these rats would have been very well practised at the task.

Research in progress by the same team is using a variety of techniques including selective lesions of hippocampus and cannabinoid treatment and blockade, ensemble (many neuron) recordings, and specific types of error and sequential dependency analyses of delayed-non-match-to-sample performance, in working toward a unified theory of cannabinoid actions on hippocampal ensemble firing, encoding of task-relevant information and receptor-mediated effects (S.A. Deadwyler, personal communication; see also Deadwyler, Bunn & Hampson, 1996; Deadwyler, Byrd et al., 1996; Deadwyler & Hampson, 1997; Deadwyler, Heyser & Hampson, 1995; Hampson & Deadwyler, 1996a; 1996b; Hampson, Byrd et al., 1996). Essentially, the data suggest that cannabinoids make the animal susceptible to proactive interference from prior trials, an interference effect so enhanced that what is sample on one trial and what was non-match on the last trial are confused and not decipherable after several trials. Thus, in the short term, exogenously administered cannabinoids affect delayed-match and non-match-to-sample performance in the same manner as a hippocampal lesion: they operate to screen out relevant "to-be-remembered" information at an inappropriate time (during the sample phase) rather than at the appropriate time (during the intertrial interval) to reduce proactive interference (S.A. Deadwyler, personal communication).

Other studies have provided evidence that cannabinoids impair working memory through a cannabinoid receptor mechanism: Lichtman, Dimen and Martin (1995) reported that intracerebral administration of cannabinoids such as CP-55,940 into the cannabinoid receptor-rich hippocampus disrupted working memory in the radial-arm maze task. Lichtman and Martin (1996) argued that more compelling support for receptor-mediated THC-induced memory impairment would be provided by the reversal of such impairment by a cannabinoid antagonist. Previously, Collins, Pertwee and Davies (1995) had shown that the inhibitory effects of the potent cannabinoid HU-210 on long-term potentiation in the rat hippocampus, a neural model for a cellular substrate underlying learning or memory processes, were blocked by SR141716A. Lichtman and Martin (1996) were able to show that SR141716A in a dose-dependent manner prevented THC-induced impairment of spatial working memory assessed by radial-arm maze performance. Furthermore, Terranova et al. (1996) have demonstrated in rats

and mice actual improvement of short-term working memory and of memory consolidation, and the abolishment of memory disturbance induced by retroactive inhibition or that associated with aging, by the administration of the above antagonist in a dose-dependent fashion in the absence of any pretreatment with cannabinoids. The authors commented that SR141716A did not enhance retrieval, but facilitated the memory processes involved immediately after acquisition and during consolidation. The results of this research suggest that the endogenous cannabinoid system is involved in forgetting and in the memory deterioration associated with aging.

However, it should be noted that this facilitation of memory was partially antagonized by scopolamine, a muscarinic antagonist that impairs memory, which implies a connection between the blockade of cannabinoid receptors and the facilitation of cholinergic transmission (Terranova, Storme et al., 1996). Gifford and Ashby (1996) have suggested that an endogenous substance might inhibit the release of acetylcholine through activation of the cannabinoid receptor (see also Gifford, Samiian et al., 1997). However, Lichtman and Martin (1996) found that SR141716A did not alleviate scopolamine-induced impairment on the radial-arm maze in rats and concluded that cannabinoids and cholinergic drugs do not impair spatial memory through a common serial pathway.

Some recent studies have reported that while THC and several other psychoactive cannabinoids impaired memory function in rats, anandamide failed to do so (Crawley, Corwin et al., 1993; Lichtman, Dimen & Martin, 1995). However, the lack of demonstrable memory impairment following administration of anandamide may be due either to the nature of the tasks employed in different studies, or to its rapid metabolism (Deutsch & Chin, 1993). When rats were pretreated with a protease inhibitor, anandamide dose-dependently impaired working memory in a delayed-non-match-to-sample task (Mallet & Beninger, 1995). The possibility also exists that endogenous ligands other than anandamide may be more specific to cognition, as anandamide may represent one member of a family of endogenous compounds.

In a series of studies described by Slikker and colleagues (1992), rhesus monkeys were trained for one year to perform five operant tasks, and were then started on one year of chronic administration of cannabis. One group was exposed daily to the smoke of one standard joint, another on weekends only and control groups received sham smoke exposure (N = 15 or 16 per group). Performance on the tasks indicated the induction of what the authors referred to as an "amotivational syndrome" during chronic exposure to cannabis, manifested in a decrease in motivation to respond, regardless of whether the monkeys were exposed daily or only on weekends. This led the authors to suggest that motivational problems can occur at relatively low or recreational levels of use (in fact, the effect was maximal with intermittent exposure). Task performance was grossly impaired for more than a week following last exposure, although performance returned to baseline levels two to three months after cessation of use. Thus, the effects of chronic exposure were slowly reversible, leaving no long-term behavioral effects. The authors concluded that persistent exposure to compounds that are very slowly cleared from the brain could account for their results. This hypothesis is consistent with the long half-life of THC in the body.

One of the problems with studies such as these is that animals are often only exposed for a relatively short period of time, for example, one year or less. Slikker and colleagues acknowledge that it remains to be determined whether longer or greater exposures would cause more severe or additional behavioral effects. It may be that chronic dysfunction is manifest only after many years of exposure, as suggested by human research (see section II, "Cognitive Functioning"). Although it is of concern that behavioral impairments have been shown to last for several months after exposure, it is reassuring that they have generally resolved over time.

A further difficulty with animal studies is a consequence of differences between animals and humans in route of cannabinoid administration. In humans the most common route of exposure to THC is via the inhalation of marijuana smoke, whereas most animal studies have relied upon the oral administration or injection of THC because of the difficulty in efficiently delivering smoke to animals and the concern about the complications introduced by carbon monoxide toxicity. While it may well be impossible to evaluate the pharmacological and toxicological consequences of exposure to the hundreds of compounds in cannabis simultaneously, it is arguably inappropriate to assess the long-term consequences of human cannabis smoking by administering THC alone (Abood & Martin, 1992). Hundreds of additional compounds are produced by pyrolysis when marijuana is smoked, which may contribute either to acute effects or to long-term toxicity. Future studies need to address these issues for comparability to human usage. Appropriate controls, including those which mimic the carbon monoxide exposure experienced during the smoking of marijuana, may be necessary.

Neurochemistry

The discovery of the cannabinoid receptor and its endogenous ligand anandamide revolutionized previous conceptions of the mode of action of the cannabinoids. However, much further research is required before the interactions between ingested cannabis, anandamide or other endogenous ligands, and the cannabinoid receptor are fully understood. Nor should the anandamide pathways be seen as responsible for all of the central effects of the psychoactive cannabinoids. There is good evidence that cannabinoids affect the concentration, turnover or release of other endogenous substances (Pertwee, 1988; 1992). Much research has been devoted to examining the interactions between cannabinoids and several neurotransmitter receptor systems (e.g., norepinephrine, dopamine, serotonin, acetylcholine, gamma-aminobutyric acid (GABA), histamine, opioid peptides and prostaglandins) (Pertwee, 1992). The results suggest that all these substances have some role in the neuropharmacology of cannabinoids, although little is known about the precise nature of this involvement. Cannabinoids may alter the activities of neurochemical systems in the central nervous system by altering the synaptic concentrations of these mediators through an effect on their synthesis, storage, release or metabolism, and/or by modulating mediator-receptor interactions. There have been numerous reports of neurotransmitter perturbations *in vitro* and after short-term administration of cannabinoids (for reviews see Dewey, 1986; Martin, 1986; Pertwee, 1988; 1992).

Relatively few studies have examined whether long-term exposure to cannabinoids results in lasting changes in brain neurotransmitter and neuromodulator levels. An early study examined cerebral and cerebellar neurochemical changes accompanying behavioral manifestations of neurotoxicity (involuntary vertical jumping) in rats exposed to marijuana smoke for up to 87 days (Luthra, Rosenkrantz & Braude, 1976). Sex differences emerged in the neurochemical consequences of chronic exposure: in females, acetylcholinesterase showed a cyclic increase and cerebellar enzyme activity declined. For both sexes, cerebellar RNA increased, but at different times for each sex, and at 87 days remained elevated only in females. Some of these neurochemical changes persisted during a 20-day recovery period, but the authors predicted the return to normality after a much longer recovery period. Cannabinoids administered prenatally not only impaired developmental processes in rats, but also produced significant decrements in RNA, DNA and protein concentrations and reductions in dopamine and norepinephrine concentrations in mice, which could be important in the role of protein and nucleic acids in learning and memory (see Fehr & Kalant, 1983b). Bloom (1984) reported that cannabinoids increase the synthesis and turnover of dopamine and norepinephrine in rat and mouse brain while producing little or no change in endogenous steady-state levels of catecholamines, but chronic exposure to cannabi-

noids leads to increased activity of tyrosine hydroxylase in rat brain (Ho, Taylor & Englert, 1973). Mailleux and Vanderhaeghen (1994) demonstrated that THC modulates gene expression of neuropeptides: a three-week treatment with THC significantly increased the messenger RNA levels for substance P and enkephalin in the rat caudate-putamen. The authors reported this as opening the possibility that cannabis abuse might induce long-term effects on the physiology of the brain. These same authors had previously shown that dopamine, glucocorticoids and glutamate regulated cannabinoid receptor gene expression in the caudate-putamen (see Mailleux & Vanderhaeghen, 1994).

Recent evidence suggests, however, that there are few, if any, irreversible effects of THC on known brain chemistry. Ali and colleagues (1989) administered various doses of THC to rats for 90 days and then assessed several brain neurotransmitter systems 24 hours or 2 months after the last drug dose. Examination of dopamine, serotonin, acetylcholine, GABA, benzodiazepine and opioid neurotransmitter systems revealed that no significant changes had occurred. A larger study with both rats and monkeys examined receptor binding of the above neurotransmitters and the tissue levels of monoamines and their metabolites (Ali, Newport et al., 1991). No significant irreversible changes were demonstrated in the rats chronically treated with THC. Monkeys, exposed to chronic treatment with marijuana smoke for one year and then sacrificed after a seven-month recovery period, were found to have no changes in neurotransmitter concentration in frontal cortex, caudate nucleus, hypothalamus or brainstem regions. The authors concluded that there are no significant irreversible alterations in major neuromodulator pathways in the rat and monkey brain following long-term exposure to the active compounds in marijuana.

Slikker et al. (1992), reporting on the same series of studies, noted that there were virtually no differences between placebo, low-dose or high-dose groups of monkeys in blood chemistry values. The general health of the monkeys was unaffected, but the exposure served as a chronic physiological stressor evidenced by increases in urinary cortisol levels that were not subject to tolerance (although plasma cortisol levels did not differ). Urinary cortisol elevation has not been demonstrated in other studies with monkeys. Slikker et al. reported a 50 per cent reduction in circulating testosterone levels in the high-dosed group with a non-significant rebound one to four weeks post cessation of treatment. It is worthy of note that these monkeys were three years of age at the commencement of the study and would have experienced hormonal changes over the course of entering adolescence during the study.

A recent pilot study compared monoamine levels in cerebrospinal fluid (CSF) in a small sample of human cannabis users and age- and sex-matched normal controls (Musselman, Haden et al., 1994). The authors' justification for the study was that THC administered to animals has been shown to produce increases in serotonin and decreases in dopamine activity. No differences were found between the user and non-user groups in the CSF concentrations of homovanillic acid, 5-hydroxyindoleacetic acid, 3-methoxy-4-hydroxyphenylglycol, adrenocorticotropic hormone (ACTH) or corticotropin releasing factor. The authors proposed a number of explanations for these results: (1) cannabis use has no chronic effect on levels of brain monoamines; (2) those who use cannabis have abnormal levels of brain monoamines that are normalized over long periods of time by cannabis use; or (3) those who use cannabis have normal levels of brain monoamines that are transiently altered with cannabis use and then return to normal. There were insufficient data in this study to permit a choice between these hypotheses. The frequency and duration of cannabis use, and the time since last use in the user group could not be determined. All users had denied using cannabis, having been drawn from a larger normative sample and identified as cannabis users by the detection of cannabinoid metabolites in urine screens. Further research is required to assess neurotransmitter levels in human cannabis users properly.

Electrophysiological Effects

Cannabis is clearly capable of causing marked changes in brain electrophysiology as determined by electroencephalographic (EEG) recordings. Long-term abnormalities in EEG tracings from cortex and hippocampus have been shown in cats (Barratt & Adams, 1972; 1973; Domino, 1981; Hockman, Perrin & Kalant, 1971), rats (see Fehr & Kalant, 1983b) and monkeys (Adams & Barratt, 1975; Harper, Heath & Myers, 1977; Heath, Fitzjarrell et al., 1980) exposed to cannabinoids. Some sleep EEG abnormalities, such as a decrease in slow-wave sleep, have also been observed. Stadnicki et al. (1974) demonstrated increased EEG synchrony and high-voltage slow-wave activity in the occipital cortex, amygdala, septum and hippocampus of rhesus monkeys with implanted electrodes, following several days' administration of oral THC, but tolerance developed to these EEG effects. Withdrawal effects are sometimes apparent in the EEG (Fehr & Kalant, 1983b) with epileptiform and spikelike activity most often seen.

Shannon and Fried (1972) related EEG changes in rat to the distribution of bound and unbound radioactive THC. Disposition of the tracer was primarily in the extrapyramidal motor system and some limbic structures and 0.8 per cent of the total injected drug that was weakly bound in the brain accounted for the EEG changes. In monkeys, serious subcortical EEG anomalies were observed in monkeys exposed to marijuana smoke for six months (Heath, Fitzjarrell et al., 1980). The septal region, hippocampus and amygdala were most profoundly affected, showing bursts of high amplitude spindles and slow-wave activity. Such early studies often lacked critical quantitative analysis. The definition of abnormal spikelike waveforms in EEG was not made to rigorous criteria and EEG frequency was not assessed quantitatively.

More recent studies have examined the effects of acute THC on extracellular action potentials recorded from the dentate gyrus of the rat hippocampus (Campbell, Foster et al., 1986a; 1986b). THC produced a suppression of cell firing patterns and a decrease in the amplitude of sensory-evoked potentials, also impairing performance on a tone discrimination task. The evoked-potential changes recovered rapidly (within four hours), but the spontaneous and tone-evoked cellular activity remained significantly depressed, indicating an abnormal state of hippocampal/limbic system operation. The authors proposed that such changes could account for decreased learning and memory function and generally impaired cognitive performance following exposure to cannabis. The long-lasting effects of prolonged cannabis administration on animal electrophysiology have not been investigated to any degree of specificity.

Most recently, the cannabinoid receptor antagonist SR141716A was shown to have arousal-enhancing properties as assessed by analysis of the sleep-waking cycle and of EEG spectra in rats (Santucci, Storme et al., 1996). There was a dose-dependent increase in time spent in wakefulness at the expense of slow-wave sleep and rapid eye movement sleep, but no change in motor behavior. The spectral power of EEG signals typical of slow-wave sleep were reduced. The authors claim their results suggest that an endogenous cannabinoid system is involved in the control of the sleep-waking cycle. Further evidence that anandamide may mediate the induction of sleep is reported by Mechoulam et al. (1997).

The waking or sleep EEG is increasingly recognized as a particularly sensitive tool for evaluating the effects of drugs in humans, especially drugs that affect the central nervous system (CNS). The recording of the EEG is one of the few reasonably direct, non-intrusive methods of monitoring CNS activity in humans. However, alterations in EEG activity are difficult to interpret in a functional sense. Struve and Straumanis (1990) provided a review of the human research dating from 1945 on the EEG and evoked potential studies of acute and chronic effects of cannabis use. Although the data have often been contradictory, the most typical human alterations in EEG patterns include an increase in alpha

activity and a slowing of alpha waves with decreased peak frequency of the alpha rhythm, and a decrease in beta activity (Fink, 1976b; Fink, Volavka et al., 1976; Heath, 1972; Rodin, Domino & Porzak, 1970; Volavka, Fink et al., 1977). In general, this is consistent with a state of drowsiness. Desynchronization, variable changes in theta activity, abnormal sleep EEG profiles and abnormal evoked responses have also been reported (Fehr & Kalant, 1983b). Cannabis has been reported to reduce the duration of REM sleep (Feinberg, Jones et al., 1976; Jones, 1980), although this may only occur early in administration studies, followed by a resolution and then an increase in REM sleep above baseline levels as smoking continues (Kales, Hanley et al., 1972).

Campbell (1971) compared EEG abnormalities observed in chronic cannabis users who had developed psychotic reactions, to the EEG patterns of schizophrenics, neurological patients and non-problematic cannabis users, and claimed that the incidence of EEG abnormalities was higher in the two groups of cannabis users than in either patient sample. These included excess sharp and theta activity, severe dysrhythmia, and epileptiform spikes in frontal and temporal regions. In contrast, Dornbush et al. (1972) reported increased EEG alpha activity in the intoxicated state, but no persistent changes following 21-day administration of cannabis to human volunteers. Koukkou and Lehmann (1976; 1977) examined EEG frequency spectra during self-reported THC-induced hallucinations and found slower alpha and more theta. Subjects with a high tendency toward "cannabis-induced experiences" exhibited resting spectra both before and after THC injection with higher modal alpha frequencies, reminiscent of subjects with high neuroticism scores, than subjects with a low tendency. Fink and colleagues (1976b) suggested that the acute effects of cannabis on EEG are similar to those of anticholinergics, but differ to those of opiates and hallucinogens. Jones (1975) reviewed the data on EEG characteristics of over 200 marijuana users from a number of studies, mostly during acute intoxication, and reported very few EEG abnormalities being detected in those studies that were well controlled.

Clinical reports have associated cannabis with triggering seizures in epileptics (Feeney, 1979) and experimental studies have shown that THC triggers abnormal spike waveforms in the hippocampus, whereas cannabidiol had the opposite effect. Yet there is suggestive evidence that cannabis may be useful in the treatment of convulsions. Feeney (1979) discusses these paradoxical effects.

A number of studies have investigated EEG in chronic cannabis users. No EEG abnormalities were found in the resting EEG of chronic users from Greek, Jamaican or Costa Rican populations compared to controls (Karacan, Fernandez-Salas et al., 1976; Rubin & Comitas, 1975; Stefanis, 1976). These early studies were flawed in many respects (see section II, "Cognitive Functioning") and only subjects who were in good health and who were functioning adequately in the community were selected, thereby systematically eliminating subjects who may have been adversely affected by cannabis use and who may therefore have shown residual EEG changes. Further, quantitative techniques for analysing EEG spectra were not applied.

The evidence from many other studies has been contradictory: users have been found to show either higher or lower percentages of alpha-components than non-users, and to have higher or lower visual evoked response amplitudes (Cohen, 1976; Deliyannakis, Panagopoulos & Huott, 1970; Richmon, Murawski et al., 1974). In a 94-day cannabis administration study (Cohen, 1976), lasting EEG abnormalities were more marked in subjects who had taken heavier doses, but it was observed that even in abstinence, cannabis users had more EEG irregularities than non-using controls. It was not determined for how long after cessation of use the EEG changes persisted. The equivocal results of many EEG studies might have been more consistent had quantitative methods been employed (early studies relied on visual inspection but by the mid-1970s power spectral analyses were sometimes being performed).

It has also been reported that chronic users develop tolerance to some of the acute EEG changes caused by cannabis (Feinberg, Jones et al., 1976). Fried (1977) reviewed the literature pertinent to the development of tolerance to EEG effects in animals and humans, which again produced many inconsistent results. The question as to why chronic cannabis users can continue to display changes in EEG when tolerance is known to develop to such alterations remains unanswered.

In a recent series of well-controlled studies, Struve and colleagues (1992; 1993; 1994; 1995) have used quantitative techniques to investigate persistent EEG changes in long-term cannabis users, characterized by a "hyperfrontality of alpha." Significant increases in absolute power, relative power and interhemispheric coherence of EEG alpha activity over the bilateral frontal-central cortex in daily marijuana users compared to non-users were demonstrated and replicated several times. The quantitative EEGs of subjects with very long cumulative exposures (> 15 years) appear to be characterized by increases in frontal-central theta activity in addition to the hyper-frontality of alpha found in cannabis users in general (or those with much shorter durations of use). These very long-term users have shown significant elevations of theta absolute power over frontal-central cortex compared to short-term users and controls, and significant elevations in relative power of frontal-central theta in comparison to short-term users. Over most cortical regions, ultra-long-term users had significantly higher levels of theta interhemispheric coherence than short-term users or controls. Thus, excessively long duration of cannabinoid exposure (15 to 30 years) appears to be associated with additional topographic quantitative EEG features not seen in subjects using cannabis for short to moderately long time periods.

These findings have led to the suspicion that there may be a gradient of quantitative EEG change associated with progressive increases in the total cumulative exposure (measured in years) of daily cannabis use. Infrequent, sporadic or occasional use did not seem to be associated with persistent quantitative EEG change. As daily use begins and continues, the topographic quantitative EEG becomes characterized by the hyperfrontality of alpha (Struve, Straumanis et al., 1993; Struve, Straumanis & Patrick, 1994). While it is not known at what point during cumulative exposure it occurs, at some stage substantial durations of daily cannabis use become associated with a downward shift in maximal EEG spectral power from the mid alpha range to the upper theta/low alpha range. Excessively long cumulative exposure of 15 to 30 years may be associated with increases of absolute power, relative power and coherence of theta activity over frontal-central cortex (Struve, Straumanis et al., 1992). One conjecture is that the EEG shift toward theta frequencies, if confirmed, may suggest organic change (Struve, Straumanis et al., 1992). These data are supplemented by neuropsychological test performance features separating long-term users from moderate users and non-users (Leavitt, Webb et al., 1993), but the relationship between neuropsychological test performance and EEG changes has not yet been investigated.

While the EEG provides little functionally interpretable information about the brain, event-related potential measures are more direct electrophysiological markers of cognitive processes. Relatively few studies have utilized event-related potential measures in research into the long-term effects of cannabis. Studies by Herning, Jones and Peltzman (1979) demonstrated that THC administered orally to volunteers alters event-related potentials according to dose, duration of administration, and the complexity of the task. Recent, well-controlled, human brain event-related potential studies have provided evidence for long-lasting functional brain impairment and subtle cognitive deficits in chronic cannabis users and ex-users in the unintoxicated state (Solowij, 1998). This research is reviewed in section II of this chapter.

Cerebral Blood Flow Studies

Brain cerebral blood flow (CBF) is closely related to brain function. The study of CBF may help to identify brain regions responsible for the behavioral changes associated with drug intoxication.

However, since psychoactive drugs may induce CBF changes through mechanisms other than alteration in brain function (e.g., by increasing carbon monoxide levels, changing blood gases or vasoactive properties, affecting blood viscosity, autonomic activation or inhibition of intraparenchymal innervation, acting on vasoactive neuropeptides), any conclusions drawn from drug-induced CBF changes must be treated with caution.

Mathew and Wilson (1992) report several studies of the effects of cannabis on cerebral blood flow. Acute cannabis intoxication in inexperienced users produced a global CBF decrease, whereas in experienced users CBF increased in both hemispheres but primarily at frontal and left temporal regions. There was an inverse relationship between anxiety and CBF. The authors attributed the decrease in CBF in naive subjects to their increased anxiety after cannabis administration, while the increased CBF in experienced users was attributed to the behavioral effects of cannabis. A further study showed that the largest increases in CBF occurred 30 minutes after smoking. The authors concluded that cannabis causes a dose-related increase in global CBF, but also appears to have regional effects, with a greater increase in the frontal region and in particular in the right hemisphere. The following variables were positively correlated with frontal CBF increases and inversely correlated with parietal flow: the "high," plasma THC levels and pulse rate, loss of time sense, depersonalization, anxiety and somatization scores.

The authors claimed their results suggested that altered brain function was mainly, if not exclusively, responsible for the CBF changes. The time course of CBF changes resembled that of mood changes more closely than plasma THC levels. Global CBF was closely related to levels of arousal mediated by the reticular activating system. High arousal states generally show CBF increases while low arousal states show CBF decreases. Of all cortical regions, the frontal lobe has the most intimate connections with the thalamus, which mediates arousal, and CBF increases after cannabis use were most pronounced in frontal lobe regions. The right hemisphere is generally associated with the mediation of emotions and the most marked changes after cannabis were seen there. Time sense and depersonalization that are associated with the temporal lobe were severely affected but there were no significant correlations between these scores and temporal flow. CBF techniques are probably not sensitive enough in terms of spatial resolution to detect such effects and may well be limited to superficial layers of cortex. The parietal lobes are associated with perception and cognition. Cannabis reduces perceptual acuity, but during intoxication subjects report increased awareness of tactile, visual and auditory stimuli. It is possible that their altered time sense and depersonalization is related to such altered awareness.

The possibility remains that the CBF changes reflect drug-induced vascular changes and not an alteration of specific brain functions. Acute administration of cannabis also increased cerebral blood velocity; however, upon prolonged standing after smoking, a dramatic reduction in cerebral blood velocity with reports of dizziness but with normal blood pressure suggested that cannabis may impair cerebral autoregulation. Carbon monoxide increased after both cannabis and placebo but did not correlate with CBF, and cannabis-induced "red eye" lasted for several hours while the increased CBF declined significantly within two hours of smoking, lending support to the hypothesis that the CBF changes are related to alterations in brain function.

There have been a few investigations of the long-term effects of cannabis on CBF. Tunving et al. (1986) demonstrated globally reduced resting levels of CBF in nine chronic heavy users (10 years), 1 to 12 hours after last use, compared to non-user controls, but no regional flow differences were observed. Four of these subjects were assessed again between 9 and 60 days later and showed a hemispheric CBF increase of 12 per cent, indicating reduced CBF in heavy users immediately after cessation of cannabis use, followed by a return to normal levels with more prolonged abstinence. This study was flawed in that some subjects were given benzodiazepines, which are known to lower CBF, prior to the first measurement. Mathew, Tant and Berger (1986) assessed chronic users of at least six months' duration (mean 83 months) after two weeks of abstinence. No differences in CBF levels were found between users and non-user controls. The subjects of this study, however, were not regular heavy users as were those in the study by Tunving et al. (1986), and they were not impaired in any identifiable way as a result of their use (Mathew & Wilson, 1992). In contrast, the experienced subjects of Mathew and Wilson's acute studies (1992) were chronic heavy users and they had also shown lower baseline CBF levels compared to the inexperienced subjects. The number of studies available on the effects of cannabis on CBF are relatively small and the findings of reduced CBF levels in chronic heavy users clearly require replication. Further application of techniques with better spatial resolution, such as positron emission tomography (PET) which also permits quantification of subcortical flow, may provide better information.

Positron Emission Tomography (PET) Studies

Positron emission tomography (PET) is a nuclear imaging technique that allows the concentration of a positron-labelled tracer to be imaged in the human brain (Raichle, 1983). PET can measure the regional distribution of positron-labelled compounds in the living human brain, and to some extent their time course. Some PET studies have used labelled oxygen and measured blood flow, while many others have utilized an analogue of glucose to measure regional brain glucose metabolism (since nervous tissue uses glucose as its main source of energy). Measurement of glucose metabolism reflects brain function since activation of a given brain area is indicated by an increase in glucose consumption. PET may be used to assess the effects of acute drug administration by using regional brain glucose metabolism to determine the areas of the brain that are activated or inhibited by a given drug. Assessment of brain glucose metabolism has been useful in identifying patterns of brain dysfunction in patients with psychiatric and neurological diseases. It is a direct and sensitive technique for identifying brain pathology since it can detect abnormalities in the functioning of brain regions in the absence of structural changes, such as may occur with chronic drug use. It is accordingly more sensitive than either computer-assisted tomography (CAT) scans or magnetic resonance imaging (MRI) in detecting early pathological changes in the brain.

Only one set of studies to date has used the PET technique to investigate the effects of acute and chronic cannabis use. Volkow et al. (1991b) reported data from a preliminary investigation comparing the regional brain metabolic effects of acute cannabis administration in three control subjects (who had used cannabis no more than once or twice per year) and in three chronic users (who had used at least twice per week for at least ten years). The regions of interest were the prefrontal cortex, the left and right dorsolateral, temporal and somatosensory parietal cortices, the occipital cortex, basal ganglia, thalamus and cerebellum. A measure of global brain metabolism was obtained using the average for the five central brain slices, and relative measures for each region were obtained using the ratios of region/global brain metabolism. Due to the small number of subjects, descriptive rather than inferential statistical procedures were used for comparison. The relation between changes in metabolism due to cannabis and the subjective sense of intoxication was tested with a regression analysis.

In the control subjects, administration of cannabis led to an increase in metabolic activity in the prefrontal cortex and cerebellum; the largest relative increase was in the cerebellum and the largest relative decrease was in the occipital cortex. The degree of increase in metabolism in the cerebellar cortex was highly correlated with the subjective sense of intoxication. The cannabis users reported less subjective effects than the controls and showed less changes in regional brain metabolism, reflecting tolerance to the actions of cannabis. However, the authors did not report comparisons of baseline levels of activity in the users and controls, perhaps due to the limitations of the small sample size. In a larger sample, such a comparison would enable an evaluation of the consequences of long-term cannabis use on resting levels of glucose metabolism. The increases in regional metabolism in the study by Volkow et al. are in accord with the increases in cerebral blood flow reported by Mathew and Wilson (1992). The regional pattern of response to cannabis in this study is consistent with the localization of cannabinoid receptors in brain.

Further studies with 8 infrequent cannabis users (range: once every two weeks to once per year) (Volkow, Gillespie et al., 1991a) or 11 subjects with a wide range of experience with cannabis (Volkow, Gillespie et al., 1995) found a variable response to acute intravenous THC administration in terms of global cerebral glucose metabolism, with some subjects showing an increase, others a decrease or no change. Nevertheless, the regional metabolic changes replicated those of their preliminary study, but the only significant changes were an increase in metabolic activity in the cerebellum, which correlated significantly with both the subjective sense of intoxication and with plasma THC concentration, and activation of prefrontal cortex, which was most prominent in those subjects with a history of frequent use of cannabis (Volkow, Gillespie et al., 1995). Interestingly, there was a negative correlation between plasma THC concentration and the degree of metabolic change in prefrontal cortex — the higher the plasma THC, the higher the metabolic values in cerebellum, but the lower the values in prefrontal cortex (Volkow, Gillespie et al., 1991a; 1991b). The authors discussed the implications of their findings in terms of the reinforcing properties of drugs of abuse, citing the role of the cerebellum in emotion and reinforcement and emphasizing its anatomical interconnections with the limbic system and prefrontal cortex.

A recently reported study by the same team (Volkow, Gillespie et al., 1996) investigated brain glucose metabolism in chronic cannabis users at baseline and during intoxication. At baseline, the eight chronic users (mean 5.5 years of use of between one and seven days per week) showed lower cerebellar metabolic activity than the eight controls, which was suggested to reflect changes in the cannabinoid receptors, possibly attributable to chronic cannabis use. Thirty to 40 minutes after intravenous administration of 2 mg THC, all subjects showed significantly increased metabolism in prefrontal cortex, left and right frontal cortices, right temporal cortex and cerebellum. Cerebellar metabolism was correlated with the degree of subjective intoxication, but not with plasma THC concentration. Chronic users showed significantly greater increases in prefrontal cortex, orbitofrontal cortex and basal ganglia, while controls showed a decrease in the latter two regions. The increased prefrontal activation during intoxication is consistent with Mathew and Wilson's (1992) findings of prefrontal CBF increases in regular but not infrequent cannabis users. Volkow et al. (1996) interpreted the altered metabolic function observed in orbitofrontal cortex and basal ganglia in their chronic users to be similar to that found in cocaine abusers, alcoholics and patients with obsessive-compulsive disorders, and postulated the importance of a dysfunction in these regions in the regulation of initiation and termination of behaviors, loss of control and compulsion. However, unlike other drugs of abuse that have consistently been shown to decrease regional brain metabolism following a single acute administration (e.g., cocaine, heroin, amphetamines, alcohol and benzodiazepines), cannabis consistently produced increases.

A further application of PET would be to label cannabinoids themselves: labelling of THC with a positron emitter has been achieved, and preliminary biodistribution studies have been carried out in mice and in the baboon (Charalambous, Marciniak et al., 1991; Marciniak, Charalambous et al., 1991). More recently, an iodinated analogue of SR141716A,

the cannabinoid receptor antagonist, has been utilized for PET or SPECT (single photon emission computerized tomography) studies in mice, but does not bind in baboons (Gatley, Gifford et al., 1996; Lan, Gatley & Makriyannis, 1996). Research in progress from this team is developing a new radiotracer with better blood brain barrier penetration that binds to the CB_1 receptor *in vivo* and does permit SPECT brain images in baboons (S.J. Gatley, personal communication). The use of PET in future human studies is promising.

Brain Histology and Morphology

Animal Studies

Early attempts to investigate the effects of chronic cannabinoid exposure on brain morphology in animals failed to demonstrate any effect on brain weight or histology under the light microscope. Electron microscopic examination, however, led to reports of alterations in septal, hippocampal and amygdaloid morphology in monkeys after chronic treatment with THC or cannabis. A series of studies from the same laboratory (Harper, Heath & Myers, 1977; Heath, Fitzjarrell et al., 1980; Myers & Heath, 1979, discussed below) reported widening of the synaptic cleft, clumping of synaptic vesicles in axon terminals, and an increase in intranuclear inclusions in the septum, hippocampus and amygdala. These findings incited a great deal of controversy and the studies were criticized for possible technical flaws (Institute of Medicine, 1982) with claims that such alterations are not easily quantifiable.

Harper and colleagues (1977) examined the brains of three rhesus monkeys seven months after the end of a six-month exposure to marijuana, THC or placebo, and two non-exposed control monkeys. In the treated group, one monkey was exposed to marijuana smoke three times each day, five days per week, another was injected with THC once each day, and the third was exposed to placebo smoke conditions. The latter two had electrode implants for EEG recording; the one receiving THC, but not the one exposed to placebo smoke, had shown persistent EEG abnormalities following the exposure. Morphological differences were not observed by light microscopy, but electron microscopy revealed a widening of the synaptic cleft in the marijuana and THC-treated animals with no abnormalities detected in the placebo or control monkeys. Further, "clumping" of synaptic vesicles was observed in pre- and postsynaptic regions in the cannabinoid-treated monkeys, and opaque granular material was present within the synaptic cleft. The authors concluded that chronic heavy use of cannabis alters the ultrastructure of the synapse and proposed that the observed EEG abnormalities may have been related to these changes.

Myers and Heath (1979) examined the septal region of the same two cannabinoid-treated monkeys and found the volume density of the organized rough endoplasmic reticulum to be significantly lower than that of the controls, and fragmentation and disorganization of the rough endoplasmic reticulum patterns, free ribosomal clusters in the cytoplasm, and swelling of the cisternal membranes was observed. The authors noted that similar lesions have been observed following administration of various toxins or after axonal damage, reflecting disruptions in protein synthesis.

Heath et al. (1980) extended the above findings by examining a larger sample of rhesus monkeys (N = 21) to determine the effects of marijuana on brain function and ultrastructure. Some animals were exposed to smoke of active marijuana, some were injected with THC and some were exposed to inactive marijuana smoke. After two to three months of exposure, those monkeys that were given moderate or heavy exposure to marijuana smoke developed chronic EEG changes at deep brain sites, which were most marked in the septal, hippocampal and amygdaloid regions. These changes persisted throughout the six- to eight-month exposure period as well as the postexposure observation period of

between one and eight months. Brain ultrastructural alterations were characterized by changes at the synapse, destruction of rough endoplasmic reticulum and development of nuclear inclusion bodies. The brains of the placebo and control monkeys showed no ultrastructural changes. The authors claimed that at the doses used, which were comparable to human usage, permanent alterations in brain function and ultrastructure were observed in these monkeys.

Brain atrophy is a major non-specific organic alteration that must be preceded by more subtle cellular and molecular changes. Rumbaugh et al. (1980) observed six human cases of cerebral atrophy in young male substance abusers of primarily alcohol and amphetamines. They then conducted an experimental study of six rhesus monkeys treated chronically with various doses of cannabis extracts orally for eight months and compared them to groups that were treated with barbiturates or amphetamines or untreated. No signs of cerebral atrophy were demonstrated in the cannabis-exposed group and light microscopy revealed no histological abnormalities in four of the animals, but gave "equivocal" results for the other two. Brains were not examined under the electron microscope. The amphetamine-treated group showed the greatest histological, cerebrovascular and atrophic changes.

More recently, McGahan et al. (1984) used high resolution computerized tomography scans in three groups of four rhesus monkeys. One was a control group, a second was given 2.4 mg/kg of oral THC per day for 2 to 10 months and a third group received a similar daily dose over a five-year period. The dosage was considered the equivalent of smoking one joint per day. The groups receiving THC were studied one year after discontinuing the drug. There was a statistically significant enlargement of the frontal horns and the bicaudate distance in the brains of the five-year treated monkeys as compared to the control and short-term THC groups. This finding suggests that the head of the caudate nucleus and the frontal areas of the brain can atrophy after long-term administration of THC in doses relevant to human exposure.

A number of rat studies have found similar results to those in rhesus monkeys described above. Investigators have reported that after high-dose cannabinoid administration there was a decrease in the mean volume of rat hippocampal neurons and their nuclei, and after low-dose administration there was a shortening of hippocampal dendritic spines. Scallet and colleagues (1987) used quantitative neuropathological techniques to examine the brains of rats seven to eight months after 90-day oral administration of 10 to 60 mg/kg THC. The anatomical integrity of the CA3 area of rat hippocampus was examined using light and electron microscopy. High doses of THC resulted in striking ultrastructural alterations, with a significant reduction in hippocampal neuronal and cytoplasmic volume, detached axodendritic elements, disrupted membranes, increased extracellular space and a reduction in the number of synapses per unit volume (i.e., decreased synaptic density). These structural changes were present up to seven months following treatment. Lower doses of THC produced a reduction in the dendritic length of hippocampal pyramidal neurons two months after the last dose, and a reduction in GABA receptor binding in the hippocampus although the ultrastructural appearance and synaptic density appeared normal. The authors suggested that such hippocampal changes may constitute a morphological basis for the persistent behavioral effects demonstrated following chronic exposure to THC in rats, effects that resemble those of hippocampal brain lesions. These findings are in accord with those of Heath et al. (1980) with rhesus monkeys and the doses administered correspond to daily use of approximately six joints in humans.

A study by Landfield, Cadwallader and Vinsant (1988) showed that chronic exposure to THC reduced the number of nucleoli per unit length of the CA1 pyramidal cell somal layer in the rat hippocampus. The brains of rats treated five times per week for four or eight months with 4 or 8 mg/kg injected subcutaneously were examined by light and electron microscopy. Significant THC-induced changes were found in hippocampal structure: pyramidal neuronal cell density

decreased and there was an increase in glial reactivity, reflected by cytoplasmic inclusions, similar to that seen during normal aging or following experimentally induced brain lesions. However, no effects were observed on ultrastructural variables such as synaptic density. Adrenal-pituitary activity increased, resulting in elevations of ACTH and corticosterone during acute stress. The authors claimed that the observed hippocampal morphometric changes produced by THC exposure were similar to glucocorticoid-dependent changes that develop in rat hippocampus during normal aging. They proposed that, given the chemical structural similarity between cannabinoids and steroids, chronic exposure to THC may alter hippocampal anatomical structure by interacting with adrenal steroid activity. More recently, Eldridge et al. (1992) reported that $\varnothing^8$-THC bound with the glucocorticoid receptors in the rat hippocampus and was displaced by corticosterone or $\varnothing^8$-THC. A glucocorticoid agonist action of $\varnothing^8$-THC injections was demonstrated. Injection of corticosterone increased hippocampal cannabinoid receptor binding. These interactions suggest that cannabinoids may accelerate brain aging. Eldridge and Landfield (1990), Eldridge, Murphy and Landfield (1991) and Landfield and Eldridge (1993) further discuss this research and its implications.

It should be noted that where THC has been administered to monkeys for six months, this represents only 2 per cent of their lifespan and may not have been long enough to detect the gradual effects that could arise from interactions with steroid systems (and affect the aging process). In contrast, eight months' administration to rats represents approximately 30 per cent of their lifespan. The differences in the ultrastructural findings of Landfield's and Scallet's studies may be due to the largely different doses administered; the 8 mg/kg of Landfield's study was not sufficient to produce any marked behavioral effects. Further, the two studies examined slightly different hippocampal areas (CA1 or CA3).

Most recently, Slikker and colleagues (1992) reported the results of their neurohistochemical and electronmicroscopic evaluation of the rhesus monkeys whose dosing regime, behavioral and histochemical data were reported above. They failed to replicate earlier findings: no effects of drug exposure were found on the total area of hippocampus, or any of its subfields, nor were there any differences in hippocampal volume, neuronal size, number, length or degree of branching of CA3 pyramidal cell dendrites. There were no effects on synaptic length or width, but there were trends toward increased synaptic density (the number of synapses per cubic millimetre), increased soma size, and decreased basilar dendrite number in the CA3 region with cannabis treatment. Slikker et al. were able to demonstrate an effect of enriched environments upon neuroanatomy: daily performance of operant tasks increased the total area of hippocampus and particularly the CA3 stratum oriens, producing longer, more highly branched dendrites and less synaptic density, while the reverse occurred in the animals deprived of the daily operant tasks. The extent of drug interaction with these changes was not clear and may explain some of the inconsistencies between this study and those described above. Clearly, the question of whether prolonged exposure to cannabis results in structural brain damage has not been fully resolved.

Human Studies

There is very little evidence from human studies of structural brain damage. In their controversial paper, Campbell et al. (1971) were the first to present evidence suggestive of structural/morphological brain damage associated with cannabis use in humans. They used air encephalography to measure cerebral ventricular size and claimed to have demonstrated evidence of cerebral atrophy in 10 young males who had used cannabis for 3 to 11 years, and who complained of neurological symptoms, including headaches, memory dysfunction and other cognitive impairment. Compared to controls, the cannabis users showed significantly enlarged lateral and third ventricular areas. Although this study was widely publicized in the media because of its serious implications, it

was heavily criticized on methodological grounds. Most subjects had also used significant quantities of LSD and amphetamines, and the measurement technique was claimed to be inaccurate, particularly since it is difficult to assess ventricular size and volume to any degree of accuracy using the air encephalographic technique (e.g., Bull, 1971; Fink, Ashworth & Brewer, 1972; Susser, 1972). Moreover, the findings could not be replicated. Stefanis (1976) reported that echoencephalographic measurements of the third ventricle in 14 chronic hashish users and 21 non-users did not support pneumoencephalographic findings of ventricular dilation reported by Campbell et al.

The introduction of more accurate and non-invasive techniques, in the form of computerized tomographic (CT) scans, (also known as computer-assisted tomographic [CAT] scans), permitted better studies of possible cerebral atrophy in chronic cannabis users (Co, Goodwin et al., 1977; Kuehnle, Mendelson & David, 1977). Co et al., for example, compared 12 cannabis users recruited from the general community, with 34 non-drug-using controls, all within the ages of 20 to 30. The cannabis users had used cannabis for at least five years at the level of at least five joints per day, and most had also consumed significant quantities of a variety of other drugs, particularly LSD. Kuehnle, Mendelson and David's subjects were 19 heavy users aged 21 to 27 years, also recruited from the general community who had used on average between 25 and 62 joints per month in the preceding year, although their duration of use was not reported. CT scans were obtained presumably at the end of a 31-day study, which included 21 days of *ad libitum* smoking of marijuana (generally five joints per day), and were compared to a separate normative sample. No evidence for cerebral atrophy in terms of ventricular size and subarachnoid space was found in either study. Although these studies could also be criticized for their research design (e.g., inappropriate control groups, and the fact that cannabis users had used other drugs), these flaws would only have biased the studies in the direction of detecting significant differences between groups, yet none were found. The results were interpreted as a refutation of the findings by Campbell et al., and supporting the absence of cortical atrophy as demonstrated by CAT scans of monkeys (Rumbaugh, Fang et al., 1980). A further study (Hannerz & Hindmarsh, 1983) investigated 12 subjects, who had smoked on average 1 gram of cannabis daily for between 6 and 20 years, by thorough clinical neurological examination and CT scans. As in the studies above, no cannabis-related abnormalities were found on any assessment measure.

Recent Research on Cannabinoid Receptor Alterations

The development of tolerance following chronic administration of psychoactive compounds is often mediated by a down-regulation of receptors. Thus, chronic exposure to THC could lead to receptor down-regulation or receptor internalization (both resulting in a decreased number of cannabinoid receptors in the brain) or to conformational changes in the receptor that produce an altered receptor structure, each of which results in decreased receptor-ligand interaction (Adams & Martin, 1996). Receptor down-regulation and reduced binding (particularly in the striatum and limbic forebrain) has been demonstrated in rats (Oviedo, Glowa & Herkenham, 1993; Rodríguez de Fonseca, Gorriti et al., 1994). However, Westlake et al. (1991) reported that cannabinoid receptor properties were not irreversibly altered in rat brain 60 days following 90-day administration of THC, nor in monkey brain seven months after one year of exposure to marijuana smoke. It was argued that these recovery periods were sufficient to allow the full recovery of any receptors that would have been lost during treatment. Abood et al. (1993) had also demonstrated the development of tolerance to THC without any alteration of cannabinoid receptor binding or mRNA levels in whole brain. More recently, Romero et al. (1995)

reported increased binding in the cerebellum and hippocampus after acute or chronic exposure to either anandamide or THC: increased binding following acute administration was attributed to changes in receptor affinity, but that following chronic administration was attributed to an increase in the density of receptors. However, following chronic exposure to THC only, a down-regulation of receptors in the striatum was observed. Mackie et al. (1997) demonstrated rapid internalization of cannabinoid receptors following agonist binding. The research suggested that longer-term treatment with cannabinoids may cause the receptor to progress to lysosomes where it is degraded and the recovery of surface receptors requires new protein synthesis. The precise parameters of any alterations in cannabinoid receptor number and function that may result from chronic exposure to cannabinoids, and the extent of reversibility following longer exposures, have not yet been determined to any degree of accuracy.

A recent study has demonstrated large decreases in G-protein activation throughout the brain following chronic treatment with THC, showing that effects on receptor function may occur without consistent changes in the number of receptor binding sites. Sim and colleagues (1996) investigated the alterations in signal transduction that mediate the production of tolerance. They pointed out that changes in receptor binding may not reflect changes in receptor function. They showed that a specific treatment regimen, which had previously been shown to produce complete adaptation to the impairing effects of large doses of cannabinoids on a delayed-matching-to-sample task (Deadwyler, Heyser & Hampson, 1995), produced a functional "uncoupling" of the cannabinoid receptor from the G-protein that links it to cyclic AMP and other cellular mechanisms. Cannabinoid-stimulated $[^{35}S]GTP\gamma S$ binding was substantially reduced in brain regions rich in cannabinoid receptors, and most dramatically in the hippocampus. This finding is consistent with the impairing effects of cannabinoids on short-term memory tasks (Heyser, Hampson & Deadwyler, 1993). The uncoupling of the receptor from the G-protein by chronic drug treatment explains the cessation of the disruptive acute effects of THC on such tasks, which may be adaptive in certain circumstances, but the receptor-G-protein uncoupling may have profound effects on potassium A channels and all other effectors downstream from the receptor-transducer coupling. The loss in agonist activity is analogous to desensitization and the findings are consistent with the concept that desensitization and down-regulation are separate processes, with the former preceding the latter. The results of this study suggested that "profound desensitization of cannabinoid-activated signal transduction mechanisms occurs after chronic Delta(9)-THC treatment" (Sim, Hampson et al., 1996, p. 8057). The chronic treatment in this study was only 21 days. Studies such as this, in combination with research investigating the role of cannabinoid receptors in memory dysfunction (e.g., Hampson, Byrd et al., 1996; Heyser, Hampson & Deadwyler, 1993; Lichtman & Martin, 1996; Terranova, Storme et al., 1996), lead the way for revolutionizing our understanding of the mechanism of action of both endogenous and exogenous cannabinoids.

Two studies of human brain postmortem have investigated changes in cannabinoid receptor binding or density with disease and normal aging. Westlake et al. (1994) showed that binding of the potent cannabinoid agonist CP-55,940 was substantially reduced in the caudate and hippocampus of brains of patients with Alzheimer's disease, with lesser reductions in the substantia nigra and globus pallidus. Reduced binding was associated also with increasing age and/or general disease processes resulting in cortical pathology and thus not specific to Alzheimer's. They claimed that receptor losses were not associated with overall decrements in levels of cannabinoid receptor gene expression. Biegon and Kerman (1995) found that increasing age is associated with a decrease in the density of cannabinoid receptors in prefrontal cortex, particularly in cingulate cortex and the superior frontal gyrus. The authors discussed their findings in terms of possible indirect modulation of dopaminergic activity by cannabi-

noids, and suggested that the age-related decline in receptor density in prefrontal regions may contribute to decreased drug-seeking behavior with increasing age. As this age-related decrease in cannabinoid receptors was found in the normal human brain, it would be interesting for further research to examine receptor density in the prefrontal cortex of chronic cannabis users. These findings reinforce the possibility of a role for the cannabinoid receptor in higher order cognitive functions and may have implications for elucidating the cognitive decline that occurs with age.

Animal research has also examined changes in cannabinoid receptors with age: Mailleux and Vanderhaeghen (1992) reported age-related losses in cannabinoid receptor binding sites and mRNA in the rat striatum. Belue et al. (1995) demonstrated progressively increased binding capacity in rat striatum, cerebellum, cortex and hippocampus from birth through to adulthood, which they interpreted as reflecting either "an increased differentiation of neurons into cells possessing cannabinoid receptors, or an increase in the number of receptors on cell bodies or projections in regions undergoing developmental changes." Once the adult levels had been reached, binding activity in a whole brain preparation neither increased nor declined with normal aging; it would be interesting to see if the same results would have been obtained had specific sites such as prefrontal cortex been examined and if rats had been chronically administered cannabinoids. These studies require replication and pave the way for further exploration of aging phenomena as they may interact with chronic exposure to the drug.

Conclusion

Overall, surprisingly few studies of neurotoxicity have been published and the results have been equivocal. There is convincing evidence that chronic administration of large doses of THC leads to residual changes in rodent behaviors that are believed to depend upon hippocampal function. There is evidence for long-term changes in hippocampal ultrastructure and morphology in rodents and monkeys. Animal neurobehavioral toxicity is characterized by long-lasting impairment in learning and memory function, EEG and biochemical alterations, impaired motivation and impaired ability to exhibit appropriate adaptive behavior. Although direct extrapolation to humans is not possible, the results of these experimental animal studies have demonstrated cannabinoid toxicity at doses comparable to those consumed by humans using cannabis several times a day. There is sufficient evidence also from human research to suggest that cannabinoids act on the hippocampal region, producing behavioral changes similar to those caused by injury to that region (e.g., Drew, Weet et al., 1980; see section II, "Cognitive Functioning").

Human research has defined a pattern of acute CNS changes following cannabis administration. EEG, CBF and PET techniques have demonstrated altered brain function and metabolism in humans following acute and chronic use. However, the cognitive, behavioral and functional responses to long-term cannabis consumption in humans continue to be the most consistent manifestation of its potential toxicity. It is possible that the extent of damage could be more pronounced at two critical stages of central nervous system development: in neonates when exposed to cannabis during intrauterine life (e.g., Fried, 1993; 1995; 1996; see section II, "Cognitive Functioning"), and in adolescence, during puberty when neuroendocrine, cognitive and affective functions and structures of the brain are in the process of integration. As discussed in the next section, research needs to investigate the possibility that more severe consequences may occur in adolescents exposed to cannabinoids, than in those who commence cannabis use at a later age.

Human studies of brain morphology have yielded generally negative results, failing to find gross signs of "brain damage" after chronic exposure to cannabis. Nevertheless, the results of many human studies are indicative of more subtle brain dysfunction. It may be that existing methods of brain imaging are not sensitive enough to demonstrate subcellular alterations produced in the CNS. Many psychoactive substances exert their action through molecular biochemical mechanisms that do not distort gross cell architecture. The most convincing evidence on brain damage would come from postmortem studies. The postmortem finding of age-related decline in the density of cannabinoid receptors in prefrontal cortex of the normal human brain (Biegon & Kerman, 1995) holds promise for interesting future research to examine such changes as they interact with the chronic use of cannabis.

In 1983, Fehr and Kalant concluded that "the state of the evidence at the present time does not permit one either to conclude that cannabis produces structural brain damage or to rule it out" (p. 602). In 1984, Nahas wrote "The brain is the organ of the mind. Can one repetitively disturb the mental function without impairing brain mechanisms? The brain, like all other organs of the human body, has very large functional reserves which allow it to resist and adapt to stressful abnormal demands. It seems that chronic use of cannabis derivatives slowly erodes these reserves" (1984, p. 299). In 1986, Wert and Raulin proposed, that on the available evidence "there are no gross structural or neurological deficits in marijuana-using subjects, although subtle neurological features may be present. However, the type of deficit most likely to occur would be a subtle, functional deficit which could be assessed more easily with either psychological or neuropsychological assessment techniques" (1986a, p. 624). By 1998, little further evidence has emerged to challenge or definitively refute these earlier conclusions.

This conclusion was anticipated as early as 1845 by the Parisian physician Moreau when he wrote of his observations of chronic hashish smokers: "unquestionably there are modifications (I do not dare use the word 'lesion') in the organ which is in charge of mental functions. But these modifications are not those one would generally expect. They will always escape the investigations of the researchers seeking alleged or imagined structural changes. One must not look for particular, abnormal changes in either the gross anatomical or the fine histological structure of the brain; but one must look for any alterations of its sensibility, that is to say, for an irregular, enhanced, diminished or distorted activity of the specific mechanisms upon which depends the performance of mental functions" (Moreau de Tours, 1845).

What Moreau was suggesting, was that we find other ways of assessing the subtle changes in cognition that occur with prolonged use of cannabis. Traditionally, this has entailed the application of neuropsychological tests and such studies are reviewed extensively in the next section. Nevertheless, the vastly advanced techniques of today ensure that research will continue to investigate the minute changes in brain ultrastructure and the functioning of the cannabinoid receptor that would no doubt underlie the cognitive and behavioral dysfunction.

II. COGNITIVE FUNCTIONING

One of the well-known acute effects of cannabis is to impair cognitive processes. It has long been suspected that cognitive dysfunction may persist well beyond the period of acute intoxication, and that chronic cannabis use may cause lasting cognitive impairments. Although considerable research has been conducted into the acute cognitive effects of cannabis, there is a paucity of well-controlled studies of the long-term effects of chronic cannabis use on cognitive function. This section reviews the literature from each of several methodological approaches that have been used to investigate the chronic effects of cannabis on human cognitive functioning. Clinical observations will only be covered very briefly, with discussion restricted to either key papers or recent research. The priority in this section will be given to those human studies that made some attempt to control scientifically for extraneous variables. These have largely concentrated on neuro-psychological assessments of brain function in chronic cannabis users.

The terms *acute, subacute* and *chronic,* when used to describe drug effects, have been defined in section I, "Brain Function and Neurotoxicity." The term *residual* is also sometimes employed in the literature and may lead to some confusion. Strictly it refers to drug effects that remain after the drug has been eliminated from the body and not, as the name might imply, to those effects due to a residue of the drug itself. Because of the slow clearance of THC and its metabolites from the body, repeated administration results in the accumulation of cannabinoids. There is no conclusive evidence for effects associated with accumulated cannabinoids, but the possibility that they continue to exert an effect remains nevertheless. To avoid confusion, the term *residual* will not be used here and any effects possibly attributable to drug residues will be discussed separately from more enduring effects.

A caveat must be borne in mind while critically assessing this literature; it is difficult to assess the long-term consequences of the use of any psychoactive drug. Many factors other than drug use must be controlled in order to attribute confidently any effects to the drug in question. In the case of assessing the long-term effects of drugs on cognitive function, these difficulties include: differentiating cognitive impairment that preceded drug use from that which may have been drug-induced; accurately determining the duration and frequency of past drug use; and taking account of the cognitive effects of multiple drug use. All these issues contribute to uncertainty in the attribution of any observed impairment to the use of a particular drug (Carlin, 1986).

Clinical Observations

Concerns about the possibility that chronic cannabis use affected mental processes were reinforced by early clinical reports of mental deterioration in long-term cannabis users. Fehr and Kalant (1983b) provide a historical review of early clinical observations. In general, the clinical literature suggests that cognitive dysfunction is most often observed in persons who have used heavily (at least daily) for more than one year (Fehr & Kalant, 1983b).

The most widely cited evidence for clinically significant impairment due to cannabis is the work of Kolansky and Moore (1971; 1972). These authors initially reported 38 cases of psychiatric symptomatology ranging from mild apathy, through personality disturbance, to psychosis that was observed in adolescents and young adults (aged 13 to 24) who had used marijuana at least twice per week. They later presented 13 case reports of adult psychiatric patients (aged 20 to 41) who had used marijuana or hashish 3 to 10 times per week or more for between 16 months and 6 years.

The clinical picture was one of poor social judgment, poor attention span, poor concentration, confusion, anxiety, depression, apathy, passivity, indifference and slowed and slurred speech (Kolansky & Moore, 1971). Various cognitive symptoms began with cannabis use and disappeared within 3 to 24 months after cessation of drug use. These included: apathetic and sluggish mental and physical responses, emotional lethargy, mental confusion, difficulties with recent memory, incapability of completing thoughts during verbal communication, loss of interest in life, and goallessness.

The course and remission of symptoms appeared to be correlated with past frequency and duration of cannabis smoking. Those with a history of less intensive use showed complete remission of symptoms within six months; those with more intensive use took between six and nine months to recover; while those with chronic intensive use were still symptomatic nine months after discontinuation of drug use. Symptoms were also more marked in users of hashish than in marijuana smokers.

Tennant and Groesbeck (1972) monitored the medical and psychiatric consultations of 720 hashish-smoking U.S. soldiers in West Germany. Just over half of the sample were occasional users who consumed between 0 to 12 grams of hashish

per month. This group only complained of respiratory ailments. The heavy-using group (N = 110), who consumed between 50 and 600 grams of hashish per month, were described as "chronically intoxicated," generally apathetic and displaying impaired memory, judgment and concentration. Tennant and Groesbeck followed up nine heavily using patients after periods of abstinence, providing one of the few prospective studies to date. Six of the nine reported improvement in memory, alertness and concentration following discontinuation of use, while the other three complained of confusion and impaired memory for many months after ceasing use of the drug.

Both Kolansky and Moore, and Tennant and Groesbeck, emphasized the similarity between the symptoms they observed in long-term heavy cannabis users and those of organic brain damage. Kolansky and Moore hypothesized that the use of cannabis "adversely affects cerebral functioning on a biochemical basis. In the mildest cases there appears to be a temporary toxic reaction when small amounts of cannabis are consumed over a short period of time. However, in those individuals who demonstrate stereotyped symptomatology after prolonged and intensive cannabis use, the possibility of structural changes in the cerebral cortex must be raised" (1972, p. 42). They called for investigation to assess structural and functional alterations in the brains of chronic cannabis users.

These clinical reports, together with a report of cerebral atrophy in young cannabis users that appeared around the same time (Campbell, Evans et al., 1971), incited substantial controversy. Critics were quick to fault the experimental designs and to raise objections to the conclusions and extrapolations based on the evidence. Among these were the lack of objective measures of impairment and the biased sampling from psychiatric patient populations. The clinical observations, however, have been largely unchallenged, and the consistency of symptoms across reports and cultures is particularly striking. For example, the clinical descriptions of chronic users in India have matched those from North America (Chopra, 1971; 1973; Chopra & Jandu, 1976; Chopra & Smith, 1974).

While clinical observations may raise concerns, they do not provide definitive evidence of causality because they are unable to rule out alternative explanations of an apparent association between drug use and symptoms. Altman and Evenson (1973), for example, examined 158 psychiatric patients and found 38 cases in which cannabis use had preceded such symptoms as confusion, depression, poor judgment, anxiety and apathy. In an exploration of possible relationships between other factors and psychiatric problems, they found 10 other events (such as use of tobacco and beer, sexual intercourse, etc.) that preceded the onset of psychiatric symptoms more frequently than did cannabis use. The authors criticized Kolansky and Moore's failure to include in their sample individuals who had used cannabis and did not develop psychiatric symptoms. They warned of the scientifically unsound practice of using the case history technique to test hypotheses about causal relationships.

The clinical observations reported in the early 1970s were not new. Reports of adverse mental effects of cannabis use have appeared throughout history (see Abel, 1980; Fehr & Kalant, 1983a; Nahas, 1984). While the frequency of clinical reports of cognitive dysfunction has diminished in the past decade, this may reflect a decline in their novelty and noteworthiness rather than any reduction in the incidence of clinical disorders resulting from the chronic use of cannabis. Kalant (1996) shows a decline in the numbers of publications on cannabis in general as indexed by the *Cumulative Index Medicus* from 1971 to 1994 and argues that this is a reflection of political trends and lack of funding. There is plenty of evidence, anecdotal and research based (e.g., Stephens, Roffman & Simpson, 1993), that chronic cannabis users continue to seek treatment (or would if they knew that it was available to them). They present with complaints primarily of dependence on the drug, but often give as their prime reason for wanting to cease using, a concern that they are experiencing mental deterioration, a "dulling" of cognitive abilities, or difficulties with concentration and memory.

In recent years, clinicians have sought to characterize the specific deficits they observe in chronic cannabis users by integrating these into cognitive theory and evidence from empirical research (e.g., Lundqvist, 1995a; 1995b; 1995c). Treatment programs for chronic cannabis users have been established that focus on specific areas of cognitive dysfunction, such as verbal and logical-analytic abilities, abstraction, psychomotility and memory (Lundqvist, 1995a; 1995c; Tunving, Lundqvist & Eriksson, 1988). Clinical observation suggests that the use of cannabis more often than every six weeks for approximately two years leads to changes in cognitive functioning, but clinical improvement in cognitive functioning can be seen within 14 days of abstinence, and following six weeks of therapy users may function normally (Lundqvist, 1995a; 1995c). The cannabis-induced cognitive dysfunction was likened to the prefrontal syndrome, which is difficult to measure due to its complex effects on human behavior (Stuss & Benson, 1986).

The clinical reports that appeared in the early 1970s served to alert the community at large to the possible risks involved in using cannabis at a time when the substance was becoming increasingly popular among the young. This in turn prompted field studies and better-controlled empirical research.

Studies of Users in Countries with a Long History of Cannabis Use Within Their Culture

A logical starting point for the investigation of cognitive function in chronic cannabis users is to assess populations of users in countries where chronic daily use of cannabis has been an integral part of the culture for many decades, if not centuries. This kind of research was pioneered by Soueif (1971) in the largest scale study to date of

850 Egyptian hashish smokers and 839 controls. In response to public anxiety about the epidemic increase in marijuana use in the late 1960s, the National Institute on Drug Abuse (NIDA) commissioned three studies in countries with long histories of cannabis use, namely, Jamaica, Greece and Costa Rica. These studies have been the most widely quoted and are considered to be comprehensive. This is not so much due to their sample sizes, which were quite small and therefore limit the conclusions that can be drawn, but mainly because each study was multidisciplinary, investigating not only cognitive function, but also medical-physiological status. However, aside from the small sample size, each of these studies suffered from a number of other methodological difficulties which limited the conclusions that could be drawn. These studies will each be briefly discussed, along with the Egyptian study and several studies conducted in India.

Egypt

Soueif's Egyptian sample was from a male prison population that was poorly educated, largely illiterate and of lower socioeconomic status and hence unrepresentative of the general cannabis-using populations in most other cultures. Significant differences were found between users and controls on 10 out of 16 measures of perceptual speed and accuracy, distance and time estimation, immediate memory (digit span backwards), reaction time and visual-motor abilities, including the Trail Making Test (Part A) and the Bender-Gestalt test (Soueif, 1971; 1975; 1976a; 1976b). These differences in performance were more marked in the youngest (< 25 years) and best-educated urban users than in the older, illiterate and rural subjects. Soueif concluded that prolonged cannabis use produces subtle deficits in the cortical level of arousal (Soueif, 1976a). He argued that high cortical levels of arousal are associated with high levels of proficiency, and "the lower the non-drug level of proficiency on tests of cognitive and psychomotor performance the smaller the size of function deficit associated with drug taking" (Soueif, 1976b).

Soueif's Egyptian study was subsequently criticized for methodological reasons (Fletcher & Satz, 1977). Soueif replied to these criticisms (Soueif, 1977) and maintained that long-term use of cannabis may lead to deficits in speed of psychomotor performance, distance and time estimation, immediate memory and visuomotor co-ordination, particularly in young, educated and urban users. The validity of these findings, however, remains under doubt because some of the tests used by Soueif do not have established neuropsychological validity (Carlin, 1986).

Jamaica

Bowman and Pihl (1973) conducted two field studies of chronic cannabis use in Jamaica, one with a small sample of 16 users and 10 controls from rural and semirural areas, and the other with a small urban slum sample of 14 users and controls. Users had been very heavy daily consumers of cannabis for a minimum of 10 years (current use of about 23 high-potency joints per day), while controls had no previous experience with cannabis. Tests were selected on the basis of having previously been shown to be sensitive to impairment following chronic heavy alcohol use (or other chemical insult). They were generally described as measures of the efficiency of concept formation and memory (Bowman & Pihl, 1973). The groups were matched for age, sex, social class, alcohol use, education and "intelligence," but most subjects were illiterate or semi-literate, with an average age of 30. No differences were found between the users and non-users of either study, nor when the rural and urban samples were combined.

A more extensive study of 60 male laborers in Jamaica (Rubin & Comitas, 1975) came to be regarded as the main Jamaican project (NIDA-funded). It was hailed as a major breakthrough in cultural drug research because it used a combination of field-based social-scientific evaluation and hospital-based clinical evaluation. The neuropsychological and personality assessments were much more extensive than those conducted in Egypt or Greece. This study compared 30 users and 30 non-users matched on age, socioeconomic status and residence. The user group, which was aged between 23 and 53 years with a mean age of 34 years, had used cannabis for an average of 17.5 years (range 7 to 37 years) at around 7 joints per day (range 1 to 24), estimated to contain 60 milligrams of THC. They had not used any other substances except alcohol and tobacco. Although it was stated that no control subject had used cannabis heavily in recent years, whether there had been heavy use in the past was not reported. At least 9 of the controls were current "occasional" users of cannabis and all but 12 of the controls had some experience with cannabis.

A battery of 19 psychological tests were administered, generally after three days of abstinence, as part of a six-day inpatient drug-free hospitalization period during which many other clinical and physiological examinations were performed. The test battery included three tests of intellectual and verbal abilities (the Wechsler Adult Intelligence Scale [WAIS], Ammons Full-Range Picture Vocabulary Test and the Reitan Modification of the Aphasia Screening Test), and 15 neuropsychological tests measuring abilities previously shown to be affected by acute cannabis intoxication. Simple and complex motor functions were tested by dynamometer, finger tapping, maze steadiness, graduated holes and pegboard. Sensory perception was assessed by tests of tactile and auditory stimulation, and tactile form and finger-tip writing recognition. Memory and attention were measured by the Tactual Performance Test (child's version), the Time-Sense-Memory Test and the Seashore Rhythm Test. The Indiana-Reitan Category Test (child's version) assessed concept formation. Portions of the WAIS, such as the Information, Vocabulary and Picture Arrangement subtests, were omitted as they were judged to be culturally inappropriate.

Comparisons of the users and non-users on 47 subtest variables failed to reveal any consistently significant differences. There was no strong suggestion of differences that failed to be detected because of a small sample size since the user group scored better than the non-user group on 29 variables, albeit non-significantly. The authors considered their results to be consistent with Bowman and Pihl's Jamaican study, and concluded that "in a wide variety of human abilities, there is no evidence that long-term use of cannabis is related to chronic impairment" (Rubin & Comitas, 1975, p. 199).

The interpretation of these null results as evidence of an absence of effect of cannabis on cognitive functioning is complicated by a number of factors that may have attenuated differences between users and controls. First, the tests used were not standardized for use in Jamaica. Second, there are problems with the interpretation of test scores with the possibility of floor and ceiling effects obscuring any drug effects (particularly as the children's version of some tests were used), and test score means were not published. Third, the inclusion of cannabis users in the control group may have further contributed to the lack of significant group differences. No attempt was made to evaluate any long-term neuropsychological effects as a function of frequency or duration of use. Fourth, a number of other cultural differences may have confounded the results of this study. Jamaican society at the time had a tradition of cannabis use within which many viewed the drug as medicinal, benign or even as a work enhancer. Cannabis users were not viewed as amotivated "drop-outs" from society, as they were in North America, for example. The cannabis users of this Jamaican sample were mainly farmers, fishermen and artisans from rural areas or casual urban laborers, who claimed to increase their work output by using cannabis to relieve the monotony of dull, repetitive and laborious work (Comitas, 1976). If only the higher cognitive functions are affected by cannabis, the work performance of rural or manual laborers would not necessarily be affected. However, this does not exclude the possibility that the long-term use of cannabis may impair the performance of workers who have more complex tasks or those who come from higher socioeconomic groups, for whom mental operations may predominate (Fink, 1976a). This sample was poorly educated, with a mean of 4.5 years of schooling (equivalent to third grade) so that if Soueif (1976a) is correct, there would only be small functional deficits associated with cannabis use.

Greece

The Greek NIDA study (Stefanis, Dornbush & Fink, 1977) examined a sample of 47 chronic hashish users and 40 controls matched for age, sex, education, demographic region, socio-economic status and alcohol consumption. The subjects were mostly refugees from Asia Minor, residing in a low-income, working class area of Athens. The average duration of use was 23 years of an estimated daily use of 200 milligrams per day, and most users had smoked hashish on the day before testing, and some had smoked several hours before the test session. Controls were slightly better educated than users.

The WAIS and Raven's Progressive Matrices were administered to assess general intelligence and mental functioning (Kokkevi & Dornbush, 1977). Subtests of the WAIS were used to evaluate the possibility of impairment in specific cognitive and perceptual functions. Although the WAIS was not standardized on a Greek population it had been used by the authors in a translated form for many years. Raven's test was considered to be a more culture-free assessment of intelligence and was used for reliability and validity purposes. The groups did not differ in global IQ score on either the WAIS or Raven's Progressive Matrices, but non-users obtained a higher verbal IQ score than users. The users' performance was worse than controls on all but one of the subtests of the WAIS (Digit Span), even if not significantly so. Significant differences in performance between the two groups were obtained in three subtests of the WAIS: Comprehension, Similarities, and Digit-Symbol Substitution. Impaired performance in the Comprehension and Similarities subtests indicates a possible defect in verbal comprehension and expression, verbal memory, abstraction and associative thinking. A low score on Digit-Symbol Substitution (consistently shown to be affected by cannabis acutely) indicates a possible defect in visual-motor co-ordination and memorizing capacity. A trend toward inferior performance in

the Picture Arrangement test may indicate a dysfunction in logical sequential thought.

The interpretation of these results was complicated by the lack of a requirement that subjects abstain from hashish prior to testing. Consequently, it was not clear whether the impairment found on these subtests was related to long-term use of hashish, or whether it was due to the persistence of an acute drug effect at the time of testing. The poorer performance by users was assumed to reflect their recent use of hashish, since the test was given within two hours of smoking hashish by some users (Kokkevi & Dornbush, 1977), an interval that coincided with increased pulse rates, a reliable sign of acute intoxication. Because the differences between verbal and performance IQ were similar in both groups the authors argued that there was no evidence of deterioration in mental abilities in the hashish users. They attributed the poorer performance by users to "acculturational and adaptational processes" rather than to "logical reasoning abilities"; however, in line with the Egyptian and Jamaican studies, they conceded that it was possible that the detection of subtle intellectual dysfunctions in groups with low levels of mental functioning was less easily observed (Kokkevi & Dornbush, 1977).

A subsample of 20 of the Greek chronic users were administered a brief psychometric battery after smoking a given dose of cannabis (Dornbush & Kokkevi, 1976). These subjects had smoked for over 25 years and were assessed on simple tests of perceptual-motor ability. This study demonstrated the acute response of chronic users to be similar to that of short-term users in the United States: psychological test performances were adversely affected by cannabis in a way similar to that observed in naive subjects or short-term users under acute intoxication. The adverse effects on mental functioning were short-lived, persisting for approximately 70 minutes after commencing smoking. Thus, no evidence was provided for tolerance or withdrawal effects. The only effect to be inferred was that practice effects, although not abolished by the consumption of marijuana, were less than those observed under placebo conditions. Further, no differences were found in the EEG changes produced by an acute dose of cannabis in this Greek sample and a group of American volunteers; nor were there differences between the two samples in resting EEG patterns.

Costa Rica

The NIDA study of chronic heavy cannabis users in Costa Rica was modelled upon the Jamaican project but with greater sensitivity to cultural issues. It involved an intensive physiological, psychological, sociological and anthropological study of matched pairs of users and non-users (Carter, Coggins & Doughty, 1980). Satz, Fletcher and Sutker (1976) reported the results of comparing 41 male long-term heavy cannabis users (on average 9.6 joints per day for 17 years) with matched controls on an extensive test battery designed to assess the impact of chronic cannabis use on neuropsychological, intellectual and personality variables. The educational level of the Costa Rican sample was slightly higher than that of either the Greek or the Jamaican populations, although more than half of the user group had not completed primary school, and both users and non-users had commenced employment at 12 years of age on average. The users were working class, mostly tradesmen with lower than "average income, who reported that they often used cannabis to augment their work performance in a similar fashion to the Jamaican sample.

The tests included Finger Localization and Finger Oscillation (tapping) Tests, the Tactual Performance Test, the Rey-Davis test of non-verbal memory and learning and the Word Learning and Delayed Recall tests from the Williams Memory Battery, Logical Memory from the Wechsler Memory Scale (WMS), the Milner Facial Recognition Memory Test, the Benton Visual Retention Test, and a short form of the WAIS. These tests were translated into Spanish and standardized on a separate sample of the Costa Rican population. They were found to be free of cultural bias, and no floor or ceiling effects were demonstrated. All data were subjected to appropriate multivariate statistical analyses.

Despite their long duration and heavy use, the Costa Rican users did not differ significantly from controls on any test. Users scored consistently lower, if not significantly so, than non-users on 11 of 16 variables in the neuropsychological test battery. These included the Word Learning, Delayed Recall and the Rey-Davis subtests of the Williams Memory Battery, the Logical Memory test of the Wechsler Memory Scale and the Facial Recognition Memory Test. Although users' performance was poorer, particularly in the mean number of errors made, learning curves were similar for both groups. A multivariate analysis of the 14 variables constituting the WAIS also revealed no significant differences between groups. Users performed slightly better on 6 of the 11 subtests and had a slightly higher verbal and full-scale IQ. An attempt to correlate test results with level of marijuana use yielded no consistent findings. The authors concluded that there was no evidence for irreversible brain damage, significant impairment of memory function or other cognitive impairment due to the chronic use of cannabis.

A 10-year follow-up of the Costa Rican sample was conducted by Page, Fletcher and True (1988). By the time of follow-up, the users had an average 30 years' experience with cannabis, but the sample size had dropped to 27 of the 41 original users and 30 of the 41 controls. The test protocol included some of the original tests, as well as a number of additional tests measuring short-term memory and attention, which were selected for their sensitivity in detecting subtle changes in cognitive functioning. The new tests included: the Rey-Osterrieth Complex-Figure Test, Buschke's Verbal Selective Reminding Test, the Self-Paced Continuous Performance and Underlining Tests, Mazes and Trail Making Test Part A.

No differences were detected on any of the original tests, but three tests from the new battery yielded significant differences between users and controls. In Buschke's Verbal Selective Reminding Test, the user group retrieved significantly fewer words from long-term storage than the non-user group, although the groups did not differ on a measure of storage. Users performed more slowly than non-users in the Underlining

Test, with particularly poor performance in the most complex subtest. Differences between groups were not a function of practice or purely motor speed. The Continuous Performance Test also revealed users to be slower than controls on measures requiring sustained attention and effortful processing, although there were no differences in correct hits nor false alarm rates.

Page et al. interpreted their results as providing evidence that long-term consumption of cannabis is associated with difficulties in sustained attention and short-term memory. They hypothesized that such tests require more mental effort than the tests used in the original study, and, as such, the results imply that long-term users of cannabis experience greater difficulties with effortful processing. They provided anthropological data to further support their hypotheses: users exhibited lower levels of mental effort at work than non-users, although this was confounded by the choice of job. Users tended to work as laborers, street vendors or in the service industry, while non-users tended to be craftsmen, store tenders or office managers. Page et al. claimed that if users found it difficult to concentrate, especially on tasks that require attention to detail, they might be expected to choose jobs that are less demanding in mental performance than the jobs chosen by non-users.

This study differs from its predecessors in that it did find differences between users and non-users in tests of information processing, sustained attention and short-term memory. Nevertheless, Page et al. emphasized that the differences they found were "quite subtle" and "subclinical." Only a small number of subjects were classified as clinically impaired. Because the differences are so small and subtle, it is difficult to exclude several other alternative explanations before concluding that they reflect the longer duration of use by the sample, or the greater sensitivity and specificity of tests used. These alternative possibilities include: that the differences were due to the inclusion of the few clinically impaired subjects within the sample; and that some of the differences were due to acute intoxication or recent use, since 24-hour abstinence was requested, but was not verified.

Most recently, a further follow-up of 17 of the original users and 30 of the original controls was reported by Fletcher and colleagues (1996). These subjects (mean age 45 years) were compared with a younger cohort (mean age 29 years) of 37 Costa Rican cannabis users (mean duration of use of 8 years) and 49 non-user controls on tests of short-term and working memory and attention following a 72-hour period of abstinence verified by the analysis of two urine samples. Older long-term users performed worse than older non-users on complex short-term memory tests involving learning lists of words and on complex tasks of selective and divided attention associated with working memory. No differences were found between younger users and non-users.

India

Studies of long-term cannabis use in India commenced with Agarwal, Sethi and Gupta's (1975) examination of chronic bhang drinkers. Bhang is a tealike infusion of cannabis leaves and stems which is drunk, sometimes for medicinal purposes. The 40 subjects had used bhang daily for about five years, were less than 45 years of age, reasonably well educated with 65 per cent having completed high school and none illiterate. There was no control group, so scores were compared to normative data on the tests used. By comparison with these norms, 18 per cent of the bhang users had memory impairment on the Wechsler Memory Scale, 28 per cent showed mild intellectual impairment on the Bhatia Battery of Intelligence (IQs less than 90), and 20 per cent showed substantial cognitive disturbances on the Bender-Gestalt Visuo-Motor Test. The authors concluded that bhang may cause mild impairment in cognitive functions.

Wig and Varma (1977) administered a test battery to 23 long-term male users of cannabis (including both daily charas [hashish] smokers and bhang drinkers of at least five years). Eleven of these were matched to a non-using control group with respect to sex, education, income, marital status and occupation. The entire sample was compared to the 11 controls on scores from Raven's Progressive Matrices, Malin's Intelligence

Scale for Indian Children (adapted from the WAIS), PGI Memory Scale (adapted from the WMS), Bender-Gestalt, speed and "H" marking tests from the General Aptitude Test Battery, a color cancellation test and a time-perception test. Users scored significantly lower on the tests of intelligence, memory, speed and accuracy, replicating the findings of Agarwal et al., and pointing to problems in memory and concentration associated with long-term cannabis use.

The results of these studies are limited by either the absence of controls or the use of poorly matched controls, inadequate consideration of premorbid variables, unreliable measurement of the duration and severity of cannabis and other drug use, and the use of culturally inappropriate psychometric tests or tests that had not been adequately validated in the sample population. Nonetheless, many of the subjects in these studies were extremely heavy users, and the differences in cognitive performance could not always be explained by the uncontrolled confounding variables.

Mendhiratta, Wig and Verma (1978) compared 50 heavy cannabis users (half bhang drinkers, half charas smokers of at least 25 days per month for a mean of 10 years) with matched controls. The entire sample was of low socioeconomic status. Tests were administered after 12 hours' abstinence, which was verified by overnight admission to a hospital ward. The tests included digit span, a recognition test, a pencil-tapping test, speed and accuracy tests, a time-perception test, a reaction-time test, a size-estimation test (most of which were not standardized for the population studied), and the Bender-Gestalt Test.

The cannabis users reacted more slowly, and performed more poorly in concentration and time estimation. The charas smokers were the poorest performers, showing impaired memory function, lowered psychomotor activity and poor size estimation. The fact that the smokers were most impaired may reflect a contribution by other compounds formed by pyrolysis in the production of cognitive impairment; on the other hand, it may simply be a function of the higher potency of charas preparations. Nine to

10 years later, Mendhiratta et al. (1988) followed up 11 of the original bhang drinkers, 19 charas smokers and 15 controls. Repeat administration of the original tests showed significant deterioration on digit span, speed and accuracy tests, reaction time and on the Bender-Gestalt.

Ray et al. (1978) assessed the cognitive functioning of 30 chronic cannabis users (aged 25 to 46 years) who had used bhang, ganja (leaf and flowering heads) or charas for a minimum of 11 times per month for at least five years, comparing their performance to that of 50 randomly selected non-user controls of similar age, occupation, socioeconomic status and educational background. Few differences were found on tests of attention (e.g., digits backwards, serial addition/subtraction), visuomotor co-ordination (e.g., the Minnesota Perceptuo-Diagnostic Test) or memory (the PGI Memory Scale). Cannabis users' performance was impaired on one of the subtests of the memory scale. However, the matching of subjects was not rigorous and the fact that all subjects were illiterate may have produced a floor effect masking differences between groups.

Varma et al. (1988) administered 13 psychological tests selected to assess intelligence, memory and other cognitive functions, to 26 heavy marijuana smokers and 26 controls matched on age, education and occupation. The average daily intake of the cannabis users was estimated as 150 mg THC, with a frequency of at least 20 times per month, and a mean duration of use of 6.8 years (minimum five years). Twelve hours' abstinence was ensured by overnight hospitalization. The tests included pencil tapping, time perception, reaction time, size estimation, Trail Making (Part A), Bender-Gestalt, Nahor and Benson visuospatial reproduction, Standard Progressive Matrices, WAIS-R Verbal Scale, Bhatia's Short Scale (measure of IQ), PGI Memory Scale, and a disability assessment schedule. Varma et al. reported that the PGI Memory Scale was a locally developed and validated adaptation of the Wechsler Memory Scale which assessed memory function in 10 different domains.

Cannabis users were found to react more slowly on perceptuomotor tasks such as the pencil-tapping and reaction-time tests, but did not differ from controls on the tests of intelligence. When the scores of all the memory tests were combined, there was no difference between the total scores of cannabis users and controls, although cannabis users scored significantly more poorly on a subtest of recent memory. There were trends toward poorer performance on subtests of remote memory, immediate and delayed recall, retention and recognition. Users suffered disability in personal, social and vocational areas. The authors concluded that impairment of cognitive functions associated with long-term heavy use of cannabis was more apparent in perceptuomotor tasks than in tests of intelligence or memory. Nevertheless, the perceptuomotor tests employed in this study were of questionable validity, with particularly poor measures of reaction time and speed of responding, while the measures of memory function may have reached significance had a larger sample been tested. This suggests that any cognitive deficits due to cannabis may be specific to particular aspects of short-term memory.

Concerns Mostly Allayed but Methodology Flawed

The results of these culture-specific studies of long-term heavy cannabis users served to allay concerns about the consequences of cannabis use since overt signs of "brain damage" as measured by psychological tests were not found among heavy long-term cannabis users. There was equivocal evidence for an association between cannabis use and more subtle long-term cognitive impairments.

Given that cognitive impairments are most likely to be found in subjects with a long history of heavy use, it is reassuring that most such studies have found few and small differences. It is unlikely that the negative results of these studies can be attributed to an insufficient duration or intensity of cannabis use within the samples studied. For example, the duration of cannabis use averaged 17.5 years and the daily THC level consumed ranged from an estimated 20 to 90 milligrams daily in Rubin and Comitas's Jamaican

study; 23 years and 120 to 200 milligrams daily in the Greek sample; and 16.9 years and 20 to 160 milligrams daily in the initial Costa Rican study.

The absence of differences is all the more unexpected since a number of factors may have biased these studies toward finding poorer performance among cannabis users. These include higher rates of polydrug use, poor nutrition, poor medical care and illiteracy among users, and the failure in many studies to ensure that subjects were not intoxicated at the time of testing, which would have increased the likelihood of detecting impairment. The use of a laboratory test to detect recent marijuana ingestion in studies with positive results would have been helpful in ruling out acute effects as the cause of the apparent impaired performance among users. Given the generally positive biases in these studies, it has been argued that if cannabis use did produce cognitive impairment, a larger number of these studies should have shown positive results (Wert & Raulin, 1986b).

The force of this argument is weakened, however, by the fact that most of these studies suffered from numerous other methodological difficulties that may have operated against finding a difference. First, the instruments most often used for assessment have been developed and standardized mostly on North American populations. Second, many of these studies were based on small samples of questionable representativeness and subject to sampling bias, since only subjects who could be reached and were willing to participate were included in the studies while others possibly not equally resistant to drug-induced impairments might have been missed. Third, a number of studies failed to include a control group while others used inappropriate controls. Fourth, generalization of the results of these studies to users in other cultures is difficult, given the predominance of illiterate, rural, older and less intelligent or less educated subjects in these studies. Fifth, the studies were limited by their investigative instrumentation which may only be capable of detecting gross deficits at a group level. Sixth, few attempts were made to examine relationships between neuropsychological test performance and frequency and duration of cannabis use. Such an evaluation would rule out possible within-group differences in chronic users.

In terms of the specific deficits reported, slower psychomotor performance, poorer perceptual motor co-ordination, and memory dysfunction were the most consistently reported deficits. Of the studies that specifically included tests of memory function, five detected persistent short-term memory and attentional deficits in chronic cannabis users (Fletcher, Page et al., 1996; Page, Fletcher & True, 1988; Soueif, 1976a; Varma, Malhotra et al., 1988; Wig & Varma, 1977), while three detected no such deficits (Bowman & Pihl, 1973; Mendhiratta, Wig & Verma, 1978; Satz, Fletcher & Sutker, 1976). Impairments were most frequently found on such tests as the Wechsler Memory Scale, the Bender-Gestalt test, Buschke's Selective Reminding Test and the Continuous Performance Test. The measures of short-term memory were often inadequate, failing to determine which processes may be impaired (e.g., acquisition, storage, encoding, retrieval) and often with an exclusion of higher mental loads and conditions of distraction. A proper evaluation of the complexity of effects of long-term cannabis use on higher cognitive functions requires greater specificity in the selection of assessment methods as well as the use of more sensitive tests.

Studies of Young American or Canadian Users with a Relatively Short History of Cannabis Use

Clinical Findings

The cognitive performance of American or Canadian cannabis users was also assessed in a number of studies in the 1970s. Most of the subjects in these studies were young and well-educated college students with relatively short-term

exposure to cannabis in comparison to the long history of use among chronic users in the studies reviewed above. In 1970, Hochman and Brill (1973) surveyed a large sample of college students (N = 1400). The sample comprised non-users (65.5 per cent), occasional users (26 per cent), and chronic users (8.5 per cent) defined as those who had used three times per week for three years or had used daily for two years. They found no evidence of an "amotivational syndrome" in terms of lethargy or social and personal deterioration, but did demonstrate significant psychosocial differences between users and non-users. Marijuana users were more rebellious, reckless, questioning and anti-authoritarian. Chronic users were less certain of long-term life plans than non-users, although there was no relationship between either frequency or duration of use and academic achievement. About 1 per cent of marijuana users were estimated to suffer from impaired ability to function due to their use, but such loss of ability was subject to large individual differences and variability.

In a follow-up of the original sample over two consecutive years (1971: N = 1133; 1972: N = 901), Brill and Christie (1974) assessed non-users, occasional users (< 2/week), frequent (2 to 4 per week), and regular users (≥ 5 per week) by a self-report questionnaire. The majority of users perceived no effect of cannabis use on most areas of psychosocial adjustment. Just over 12 per cent reported that their academic performance had declined and they were more likely to reduce their frequency of use or to quit. There were no significant differences found between users, non-users or former users in grade point average. Cannabis users were more likely to drop out of college and had greater difficulty formulating life and career goals; fewer users planned to seek advanced academic degrees and more considered themselves to have poorer academic adjustment. Whether these attributes preceded cannabis use or were caused by it, is impossible to determine. It may be argued that such differences do not necessarily reflect impairment nor are they harmful. Indeed, the authors concluded that in a functioning, intelligent undergraduate university population, few deleterious effects could be attributed to the use of the drug.

Entin and Goldzung (1973) conducted two studies of the residual impact of cannabis use on memory processes. In the first study, verbal memory was assessed by the use of paired-associate nonsense syllable (CVC) learning lists. Twenty-six cannabis users (defined as daily for at least six months, but the range of use was not reported) were compared to 37 non-users drawn from a student population. Cannabis users scored significantly more poorly on both free recall (the number of syllables recalled after a delay) and on acquisition, measured as improvement in recall over repeated trials.

In the second study, verbal and numerical memory were tested by the presentation of word lists, interspersed with Wendt three-step arithmetic problems prior to recall. Cannabis users (N = 37) recalled significantly fewer words than non-users (N = 37), but did not differ from controls on arithmetic test scores. The lack of an effect on the arithmetic tests was interpreted as a function of the short length of time during which numeric information must be stored for further manipulation, rather than being due to any numerical memory functions per se. That is, the verbal memory tasks required longer term storage of information prior to retrieval.

These findings were interpreted as residual impairment of both the acquisition and recall phases of long-term memory processes. The authors attributed the impairments to either an enduring residual pharmacological effect on the nervous system, or to an altered learning or attention pattern due to repeated exposure to cannabis. No details were provided with regard to the length of abstinence prior to testing, however. The authors stated that subjects were assumed "not to be under the influence of marihuana or any other drug during the testing situation. Any who were suspected were asked to return at another time for testing" (Entin & Goldzung, 1973, p. 171).

Grant et al. (1973) studied the effects of cannabis use on test performance using eight measures from the Halstead-Reitan Battery among medical students. They found no differences between 29 cannabis users (of median four-year duration and frequency three times per month) and 29 age- and intelligence-matched non-users on seven of the eight measures. Users performed more poorly on the localization subtest of the Tactual Performance Test. These subjects were very select in that they were only light users, and as medical students were obviously functioning well. The failure to find any difference in sensory-motor integration or immediate sensory memory was later replicated by Rochford, Grant and LaVigne (1977) in a comparison of 25 users (of at least 50 times over a mean 3.7 years) and 26 controls matched on sex, age and scholastic aptitude scores. By limiting their samples to populations of successful students, these studies are flawed in the reverse direction to the reports of Kolansky and Moore (1971; 1972).

Weckowicz and Janssen (1973) compared 11 male college students who smoked cannabis three to five times per week for at least three years with non-users who were matched on age, education, socioeconomic and cultural backgrounds. They were assessed on a variety of tasks designed to measure field dependence, personality traits, social attitudes and values, as well as cognitive function. Users performed better than controls on 8 of the 11 cognitive tests but performed more poorly on the Guilford Number Facility test, suggesting that chronic use may affect sequential information processing. Otherwise, there was no evidence of organic brain damage or gross impairment of cognitive functioning. Weckowicz and Janssen interpreted their findings in terms of social deviance, lack of conformity, rebelliousness and alienation.

In a cross-validation of their previous findings, Weckowicz, Collier and Spreng (1977) compared 24 heavy smokers (at least daily for three years) belonging to the "hippie subculture" with non-user controls matched for age (mean 22.5), education (mean 13.5 years) and social background. Cognitive functioning, personality traits and social values were assessed using the same test battery as used previously, with addition of a selective listening task, the Wechsler Memory Scale, Miller Analogies Test, Utility Test, Word Association Test and Association Test. Cannabis users once again performed better on tests of "originality and cognitive ability," and scored significantly better on the selective listening task, leading the authors to interpret this as users having "better control of attention processes" and showing no signs of cognitive impairment. The measures analysed in the selective listening task were not reported. The cannabis users were also more likely to be current polydrug users, and to have used LSD, psilocybin, cocaine, amphetamines and heroin.

Culver and King (1974) used the Halstead-Reitan Battery, the WAIS, the Trail Making Test, the Laterality Discrimination Test and three tests of spatial-perceptual abilities to examine the neuropsychological performance of three groups of undergraduates (N = 14) from classes in two successive years. These were: marijuana users (of at least twice per month for 12 months), marijuana plus LSD users (LSD use of at least once per month for 12 months), and non-drug users. Significant differences appeared, disappeared and reappeared among the groups and classes in different years. The only consistent difference was on the Trail Making Test, in which the cannabis group performed significantly better than the cannabis plus LSD group, who also used more cannabis, but cannabis users did not differ from non-users.

Gianutsos and Litwack (1976) compared the verbal memory performance of 25 cannabis smokers who had used for two to six years and at least twice per week for the last three months, with 25 non-smokers who had never smoked cannabis. Subjects were drawn from an undergraduate university student population and were matched on age, sex, year at university, major and grade average. Cannabis users were "asked not to smoke before the experiment" and gave verbal report that they had not "smoked recently" prior to the time of testing, although the length of abstinence was not reported.

The task was a modification of the Peterson-Peterson paradigm that allows examination of short- versus long-term storage of verbal

information. In the original version of the task, arithmetic manipulations intervened between word presentation and recall. The modified task substituted further word reading for the arithmetic, arguing that such an interference task would prevent rehearsal of words and displace the to-be-recalled words from short- to long-term storage. In interference tasks of this kind, the number of words recalled is a function of the number of postlist interference task words. Subjects were required to recall the first 3 words from a list of 5, 9 or 13 words read aloud, and the forced reading of 2, 6 or 10 words constituted the postlist reading task. Cannabis users recalled significantly fewer words overall than non-users, and the difference in performance increased as a function of the number of postlist words. Users also generated significantly more intrusion errors than non-users. The authors concluded that the chronic use of cannabis interfered with the transfer of information from short- to long-term storage.

Carlin and Trupin (1977) assessed 10 normal subjects who smoked marijuana daily for at least two years (range 2.5 to 8, mean 5; mean age 24; mean years education 14.6) and who denied other drug use. They administered the Halstead Neuropsychological Test Battery after 24 hours abstinence. No significant impairment was found by comparison with non-smoking subjects matched for age, education and full-scale IQ. Cannabis users performed faster on the Trail Making Test Part B, a test sensitive to frontal damage. The authors concluded that "relatively long-term chronic marijuana use does not impair an individual's ability to solve complex cognitive tasks requiring recurrent observations of subtle stimulus characteristics, to manipulate complex visual motor problems, to answer questions dependent on prior learning, and to be accurate in identifying sensory stimulations, both unilateral and bilateral" (Carlin & Trupin, 1977, p. 622). They acknowledged, however, that their sample was small and that perhaps less bright individuals may be at greater risk of developing impairments.

In 1981, Schaeffer, Andrysiak and Ungerleider reported no impairment of cognitive function in one of the first studies of a prolonged heavy cannabis-using population in the United States. They assessed 10 long-term heavy users of ganja, aged between 25 and 36 years, all of whom were Caucasian and had been born, raised and educated in the United States (mean years of education 13.5). All had smoked between 30 and 60 grams of cannabis (> 8 per cent THC) per day for a mean of 7.4 years for religious reasons and were active members of a religious sect. They had not consumed alcohol or other psychoactive substances. Although this sample contained cannabis users who had not used any other substances, it is not known what other confounding variables may have been introduced as a result of the peculiarities of belonging to a religious sect. Such a sample may not be representative of the general cannabis-using population.

This study was also one of the first to use a laboratory test to assess levels of cannabinoids in body fluids. Schaeffer et al. (1981) reported that at the time of testing, all subjects had at least 50 ng/mL cannabinoids in their urines but they also stated that subjects smoked continuously, even during the testing session. It is expected that heavy users such as these would have developed tolerance to many of the effects of cannabis. The tests that were selected to assess intellectual function included the WAIS, the Benton Visual Retention Test, the Rey Auditory-Verbal Learning Test, Symbol-Digits Modalities Test, Hooper Visual Organization Test, Raven's Progressive Matrices and Trail Making (Parts A and B). Since there was no control group, the data was compared with the standardized-normative information available for each test. An attempt was also made to obtain a measure of premorbid intellectual functioning. The authors obtained IQ measures from school assessments for two of the subjects, which were virtually identical to those measured in the study. Overall, WAIS IQ scores were in the superior to very superior range, and the scores of all other tests were within normal limits for age.

Despite the heavy and prolonged use of cannabis, there was no evidence of impairment in the cognitive functions assessed, namely, language function, non-language function, auditory and visual remote, recent and immediate memory, or complex multimodal learning. The authors suggested that tolerance may develop to one or more of the constituents of cannabis, explaining the lack of impairment. Further, it is possible that the superior to very superior intellect of these subjects may have allowed them to compensate for the effects of cannabis, and perhaps they would have performed not merely within normal limits, but at a superior level had they not smoked cannabis.

Interpretation

The results of these empirical studies served to further allay fears that cannabis smoking caused gross impairment of cognition and cerebral function. The lack of consistent findings failed to support Kolansky and Moore's (1971; 1972) clinical reports of an organiclike impairment. However, some critics (e.g., Cohen, 1982) have argued that the lack of evidence for impairment in these studies may be a function of their small sample sizes and potentially biased sampling techniques. By focusing on college students, it is suggested, these studies have sampled from a population unlikely to contain many impaired persons. The samples of younger, brighter and "successful" users may reflect the survivors whereas Kolansky and Moore reported on the casualties.

Such hypotheses, however, conflict with the explanations provided for the lack of evidence of impairment in the culture-specific studies reviewed above. Soueif's proposition, for example, was that the lower the non-drug level of proficiency, the smaller the size of functional deficit associated with drug usage. This would imply maximal differences at the high end of cognitive ability. Perhaps the argument could be rephrased in terms of maximizing the possibility of detecting impairment by sampling from a broader range of ability, minimizing the possibility of sampling bias and floor and ceiling effects. In any case, Soueif's claim that the greatest drug-induced impairment would occur in users with the highest levels of arousal, i.e., those for whom mental operations predominate (Fink, 1976a), was not supported by these studies of college students.

A more pertinent explanation for the lack of impairment is that the duration of cannabis use in these samples was quite brief, generally less than five years. It has been argued that at the time, cannabis smoking in North America had not existed long enough for impairments to emerge. Further, when psychometric testing was used as a metric of cognitive function as opposed to self-report questionnaires, sample sizes were often too small to permit the detection of any but very large differences between groups.

However, not all studies found negative results. A small number of studies did find significant impairments in their cannabis-using populations. What distinguished those studies that found differences between users and non-users from those that did not? The answer may lie in the specificity of assessment methods. Rather than administering a standard psychometric test battery or tests of general intelligence, the studies that found differences selected tests to assess a specific cognitive function (memory), and attempted to determine the specific stages of processing where dysfunction occurred. Entin and Goldzung (1973), for example, found that users were impaired on both verbal recall and acquisition of long-term storage memory tasks, but not on arithmetic manipulations which require short-term storage of information. Gianutsos and Litwack (1976) used an interference condition in their verbal recall memory paradigm, thereby increasing the complexity of the task. Impairments became more apparent in the users as the interference increased, suggesting that cannabis use may affect the transfer of information from short- to long-term storage.

Given the lack of self-awareness of such specific deficits, self-report questionnaires would probably not be able to detect such an impairment. In the other studies, the only assessment of memory function was the inherent components of memory, alertness and concentration throughout all tests of the Halstead-Reitan Battery. Reitan himself acknowledged that this test battery "is probably not as specifically represented in terms of the memory factor as it might be" and that "it might be of value to include supplementary tests of memory" for proper evaluation (Reitan, 1986, p. 10).

Controlled Laboratory Studies

A different approach to the investigation of the cognitive consequences of chronic cannabis use was taken in laboratory studies of the effects of daily administration of cannabis over periods of weeks to months. These studies have attempted to control for variation in quantity, frequency and duration of use, as well as other confounding factors such as nutrition and other drug use, by having select samples of subjects reside in a hospital ward while receiving known quantities of cannabis. All of these studies employed pre- and postdrug observation periods, and could be thought of as a short form of longitudinal research. Because of the expense of such studies, sample sizes have generally been small and the duration of cannabis administration has ranged from 21 to 64 consecutive days.

Dornbush et al. (1972) administered 1 gram of marijuana containing 14 milligrams THC to five regular smokers (all healthy young students) for 21 consecutive days. The subjects were tested immediately before and 60 minutes after drug administration. Data were collected on subjective ratings of mood, clinical observations, short-term memory and digit-symbol substitution tests, and physiological signal recordings. Four subjects demonstrated partial tolerance to the euphoric effects of cannabis after the first week. Performance on the short-term memory test decreased on the first day of drug administration but gradually improved until by the last day of the study performance had returned to baseline levels. On the postexperimental day baseline performance was surpassed. Performance on the digit-symbol substitution test was unaffected by drug administration and also improved with time, suggesting a practice effect. The authors interpreted their results as showing the apparent safety of smoking 14 mg/day THC for 3 weeks.

Mendelson, Rossi and Meyer (1974) reported a 31-day cannabis administration study in which 20 healthy, young male subjects (10 casual and 10 heavy users, mean age 23) were confined in a research ward and allowed 21 days of *ad libitum* marijuana smoking. A multidisciplinary battery of tests (psychiatric, psychological, physiological, biochemical and sociological) were administered during: a 5-day drug-free baseline phase, the 21-day smoking period, and a 5-day drug-free recovery phase. Acute and repeat dose effects of marijuana on cognitive function were studied with a battery of psychological tests known to be sensitive to organic brain dysfunction (WAIS, Halstead Category Test, Tactual Performance Test, Seashore Rhythm Test, Finger Tapping Test, Trail Making Test). Overall, there was no overt impairment of performance prior to or following cannabis smoking nor was there any difference between the performance of the heavy and the casual users. Short-term memory function, as assessed by digit span forwards and backwards, was impaired during intoxication and there was a relationship between performance and time elapsed since smoking. An interesting finding was that subjects performed better when they were aware that the effects of cannabis smoking on memory were being assessed, than when they were not. This was interpreted as evidence that the: "acute deleterious effect of marihuana on ability to perform on a memory task may not be a reflection of direct impairment of neuronal systems subserving memory, but rather a reflection of what a person chooses to attend to while under the influence of the drug" (Mendelson, Rossi & Meyer, 1974, p. 180).

Reed (1974) reported that two of the subjects in each group from the above study showed "unequivocal evidence of impairment" in some aspect of cognitive or motor functioning. Two of the heavy users performed quite poorly on the Trail Making Test, and they and two casual users showed no consistent patterns of improvement on other tests. Their scores were lower than

would have been predicted on the basis of their IQ scores and educational background. The probability of detecting such impairment in the normal population of healthy young adults would be low but it was not possible to find any relationship to prior history of cannabis use. The authors claimed that tolerance did not develop to the impairing effect of cannabis over the 21-day period, but there were no indications that cannabis interfered with the ability of subjects to improve their performance with practice.

Rossi and O'Brien (1974) assessed memory and time estimation in the same sample of subjects. They aimed to explore the possible mechanisms of the observation that marijuana produces a subjective impression that time is passing slowly. One hypothesis is that of a direct pharmacological action on neuronal systems serving as a "biological clock." Another possibility is that altered time perception is incidental to the effects of cannabis on perception, memory and organization of thought, with a loosening of associations and the rapid flow of ideas speeding up the subjective sense of time. A further possibility is that short-term memory impairment may interfere with a sense of temporal continuity, which is an essential element in time perception. The results of the study suggested that the effect on time perception was mediated directly through the action of THC on the central nervous system. They found a short-term acute effect on time perception (speeding up of the internal clock), and a longer-lasting compensatory effect (slowing of the internal clock) that paralleled the stimulatory and depressant effects of the drug. Tolerance to the acute effect on time perception developed during the 21-day period.

Similar failures to detect cognitive effects have been reported by three other groups of investigators. Frank et al. (1976) assessed short-term memory and goal-directed serial alternation and computation in healthy young males over 28 days of cannabis administration. Harshman, Crawford and Hecht (1976) and Cohen (1976) conducted a 94-day cannabis study in which 30 healthy moderate-to-heavy male cannabis users, aged 21 to 35, were administered on average

5.2 joints per day (mean 103 mg THC, range 35 to 198 mg) for 64 days and were assessed on brain hemisphere dominance before, during and after cannabis administration. Psychometric testing was not employed, but subjects were given two work assignments with financial incentive: a "psychomotor" task involving the addition of two columns of figures on a calculator and a "cognitive task" of learning a foreign language. No long-term impairments were detected with these somewhat inadequate assessment materials.

The experimental studies of daily cannabis usage for periods of up to three months in young adult male volunteers have consistently failed to demonstrate a relationship between marijuana use and neuropsychological dysfunction. This is not surprising given the short periods of exposure to the drug in these studies. Furthermore, since subjects served as their own controls, and had all used cannabis for at least one year prior to the study, it would be surprising if an additional few months of cannabis produced any significant decrements in performance. It may take many years for subtle impairments to be detected.

Studies of Carry-Over Effects

Most investigations of the acute effects of cannabis monitored performance on psychomotor tasks for a few hours following the onset of smoking on the assumption that performance decrements would last only for the duration of subjective intoxication. Impaired performance, particularly on tasks requiring divided attention among other cognitive abilities, has been reported to last from two to eight hours following moderate doses (e.g., Barnett, Licko & Thompson, 1985; Heishman, Stitzer & Yingling, 1989; Marks & MacAvoy, 1989; Perez-Reyes, Hicks et al., 1988). Chait et al. (1985) reported minimal evidence for a "hangover" effect the morning after smoking (nine hours later) on hand-eye co-ordination tasks, free recall and time perception. Few studies have investigated effects

beyond eight hours, nor attempted to determine the actual duration of the impairments observed.

By the mid-1980s, new evidence was mounting for lingering effects of cannabis beyond the period of acute intoxication. In particular, a report suggesting that cannabis may have residual detrimental effects on the performance of psychomotor tasks for up to 24 hours after smoking (Yesavage, Leirer et al., 1985) aroused some concern. This study monitored the performance of 10 pilots on a flight simulator task after smoking a single moderate dose of cannabis. Despite the pilots' lack of subjective awareness of any residual intoxicating effects or decrements in performance, they showed definite trends toward impairment on all variables measured 24 hours later. One of the criticisms of this study was that it failed to include a placebo control condition or group. In a follow-up study, the task was modified somewhat and impairment was only manifest for up to 4 hours after smoking, leading the authors to suggest that performance decrements may only be apparent on more complex, as opposed to simple, psychomotor tasks (Leirer, Yesavage & Morrow, 1989). More recently, these authors replicated their original findings using a more difficult but realistic simulator task in a double-blind experiment (Leirer, Yesavage & Morrow, 1991). Those pilots who had smoked marijuana still experienced significant difficulty in aligning the computerized landing simulator and in landing the plane at the centre of the runway 24 hours later, with no subjective awareness of any carry-over effects on their performance, mood or alertness. The authors interpreted their findings in terms of Baddeley and Hitch's (1974) framework of working memory as a "limited capacity work space for the temporary storage and processing of information coming from sensory input or from long-term memory" (Leirer, Yesavage & Morrow, 1991, p. 221), and suggested the carry-over effects from cannabis may occur whenever "our limited capacity working memory is presented with more information than it is able to process" (p. 226). The concept of working memory encompasses various other cognitive functions that require conscious integration and manipulation of information, such as divided and focused attention, short-term retention of information and reasoning (Baddeley, 1986).

Heishman et al. (1990) also reported preliminary findings to suggest that smoked marijuana can impair performance on cognitive tasks for up to 24 hours. Although based on a very small sample (N = 3), decreased accuracy and increased response time on serial addition/subtraction and digit recall tasks indicated that performance remained impaired the day after smoking, but the decrements were not as severe as they were whilst subjects were acutely intoxicated. They have since reported an extension of that study with nine subjects with a moderate history of cannabis use in a double-blind experimental procedure with minimal exposure (eight puffs only) to two active doses (1.8 per cent or 3.6 per cent THC) (Heishman, Pickworth et al., 1993). Psychomotor and cognitive performance measures included a circular lights (hand-eye co-ordination) task, serial addition/subtraction, logical reasoning, digit recall, and a manikin (spatial skills) task, and these were administered at nine set intervals before and up to 25 hours after smoking. Results indicated minimal acute performance impairment: response rate decreased, whilst response times increased on the serial addition/subtraction task, with a trend towards decreased accuracy, and similar effects on the logical reasoning and digit recall tasks. Not surprisingly, there was no evidence of residual impairment on any task the day after marijuana smoking. Few conclusions can be drawn from Heishman's studies, given the small sample size and the minimal exposure to low dose minimally impairing cannabis preparations, and the authors made no attempt to reconcile the likely effects of practice in their experimental design.

At best, these reports have provided some evidence for lingering impairments on complex cognitive tasks following the acute ingestion of cannabis.

Recent Research

The equivocal results of the early investigations into the long-term effects of cannabis on cognitive function, together with the problem of relatively short exposure to the drug in many countries, led to something of a hiatus in research on the long-term cognitive effects of cannabis in the 1980s. Although the accumulated evidence indicated that cannabis did not severely affect intellectual functioning, uncertainty remained about more subtle impairments. Their study required advances in methodology and assessment techniques. Instances of mental deterioration and impaired cognitive functioning in cannabis users continued to be reported in the clinical literature (e.g., National Institute on Drug Abuse, 1982) and anecdotally.

In the meantime, considerable advances were made in the field of cognitive psychology and neuropsychology. There were substantial theoretical developments in the fields of cognition, memory function and information processing, and more sensitive measures of cognitive processes were developed. Moreover, by the late 1980s, cannabis use had become sufficiently widespread and at a progressively younger age to revive interest in the issue.

Attentional and Memory Processes

Research from the late 1980s through the 1990s improved upon the design and methodology of previous studies in a number of ways. It ensured the use of adequate control groups, attempted to verify abstinence from cannabis prior to testing and attempted to quantify precisely the levels of cannabis use. In addition, there has to some extent been a narrowing of focus on the cognitive functions assessed, with greater attention to investigating specific cognitive processes and relating impairments in them to the quantity, frequency and duration of cannabis use.

Greater specificity in the focus of research was prompted by accumulating evidence from previous research and advances in pharmacology and biochemistry that suggest that cannabis primarily exerts its effect upon those areas of the brain responsible for attentional and memory functioning. Miller and Branconnier

(1983), for example, reviewed the literature and concluded that the detrimental effect of cannabis on human memory is the single most consistently reported psychological deficit produced by cannabinoids acutely, and the most consistently detected impairment in studies of long-term cannabis use. They proposed that the observed deficits in attention, memory consolidation and sequential-integration behaviors were mediated by the cholinergic limbic system, particularly in the septal-hippocampal pathway.

This proposal was supported by an earlier study that reported the similarity between cannabis-induced impairments of memory and those due to hippocampal damage (Drew, Weet et al., 1980). Performance of hippocampally lesioned patients on a battery of psychometric tests thought to assess various aspects of auditory and visual recent memory and mental set shifting, were compared to retrospective data from cannabis-intoxicated subjects. Tests for comparison included the Babcock Story Recall, digit span, paired-associate learning, and the Benton Visual Retention Test (for patients) or the similar Army Designs task (for marijuana-intoxicated subjects). When compared to controls, the two groups exhibited similar impairments of memory function, although the cannabis-intoxicated subjects produced significantly more intrusion errors.

Intrusion errors are among the most robust phenomena of cannabis-induced memory deficits in tasks of both recall and recognition (Miller & Branconnier, 1983). Such errors involve the introduction of extraneous items, word associations or new material during free recall of words, or the identification of false or previously unseen items in recognition. Miller and Branconnier conjectured that the mechanism causing intrusion errors was the failure to exclude irrelevant associations or extraneous stimuli during concentration of attention, a process in which the hippocampus may play a major role (Douglas, 1967; Eichenbaum & Cohen, 1988; Kimble, 1968). The finding of high densities of the cannabinoid receptor in the cerebral cortex and hippocampus (Herkenham, Lynn et al., 1990) is consistent with the hypothesis that cannabinoids are involved in attentional and memory processes. Past studies of the long-term effects of cannabis have not used sufficiently specific nor sensitive measures of such processes.

It is also important to note that most past studies have been conducted on adults, while the effects of long-term cannabis use on the young have not been adequately addressed. With an increase in the prevalence of cannabis use among adolescents and young adults, there has been a growing concern about its possible impact on the psychological development of young people. This is important because of the possibly deleterious effects of such a psychoactive substance upon psychosocial adaptation and maturation during their formative years, and the effects on cognition, learning and scholastic achievement.

In the first study of its kind with adolescents, Schwartz et al. (1989) reported the results of a small but carefully controlled pilot study of persistent short-term memory impairment in 10 cannabis-dependent adolescents (aged 14 to 16 years). Schwartz's clinical observations of adolescents in a drug-abuse treatment program suggested that memory deficits were a major problem, which according to the adolescents persisted for at least three to four weeks after cessation of cannabis use. His sample was middle class, North American, matched for age, IQ and absence of any previous learning disabilities with 17 controls, 8 of whom were drug abusers who had not been long-term users of cannabis, and another 9 who had never abused any drug. The cannabis users consumed approximately 18 grams per week, smoking at a frequency of at least 4 days per week (mean 5.9) for at least 4 consecutive months (mean 7.6 months but the range was not reported). Subjects with a history of excessive alcohol or phencyclidine use were excluded from the study. Cannabinoids were detected in the urines of 8 of the 10 users over two to nine days.

Users were initially tested between two and five days after entry to the treatment program, this length of time allowing for dissipation of any obvious short-term effects of cannabis intoxication on cognition and memory. Subjects were assessed by a neuropsychological battery which included the Wechsler Intelligence Scale for Children, and six tests "to measure auditory/verbal and visual/spatial immediate and short-term (delayed) memory and praxis (construction ability)" (Schwartz, Gruenewald et al., 1989, p. 1215). These were the Peterson-Peterson short-term Memory Paradigm, Buschke's Selective Remembering Test, the Benton Visual Retention Test, Wechsler Memory Scale Prose Passages, Rey-Osterrieth or Taylor's Complex Figure Drawing, and a Paired-Associate Learning Test. After six weeks of supervised abstinence with bi-weekly urine screens for drugs of abuse, a parallel test battery was administered.

On the initial testing, there were statistically significant differences between groups on two tests: cannabis users were selectively impaired on the Benton Visual Retention Test and the Wechsler Memory Scale Prose Passages. The differences were smaller but were still detectable six weeks later. Analysis of test measures showed cannabis users to commit significantly more errors than controls initially on the Benton Visual Retention Test for both immediate and delayed conditions, but differences in the six-week posttest were not significant. Users scored lower than controls on both immediate and delayed recall in the Wechsler Memory Prose Passages Test in both test sessions. The authors concluded that "cannabis-dependent adolescents have selective short-term memory deficits that continue for at least six weeks after the last use of marijuana" (1989, p. 1214). Further testing beyond six weeks, while not possible in this study, would have provided useful information on the recovery of function. The fact that there was a trend towards improvement in the scores of cannabis users suggests that the deficits observed were related to their past cannabis use and that functioning may return to normal following a longer period of abstinence.

The authors discussed the clinical implications of their results in terms of the need to develop treatment strategies that address the possible long-lasting cognitive deficits that affect both performance of complex tasks and the ability to learn. They referred to investigations which suggest that adolescents with learning disabilities are at high risk of cannabis abuse. Their own results heighten concerns about the effects of long-term cannabis use on learning-impaired adolescents. For such individuals, regular use of cannabis, even to a lesser degree than that used by Schwartz's sample, may significantly contribute to worsening school performance. Further, they suggest that individuals with learning disabilities and those who have a borderline or low IQ might be even more susceptible to cannabis-induced deficits of short-term or recent memory.

Schwartz's study was the first well-controlled study to demonstrate cognitive dysfunction in cannabis-using adolescents with a brief mean duration of use. The implications of these results are that young people may be more vulnerable to any impairments resulting from cannabis use. Unfortunately, like many of its predecessors, Schwartz's team made little effort to interpret the significance of the selectivity of their results. There was nothing to suggest which specific elements of memory formation or retrieval were disrupted. The two tasks represented two different types of information processing. The Benton requires the retention of visual information in iconic or unprocessed form over very brief periods, whereas the Wechsler task requires the extraction of abstractions from stories, encoding these abstractions, retrieving information and complex responding. The authors acknowledged that their "data provide little guidance on which to formulate hypotheses concerning the neurologic substrates of the observed results" and suggested that the "isolation of the location and types of disruptions that account for the current results should, therefore, be one goal of future research in this area" (1989, p. 1218).

A more recent examination of memory and intellectual function in adolescents (Millsaps, Azrin & Mittenberg, 1994) supported the findings of Schwartz et al. (1989). The Wechsler Memory Scale-Revised and the WAIS-R were administered to 15 adolescent users (mean age 16.9 years) who had used on average 8.9 grams of cannabis per week for over two years (mean 29.1 months). They had completed a mean of 9.5 years of education, although some had fallen behind in their schooling due to delinquent behavior. Subjects were excluded on the basis of abuse of or dependence on any other substances, ever having used phencyclidine (PCP), or any history of neurologic illness, seizures or head injury. All subjects met the criteria for cannabis dependence according to the *Diagnostic and Statistical Manual of Mental Disorders, Third Edition, Revised (DSM-III-R)* (American Psychiatric Association, 1987). They were abstinent for a mean of 27 days prior to testing. Most, but not all, subjects underwent urine drug screens, but for those who did not, information from collaterals was obtained to verify abstinence.

Each subject's premorbid IQ was calculated using a demographically based prediction equation. Subjects were then used as their own controls, comparing the premorbid estimated IQ to the obtained full-scale IQ. Difference scores for each individual subject were also calculated by subtracting each of the WMS-R General Memory Index and the Delayed Memory Index from the full-scale IQ, and the former two measures from the Attention/Concentration Index. The authors reported that memory impairment due to central nervous system dysfunction has been investigated in this manner in the recent neuropsychological literature. Full-scale IQ was found not to be lower than the premorbid IQ estimate, consistent with all other findings to date that suggest that general intellectual function is not impaired by chronic cannabis use. In contrast, both the General and Delayed Memory Indices were significantly reduced when compared to full-scale IQ, although they remained in the low-average range. Attention/concentration was found to be relatively intact. These results suggest that long-term marijuana use in adolescents leads to subtle impairment of memory functions, still detectable following abstinence of about one month. Once again, this study made no attempt to identify the precise memory processes that might be impaired.

Leon-Carrion (1990) used the subscales of the WAIS to compare an older group of 23 male chronic cannabis users (aged 18 to 27 years,

2.5 joints per day for 4.5 years) to a matched control group. The cannabis users had significantly lower scores than controls on six of the eleven subscales: Comprehension, Similarities, Vocabulary, Block Design, Picture Arrangement and Object Assembly. Overall, the cannabis users' scores were lower than would be expected for their age. Their full-scale IQ, and both verbal and performance IQs, were lower than those of the controls. These results suggest that the cannabis users may well have differed in ability from controls prior to their having commenced using cannabis, even though the author argues against this on the basis of socioeconomic, cultural and educational status. A vocabulary score alone is perhaps the single best indicator of original intellectual endowment, being the the most resilient to insult. Nevertheless, the author's interpretation of the results is in accord with many other observations: users were most impaired in their ability to learn from experience, their capacity for compromise, elaboration of adequate judgments and situational adaptation, and organizational, verbal and communication skills. Many of these abilities are thought to be under the control of the frontal lobes.

It appears that the same group of subjects were assessed on an eight-hour-long version of the Trail Making Test to investigate cognitive styles and relations between the two cerebral hemispheres (Leon-Carrion & Vela-Bueno, 1991). Cannabis users exhibited great fluctuation between cognitive styles and weaker dominance-subdominance hemispheric alternation that was clearly maintained over time in control subjects. The authors interpreted these findings to suggest that chronic consumption of cannabis can affect cognitive styles and the brain, altering the basic rest/activity cycle between the hemispheres. The significance of these findings is open to interpretation, although the tests may be tapping some aspect of frontal lobe function.

One crucial requirement for evaluating the performance of chronic marijuana users is comparison with an appropriately matched group of non-using subjects. Although most studies have made substantial progress in this regard, one concern remains that some of the impairments found may have been present in the cannabis users prior to their cannabis use. Short of an expensive longitudinal study that follows children over many years, the most desirable procedure is to match groups of users and non-users on some measure of intellectual functioning, preferably obtained before the onset of drug use, or otherwise to obtain a valid measure that can be used to estimate the premorbid level of intellectual functioning, as was used in Millsaps, Azrin and Mittenberg's (1994) study with adolescents.

Block and colleagues (1990; 1993) conducted a study in which they used scores on the Iowa Tests of Basic Skills collected in the fourth grade of grammar school. These are standardized ability tests that have been administered to almost all grammar school children in Iowa for several decades. Block et al. used these scores to establish that their user and non-user samples were comparable in intellectual functioning before they began using marijuana. The study's aim was to determine whether chronic marijuana use produced specific cognitive impairments, and if so, whether these impairments depend on the frequency of use. Block and colleagues assessed 144 cannabis users (aged 18 to 42 years), 64 of whom were light users (1 to 4 times per week for 5.5 years) and 80 heavy users (≥ 5 times per week for 6.0 years) (range 2 to 10+ years use), and compared them with 72 controls. Twenty-four hours of abstinence was required prior to testing.

Subjects participated in two sessions. In the first session they completed the 12th grade version of the Iowa Tests of Educational Development, which emphasize basic, general intellectual abilities and academic skills and effective utilization of previously acquired information in verbal and mathematical areas (subtests include Vocabulary, Correctness and Appropriateness of Expression, Ability To Do Quantitative Thinking and Ability To Interpret Literary Materials plus a Short Test of Educational Ability). In the second session, subjects were administered computerized tests that emphasized learning and remembering new information, associative processes and semantic memory retrieval (e.g., free and constrained

associations, paired-associate learning, text learning, Buschke's Selective Reminding Task), concept formation and psychomotor performance (e.g., discriminant reaction time and critical flicker fusion). The tasks selected had been previously shown to be sensitive to the acute or chronic effects of cannabis. They were also relevant to the skills required in school and work performance.

The results showed that while users and non-users were matched on 4th grade Iowa scores, heavy users showed impairment in two areas when tested on the 12th grade Iowa Test: verbal expression (Correctness and Appropriateness of Expression) and mathematical skills (Ability To Do Quantitative Thinking). The results of the computerized tests (Block & Ghoneim, 1993), showed that heavy, chronic marijuana use of at least 7 times per week did not produce overall impairments in Buschke's Test but selectively impaired the retrieval of words that were easy to visualize. The impairments in heavy users remained significant after controlling for the effects of lifetime and recent use of other drugs and alcohol. One test of abstraction (Concept Formation) showed superior performance in a particular test condition (fuzzy concepts) in users of moderate frequency (5 to 6 times per week). The authors were also able to show reasonable, albeit imperfect, agreement between acute and chronic effects of marijuana on cognition by comparison with the results of another study examining the acute effects of cannabis on the same battery of tests (Block, Farinpour & Braverman, 1992). The impairments associated with heavy, chronic use were much less pervasive than the immediate effects of marijuana smoking. Two tests showing a large degree of impairment acutely (Ability To Interpret Literary Materials, and Text Learning) showed no long-term adverse effect. This research has been among the first to compare directly the acute and chronic effects of cannabis on the same test battery, and the authors point out that while acute and chronic effects of drugs are sometimes similar, they can also be markedly different.

Event-related Potentials

In an attempt to isolate with greater specificity the nature of cognitive dysfunction in long-term cannabis users, Solowij and co-authors (Solowij, 1995; Solowij, Grenyer et al., 1995; Solowij, Michie & Fox, 1991; 1995a; 1995b; 1998), conducted a series of studies that examined specific stages of information processing, focusing on attentional mechanisms. As noted by Miller and Branconnier (1983), many of the observed memory deficits may occur because cannabinoids disinhibit septal-hippocampal inputs to the reticular activating system resulting in failure to habituate to irrelevant stimuli. Solowij and colleagues accordingly assessed the integrity of attentional processes in long-term cannabis users using a combination of performance and brain event-related potential measures, which together can provide insight into the nature of attentional dysfunction. Event-related potential (ERP) measures, extracted from the EEG, are sensitive markers of covert cognitive processes underlying overt behavior; the amplitude and latency of various ERP components have been shown to reflect various stages of information processing.

In each study, cannabis users were recruited from the general community and matched on age, sex, years of education and alcohol consumption with non-user controls who had either never used or had limited experience with cannabis (e.g., maximum use 15 times). Strict exclusion criteria were applied to any subjects with a history of head injury, neurological or psychiatric illness, significant use of other drugs, or high levels of alcohol consumption. The National Adult Reading Test (Nelson, 1982) was used to estimate premorbid full-scale IQ that did not differ between groups. Subjects were instructed to abstain from cannabis and alcohol for 24 hours prior to testing, and two urine samples were analysed to ensure that subjects were not acutely intoxicated at the time of testing. The criterion on which this assertion was based was that cannabinoid levels detected in a sample provided on the day of testing be lower than those detected in a sample taken from the night before testing. Any subject returning a urine

sample positive for other drugs was excluded. Subjects completed a multidimensional auditory selective attention task, in which random sequences of tones varying in location, pitch and duration were delivered through headphones while brain electrical activity (EEG) was recorded. They were instructed to attend to a particular ear and a particular pitch, and to respond to the long duration tones with a button press. This procedure enabled an examination of the brain's response to tones when attended and unattended.

The first study (Solowij, Michie & Fox, 1991) assessed a small and heterogeneous group of long-term cannabis users (N = 9), aged 19 to 40, who had used cannabis for a mean of 11.2 years (range 3 to 20 years) at the level of 4.8 days per week (range twice per week to daily use). Users performed significantly more poorly than controls, with fewer correct detections, more errors (false alarms) and slightly longer reaction times. Analysis of the ERP measures showed that cannabis users had reduced P300 amplitudes compared to controls, reflecting dysfunction in the allocation of attentional resources and stimulus evaluation strategies. Further, cannabis users showed an inability to filter out complex irrelevant information, as evidenced by increased frontal processing negativity to stimuli of the irrelevant pitch, while controls were able to reject this irrelevant information from further processing at an early stage. The results suggested that long-term use of cannabis may impair the ability to process complex information efficiently.

A second study was conducted with a larger sample in order to examine the effects of frequency and duration of use (Solowij, Michie & Fox, 1995a). Thirty-two cannabis users were split at the median on both frequency (light: ≤ twice per week versus heavy: ≥ 3 times per week) and duration (short: 3 to 4 years versus long: ≥ 5 years) of cannabis use. Equal numbers of heavy and light cannabis users contributed to the long- and short-duration user groups and vice versa. The mean number of years of use for the long-duration users was 10.1, and it was 3.3 for short-duration users (range 3 to 28 years). The mean frequency of use was 18 days per month for the heavy group and 6 for the light group (range: once per month to daily use). Subjects were matched to a group of non-user controls (N = 16) according to the criteria of the first study and a similar methodology was employed.

Once again cannabis users' performance was worse than that of controls, with the greatest impairment observed in the heavy user group. The results of this study replicated the original ERP findings but indicated that different cognitive processes were differentially affected by frequency and duration of cannabis use. The long-duration user group showed significantly larger frontal processing negativity to pitch irrelevant stimuli than did short-duration users and controls. There were no differences in processing negativity between groups defined on frequency of use. A significant correlation between this ERP measure and duration of cannabis use indicated that the ability to focus attention and filter out complex irrelevant information was progressively impaired with the number of years of use, but was unrelated to frequency of use. Frequency of use affected the speed of information processing, as reflected in a delay in P300 latency in the heavy user group compared to light users and controls. P300 latency reflects the time taken to evaluate a stimulus. There was a significant correlation between P300 latency and increasing frequency of use, but this measure was unrelated to duration of use.

These results were interpreted by the authors to reflect different mechanisms of short-lasting and long-lasting action of cannabinoids. The slowing of information processing in the brain was interpreted as a function of a chronic build-up of cannabinoids, and hence as a subacute effect that, it was hypothesized, would be eliminated by decreasing frequency of use. The inability to focus attention and reject irrelevant information was interpreted as reflecting long-term changes, possibly at the cannabinoid receptor site. These hypotheses were supported by a third study that examined the reversibility of these impairments in a group of ex-cannabis users (Solowij, 1995). The 32 ex-users had used for a mean of 9 years (range 3 to 20 years) and

had given up using between 3 months and 6 years ago (mean 2 years abstinence). The speed of information processing, as reflected by P300 latency, was not reduced in the ex-users, but the inability to focus attention and reject irrelevant information, evidenced by large processing negativity to irrelevant stimuli, increased as a function of past duration of cannabis use and did not resolve as a function of the duration of abstinence. These results were discussed in terms of possible partial recovery of function in some individuals but not others (see also Solowij, Michie & Fox, 1995b). A single case pilot study reported by the same group (Solowij, Grenyer et al., 1995) further investigated the parameters of recovery by testing the subject on multiple occasions before and after quitting cannabis use. In this individual there was no indication of resolution of the large processing negativity to irrelevant stimuli by six weeks of abstinence. An interesting observation from the ERPs recorded from this individual whilst acutely intoxicated led the authors to speculate that cannabis might serve to normalize information processing in highly dependent individuals.

The series of studies by Solowij and colleagues provide a substantial advance in terms of rigor of methodology, specificity of assessment techniques and sensitivity of the measures used to investigate cognitive functioning in long-term cannabis users. The results provide further evidence of subtle but enduring impairments in specific cognitive processes, which the authors relate to both attention and memory function. The implications for functioning in the real world are difficult to extrapolate, but one could speculate that higher levels of distractibility may subtly affect driving, operating complex machinery, learning in the classroom, and efficient work performance in any situation where concentration is essential. The ability to attend selectively to one source of information while actively rejecting another is a function attributed to the frontal lobes. Such attentional deficits would impair memory and other higher-order cognitive functions. There was some evidence that cannabis users of higher IQ may be better able to compensate for its impairing effects (Solowij, 1995; Solowij, Michie & Fox, 1995a). The studies demonstrated the insensitivity of performance measures alone to cannabinoid effects, emphasizing the need to use more sensitive measures to examine otherwise inaccessible, covert cognitive processes. The demonstration of differential impairments due to frequency and duration of use are important in terms of assessing subacute versus more long-lasting impairments as a function of long-term use of cannabis.

Other Tests of Frontal Lobe Function

Another recent study detected specific impairments of attention, memory and frontal lobe function in heavy marijuana-using college students by means of selected neuropsychological tests (Pope & Yurgelun-Todd, 1996). This well-controlled research used self-reported high school Scholastic Aptitude Test scores as a measure of premorbid intellectual ability. Pope and Yurgelun-Todd tested two samples of undergraduate college students: 64 light and 65 heavy cannabis users of median age 21 (range 18 to 28), and comprising equivalent numbers of males and females. Light users were those who reported using cannabis only occasionally (a maximum of 9 days in the past 30 days), while heavy users reported using regularly (a minimum of 22 days in the past 30 days). The duration of cannabis use was not reported nor were its effects investigated. Subjects were hospitalized overnight to ensure abstinence from cannabis of at least 19 hours prior to testing. The tests administered were the vocabulary subtest of the WAIS-R to obtain a measure of verbal IQ, digit span, the Stroop test, the Wisconsin Card Sorting Test (WCST), the Benton Verbal Fluency Test, the Wechsler Memory Scale (WMS), the California Verbal Learning Test (CVLT) and the Rey-Osterreith Complex Figure Test.

Heavy users and light users were equivalent on the verbal portion of the Scholastic Aptitude Test, but heavy users had lower scores on the quantitative portion and on the total score, as

well as a lower verbal IQ. These variables were used as covariates in the analyses. No differences between the two groups were found on digit span. Male heavy users were slower than light users in the interference condition of the Stroop test. Heavy users of both sexes made more perseverative responses on the WCST than light users. On the verbal fluency test, heavy users of low verbal IQ produced significantly fewer words than light users of low verbal IQ, and five of the heavy users scored below the threshold of low normal scores. The memory quotient on the WMS did not differ between groups, nor did any of the subtests except that male heavy users performed significantly more poorly on the delayed recall of figures. Male heavy users also recalled significantly fewer elements of the Rey figure on immediate recall. Heavy and light users differed significantly on recall of the first administration of the CVLT word list, and on each subsequent administration over five trials and in an interference condition involving short delay. There was a trend also toward poorer performance following a long delay. The sex differences found on certain subtests of this study are interesting in that they suggest that there may be differential effects of cannabis use on males and females. Sex differences have rarely been investigated in the research to date on the cognitive effects of cannabis.

The investigators performed a number of careful *post hoc* analyses in an attempt to establish that the poorer performance of the heavy users was an effect of cannabis and not attributable to, say, premorbid deficits or use of other substances. Although these confounds were ruled out, the authors were unable to attribute their findings to either a temporary effect due either to drug residues lingering in the brain or to an abrupt withdrawal from heavy use, or to a lasting alteration of central nervous system function as a result of lifetime exposure to cannabis. The authors have previously argued, quite correctly, that this attributional problem applies to all studies of cognitive function in long-term cannabis users (Pope, Gruber & Yurgelun-Todd, 1995). Further analyses failed to support the hypothesis that poorer performance was related to total lifetime consumption of cannabis. However, no correlational analysis was reported nor were any effects associated with the actual duration of use tested. In fact, the mean duration of cannabis use of their samples was not reported and it is unlikely that their subjects had used for an extensive period of time as they were all college students with a mean age of 20 to 21 years. In fact the authors did state that "many" subjects had used for two years or more, and that none had used for more than a decade. It is possible that their heavy users had in fact used for a greater number of years than their light users. This is proposed in the light of recent data collected by this author that suggest an effect of duration of cannabis use on perseverative responding and verbal learning, but no effect of frequency of use (Solowij, Grenyer et al., 1997).

The sample of the Solowij et al. (1997) study differed substantially from that of Pope and Yurgelun-Todd: they were a cohort of long-term cannabis users (n = 100) who responded to an advertisement offering treatment for cannabis users who wanted to quit. The mean age of the respondents was about 33 and the mean duration of cannabis use was approximately 14 years (range 5 to 32). Long-term users made significantly more perseverative responses on the WCST than age-matched norms, and these increased as a function of the number of years of cannabis use. As this group were almost all daily users of cannabis, effects of frequency of use were examined as a quantity/frequency measure, but no significant frequency effects or correlations were found. The Rey Auditory Verbal Learning Test (RAVLT), which is very similar to the CVLT, was also administered. Once again, no relationship was found between performance on this task and quantity/frequency of cannabis use, but long-term users recalled fewer words on every measure of memory function from the RAVLT than age-matched norms. Performance on the RAVLT did not correlate significantly with duration of cannabis use, but a significantly larger proportion of longer-term users than shorter-term users lost more than three words from trial V to VI (an abnormal amount of shrinkage for delayed recall

following interference). These results, which come from a much more entrenched group of cannabis users than those of Pope and Yurgelun-Todd's study, provide support for a subtle yet progressive impairment related to the number of years of cannabis use. This implies that gradual changes may occur in the brain as a result of cumulative exposure, and that these changes are related more to "how long" as opposed to "how much" cannabis is used. The ERP studies by Solowij and colleagues reviewed above lend further credence to this hypothesis.

Pope and Yurgelun-Todd's study was important in identifying with much greater precision and specificity those aspects of cognitive functioning that may be impaired by even relatively short-term but heavy use of cannabis. Their results suggested that heavy cannabis use "was associated with reduced function of the attentional/executive system, as exhibited by decreased mental flexibility and increased perseveration on the WCST, and reduced learning on the CVLT" (1996, p. 526). They claimed that cannabis use may compromise some memory functions, but the principal effect is on the attentional/executive system, while recall per se remains relatively intact. They further claimed that the most pronounced effects may be on the abilities to shift and/or sustain attention, functions associated with the prefrontal cortex. A similar conclusion was drawn by the recently reported Costa Rican follow-up (Fletcher, Page et al., 1996; see above).

The Ottawa Prenatal Prospective Study (OPPS)

Converging evidence for frontal involvement comes from a very different approach to assessing the long-term consequences of exposure to cannabis. The Ottawa Prenatal Prospective Study (OPPS) is an exceptionally well-controlled longitudinal study of children who had been prenatally exposed to cannabis *in utero*. Summaries of the findings to date and a discussion of their interpretation and implications are presented by Fried (1993; 1995; 1996; see also chapter 12 in this volume). For the purposes of this chapter, only assessments of the cognitive and central nervous system development of the children, and only those effects that remained statistically significant after controlling for many potentially confounding variables, such as birthweight, other drug use, socioeconomic status and nutrition, will be discussed.

The levels of exposure to cannabis in the sample were approximately as follows: 60 per cent of the mothers used cannabis irregularly, 10 per cent reported smoking two to five joints per week, and 30 per cent smoked a greater amount during each trimester of pregnancy. Prenatal exposure to cannabis was associated with high-pitched cries, disturbed sleep cycles, increased tremors and exaggerated startle responses to minimal stimulation in newborn to 30-day-old babies. The babies showed poorer habituation to visual stimuli, consistent with the sensitivity of the visual system to the teratogenic effects of cannabis demonstrated in rhesus monkeys and rats (e.g., Fried & Charlebois, 1979). Fried's interpretation of these findings was that exposure to cannabis may affect the rate of development of the central nervous system, with particularly slow rate of maturation of the visual system. This hypothesis was supported by visual evoked potential studies of the children at four years of age. Children who had been exposed to cannabis *in utero* showed greater variability and longer latency of the evoked potential components, indicating immaturity in the system.

From one to three years of age, no adverse effects of prenatal exposure were found on the Bayley Scales, which provide mental and psycho-motor developmental indices and assess infant behavior. At two years, it appeared that the children were impaired on tests of language comprehension as assessed by the Reynell Developmental Language Scale, but this effect did not persist after controlling for other factors such as ratings of the home environment. At three years of age, the McCarthy Scales of Children's Abilities also failed to detect any negative associations with prenatal exposure to cannabis. At four years of age, however, the children of cannabis-using mothers were significantly inferior to controls on tests of verbal ability and memory as assessed by the McCarthy scale and the Peabody test of receptive vocabulary. The explanation for the gap in detecting impairments in the preceding age range was that the degree and types of deficits observed may only be identifiable when cognitive development has proceeded to a certain level of maturity and when complex behavior can be examined at a more specific rather than global level (Fried, 1996). It has been suggested that it is around this age that the frontal lobes begin to function.

At five and six years of age, the children were not impaired on global tests of cognition and language, and the investigators speculate on the possible influence of schooling as an explanation for the "catching up" of the exposed children. By age six, however, a deficit in sustained attention was detected in a computerized task that differentiated between impulsivity and vigilance. Fried (1993) proposed that "instruments that provide a general description of cognitive abilities may be incapable of identifying nuances in neurobehavior that may discriminate between the marijuana-exposed and non-marijuana-exposed children" (p. 332). He suggested the need for tests that examine specific cognitive characteristics and strategies, such as the test of sustained attention. From six to nine years of age the children continued to be assessed on a battery of neurobehavioral tests. Preliminary analyses have suggested that cannabis-exposed children scored more poorly than non-exposed children on parental behavioral ratings, visual perceptual and memory tasks, language comprehension and distractibility, although the extent to which these differences remain clinically significant following statistical control of (possibly inappropriate) confounding variables is uncertain (Fried, 1996). Fried warns that his sample came from a middle-class, low-risk population and that his results might therefore be interpreted as a somewhat conservative estimate of the potential risk, but also notes that any effects associated with prenatal exposure to cannabis are likely to be subtle and yet to affect the complex executive functioning that develops throughout childhood (Fried, 1995; 1996). Fried (1993) suggested that cannabis "may affect a number of neonatal behaviors and facets of cognitive behavior under conditions in which complex demands are placed on nervous system functions" (p. 332). Most recently, Fried (1995; 1996) concludes that the areas of vulnerability that have emerged from this course of study are consistent with the cognitive construct termed *executive function* — the ability to maintain an appropriate problem-solving set for attainment of a future goal, which involves the integration of a variety of cognitive processes and which is thought to be subserved by the prefrontal lobes.

Further evidence for an enduring deficit comes from a NIDA-funded project (principal investigator, F. Struve) to investigate persistent central nervous system sequelae of chronic cannabis exposure. This research has utilized both neuropsychological tests and quantitative EEG techniques. The latter determined significant increases in absolute power, relative power and interhemispheric coherence of EEG alpha and theta activity, primarily in frontal-central cortex, in daily cannabis users of up to 30 years' duration compared to short-term users and non-users (e.g., Struve, Straumanis & Patrick, 1994; see section I, "Brain Function and Neurotoxicity"). The results suggest that there may be a gradient of quantitative EEG change associated with progressive increases in the total cumulative exposure (duration in years) of daily cannabis use that may indicate organic change. To date, correlations between the EEG changes and neuropsychological test performance have not been reported.

Preliminary analyses of the neuropsychological test data have been presented at conferences (e.g., Leavitt, Webb et al., 1992; 1993). These investigations have been exceptionally well controlled. Subjects were extensively screened for current or past psychiatric or medical disease or CNS injury, and underwent extensive drug history assessments with eight weeks of twice weekly drug screens. Groups were matched for age and sex. Daily cannabis users who had at least 3 to 6 years of use were compared to a group who had used for 6 to 14 years, a special interest group who had used on a daily basis for 15 years or more, and a non-user control group. Sample sizes varied from study to study, but averaged approximately 15 per group.

An extensive battery of psychological tests included measures of simple and complex reaction time (using Sternberg's procedure), attention and memory span (e.g., digits forwards and backwards, continuous performance task, trail making, serial addition/subtraction, divided attention [Paced Auditory Serial Addition Test — PASAT], Stroop interference task), language and comprehension tasks, construction (complex Rey figure), verbal and visual learning/memory (Wechsler Memory Scale and California Verbal Learning Test [CVLT]) and "higher" mental abilities/concept formation/logical reasoning (WAIS-R, Category Test and Conceptual Level Analogies Test [CLAT]). The effects of age and education were addressed through a multiple regression procedure that removed expected values computed using only age and education from all outcome variables. Only non-users were used to estimate regression weights and these were "jackknifed."

Preliminary analyses have shown test scores in general to show a gradation, with the best performance characterizing non-user controls, followed by the daily cannabis users and the worst mean scores shown by the ultra long-term special interest group (Leavitt, Webb et al., 1992; 1993; J. Leavitt, personal communication). Neuropsychological measures that would not be expected to be affected by cannabis use (e.g., information and vocabulary subtests of the WAIS-R) were not significantly different between groups. Selected WAIS-R subtests did show significant differences between groups, with, in each case, the daily cannabis users performing more poorly than controls and the greatest level of impairment being found in the ultra long-term group. Select subscales of the Revised Wechsler Memory Scale showed similar trends. Long-duration users performed more poorly than short-term users and controls, and there were few differences between the latter two groups, on complex reaction time, verbal learning/recall (CVLT), complex reasoning/conceptual abilities (category,

CLAT) and short-term memory (verbal, visual, delayed Wechsler Memory Scale subtests). There was a trend toward poorer performance on the complex mental tracking task (PASAT). The investigators claimed that duration of use was related to impaired performance, but did not report any correlations. Tests sensitive to mild cortical dysfunction were those most affected in the long-term user groups. The results attest to the importance of taking cumulative duration of exposure to cannabis into account when studying the cognitive functioning of chronic cannabis users.

One of the robust sequelae of acute intoxication is altered time sense, and the underproduction of time estimations has been demonstrated and replicated in many studies (e.g., Melges, Tinklenberg et al., 1970; Tinklenberg, Kopell et al., 1972). A further study from this group has investigated time production in chronic users after 24 hours' abstinence (Webb, Struve et al., 1993). Twenty-eight daily users (≥ seven joints per week for ≥ three years) displayed greater time underproduction than 32 controls, suggesting that time distortion may persist beyond the acute phase of intoxication. Additional analyses suggested that time distortions were greater for long-term than short-term users.

Overall, this series of studies made an important advance in terms of its rigorous methodology, extensive range of neuropsychological assessment tests and the analyses and interpretations of the results. The results suggested that long-duration users seem to process some kinds of information more slowly than non-users, and that the effects of long-term cannabis use are most likely to surface under conditions of moderately heavy cognitive load. The authors acknowledge that small sample sizes dictate caution and that there were no data available to assess the premorbid cognitive capacity of these subjects. Nevertheless, the results allowed the following conclusions to be drawn (J. Leavitt, personal communication):

1. although basic attentional processes appear to be intact, long-term cannabis users are less efficient when performing complex cognitive tasks or attempting to resist distraction;

2. long-term users' ability to process information efficiently declines more rapidly under a moderate cognitive load when compared with controls or short duration users;

3. although remote memory appears unaffected, long-term users are inefficient at learning and recalling information over the short term, especially when the task is unfamiliar or complex; they show increased susceptibility to retroactive interference, whereby new information interferes with the retrieval of old information (which is consistent with difficulty in resisting distraction);

4. long-term users are inefficient at performing complex tasks that require cognitive flexibility, recognition of unproductive planning strategies, and learning from experience, functions that have been clinically associated with the frontal area;

5. because language and verbal intellectual abilities appear unaffected, long-term cannabis users may cope reasonably well with routine tasks of everyday life, but they may have difficulties with verbal tasks that are novel and/or which cannot be solved by automatic application of previous knowledge.

Further specific assessments are required to fully explore the scope and nature of deficits in long-term user populations.

Discussion

Previous reviewers have generally concluded that there is insufficient evidence to conclude that cannabis produces any long-term cognitive deficits (e.g., Wert & Raulin, 1986a; 1986b). This is probably a reasonable conclusion when gross deficits are considered: the weight of evidence suggests that the long-term use of cannabis does not result in any severe or grossly debilitating impairment of cognitive function. However, recent reviewers agree that there is now sufficient evidence that the long-term use of cannabis leads to a more subtle and selective impairment of cognitive functioning (Block, 1996; Hall, Solowij & Lemon, 1994; Pope, Gruber & Yurgelen-Todd, 1995; Solowij, 1998). The findings from recent methodologically rigorous research provide evidence for complex but subtle impairments that include the organization and integration of complex information involving various mechanisms of attention and memory processes. These cognitive impairments are either associated with the frequency of cannabis use or increase with duration of cannabis use. There is evidence that impairment on some standard neuropsychological tests may become apparent only after 10 to 15 years of use (e.g., Leavitt, Webb et al., 1993). But very sensitive measures of brain function (e.g., ERPs) are capable of detecting specific attentional impairments after five years of use and cannabis users of only three to four years showed early signs of impairment (Solowij, Michie & Fox, 1995a). Consistent with these findings, other recent well-controlled research has demonstrated impaired executive/attentional function and learning in relatively short-term but heavy users of cannabis by means of specific and sensitive neuropsychological tests (Pope & Yurgelen-Todd, 1996).

Impairments appear to be specific to higher cognitive functions, which include the organization and integration of complex information involving various mechanisms of attention and memory processes. The similarity between the kinds of subtle impairments associated with long-term cannabis use and with frontal lobe dysfunction is becoming more apparent (e.g., short-term memory deficits, increased susceptibility to interference, lack of impairment on general tests of intelligence or IQ). Frontal lobe function is difficult to measure as indicated by the fact that patients with known frontal lobe lesions do not differ from controls on a variety of neuropsychological tests (Stuss, 1991). Thus, the difficulty of assessing frontal lobe functions is not unique to research into the long-term effects of cannabis.

One of the functions of the frontal lobes is the temporal organization of behavior, a key process in efficient memory function, self-awareness and planning. The frontal lobe hypothesis of impairments due to long-term use of cannabis is consistent with the altered perception of time demonstrated in cannabis users and with cerebral blood flow studies that demonstrate greatest alterations in the region of the frontal lobes (see section I, "Brain Function and Neurotoxicity"). There is also sound electrophysiological evidence of altered functioning in the region of the frontal lobes. The frontal lobes are important in organizing, manipulating and integrating a variety of information, and in structuring and segregating events in memory. Further research incorporating better measures of frontal lobe function in long-term cannabis users is clearly indicated.

The equivocal results of previous studies of cognitive functioning in long-term cannabis users appear to be due primarily to poor methodology and insensitive test measures. Wert and Raulin (1986b) had rejected the possibility that tests used previously were not sensitive enough to detect impairments, on the grounds that the same tests had demonstrated impairment in alcoholics and heavy social drinkers. However, the cognitive deficits produced by chronic alcohol consumption are most likely very different to those produced by cannabis. The mechanisms of action of the two substances are vastly different with cannabis acting upon a specific receptor. Both Solowij, Michie and Fox (1995a) and Pope and Yurgelen-Todd (1996) were able to show that the cognitive impairments detected in their cannabis-using samples were not related to their alcohol consumption. Thus, not only have tests used previously not been sensitive enough, they have probably not been specific enough to detect impairments peculiar to cannabis. Furthermore, tests may have been selected inappropriately because they were previously shown to be affected by acute intoxication, when the consequences of chronic use may be very different. The patterns of cognitive deficit associated with long-term cannabis use have still not been entirely characterized. A priority for future research would be the identification of specific mechanisms of impairment by making direct comparisons with the acute effects of cannabis and the long-term effects of alcohol and a variety of other substances.

Recent research has aimed at identifying specific cannabis effects by using strict exclusion criteria and matching control groups on numerous variables to ensure that any deficits observed may be directly attributable to cannabis use. Nevertheless, interactions between the effects of long-term cannabis use and those of other substances used concurrently need to be further explored, particularly since many regular cannabis users also use alcohol and other substances to a greater degree than the rest of the population, and the cumulative effects of poly-drug use may be additive. Further, subjects have tended to be excluded if they have had a history of childhood illness, learning disabilities, brain trauma or other neurological or psychiatric illness. The effects of long-term cannabis use on such individuals may be worthy of further investigation, especially as evidence suggests that such individuals are more likely to use cannabis (e.g., Mathers, Ghodse et al., 1991).

When comparisons are made between groups of users and non-users, differences may not always reach statistical significance due to large individual variability, particularly when small sample sizes are used. Carlin (1986) proposed that studies that rely on analysis of central tendency are likely to overlook impairment by averaging away the differences among subjects with very different patterns of disability. Individual differences in vulnerability to the acute effects of cannabis are well recognized and are likely to be a factor in determining susceptibility to a variety of cognitive dysfunctions associated with prolonged use of cannabis.

Cognitive deficits may not be an inevitable consequence of cannabis use. The long-term effects of cannabis on healthy individuals may differ from those in individuals with co-existing mental illness or pre-existing cognitive impairments. As a clinical example, cannabis may trigger psychotic episodes in those already predisposed to psychiatric disturbances (e.g., Andreasson,

Allebeck et al., 1987). On the other hand, some individuals appear to function well even in cognitively demanding occupations despite their long-term use. To what extent their mental proficiency would improve further if possible subtle cognitive deficits were resolved by discontinuing cannabis use is unknown. Wert and Raulin (1986b) suggested that some individuals may adapt and overcome some forms of cognitive impairment by a process of relearning: "it is well known that a chronic or slow-developing lesion will often be masked by the adaptation of the patient to the deficits produced by the lesion" (p. 636).

There has been virtually no research designed specifically to identify predispositions or individual differences in susceptibility to the adverse effects of cannabis. A predisposition may be due to structural, biochemical or psychological factors, or as Wert and Raulin (1986b) suggested, to lack of the "cerebral reserve that most of us call on when we experience mild cerebral damage" (p. 636), for example, after a night of heavy drinking. They propose that "that functional reserve can mask very real cerebral damage." Wert and Raulin suggested that prospective studies are the ideal way to identify those subjects who show real impairment in functioning by comparing pre- and postcannabis performance scores. However, even in a retrospective design it is possible to compare retrospectively the characteristics of subjects who show impairment with those who do not, thereby identifying possible risk factors. Insufficient consideration has been given to gender, age, IQ and personality differences in the long-term consequences of cannabis use. Pope and Yurgelun-Todd (1996) found some evidence of gender differences in the performance of heavy cannabis users on a number of neuropsychological tests with males being more impaired than females. A recent study has reported an early age of onset of cannabis use to be a potent predictor of reduced speed of information processing in adult users (Kunert, Rinn et al., 1997).

Virtually all of the studies reviewed here have been retrospective studies of naturally occurring groups (users versus non-users). Although the matching of control groups has become more stringent, and attempts to obtain estimates of premorbid functioning have increased, prospective studies in which each subject is used as his/her own control would eliminate the possibility of cannabis users having demonstrated poorer performance before commencing their use of cannabis. A longitudinal study in which several cohorts at risk for drug abuse are followed over time would certainly be an excellent, albeit expensive, approach to addressing many of the issues surrounding the detrimental effects of long-term cannabis use on cognition and behavior. Recommendations that prospective studies be carried out using measures of greater sensitivity and specificity have been made in almost every review of the topic since the early 1970s. Unfortunately, actual research has been slow to adopt this design and incorporate such measures.

Carlin (1986) has suggested as an alternate approach that a "meta-analysis" be conducted of the studies to date. Such an analysis would estimate effect size in order to cumulate research findings across studies, perhaps allowing the apparently conflicting findings of the studies to be reconciled. The adequacy of control groups, entry criteria, health factors and other possible contaminating variables could be coded and entered into the analysis. He states that a determination can be made of the extent of the relationship between consumption of a substance and measures of impairment, which is independent of traditional statistical significance. Such an analysis would be of particular importance if the impact of the drug on neuropsychological function is modest, as appears to be the case with cannabis. A modest or even small effect size may have major public health implications. To date, no such research has been applied to the cannabis literature, perhaps because of the limited number of studies. The absence of similar methodology and outcome measures may indeed preclude the application of a meta-analytic approach. Nevertheless, the substantial advances that have been made in recent years justify the continuation of retrospective studies.

Future research should adhere to rigorous methodology. This should include the use of the best available techniques of detecting the presence of cannabinoids in the body to provide greater precision in the investigation of the influence of length of abstinence on performance. This would permit a distinction to be made between those impairments that may be subacute or an effect of accumulated cannabinoids and likely to resolve with abstinence over time, from those of a more enduring or chronic nature, which would be associated with cumulative duration of use.

Given that recent research has identified cognitive impairments that are associated with cumulative exposure, it is a priority to investigate further the recovery of function and rate of resolution following cessation of cannabis use. Furthermore, the parameters of drug use require careful scrutiny in terms of evaluating how much cannabis must be smoked and for how long before impairments are manifest in what kinds of individuals. One of the problems in assessing the cannabis literature is the arbitrariness with which various groups of users have been described as "heavy," "moderate" or "light," "long-term " or "short-term." Is a light user someone who uses once, twice or 10 times per month? Is a heavy user one who uses daily or at least 10 times per day? The other great source of variability is the dose of THC consumed, and to what extent the potency of the cannabis may contribute to the development of cognitive impairments has not been thoroughly investigated.

The use of very sensitive measures of cognitive function is important for the detection of early signs of impairment that may permit a harm minimization approach to be applied to cannabis use. With further research, it may be possible to specify levels of cannabis use that were "safe," "hazardous" and "harmful" in terms of the risk of cognitive impairment. These could be used in health education in the same way similar guidelines have been used in advising people about safe levels of alcohol consumption.

Given the growing prevalence of cannabis use, and proposals to reduce legal restrictions on cannabis use, it is essential that research into cognitive functioning of long-term cannabis users continue. According to U.S. survey data (Deahl,

1991), more than 29 million people in the United States may be using cannabis, and more than 7 million of these use on a daily basis. While there is some controversy surrounding the issue, it seems likely that the mean potency of cannabis has increased over the years as more potent strains have been developed for the black market. Increased THC potency combined with decreased age of onset of use may result in more marked cognitive impairments in larger numbers of individuals in future years.

While it may be true that "real and substantial inconsistencies in the literature have been magnified by those who tend to cite selected pieces of evidence in support of their own ideological beliefs" (Fehr & Kalant, 1983b, p. 501), it is essential that "any new evidence implicating cannabis with persistent harmful effects is subject to critical scrutiny and careful replication if accusations of prejudice and moral bias are to be avoided" (Deahl, 1991, p. 249). It appears that the onus of proof is on researchers to prove impairment rather than on the proponents of cannabis use to prove safety. In the case of cognitive impairments in young people, "safe until proven unsafe" may be a dangerous stance to take since cannabis, like all psychoactive substances could never be labelled entirely "safe." Further research examining the consequences of its use in comparison to other substances is clearly warranted. The dissemination of research findings in a realistic and non-sensational manner would provide users with the ability to make an informed decision about whether or not to use the drug, and if they use, how much, how long and how often to use.

Conclusion

The weight of evidence suggests that the long-term use of cannabis does not result in any severe or grossly debilitating impairment of cognitive function. However, there is sufficient evidence from the studies reviewed above that the long-term use of cannabis leads to a more subtle and selective impairment of cognitive functioning. Impairments appear to be specific to higher cognitive functions, which include the organization and integration of complex information involving various mechanisms of attention and memory processes. There is evidence that prolonged use may lead to progressively greater impairment, which may not recover with cessation of use. While these impairments may be subtle, they could potentially affect functioning in daily life.

It is apparent that not all individuals are affected equally by prolonged exposure to cannabis. Individual differences in susceptibility need to be identified and examined. For those who are dysfunctional, there is a need to develop appropriate treatment programs which address the subtle impairments in cognition and work toward their resolution. There has been insufficient research to address the impact of long-term cannabis use on cognitive functioning in adolescents and young adults, as well as examining the effects of chronic use on the cognitive decline that occurs with normal aging. Gender differences have not been thoroughly investigated and may be important given that such differences have become apparent in differential responses to alcohol.

The existence of a naturally occurring cannabinoidlike substance in the human brain (anandamide) signifies that this substance plays some role in our normal functioning. It has been suggested that anandamide may play a role in movement or motor control (Mechoulam, Hanus & Martin, 1994), in sleep (Mechoulam, Fride et al., 1997) and in the modulation of attention (Solowij, 1998; Solowij, Michie & Fox, 1995a). Recent animal research reviewed in section I of this chapter has made advances towards elucidating the role of cannabinoid receptors in memory dysfunction. It has been suggested that endogenous cannabinoids are involved in the selective forgetting or elimination of certain information at the encoding stage of short-term memory and that exogenous cannabinoids (e.g., THC) override the normal function of the endogenous cannabinoids by disrupting the encoding of information when it is not appropriate nor advantageous to do so (S.A. Deadwyler, personal communication). The neurotransmitters and peptides that govern our behavior are finely balanced and any surplus or depletion generally results in dysfunction. With long-term use of cannabis, prolonged or continual binding to the cannabinoid receptor may alter its properties also in the long term (see section I, "Brain Function and Neurotoxicity"). There is a need to elucidate these physiological mechanisms and the interactions between ingested cannabis, anandamide and the cannabinoid receptor.

Future research should continue to identify with greater specificity those aspects of cognitive functioning that are affected by long-term use of cannabis and to examine the degree to which they are reversible. There is converging evidence that dysfunction due to chronic cannabis use lies in the realm of the higher cognitive functions that appear to be subserved by the frontal lobes; these are important in organizing, manipulating and integrating a variety of information, and in structuring and segregating events in memory.

Until better measures have been developed to investigate the subtleties of dysfunction produced by chronic cannabis use, cannabis may be viewed as posing a lower level threat to cognitive function than other psychoactive substances such as alcohol. Nevertheless, the fact remains that in spite of its illegal status, use of cannabis is widespread. We therefore have a continuing responsibility to minimize drug-related harm by identifying potential risks, subtle though they may be, and communicating the necessary information to the community.

References

Abel, E.L. (1980). *Marijuana: The First Twelve Thousand Years*. New York: Plenum Press.

Abood, M.E. & Martin, B.R. (1992). Neurobiology of marijuana abuse. *Trends in Pharmacological Science, 13*, 201–206.

Abood, M.E., Sauss, C., Fan, F., Tilton, C.L. & Martin, B.R. (1993). Development of behavioral tolerance to $\varnothing$-THC without alteration of cannabinoid receptor binding or mRNA levels in whole brain. *Pharmacology, Biochemistry and Behavior, 46*, 575–579.

Adams, I.B. & Martin, B.R. (1996). Cannabis: Pharmacology and toxicology in animals and humans. *Addiction, 91*, 1585–1614.

Adams, P.M. & Barratt, E.S. (1975). Effect of chronic marijuana administration on stages of primate sleep-wakefulness. *Biological Psychiatry, 10*, 315–322.

Agarwal, A.K., Sethi, B.B. & Gupta, S.C. (1975). Physical and cognitive effects of chronic bhang (cannabis) intake. *Indian Journal of Psychiatry, 17* (1), 1–7.

Ali, S.F., Newport, G.D., Scallet, A.C., Gee, K.W., Paule, M.G., Brown, R.M. & Slikker, W., Jr. (1989). Effects of chronic delta-9-tetrahydrocannabinol (THC) administration on neurotransmitter concentrations and receptor binding in the rat brain. *Neurotoxicology, 10*, 491–500.

Ali, S.F., Newport, G.D., Scallet, A.C., Paule, M.G., Bailey, J.R. & Slikker, W., Jr. (1991). Chronic marijuana smoke exposure in the rhesus monkey. IV: Neurochemical effects and comparison to acute and chronic exposure to delta-9-tetrahydrocannabinol (THC) in rats. *Pharmacology, Biochemistry and Behavior, 40*, 677–682.

Altman, H. & Evenson, R.C. (1973). Marijuana use and subsequent psychiatric symptoms. *Comprehensive Psychiatry, 14*, 415–420.

American Psychiatric Association. (1987). *Diagnostic and Statistical Manual of Mental Disorders* (3rd ed., rev.). Washington, DC: American Psychiatric Association.

Andreasson, S., Allebeck, P., Engstrom, A. & Rydberg, U. (1987). Cannabis and schizophrenia: A longitudinal study of Swedish conscripts. *Lancet, 2*, 1483–1486.

Baddeley, A.D. (1986). *Working Memory*. Oxford: Oxford University Press.

Baddeley, A.D. & Hitch, G. (1974). Working memory. In G. Bower (Ed.), *The Psychology of Learning and Motivation*. San Diego: Academic Press.

Barnett, G., Licko,V. & Thompson, T. (1985). Behavioral pharmacokinetics of marijuana. *Psychopharmacology, 85*, 51–56.

Barratt, E.S. & Adams, P.M. (1972). The effects of chronic marijuana administration on brain functioning in cats. *Clinical Toxicology, 5*, 36.

Barratt, E.S. & Adams, P.M. (1973). Chronic marijuana usage and sleep-wakefulness cycles in cats. *Biological Psychiatry, 6*, 207–214.

Belue, R.C., Howlett, A.C., Westlake, T.M. & Hutchings, D.E. (1995). The ontogeny of cannabinoid receptors in the brain of postnatal and aging rats. *Neurotoxicology and Teratology, 17*, 25–30.

Biegon, A. & Kerman, I. (1995). Quantitative autoradiography of cannabinoid receptors in the human brain post-mortem. In A. Biegon & N.D. Volkow, (Eds.), *Sites of Drug Action in the Human Brain* (pp. 65–74). Boca Raton, FL: CRC Press.

Block, R.I. (1996). Does heavy marijuana use impair human cognition and brain function? *Journal of the American Medical Association, 275*, 560–561.

Block, R.I., Farinpour, R. & Braverman, K. (1992). Acute effects of marijuana on cognition: Relationships to chronic effects and smoking techniques. *Pharmacology, Biochemistry and Behavior, 43*, 907–917.

Block, R.I., Farnham, S., Braverman, K., Noyes, R., Jr. & Ghoneim, M.M. (1990). Long-term marijuana use and subsequent effects on learning and cognitive functions related to school achievement: Preliminary study. In J.W. Spencer & J.J. Boren (Eds.), *Residual Effects of Abused Drugs on Behavior* (NIDA Research Monograph No. 101). Rockville, MD: U.S. Department of Health and Human Services.

Block, R.I. & Ghoneim, M.M. (1993). Effects of chronic marijuana use on human cognition. *Psychopharmacology, 110*, 219–228.

Bloom, A.S. (1984). Effects of cannabinoids on neurotransmitter receptors in the brain. In S. Agurell, W.L. Dewey & R.E. Willette (Eds.), *The Cannabinoids: Chemical, Pharmacologic and Therapeutic Aspects* (pp. 575–589). New York: Academic Press.

Bowman, M. & Pihl, R.O. (1973). Cannabis: Psychological effects of chronic heavy use. A controlled study of intellectual functioning in chronic users of high potency cannabis. *Psychopharmacologia (Berl), 29*, 159–170.

Brill, N.Q. & Christie, R.L. (1974). Marijuana use and psychosocial adaptation: Follow-up study of a collegiate population. *Archives of General Psychiatry, 31*, 713–719.

Bull, J. (1971). Cerebral atrophy in young cannabis smokers. *Lancet, 2*, 1420.

Campbell, A.M.G., Evans, M., Thomson, J.L.G. & Williams, M.J. (1971). Cerebral atrophy in young cannabis smokers. *Lancet, 2*, 1219–1224.

Campbell, D.R. (1971). The electroencephalogram in cannabis associated psychosis. *Canadian Psychiatric Association Journal, 16*, 161–165.

Campbell, K.A., Foster, T.C., Hampson, R.E. & Deadwyler, S.A. (1986a). $\varnothing$-Tetrahydrocannabinol differentially affects sensory-evoked potentials in the rat dentate gyrus. *The Journal of Pharmacology and Experimental Therapeutics, 239*, 936–940.

Campbell, K.A., Foster, T.C., Hampson, R.E. & Deadwyler, S.A. (1986b). Effects of $\varnothing$-tetrahydrocannabinol on sensory-evoked discharges of granule cells in the dentate gyrus of behaving rats. *The Journal of Pharmacology and Experimental Therapeutics, 239*, 941–945.

Carlin, A.S. (1986). Neuropsychological consequences of drug abuse. In I. Grant & K.M. Adams (Eds.), *Neuropsychological Assessment of Neuropsychiatric Disorders* (pp. 478–497). New York: Oxford University Press.

Carlin, A.S. & Trupin, E.W. (1977). The effect of long-term chronic marijuana use on neuropsychological functioning. *International Journal of the Addictions, 12*, 617–624.

Carter, W.E., Coggins, W. & Doughty, P.L. (1980). *Cannabis in Costa Rica: A Study of Chronic Marihuana Use.* Philadelphia: Institute for the Study of Human Issues.

Chait, L.D., Fischman, M.W. & Schuster, C.R. (1985). "Hangover" effects the morning after marijuana smoking. *Drug and Alcohol Dependence, 15*, 229–238.

Charalambous, A., Marciniak, G., Shiue, C.-Y., Dewey, S.L., Schlyer, D.J., Wolf, A.P. & Makriyannis, A. (1991). PET studies in the primate brain and biodistribution in mice using (–)-5^1-18F-$\varnothing$-THC. *Pharmacology, Biochemistry and Behavior, 40*, 503–507.

Chopra, G.S. (1971). Marijuana and adverse psychotic reactions: Evaluation of different factors involved. *Bulletin on Narcotics, 23* (3), 15–22.

Chopra, G.S. (1973). Studies on psycho-clinical aspects of long-term marihuana use in 124 cases. *International Journal of the Addictions, 8*, 1015–1026.

Chopra, G.S. & Jandu, B.S. (1976). Psychoclinical effects of long-term marijuana use in 275 Indian chronic users: A comparative assessment of effects in Indian and USA users. *Annals of the New York Academy of Sciences, 282*, 95–108.

Chopra, G.S. & Smith, J.W. (1974). Psychotic reactions following cannabis use in East Indians. *Archives of General Psychiatry, 30*, 24–27.

Co, B.T., Goodwin, D.W., Gado, M., Mikhael, M. & Hill, S.Y. (1977). Absence of cerebral atrophy in chronic cannabis users: Evaluation by computerized transaxial tomography. *Journal of the American Medical Association, 237*, 1229–1230.

Cohen, S. (1976). The 94-day cannabis study. *Annals of the New York Academy of Sciences, 282*, 211–220.

Cohen, S. (1982). Cannabis effects upon adolescent motivation. *In Marijuana and Youth: Clinical Observations on Motivation and Learning* (pp. 2–9). Rockville, MD: National Institute on Drug Abuse.

Collins, D.R., Pertwee, R.G. & Davies, S.N. (1995). Prevention by the cannabinoid antagonist, SR141716A, of cannabinoid-mediated blockade of long-term potentiation in the rat hippocampal slice. *British Journal of Pharmacology, 115*, 869–870.

Comitas, L. (1976). Cannabis and work in Jamaica: A refutation of the amotivational syndrome. *Annals of the New York Academy of Sciences, 282*, 24–32.

Cox, B. (1990). Drug tolerance and physical dependence. In W. Pratt & P. Taylor (Eds.), *Principles of Drug Action: The Basis of Pharmacology* (pp. 639–690). New York: Churchill Livingstone.

Crawley, J., Corwin, R., Robinson, J., Felder, C., Devane, W. & Axelrod, J. (1993). Anandamide, an endogenous ligand of the cannabinoid receptor, induces hypomotility and hyperthermia in vivo in rodents. *Pharmacology, Biochemistry and Behavior, 46*, 967–972.

Culver, C.M. & King, F.W. (1974). Neuropsychological assessment of undergraduate marihuana and LSD users. *Archives of General Psychiatry, 31*, 707–711.

Deadwyler, S.A., Bunn, T. & Hampson, R.E. (1996). Hippocampal ensemble activity during spatial delayed-nonmatch-to-sample performance in rats. *Journal of Neuroscience, 16*, 354–372.

Deadwyler, S.A., Byrd, D.R., Konstantopoulos, J.A., Evans, G.J.O., Rogers, G. & Hampson, R.E. (1996). Enhancement of rat hippocampal ensemble activity by CX516 protects against errors in spatial DNMS. *Society for Neuroscience Abstracts, 22*, 1131.

Deadwyler, S.A. & Hampson, R.E. (1997). The significance of neural ensemble codes during behavior and cognition. *Annual Review of Neuroscience, 20*, 217–244.

Deadwyler, S.A., Heyser, C.J. & Hampson, R.E. (1995). Complete adaptation to the memory disruptive effects of delta-9-THC following 35 days of exposure. *Neuroscience Research Communications, 17*, 9–18.

Deahl, M. (1991). Cannabis and memory loss. *British Journal of Addiction, 86*, 249–252.

Deliyannakis, E., Panagopoulos, C. & Huott, A.D. (1970). The influence of hashish on human EEG. *Clinical Electroencephalography, 1*, 128–140.

Deutsch, D.G. & Chin, S.A. (1993). Enzymatic synthesis and degradation of anandamide, a cannabinoid receptor agonist. *Biochemical Pharmacology, 46*, 791–796.

Dewey, W.L. (1986). Cannabinoid pharmacology. *Pharmacological Reviews, 38*, 151–178.

Domino, E.F. (1981). Cannabinoids and the cholinergic system. *Journal of Clinical Pharmacology, 21*, 249S–255S.

Dornbush, R.L. & Kokkevi, A. (1976). The acute effects of various cannabis substances on cognitive, perceptual, and motor performance in very long-term hashish users. In M.C. Braude & S. Szara (Eds.), *Pharmacology of Marihuana* (pp. 421–428). New York: Raven Press.

Dornbush, R.L., Clare, G., Zaks, A., Crown, P., Volavka, J. & Fink, M. (1972). Twenty-one day administration of marijuana in male volunteers. In M.F. Lewis (Ed.), *Current Research in Marihuana* (pp. 115–127). New York: Academic Press.

Douglas, R.J. (1967). The hippocampus and behavior. *Psychological Bulletin, 67*, 416–442.

Drew, W.G., Weet, C.R., De Rossett, S.E. & Batt, J.R. (1980). Effects of hippocampal brain damage on auditory and visual recent memory: Comparison with marijuana-intoxicated subjects. *Biological Psychiatry, 15*, 841–858.

Eichenbaum, H. & Cohen, N.J. (1988). Representation in the hippocampus: What do hippocampal neurons encode? *Trends in Neuroscience, 11*, 244–248.

Eldridge, J.C., Hu, H.-Y., Extrom, P.C. & Landfield, P.W. (1992). Interactions between cannabinoids and steroids in the rat hippocampus. *Society for Neuroscience Abstracts, 18*, 789.

Eldridge, J.C. & Landfield, P.W. (1990). Cannabinoid interactions with glucocorticoid receptors in rat hippocampus. *Brain Research, 534*, 135–141.

Eldridge, J.C., Murphy, L.L. & Landfield, P.W. (1991). Cannabinoids and the hippocampal glucocorticoid receptor: Recent findings and possible significance. *Steroids, 56*, 226–231.

Entin, E.E. & Goldzung, P.J. (1973). Residual effects of marihuana use on learning and memory. *Psychological Record, 23*, 169–178.

Feeney, D.M. (1979). Marihuana and epilepsy: Paradoxical anticonvulsant and convulsant effects. In G.G. Nahas & W.D.M. Paton (Eds.), *Marihuana: Biological Effects: Analysis, Metabolism, Cellular Responses, Reproduction and Brain, Advances in the Biosciences* (pp. 643–657). Oxford: Pergamon Press.

Fehr, K.O. & Kalant, H. (Eds.). (1983a). *Cannabis and health hazards. Proceedings of an ARF/WHO Scientific Meeting on Adverse Health and Behavioural Consequences of Cannabis Use.* Toronto: Addiction Research Foundation.

Fehr, K.O. & Kalant, H. (1983b). Long-term effects of cannabis on cerebral function: A review of the clinical and experimental literature. In K.O. Fehr & H. Kalant (Eds.), *Cannabis and Health Hazards* (pp. 501–576). Toronto: Addiction Research Foundation.

Feinberg, I., Jones, R., Walker, J., Cavness, C. & Floyd, T. (1976). Effects of marijuana extract and tetrahydrocannabinol on electroencephalographic sleep patterns. *Clinical Pharmacology and Therapeutics, 19,* 782–794.

Fink, D.J., Ashworth, B. & Brewer, C. (1972). Cerebral atrophy in young cannabis smokers. *Lancet, 1,* 143.

Fink, M. (1976a). Conference summary. *Annals of the New York Academy of Sciences, 282,* 427–430.

Fink, M. (1976b). Effects of acute and chronic inhalation of hashish, marijuana, and $\varnothing$-tetrahydrocannabinol on brain electrical activity in man: Evidence for tissue tolerance. *Annals of the New York Academy of Sciences, 282,* 387–398.

Fink, M., Volavka, J., Panayiotopoulos, C.P. & Stefanis, C. (1976). Quantitative EEG studies of marijuana, $\varnothing$-tetrahydrocannabinol, and hashish in man. In M.C. Braude & S. Szara (Eds.), *Pharmacology of Marihuana* (Vol. 1) (pp. 383–391). New York: Raven Press.

Fletcher, J.M., Page, J.B., Francis, D.J., Copeland, K., Naus, M.J., Davis, C.M., Morris, R., Krauskopf, D. & Satz, P. (1996). Cognitive correlates of long-term cannabis use in Costa Rican men. *Archives of General Psychiatry, 53,* 1051–1057.

Fletcher, J.M. & Satz, P. (1977). A methodological commentary on the Egyptian study of chronic hashish use. *Bulletin on Narcotics, 29* (2), 29–34.

Frank, I.M., Lessin, P.J., Tyrell, E.D., Hahn, P.M. & Szara, S. (1976). Acute and cumulative effects of marihuana smoking in hospitalized subjects: A 36 day study. In M.C. Braude & S. Szara (Eds.), *Pharmacology of Marihuana* (Vol. 2). New York: Raven Press.

Fried, P. (1977). Behavioral and electroencephalographic correlates of the chronic use of marijuana — A review. *Behavioral Biology, 21,* 163–196.

Fried, P.A. (1993). Prenatal exposure to tobacco and marijuana: Effects during pregnancy, infancy, and early childhood. *Clinical Obstetrics and Gynecology, 36,* 319–337.

Fried, P. (1995). The Ottawa Prenatal Prospective Study (OPPS): Methodological issues and findings — It's easy to throw the baby out with the bath water. *Life Sciences, 56,* 2159–2168.

Fried, P. (1996). Behavioural outcomes in preschool and school-age children exposed prenatally to marijuana: A review and speculative interpretation. In C.L. Wetherington, V.L. Smeriglio & L.P. Finnegan (Eds.), *Behavioral Studies of Drug Exposed Offspring: Methodological Issues in Human and Animal Research* (NIDA Research Monograph No. 164, pp. 242–260). Washington, DC: U.S. Government Printing Office.

Fried, P.A. & Charlebois, A.T. (1979). Cannabis administered during pregnancy: First- and second-generation effects in rats. *Physiological Psychology, 7,* 307–310.

Gatley, S.J., Gifford, A.N., Volkow, N.D., Lan, R. & Makriyannis, A. (1996). Iodine-123 labeled AM251: A radioiodinated ligand which binds in vivo to the mouse brain CB1 cannabinoid receptor. *European Journal of Pharmacology, 307,* 301–308.

Gianutsos, R. & Litwack, A.R. (1976). Chronic marijuana smokers show reduced coding into long-term storage. *Bulletin of the Psychonomic Society, 7* (3), 277–279.

Gifford, A.N. & Ashby, C.R.J. (1996). Inhibition of acetylcholine release from hippocampal slices by the cannabimimetic aminoalkylindole WIN 55212-2, and evidence for the release of an endogenous cannabinoid inhibitor. *Journal of Pharmacology and Experimental Therapeutics, 277,* 1431–1436.

Gifford, A.N., Samiian, L., Gatley, S.J. & Ashby, C.R.J. (1997). Examination of the effect of the cannabinoid agonist, CP 55,940, on electrically-evoked transmitter release from rat brain slices. *European Journal of Pharmacology, 324,* 187–192.

Grant, I., Rochford, J., Fleming, T. & Stunkard, A. (1973). A neuropsychological assessment of the effects of moderate marihuana use. *Journal of Nervous and Mental Disease, 156,* 278–280.

Hall, W., Solowij, N. & Lemon, J. (1994). *The Health and Psychological Consequences of Cannabis Use* (National Drug Strategy Monograph No. 25). Canberra: Australian Government Publishing Service.

Hampson, R.E., Byrd, D.R., Konstantopoulos, J.K., Bunn, T. & Deadwyler, S.A. (1996). Delta-9-Tetrahydrocannabinol influences sequential memory in rats performing a delayed-nonmatch-to-sample task. *Society for Neuroscience Abstracts, 22,* 1131.

Hampson, R.E. & Deadwyler, S.A. (1996a). Ensemble codes involving hippocampal neurons are at risk during delayed performance tests. *Proceedings of the National Academy of Sciences of the United States of America, 93,* 13487–13493.

Hampson, R.E. & Deadwyler, S.A. (1996b). LTP and LTD and the encoding of memory in small ensembles of hippocampal neurons. In M. Baudry & J. Davis (Eds.), *Long-Term Potentiation* (Vol. 3) (pp. 199–214). Cambridge, MA: MIT Press.

Hannerz, J. & Hindmarsh, T. (1983). Neurological and neuroradiological examination of chronic cannabis smokers. *Annals of Neurology, 13,* 207–210.

Harper, J.W., Heath, R.G. & Myers, W.A. (1977). Effects of cannabis sativa on ultrastructure of the synapse in monkey brain. *Journal of Neuroscience Research, 3,* 87–93.

Harshman, R.A., Crawford, H.J. & Hecht, E. (1976). Marihuana, cognitive style, and lateralized hemisphere. In S. Cohen & R.C. Stillman (Eds.), *The Therapeutic Potential of Marihuana.* New York: Plenum Press.

Heath, R.G. (1972). Marihuana: Effects on deep and surface electroencephalograms in man. *Archives of General Psychiatry, 26,* 577–584.

Heath, R.G., Fitzjarrell, A.T., Fontana, C.J. & Garey, R.E. (1980). Cannabis sativa: Effects on brain function and ultrastructure in rhesus monkeys. *Biological Psychiatry, 15*, 657–690.

Heishman, S.J., Huestis, M.A., Henningfield, J.E. & Cone, E.J. (1990). Acute and residual effects of marijuana: Profiles of plasma THC levels, physiological, subjective and performance measures. *Pharmacology, Biochemistry and Behavior, 37*, 561–565.

Heishman, S.J., Pickworth, W.B., Bunker, E.B. & Henningfield, J.E. (1993). Acute and residual effects of smoked marijuana on human performance. In L. Harris (Ed.), *Problems of Drug Dependence 1992* (NIDA Research Monograph No. 132, p. 270). Washington, DC: U.S. Government Printing Office.

Heishman, S.J., Stitzer, M.L. & Yingling, J.E. (1989). Effects of tetrahydrocannabinol content on marijuana smoking behavior, subjective reports, and performance. *Pharmacology, Biochemistry and Behavior, 34*, 173–179.

Herkenham, M., Lynn, A.B., Little, M.D., Johnson, M.R., Melvin, L.S., De Costa, B.R. & Rice, K.C. (1990). Cannabinoid receptor localization in brain. *Proceedings of the National Academy of Sciences of the United States of America, 87*, 1932–1936.

Herning, R.I., Jones, R.T. & Peltzman, D.J. (1979). Changes in human event-related potentials with prolonged delta-9-tetrahydrocannabinol (THC) use. *Electroencephalography and Clinical Neurophysiology, 47*, 556–570.

Heyser, C.J., Hampson, R.E. & Deadwyler, S.A. (1993). Effects of $\varnothing^9$-tetrahydrocannabinol on delayed match-to-sample performance in rats: Alterations in short-term memory associated with changes in task specific firing of hippocampal cells. *The Journal of Pharmacology and Experimental Therapeutics, 264*, 294–307.

Ho, B.T., Taylor, D. & Englert, L.F. (1973). The effect of repeated administration of (–)-delta-9-tetrahydrocannabinol on the biosynthesis of brain amines. *Research Communications on Chemical Pathology and Pharmacology, 5*, 851–854.

Hochman, J.S. & Brill, N.Q. (1973). Chronic marijuana use and psychosocial adaptation. *American Journal of Psychiatry, 130*, 132–140.

Hockman, C.H., Perrin, R.G. & Kalant, H. (1971). Electroencephalographic and behavioral alterations produced by $\varnothing$-tetrahydrocannabinol. *Science, 172*, 968–970.

Institute of Medicine. (1982). *Marijuana and Health.* Washington, DC: National Academy Press.

Jones, R.T. (1975). Effects of marijuana on the mind. In J.R. Tinklenberg (Ed.), *Marijuana and Health Hazards* (pp. 115–120). New York: Academic Press.

Jones, R.T. (1980). Human effects: An overview. In R.C. Petersen (Ed.), *Marijuana Research Findings: 1980* (NIDA Research Monograph No. 31, pp. 54–80)(DHHS Publication No. ADM 80-1001). Washington, DC: U.S. Government Printing Office.

Kalant, H. (1996). Good report but scanty research. Comments on Hall et al.'s Australian National Drug Strategy Monograph No. 25 The Health and Psychological Consequences of Cannabis Use. *Addiction, 91*, 759–773.

Kales, A., Hanley, J., Rickles, W., Kanas, N., Baker, M. & Goring, P. (1972). Effects of marijuana administration and withdrawal in chronic users and naive subjects. *Psychophysiology, 9*, 92.

Karacan, I., Fernandez-Salas, A., Coggins, W.J., Carter, W.E., Williams, R.L., Thornby, J.I., Salis, P.J., Okawa, M. & Villaume, J.P. (1976). Sleep electroencephalographic-electrooculographic characteristics of chronic marijuana users. *Annals of the New York Academy of Sciences, 282*, 348–374.

Kimble, D.P. (1968). Hippocampus and internal inhibition. *Psychological Bulletin, 70*, 285–295.

Kokkevi, A. & Dornbush, R. (1977). Psychological test characteristics of long-term hashish users. In C. Stefanis, R. Dornbush & M. Fink (Eds.), *Hashish: Studies of Long-Term Use* (pp. 43–48). New York: Raven Press.

Kolansky, H. & Moore, R.T. (1971). Effects of marihuana on adolescents and young adults. *Journal of the American Medical Association, 216*, 486–492.

Kolansky, H. & Moore, R.T. (1972). Toxic effects of chronic marihuana use. *Journal of the American Medical Association, 222*, 35–41.

Koukkou, M. & Lehmann, D. (1976). Human EEG spectra before and during cannabis hallucinations. *Biological Psychiatry, 11*, 663–677.

Koukkou, M. & Lehmann, D. (1977). EEG spectra indicate predisposition to visual hallucinations under psilocybin, cannabis, hypnagogic and daydream conditions. *Electroencephalography and Clinical Neurophysiology, 43*, 499–500.

Kuehnle, J., Mendelson, J.H. & David, K.R. (1977). Computed tomographic examination of heavy marijuana users. *Journal of the American Medical Association, 237*, 1231–1232.

Kunert, H.J., Rinn, T., Moeller, M.R., Poser, W., Hoehe, M.R. & Ehrenreich, H. (1997). Early onset of cannabis use is associated with specific attentional dysfunctions in adult moderate users. In *1997 Symposium on the Cannabinoids* (p. 82). Burlington, VT: International Cannabinoid Research Society.

Lan, R., Gatley, S.J. & Makriyannis, A. (1996). Preparation of iodine-123 labelled AM251, a potential SPECT radioligand for the brain cannabinoid CB1 receptor. *Journal of Labelled Compounds and Radiopharmaceuticals, 38*, 875–881.

Landfield, P.W., Cadwallader, L.B. & Vinsant, S. (1988). Quantitative changes in hippocampal structure following long-term exposure to $\emptyset$-tetrahydrocannabinol: Possible mediation by glucocorticoid systems. *Brain Research, 443*, 47–62.

Landfield, P.W. & Eldridge, J.C. (1993). Neurotoxicity and drugs of abuse: Cannabinoid inter-action with brain glucocorticoid receptors. In L. Erinoff (Ed.), *Assessing Neurotoxicity of Drugs of Abuse* (NIDA Research Monograph No. 136, pp. 242–256). Washington, DC: U.S. Government Printing Office.

Leavitt, J., Webb, P., Norris, G., Struve, F., Straumanis, J., Fitz-Gerald, M., Nixon, F., Patrick, G. & Manno, J. (1993). Performance of chronic daily marijuana users on neuropsycho-logical tests. In L. Harris (Ed.), *Problems of Drug Dependence 1992* (NIDA Research Monograph No. 132, p. 179). Washington, DC: U.S. Government Printing Office.

Leavitt, J., Webb, P., Norris, G., Struve, F., Straumanis, J., Patrick, G., Fitz-Gerald, M.J. & Nixon, F. (1992). Differences in complex reaction time between THC users and non-user controls. In L. Harris (Ed.), *Problems of Drug Dependence 1991* (NIDA Research Monograph No. 119, p. 452). Washington, DC: U.S. Government Printing Office.

Leirer, V.O., Yesavage, J.A. & Morrow, D.G. (1989). Marijuana, aging and task difficulty effects on pilot performance. *Aviation, Space and Environmental Medicine, 60,* 1145–1152.

Leirer, V.O., Yesavage, J.A. & Morrow, D.G. (1991). Marijuana carry-over effects on aircraft pilot performance. *Aviation, Space and Environmental Medicine, 62,* 221–227.

Leon-Carrion, J. (1990). Mental performance in long-term heavy cannabis use: A preliminary report. *Psychological Reports, 67,* 947–952.

Leon-Carrion, J. & Vela-Bueno, A. (1991). Cannabis and cerebral hemispheres: A chrono-neuropsychological study. *International Journal of Neuroscience, 57,* 251–257.

Lichtman, A.H., Dimen, K.R. & Martin, B.R. (1995). Systemic or intrahippocampal cannabinoid administration impairs spatial memory in rats. *Psychopharmacology, 119,* 282–290.

Lichtman, A.H. & Martin, B.R. (1996). Delta-9-Tetrahydrocannabinol impairs spatial memory through a cannabinoid receptor mechanism. *Psychopharmacology, 126,* 125–131.

Lundqvist, T. (1995a). Specific thought patterns in chronic cannabis smokers observed during treatment. *Life Sciences, 56,* 2141–2144.

Lundqvist, T. (1995b). Chronic cannabis use and the sense of coherence. *Life Sciences, 56,* 2145–2150.

Lundqvist, T. (1995c). *Cognitive Dysfunctions in Chronic Cannabis Users Observed During Treatment: An Integrative Approach.* University of Lund and Stockholm: Almqvist and Wiksell International.

Luthra, Y.K., Rosenkrantz, H. & Braude, M.C. (1976). Cerebral and cerebellar neurochemical changes and behavioral manifestations in rats chronically exposed to marijuana smoke. *Toxicology and Applied Pharmacology, 35,* 455–465.

Mackie, K., Hsieh, C. & Law, J. (1997). Rapid internalization of the CB1 cannabinoid receptor following agonist binding. In *1997 Symposium on the Cannabinoids* (p. 55). Burlington, VT: International Cannabinoid Research Society.

Mailleux, P. & Vanderhaeghen, J.J. (1992). Age-related loss of cannabinoid receptor binding sites and mRNA in the rat striatum. *Neuroscience Letters, 147,* 179–181.

Mailleux, P. & Vanderhaeghen, J.J. (1994). Delta-9-Tetrahydrocannabinol regulates substance P and enkephalin mRNA levels in the caudate-putamen. *European Journal of Pharmacology, 267,* R1–R3.

Mallet, P.E. & Beninger, R.J. (1995). The endogenous cannabinoid receptor agonist anandamide impairs working memory but not reference memory in rats. *Society for Neuroscience Abstracts, 21,* 167.

Marciniak, G., Charalambous, A., Shiue, C.-Y., Dewey, S.L., Schlyer, D.J., Makriyannis, A. & Wolf, A.P. (1991). 18F-Labeled tetrahydrocannabinol: Synthesis; and PET studies in a baboon. *Journal of Laboratory and Comparative Radiophysiology, 30,* 413–415.

Marks, D.F. & MacAvoy, M.G. (1989). Divided attention performance in cannabis users and non-users following alcohol and cannabis separately and in combination. *Psychopharmacology, 99,* 397–401.

Martin, B.R. (1986). Cellular effects of cannabinoids. *Pharmacological Reviews, 38,* 45–74.

Mathers, D.C., Ghodse, A.H., Caan, A.W. & Scott, S.A. (1991). Cannabis use in a large sample of acute psychiatric admissions. *British Journal of Addiction, 86,* 779–784.

Mathew, R.J., Tant, S. & Berger, C. (1986). Regional cerebral blood flow in marijuana smokers. *British Journal of Addiction, 81,* 567–571.

Mathew, R.J. & Wilson, W.H. (1992). The effects of marijuana on cerebral blood flow and metabolism. In L. Murphy & A. Bartke (Ed.), *Marijuana/Cannabinoids: Neurobiology and Neurophysiology* (pp. 337–386). Boca Raton, FL: CRC Press.

McGahan, J.P., Dublin, A.B. & Sassenrath, E. (1984). Long-term delta-9-tetrahydrocannabinol treatment: Computed tomography of the brains of rhesus monkeys. *American Journal of Diseases of Children,* 138, 1109–1112.

Mechoulam, R., Fride, E., Hanus, L., Sheskin, T., Bisogno, T., Di Marzo, V., Bayewitch, M. & Vogel, Z. (1997). Anandamide may mediate sleep induction. *Nature, 389,* 25–26.

Mechoulam, R., Hanus, L. & Martin, B.R. (1994). The search for endogenous ligands of the cannabinoid receptor. *Biochemical Pharmacology, 48,* 1537–1544.

Melges, F.T., Tinklenberg, J.R., Hollister, L.E. & Gillespie, H.K. (1970). Marihuana and temporal disintegration. *Science, 168,* 1118–1120.

Mendelson, J.H., Rossi, A.M. & Meyer, R.E. (Eds.). (1974). *The Use of Marihuana: A Psychological and Physiological Inquiry.* New York: Plenum Press.

Mendhiratta, S.S., Varma, V.K., Dang, R., Malhotra, A.K., Das, K. & Nehra, R. (1988). Cannabis and cognitive functions. *British Journal of Addiction, 83*, 749–753.

Mendhiratta, S.S., Wig, N.N. & Verma, S.K. (1978). Some psychological correlates of long-term heavy cannabis users. *British Journal of Psychiatry, 132*, 482–486.

Miller, L.L. & Branconnier, R.J. (1983). Cannabis: Effects on memory and the cholinergic limbic system. *Psychological Bulletin, 93* (3), 441–456.

Millsaps, C.L., Azrin, R.L. & Mittenberg, W. (1994). Neuropsychological effects of chronic cannabis use on the memory and intelligence of adolescents. *Journal of Child and Adolescent Substance Abuse, 3*, 47–55.

Moreau (de Tours), J.J. (1845). *Du Haschich et de l'aliénation mentale: Etudes psychologiques.* Paris: Librairie de Fortin, Masson. (English edition: New York: Raven Press, 1972).

Musselman, D.L., Haden, C., Caudle, J. & Kalin, N.H. (1994). Cerebrospinal fluid study of cannabinoid users and normal controls. *Psychiatry Research, 52*, 103–105.

Myers, W.A. & Heath, R.G. (1979). Cannabis sativa: Ultrastructural changes in organelles of neurons in brain septal region of monkeys. *Journal of Neuroscience Research, 4*, 9–17.

Nahas, G.G. (Ed.). (1984). *Marihuana in Science and Medicine.* New York: Raven Press.

Nakamura, E.M., da Silva, E.A., Concilio, G.V., Wilkinson, D.A. & Masur, J. (1991). Reversible effects of acute and long-term administration of $\emptyset$-tetrahydrocannabinol (THC) on memory in the rat. *Drug and Alcohol Dependence, 28*, 167–175.

National Institute on Drug Abuse. (1982). *Marijuana and Youth: Clinical Observations on Motivation and Learning.* Rockville, MD: National Institute on Drug Abuse.

Nelson, H.E. (1982). *The National Adult Reading Test: Test Manual.* Windsor, UK: NFER-Nelson.

Oviedo, A., Glowa, J. & Herkenham, M. (1993). Chronic cannabinoid administration alters cannabinoid receptor binding in rat brain: A quantitative autoradiographic study. *Brain Research, 616*, 293–302.

Page, J.B., Fletcher, J. & True, W.R. (1988). Psychosociocultural perspectives on chronic cannabis use: The Costa Rican follow-up. *Journal of Psychoactive Drugs, 20*, 57–65.

Perez-Reyes, M., Hicks, R.E., Bumberry, J., Jeffcoat, A.R. & Cook, C.E. (1988). Interaction between marihuana and ethanol: Effects on psychomotor performance. *Alcoholism: Clinical and Experimental Research, 12*, 268–276.

Pertwee, R.G. (1988). The central neuropharmacology of psychotropic cannabinoids. *Pharmacology and Therapeutics, 36*, 189–261.

Pertwee, R.G. (1992). In vivo interactions between psychotropic cannabinoids and other drugs involving central and peripheral neurochemical mechanisms. In L. Murphy & A. Bartke (Eds.), *Marijuana/Cannabinoids: Neurobiology and Neurophysiology* (pp. 165–218). Boca Raton, FL: CRC Press.

Pope, H.G., Gruber, A.J. & Yurgelun-Todd, D. (1995). The residual neuropsychological effects of cannabis: The current status of research. *Drug and Alcohol Dependence, 38*, 25–34.

Pope, H.G. & Yurgelun-Todd, D. (1996). The residual cognitive effects of heavy marijuana use in college students. *Journal of the American Medical Association, 275*, 521–527.

Raichle, M.E. (1983). Positron emission tomography. *Annual Review of Neuroscience, 6*, 249–267.

Ray, R., Prabhu, G.G., Mohan, D., Nath, L.M. & Neki, J.S. (1978). The association between chronic cannabis use and cognitive functions. *Drug and Alcohol Dependence, 3*, 365–368.

Reed, H.B.C., Jr. (1974). Cognitive effects of marihuana. In J.H. Mendelson, A.M. Rossi & R.E. Meyer (Eds.), *The Use of Marihuana: A Psychological and Physiological Inquiry* (pp. 107–114). New York: Plenum Press.

Reitan, R.M. (1986). Theoretical and methodological bases of the Halstead-Reitan Neuropsychological Test Battery. In I. Grant & K.M. Adams (Eds.), *Neuropsychological Assessment of Neuropsychiatric Disorders* (pp. 3–30). New York: Oxford University Press.

Richmon, J., Murawski, B., Matsumiya, Y., Duffy, F.H. & Lombroso, C.T. (1974). Long term effects of chronic marihuana smoking. *Electroencephalography and Clinical Neurophysiology, 36*, 223–224.

Rochford, J., Grant, I. & LaVigne, G. (1977). Medical students and drugs: Further neuropsychological and use pattern considerations. *International Journal of the Addictions, 12*, 1057–1065.

Rodin, E.A., Domino, E.F. & Porzak, J.P. (1970). The marihuana-induced "social high": Neurological and electroencephalographic concomitants. *Journal of the American Medical Association, 213*, 1300–1302.

Rodríguez de Fonseca, F., Gorriti, M., Fernández-Ruiz, J.J., Palomo, T. & Ramos, J.A. (1994). Downregulation of rat brain cannabinoid binding sites after chronic Δ^9-tetrahydrocannabinol treatment. *Pharmacology, Biochemistry and Behavior, 47*, 33–40.

Romero, J., Garcia, L., Fernández-Ruiz, J., Cebeira, M. & Ramos, J. (1995). Changes in rat brain cannabinoid binding sites after acute or chronic exposure to their endogenous agonist, anandamide, or to Δ^9-tetrahydrocannabinol. *Pharmacology, Biochemistry and Behavior, 51*, 731–737.

Rosenkrantz, H. (1983). Cannabis, marihuana, and cannabinoid toxicological manifestations in man and animals. In K.O. Fehr & H. Kalant (Eds.), *Cannabis and Health Hazards: Proceedings of an ARF/WHO Scientific Meeting on Adverse Health and Behavioral Consequences of Cannabis Use* (pp. 91–175). Toronto: Addiction Research Foundation.

Rossi, A.M. & O'Brien, J. (1974). Memory and time estimation. In J.H. Mendelson, A.M. Rossi & R.E. Meyer (Eds.), *The Use of Marihuana: A Psychological and Physiological Inquiry* (pp. 89–106). New York: Plenum Press.

Rubin, V. & Comitas, L. (1975). *Ganja in Jamaica: A Medical Anthropological Study of Chronic Marihuana Use.* The Hague: Mouton.

Rumbaugh, C.L., Fang, H.C.H., Wilson, G.H., Higgins, R.E. & Mestek, M.F. (1980). Cerebral CT findings in drug abuse: Clinical and experimental observations. *Journal of Computer Assisted Tomography, 4,* 330–334.

Santucci, V., Storme, J.J., Soubrie, P. & Le Fur, G. (1996). Arousal-enhancing properties of the CB1 cannabinoid receptor antagonist SR 141716A in rats as assessed by electroencephalographic spectral and sleep-waking cycle analysis. *Life Sciences, 58,* 103–110.

Satz, P., Fletcher, J.M. & Sutker, L.S. (1976). Neuropsychologic, intellectual and personality correlates of chronic marijuana use in native Costa Ricans. *Annals of the New York Academy of Sciences, 282,* 266–306.

Scallet, A.C., Uemura, E., Andrews, A., Ali, S.F., McMillan, D.E., Paule, M.G., Brown, R.M. & Slikker, W., Jr. (1987). Morphometric studies of the rat hippocampus following chronic ∅⁹-tetrahydrocannabinol (THC). *Brain Research, 436,* 193–198.

Schaeffer, J., Andrysiak, T. & Ungerleider, J.T. (1981). Cognition and long-term use of Ganja (cannabis). *Science, 213,* 465–466.

Schwartz, R.H., Gruenewald, P.J., Klitzner, M. & Fedio, P. (1989). Short-term memory impairment in cannabis-dependent adolescents. *American Journal of Diseases of Children, 143,* 1214–1219.

Shannon, M.E. & Fried, P.A. (1972). The macro- and microdistribution and polymorphic electroencephalographic effects of ∅⁹-tetrahydrocannabinol in the rat. *Psychopharmacologia, 27,* 141–156.

Sim, L.J., Hampson, R.E., Deadwyler, S.A. & Childers, S.R. (1996). Effects of chronic treatment with ∅⁹-tetrahydrocannabinol on cannabinoid-stimulated [^{35}S]GTPγS autoradiography in rat brain. *Journal of Neuroscience, 16,* 8057–8066.

Slikker, W., Jr., Paule, M.G., Ali, S.F., Scallet, A.C. & Bailey, J.R. (1992). Behavioral, neurochemical, and neurohistological effects of chronic marijuana smoke exposure in the nonhuman primate. In L. Murphy & A. Bartke (Eds.), *Marijuana/Cannabinoids: Neurobiology and Neurophysiology* (pp. 219–273). Boca Raton, FL: CRC Press.

Solowij, N. (1995). Do cognitive impairments recover following cessation of cannabis use? *Life Sciences, 56,* 2119–2126.

Solowij, N. (1998). *Cannabis and Cognitive Functioning.* Cambridge: Cambridge University Press.

Solowij, N., Grenyer, B.F.S., Chesher, G. & Lewis, J. (1995). Biopsychosocial changes associated with cessation of cannabis use: A single case study of acute and chronic cognitive effects, withdrawal and treatment. *Life Sciences, 56,* 2127–2134.

Solowij, N., Grenyer, B.F.S., Peters, R. & Chesher, G. (1997). Long term cannabis use impairs memory processes and frontal lobe function. In *1997 Symposium on the Cannabinoids* (p. 84). Burlington, VT: International Cannabinoid Research Society.

Solowij, N., Michie, P.T. & Fox, A.M. (1991). Effects of long-term cannabis use on selective attention: An event-related potential study. *Pharmacology, Biochemistry and Behavior, 40,* 683–688.

Solowij, N., Michie, P.T. & Fox, A.M. (1995a). Differential impairments of selective attention due to frequency and duration of cannabis use. *Biological Psychiatry, 37,* 731–739.

Solowij, N., Michie, P.T. & Fox, A.M. (1995b). ERP indices of selective attention in ex-cannabis users. *Biological Psychology, 39,* 201.

Soueif, M.I. (1971). The use of cannabis in Egypt: A behavioural study. *Bulletin on Narcotics, 23* (4), 17–28.

Soueif, M.I. (1975). Chronic cannabis users: Further analysis of objective test results. *Bulletin on Narcotics, 27* (4), 1–26.

Soueif, M.I. (1976a). Differential association between chronic cannabis use and brain function deficits. *Annals of the New York Academy of Sciences, 282,* 323–343.

Soueif, M.I. (1976b). Some determinants of psychological deficits associated with chronic cannabis consumption. *Bulletin on Narcotics, 28* (1), 25–42.

Soueif, M.I. (1977). The Egyptian study of chronic cannabis use: A reply to Fletcher and Satz. *Bulletin on Narcotics, 29* (2), 35–43.

Stadnicki, S.W., Schaeppi, U., Rosenkrantz, H. & Braude, M.C. (1974). Crude marihuana extract: EEG and behavioral effects of chronic oral administration in rhesus monkeys. *Psychopharmacologia, 37,* 225–233.

Stefanis, C. (1976). Biological aspects of cannabis use. In R.C. Petersen (Ed.), *The International Challenge of Drug Abuse* (pp. 149–178). Rockville, MD: National Institute on Drug Abuse.

Stefanis, C., Dornbush, R. & Fink, M. (Eds.). (1977). *Hashish: Studies of Long-Term Use.* New York: Raven Press.

Stephens, R.S., Roffman, R.A. & Simpson, E.E. (1993). Adult marijuana users seeking treatment. *Journal of Consulting and Clinical Psychology, 61*, 1100–1104.

Stiglick, A. & Kalant, H. (1982a). Learning impairment in the radial-arm maze following prolonged cannabis treatment in rats. *Psychopharmacology, 77*, 117–123.

Stiglick, A. & Kalant, H. (1982b). Residual effects of prolonged cannabis administration on exploration and DRL performance in rats. *Psychopharmacology, 77*, 124–128.

Struve, F., Patrick, G. & Leavitt, J. (1995). Development of a "composite" measure of alpha hyperfrontality for use in THC research. In L.S. Harris (Ed.), *Problems of Drug Dependence 1994* (NIDA Research Monograph No. 153, p. 505). Washington DC: U.S. Government Printing Office.

Struve, F. & Straumanis, J.J. (1990). Electroencephalographic and evoked potential methods in human marihuana research: Historical review and future trends. *Drug Development Research, 20*, 369–388.

Struve, F., Straumanis, J.J. & Patrick, G. (1994). Persistent topographic quantitative EEG sequelae of chronic marihuana use: A replication study and initial discriminant function analysis. *Clinical Electroencephalography, 25*, 63–75.

Struve, F., Straumanis, J., Patrick, G., Norris, G., Leavitt, J. & Webb, P. (1992). Topographic quantitative EEG findings in subjects with 15+ years of cumulative daily THC exposure. In L. Harris (Ed.), *Problems of Drug Dependence 1991* (NIDA Research Monograph No. 119, p. 451). Washington DC: U.S. Government Printing Office.

Struve, F., Straumanis, J., Patrick, G., Norris, G., Nixon, F., Fitz-Gerald, M., Manno, J., Leavitt, J. & Webb, P. (1993). Altered quantitative EEG topography as sequelae of chronic THC exposure: A replication using screened normal Ss. In L. Harris (Ed.), *Problems of Drug Dependence 1992* (NIDA Research Monograph No. 132, p. 178). Washington DC: U.S. Government Printing Office.

Stuss, D.T. (1991). Interference effects on memory function in postleukotomy patients: An attentional perspective. In H.S. Levin, H.M. Eisenberg & A.L. Benton (Eds.), *Frontal Lobe Function and Dysfunction* (pp. 157–172). New York: Oxford University Press.

Stuss, D.T. & Benson, D.F. (Eds.). (1986). *The Frontal Lobes*. New York: Raven Press.

Susser, M. (1972). Cerebral atrophy in young cannabis smokers. *Lancet, 1*, 41–42.

Tennant, F.S. & Groesbeck, C.J. (1972). Psychiatric effects of hashish. *Archives of General Psychiatry, 27*, 133–136.

Terranova, J.P., Storme, J.J., Lafon, N., Pério, A., Rinaldi-Carmona, M., Le Fur, G. & Soubrié, P. (1996). Improvement of memory in rodents by the selective CB1 cannabinoid receptor antagonist, SR 141716. *Psychopharmacology, 126*, 165–172.

Tinklenberg, J.R., Kopell, B.S., Melges, F.T. & Hollister, L.E. (1972). Marihuana and alcohol: Time production and memory functions. *Archives of General Psychiatry, 27*, 812–815.

Tunving, K., Lundqvist, T. & Eriksson, D. (1988). "A way out of the fog": An outpatient program for cannabis users. In G. Chesher, P. Consroe & R. Musty (Eds.), *Marijuana: An International Research Report*. Canberra: Australian Government Publishing Service.

Tunving, K., Thulin, S.O., Risberg, J. & Warkentin, S. (1986). Regional cerebral blood flow in long-term heavy cannabis use. *Psychiatry Research, 17*, 15–21.

Varma, V.J., Malhotra, A.K., Dang, R., Das, K. & Nehra, R. (1988). Cannabis and cognitive functions: A prospective study. *Drug and Alcohol Dependence, 21*, 147–152.

Volavka, J., Fink, M., Stefanis, C., Panayiotopoulos, C. & Dornbush, R. (1977). EEG effects of cannabis in chronic hashish users. *Electroencephalography and Clinical Neurophysiology, 42*, 730.

Volkow, N.D., Gillespie, H., Mullani, N., Tancredi, L., Grant, C., Ivanovic, M. & Hollister, L. (1991a). Cerebellar metabolic activation by delta-9-tetrahydrocannabinol in human brain: A study with positron emission tomography and 18F-2-fluoro-2-deoxyglucose. *Psychiatry Research: Neuroimaging, 40*, 69–78.

Volkow, N.D., Gillespie, H., Mullani, N., Tancredi, L., Grant, C., Valentine, A. & Hollister, L. (1996). Brain glucose-metabolism in chronic marijuana users at baseline and during marijuana intoxication. *Psychiatry Research: Neuroimaging, 67*, 29–38.

Volkow, N.D., Gillespie, H., Mullani, N., Tancredi, L., Hollister, L., Ivanovic, M. & Grant, C. (1991b). Use of positron emission tomography to investigate the action of marihuana in the human brain. In G. Nahas & C. Latour (Eds.), *Physiopathology of Illicit Drugs: Cannabis, Cocaine, Opiates* (pp. 3–11). Oxford: Pergamon Press.

Volkow, N.D., Gillespie, H., Tancredi, L. & Hollister, L. (1995). The effects of marijuana in the human brain measured with regional brain glucose metabolism. In A. Biegon & N.D. Volkow (Eds.), *Sites of Drug Action in the Human Brain* (pp. 75–86), Boca Raton, FL: CRC Press.

Webb, P., Struve, F., Leavitt, J., Norris, G., Fitz-Gerald, M., Nixon, F. & Straumanis, J. (1993). Time distortion as a persistent sequela of chronic THC use. In L. Harris (Ed.), *Problems of Drug Dependence 1992* (NIDA Research Monograph No. 132, p. 177). Washington, DC: U.S. Government Printing Office.

Weckowicz, T.E., Collier, G. & Spreng, L. (1977). Field dependence, cognitive functions, personality traits, and social values in heavy cannabis users and non-user controls. *Psychological Reports, 41*, 291–302.

Weckowicz, T.E. & Janssen, D.V. (1973). Cognitive functions, personality traits, and social values in heavy marijuana smokers and non-smoker controls. *Journal of Abnormal Psychology, 81*, 264–269.

Wert, R.C. & Raulin, M.L. (1986a). The chronic cerebral effects of cannabis use: I. Methodological issues and neurological findings. *The International Journal of the Addictions, 21*, 605–628.

Wert, R.C. & Raulin, M.L. (1986b). The chronic cerebral effects of cannabis use: II. Psychological findings and conclusions. *The International Journal of the Addictions, 21*, 629–642.

Westlake, T.M., Howlett, A.C., Ali, S.F., Paule, M.G., Scallet, A.C. & Slikker, W., Jr. (1991). Chronic exposure to $\varnothing$-tetrahydrocannabinol fails to irreversibly alter brain cannabinoid receptors. *Brain Research, 544*, 145–149.

Westlake, T.M., Howlett, A.C., Bonner, T.I., Matsuda, L.A. & Herkenham, M. (1994). Cannabinoid receptor binding and messenger RNA expression in human brain: An in vitro receptor autoradiography and in situ hybridization histochemistry study of normal aged and Alzheimer's brains. *Neuroscience, 63*, 637–652.

Wig, N.N. & Varma, V.K. (1977). Patterns of long-term heavy cannabis use in North India and its effects on cognitive functions: A preliminary report. *Drug and Alcohol Dependence, 2*, 211–219.

Yesavage, J.A., Leirer, V.O., Denari, M. & Hollister, L.E. (1985). Carry-over effects of marijuana intoxication on aircraft pilot performance: A preliminary report. *American Journal of Psychiatry, 142*, 1325–1329.

Mental and Behavioral Disorders Due to Cannabis Use

Mental and Behavioral Disorders Due to Cannabis Use

S.M. CHANNABASAVANNA, MEHDI PAES AND
WAYNE HALL

A number of psychiatric syndromes and behavioral disorders have been linked to cannabis use. These include specific disorders such as an amotivational syndrome, a dependence syndrome, and cannabis-induced psychoses. They also include the possible contribution of cannabis use to the initiation and exacerbation of schizophrenia. Evidence on the status of each of these disorders and their relationship to cannabis use is reviewed in this chapter. No attempt is made to consider all possible cannabis-related psychiatric and behavioral disorders considered in the *International Classification of Diseases, 10th edition* (*ICD-10;* WHO, 1992). Instead, discussion is confined to those disorders that have been most extensively researched and discussed in the clinical and research literature. We begin with the dependence syndrome and cannabis-induced psychoses, before briefly discussing other psychiatric disorders. We conclude by reviewing the evidence on the possible role of cannabis use in precipitating and exacerbating schizophrenia.

Cannabis Dependence

In societies with long traditions of cannabis use, such as India and Morocco, it has been rare for clinical observers to report cases of cannabis dependence, or for cannabis users to seek help in stopping their cannabis use (Paes, 1986). This is probably because traditional patterns of cannabis use have been intermittent rather than regular and often regulated by cultural practices (Machado, 1994). Those small subgroups within these cultures who have been heavy cannabis users are also often users of other drugs, such as alcohol and opiates, which makes it difficult to attribute dependence or other symptoms to cannabis (Machado, 1994). The absence of a clearly defined withdrawal syndrome under these conditions of use has supported the view in these cultures that cannabis dependence is a rare event, if it occurs at all.

For much of the 1970s, experience with cannabis in Western cultures was consistent with that in traditional cannabis-using cultures. Given the predominantly intermittent use of relatively low-potency forms of cannabis, and the apparent absence of tolerance and a withdrawal syndrome, the professional consensus was that cannabis was not a drug of dependence. However, expert views on the nature of drug dependence changed during the early 1980s with the introduction of a broader concept of drug dependence modelled on the alcohol dependence syndrome (Edwards & Gross, 1976). This syndrome concept of dependence reduced the importance of tolerance and withdrawal as defining characteristics of addiction. More emphasis was placed on symptoms such as a compulsion to use, a narrowing of the drug-using repertoire, a rapid reinstatement of dependence symptoms after a period of abstinence, and the high salience of drug use in the user's life.

Around the same time, evidence was provided in animals and humans that tolerance can develop and that withdrawal symptoms can occur under certain conditions of cannabis use. Since the middle 1970s, evidence emerged in human and animal studies that chronic administration of high doses of $\varnothing$-tetrahydrocannabinol (THC) produced marked tolerance to a wide variety of cannabinoid effects, such as the cardiovascular effects, and subjective high in humans (Compton, Dewey & Martin, 1990; Fehr & Kalant, 1983; Hollister, 1986; Institute of Medicine, 1982; Jones, Benowitz & Herning, 1981). The abrupt cessation of chronic high doses of THC also produced a mild withdrawal syndrome like that produced by other long-acting sedative drugs (Compton, Dewey & Martin, 1990; Jones & Benowitz, 1976; Jones, Benowitz & Herning, 1981). What remains uncertain is how significant withdrawal symptoms, and the use of cannabis for withdrawal relief, are in maintaining cannabis dependence — see the *Diagnostic and Statistical Manual of Mental Disorders, Fourth Edition (DSM-IV)* (American Psychiatric Association, 1994).

Clinical and Observational Evidence

The existence of a cannabis dependence syndrome among some heavy and long-term cannabis users can be inferred from data on the prevalence and characteristics of persons seeking professional help to stop using cannabis, from observational studies of problems reported by non-treatment samples of long-term cannabis users, and from clinical research on the validity of the cannabis dependence syndrome as embodied in *DSM-III-R* (American Psychiatric Association, 1987) and other classification systems.

During the 1980s, a number of countries reported an increase in the number of persons seeking help for cannabis as their primary or major drug problem. Jones (1984), for example, reported that 35,000 patients sought treatment in the United States in 1981 for drug problems in which "cannabis was their primary drug," an increase of 50 per cent over three years. Many of these patients behaved "as if they were addicted to cannabis" and they presented "some of the same problems as compulsive users of other drugs." Roffman and colleagues (1988; 1993) reported a strong response to community advertisements for people who wanted help to stop using marijuana. Sweden also experienced an increase in numbers of heavy hashish users presenting to treatment services for help with problems caused by its use (Engstrom, Allebeck et al., 1985).

During the 1990s, treatment services in Australia, Europe and the United States reported increases in numbers seeking help with cannabis use. In Australia in 1995 (Torres, Mattick et al., 1995), 6 per cent of persons presenting to specialist treatment agencies had a primary cannabis problem. Between 11 and 26 per cent of U.S. treatment presentations in 1994 and 1996 had a primary cannabis problem (United States Office of National Drug Control Policy, 1994; 1996). In the European Union in 1995, between 4 and 20 per cent of treatment presentations reported cannabis as a problem (European Monitoring Centre for Drugs and Drug Addiction, 1996).

Suggestive evidence of a cannabis dependence syndrome emerged from a small number of observational studies of regular cannabis users. Weller, Halikas and Morse (1984), for example, followed up a cohort of 100 regular marijuana users, first identified in 1970–71, and assessed them for alcohol and marijuana abuse using Feighner's criteria for alcoholism and an analogous set of criteria for marijuana (see Weller & Halikas, 1980). They found that 9 per cent of subjects were alcoholic and 9 per cent were "abusers" of marijuana.

Hendin et al. (1987) reported on 150 long-term daily cannabis users who had been recruited through newspaper advertisements. Substantial proportions of their sample reported various adverse effects of long-term cannabis use, despite which they continued to use the drug. These included impaired memory (67 per cent), impaired ability to concentrate on complex tasks (49 per cent), difficulty getting things done (48 per cent), or thinking clearly (43 per cent), reduced energy (43 per cent), ill health (36 per cent), and accidents (23 per cent). Half of the subjects reported that they would like to cut down or stop their use.

These findings have been broadly supported by Kandel and Davies (1992) in a study of problems reported by near-daily cannabis users (aged 28 to 29 years) who were identified in a prospective study of adolescent drug use. The major adverse consequences of use were subjective cognitive deficits, reduced energy, depression and problems with spouses. Stephens and Roffman's (1993) sample of cannabis users complained of "feeling bad about using," procrastinating because of their use, memory impairment, loss of self-esteem, withdrawal symptoms and spousal complaints about their use.

More direct support for the validity of the cannabis abuse dependence syndrome comes from studies of diagnostic criteria for substance dependence. Kosten et al. (1987) tested the extent to which the *DSM-III-R* psychoactive substance dependence disorders for alcohol, cannabis, cocaine, hallucinogens, opioids, sedatives and stimulants constituted syndromes. A sample of 83 persons was interviewed using a standardized psychiatric interview schedule to assess symptoms of dependence as defined in the *DSM-III-R* for each of the drug classes. Multiple diagnoses were allowed so many individuals qualified for more than one type of drug dependence.

There was consistent support for a unidimensional dependence syndrome for alcohol, cocaine and opiates. The results were more equivocal in the case of cannabis. All the items were moderately positively correlated, had good internal consistency and seemed to comprise a Guttman scale, but a Principal Components Analysis suggested that there were three dimen-

sions of cannabis dependence: (1) *compulsion,* indicated by impaired social activity attributable to drug use, preoccupation with drug use, giving up other interests, and using more than intended; (2) *inability to stop,* indicated by inability to cut down, rapid reinstatement after abstinence, and tolerance to drug effects; and (3) *withdrawal,* identified by withdrawal symptoms, use of cannabis to relieve withdrawal symptoms and continued use despite problems.

Didcott et al. (1997) reported the prevalence of cannabis dependence, according to both *ICD-10* and *DSM-III-R* criteria, in a sample of 243 long-term cannabis users who had not sought treatment and were recruited from an area where there was known to be a high prevalence of heavy cannabis use. They found that 57 per cent of the group met criteria for dependence on each set of criteria and there was moderate though not perfect agreement between the two sets of criteria. Only about half of those who met criteria for cannabis dependence believed that they had a problem with cannabis use. Factor analyses did not find strong support for unidimensionality of either set of criteria.

Similar results were obtained in a study of 200 long-term cannabis users in Sydney, Australia, by Swift et al. (1997). They used the *Composite International Diagnostic Interview – Substance Abuse Module (CIDI-SAM)* to assess *DSM-III-R* and *ICD-10* criteria for dependence. Agreement between the criteria was poorer than in Didcott et al. (1997). There was a much higher prevalence of dependence diagnoses (90 per cent), and there was weak evidence of unidimensionality of dependence symptoms.

Two studies have provided stronger support for a unidimensional cannabis dependence syndrome. Newcombe (1992) performed a factor analysis on 29 questionnaire items designed to measure *DSM-III-R* abuse and dependence in a community sample of 614 young adults. He reported a strong common factor for all three drug types, which accounted for 36 to 40 per cent of the item variance. Rounsaville et al. (1993) reported similar results in factor analyses of symptoms of dependence for each of six drug classes (alcohol, cocaine, marijuana, opiates, sedatives and stimulants) in a sample of 521 persons recruited from inpatient and outpatient drug treatment, psychiatric treatment services and the general community. They found that a single common factor explained the variation between symptoms for all drug types.

Epidemiological Evidence

The prevalence of cannabis abuse and dependence in the United States has been estimated in the Epidemiological Catchment Area (ECA) study (Robins & Regier, 1991) and the National Comorbidity Survey (Kessler, McGonagh et al., 1994). The ECA study involved face-to-face interviews with 20,000 Americans in five catchment areas (Baltimore, Maryland; Los Angeles, California; New Haven, Connecticut; Durham, North Carolina; and St. Louis, Missouri) using a standardized and validated interview schedule to make a *DSM-III* (American Psychiatric Association, 1980) diagnosis of drug abuse and dependence, among other psychiatric diagnoses (Anthony & Helzer, 1991).

Individuals had to have used an illicit drug on more than five occasions before they were asked about any symptoms of drug dependence. The criteria used to define cannabis abuse and dependence were derived from the *DSM-III*. They required symptoms of pathological use or impaired social functioning, in addition to signs of either tolerance or withdrawal. The problem had to have been present for at least one month.

Diagnostic criteria for cannabis abuse and dependence were met by 4.4 per cent of the population at some time in their lives. The highest prevalence (13.5 per cent) was in the 18- to 29-year age group (16.0 per cent among men and 10.9 per cent among women), declining steeply thereafter in both sexes. Two-thirds of these cases had used cannabis within the past year, and half had used the drug within the past month. A third of those with a lifetime history of cannabis abuse and/or dependence (38 per cent) reported active problems in the prior year (Anthony & Helzer, 1991).

Similar estimates of the population prevalence of cannabis dependence were produced in a community survey of psychiatric disorders conducted in Christchurch, New Zealand, in 1986 (Wells, Bushnell et al., 1992). This study surveyed 1,498 adults aged 18 to 64 years of age using the same sampling strategy and diagnostic interview as the ECA study. The proportion who met *DSM-III* criteria for marijuana abuse or dependence was 4.7 per cent. The fact that this survey largely replicated the ECA findings for most other diagnoses, including alcohol abuse and dependence, enhances confidence in the validity of the ECA study findings.

The National Comorbidity Survey (NCS) was a population survey that was undertaken between 1990 and 1992 to estimate comorbidity between substance use and non-substance use disorders in achieving a nationally representative sample of the U.S. population. It provided prevalence estimates of disorders as defined in the newly revised *DSM-III-R* classification using a modified version of the *Composite International Diagnostic Interview (CIDI)* schedule, a derivative of the *Diagnostic Interview Schedule (DIS)* which is sponsored by the World Health Organization (WHO), to make the same diagnoses as in the ECA.

The NCS produced a higher lifetime prevalence of any mental disorder than the ECA (48 per cent versus 32 per cent). The major reasons for this seem to have been that the NCS sample was younger and thus contained more persons with mental disorders that generally commence in early adult life; the NCS estimates were corrected for non-response, which increased the overall rates; and a number of changes were made to the way in which the *CIDI* inquired about symptoms of phobias and depressive disorder that were likely to increase the rate of reporting.

In most other respects the agreement between the ECA and NCS was impressive. There was a consistent gender difference in pattern of disorders, for example, a male excess for substance use disorders (35 per cent versus 18 per cent lifetime; 16 per cent versus 7 per cent past year) and antisocial personality disorder (ASPD) (6 per cent versus 1 per cent lifetime), and a female excess in affective disorders (24 per cent versus 15 per cent lifetime; 14 per cent versus 9 per cent in the past year) and anxiety disorders (31 per cent versus 19 per cent lifetime; 25 per cent versus 12 per cent in the past year).

The NCS assessed dependence symptoms in any person who had ever used any of the drug types once (as against five or more times in the ECA). It estimated that 4 per cent of the U.S. population had met lifetime criteria for cannabis dependence, compared to 24 per cent for tobacco, 14 per cent for alcohol, 3 per cent for cocaine and 0.4 per cent for heroin, while correlates of cannabis dependence in the NCS were similar to those reported in the ECA (Anthony, Warner & Kessler, 1994).

The Risk of Cannabis Dependence

Persons who use cannabis on a daily basis over periods of weeks to months are at greatest risk of becoming dependent. In the ECA study approximately half of those who used any illicit drug on a daily basis satisfied *DSM-III* criteria for abuse or dependence (Anthony & Helzer, 1991). Kandel and Davis (1992) estimated the risk of dependence among near-daily cannabis users (according to approximated *DSM-III* criteria) at one in three.

The risk of developing dependence among less frequent users of cannabis is substantially less. In the ECA study 20 per cent of those who used any illicit drug more than five times met criteria for drug abuse and dependence at some time in their lives. The percentage of users who developed dependence and abuse in the Christchurch study (Wells, Bushnell et al., 1992) was 30 per cent. Newcombe estimated that 25 per cent of young adults who had ever used cannabis met criteria for dependence and abuse, while Kandel and Davies (1992) estimated that around a third (39 per cent) of those who had used cannabis 10 or more times developed dependence.

The NCS estimated the proportion of those who had ever used a drug who had met criteria for dependence on that drug during their lifetime. The estimates were (in decreasing order of prevalence): tobacco (32 per cent), opiates (23 per cent), cocaine (17 per cent), alcohol (15 per cent), psychostimulants (11 per cent), anxiolytics (9 per cent) and cannabis (9 per cent). This, and other formal comparisons of the dependence potential of cannabis with that of other drugs (Woody, Cottler & Caciola, 1993), suggest that the dependence risks of cannabis use are probably more like those of alcohol than those of tobacco and opiates.

Psychotic Disorders

There are good reasons for suspecting that cannabis use may be a contributory cause of psychotic disorders, i.e., illnesses in which symptoms of hallucinations, delusions and impaired reality testing are predominant features. THC is a psychoactive substance that produces euphoria, distorted time perception and cognitive and memory impairments (Brill & Nahas, 1984; Halikas, Goodwin & Guze, 1971; Thornicroft, 1990). Under laboratory conditions, high doses of THC have been reported to produce visual and auditory hallucinations, delusional ideas, thought disorder and symptoms of hypomania in normal volunteers (Georgotas & Zeidenberg, 1979; Institute of Medicine, 1982). A putative "cannabis psychosis" has been identified by clinicians in regions of the world with a high prevalence of chronic, heavy cannabis use, for example, in India, Egypt and the Caribbean (Brill & Nahas, 1984; Ghodse, 1986).

Toxic Psychosis

The literature on cannabis psychoses largely consists of case studies (e.g., Carney, Bacelle & Robinson, 1984; Drummond, 1986; Edwards, 1983; Weil, 1970) and case-series (e.g., Bernardson & Gunne, 1972; Cohen & Johnson,

1988; Kolansky & Moore, 1971; Onyango, 1986) of individuals who developed psychotic symptoms and disorders after cannabis use. These disorders were attributed to cannabis use because the onset of the symptoms followed closely on ingestion of cannabis, and unlike the symptoms of other psychotic disorders, the symptoms rapidly remitted after a period of enforced abstinence from cannabis use, usually within several days to several weeks.

Chopra and Smith (1974), for example, described 200 East Indian patients who were admitted to a psychiatric hospital in Calcutta between 1963 and 1968 with psychotic symptoms following the use of cannabis preparations. The most common symptoms "were sudden onset of confusion, generally associated with delusions, hallucinations (usually visual) and emotional lability . . . amnesia, disorientation, depersonalisation and paranoid symptoms" (p. 24). Most psychoses were preceded by the ingestion of a large dose of cannabis and there was amnesia for the period between ingestion and hospitalization. Chopra and Smith argued that it was unlikely that excessive cannabis use was a sign of pre-existing psychopathology because a third of their cases had no prior psychiatric history, the symptoms were remarkably uniform regardless of prior psychiatric history, and those who used the most potent cannabis preparations experienced psychotic reactions after the shortest period of use.

The findings of Chopra and Smith (1974) have received some support from case-series published in other countries (e.g., Bernardson & Gunne, 1972; Onyango, 1986; Tennant & Groesbeck, 1972). Bernardson and Gunne (1972) reported on 46 cases of "cannabis psychosis" admitted to Swedish psychiatric hospitals between 1966 and 1970. These were primary cannabis users who had no history of psychosis prior to their cannabis use and who presented with a clinical picture of paranoid delusions, motor restlessness, auditory and visual hallucinations, hypomania, aggression, anxiety and clouded consciousness. Their symptoms usually remitted within five weeks of admission, and those who returned to cannabis use after discharge were most likely to relapse.

Onyango (1986) reported one of the few case-series in which biochemical measures of recent cannabis use were used to identify cases of toxic cannabis psychosis. He screened the urines of 25 young adults who presented to a London psychiatric hospital with psychotic symptoms and found only 4 cases who had cannabinoid metabolites in their urines. In three cases, the patients had a prior history of psychosis, their phenomenology was unremarkable, and they did not respond rapidly to treatment. Only one case seemed to fit the picture of a cannabis psychosis. He had no prior history of psychosis and a history of chronic, heavy cannabis use prior to admission. He presented with hallucinations, delusions and labile, elated mood which responded rapidly to haloperidol, and he had no further episodes during a two-year follow-up.

There are skeptics who are unimpressed by this clinical evidence (e.g., Gruber & Pope, 1994; Lewis, 1968; Poole & Brabbins, 1996). They criticize the poor quality of information on cannabis use and its relationship to the onset of psychosis, and the person's premorbid adjustment and their family history of psychosis. They also emphasize the wide variety of clinical pictures of cannabis psychoses reported by different observers, arguing that these problems impair the evidential value of these case-series.

All considered, there is a reasonable clinical evidence that large doses of potent cannabis products can be followed by a "toxic" psychotic illness (i.e., with "organic" features of amnesia and confusion) that occurs in persons who do not have a personal history of psychotic illness (Edwards, 1976; Negrete, 1983; Thomas, 1993). Such psychoses are characterized by symptoms of confusion and amnesia, paranoid delusions and auditory and visual hallucinations, and they have a relatively benign course in that they typically remit within a week of abstinence (Chaudry, Moss et al., 1991; Thomas, 1993). They seem most likely to occur in populations that use high doses of THC, and probably occur rarely otherwise (Smith, 1968).

Functional Psychosis

Some investigators have argued that heavy cannabis use may also produce an acute functional psychosis, that is, a psychotic illness that does not reflect an organic state produced by drug intoxication. Thacore and Shukla (1976), for example, reported a case-control study comparing cases with a putatively functional cannabis psychosis with controls diagnosed as having paranoid schizophrenia. Their 25 cases of cannabis psychosis had a paranoid psychosis resembling schizophrenia in which "a clear temporal relationship between the prolonged use of cannabis and the development of psychosis has been observed on more than two occasions" (p. 384). Their 25 age- and sex-matched controls were individuals with paranoid schizophrenia who had no history of cannabis use.

The patients with a cannabis psychosis displayed more odd and bizarre behavior, violence, panic affect, and insight and less evidence of thought disorder. They also responded swiftly to neuroleptic drugs and recovered completely. According to Thacore and Shukla (1976), this functional psychotic disorder differed from a toxic cannabis psychosis because there was no confusion and amnesia; and the major presenting symptoms were delusions of persecution, and auditory and visual hallucinations occurring in a state of clear consciousness.

Rottanburg et al. (1982) conducted a case-control study in which 20 psychotic patients with cannabinoids in their urines were compared with 20 psychotic patients who did not have cannabinoids in their urines. Both groups were assessed shortly after admission, and seven days later, by psychiatrists who used a standardized psychiatric interview schedule (PSE) and who were blind as to the presence or absence of cannabinoids in the patient's urine. Compared to controls, psychotic patients with cannabinoids in their urine had more symptoms of hypomania and agitation, and fewer symptoms of auditory hallucinations, flattening of affect, incoherent speech and hysteria. They also showed strong improvements in symptoms by the end of a week, as against no change in the controls despite receiving comparable amounts of antipsychotic drugs.

Chaudry et al. (1991) reported a comparison of 15 psychotic "bhang" users with 10 bhang users without psychosis. They found that their cases were more likely to have a history of chronic cannabis use and past psychotic episodes. They also were more likely to be unco-operative and to have symptoms of excitement, hostility, grandiosity, hallucinations, disorientation and unusual thought content. All cases remitted within five days and had no residual psychotic symptoms.

Mathers et al. (1991) reported a study of patients presenting to two London hospitals. They found a relationship between the presence of cannabinoids in urine and having a psychotic diagnosis. Rolfe et al. (1993) reported a similar association between urinary cannabinoids and psychosis in 234 patients admitted to a Gambian psychiatric unit.

Tien and Anthony (1990) used data from the ECA study to compare the drug use of individuals who reported "psychotic experiences" during a twelve-month period. These psychotic experiences comprised four types of hallucinations and seven types of delusional belief. The researchers compared 477 cases who reported one or more psychotic symptoms in the one-year follow-up with 1,818 controls who did not. Cases and controls were matched for age and social and demographic characteristics. Daily cannabis use was found to double the risk of reporting psychotic symptoms (after statistical adjustment for alcohol use and psychiatric diagnoses at baseline).

In contrast to these positive findings, a number of controlled studies have not found such a clear association. Imade and Ebie (1991) compared the symptoms of 70 patients with cannabis-induced functional psychoses, 163 patients with schizophrenia and 39 patients with mania. They reported that there were no symptoms that were unique to cannabis psychosis, and none that enabled them to distinguish a cannabis psychosis from schizophrenia.

Thornicroft et al. (1992) compared 45 cases who had a psychosis and showed a positive urine test for cannabinoids with 45 controls who had a psychosis but either had a urine test negative for cannabinoids or reported no cannabis use. They found very few demographic or clinical differences between the groups.

McGuire et al. (1994; 1995) compared 23 cases of psychoses occurring in persons whose urines were positive for cannabinoids with 46 psychotic patients whose urines were negative for cannabinoids or who reported no cannabis use. The two groups did not differ in their psychiatric histories or symptoms profile, as assessed by "blind" ratings of clinical files using the PSE (McGuire, Jones et al., 1994). The cases, however, were more likely to have a family history of schizophrenia.

All considered, the clinical evidence for the hypothesis that cannabis use can produce a functional paranoid illness is better controlled but more mixed than that for a toxic psychosis. Experienced investigators remain skeptical (Thomas, 1993; Thornicroft, 1990), arguing that proponents of this hypothesis have not presented evidence that satisfactorily distinguishes the putatively cannabis-induced functional psychosis from schizophrenia and other functional psychoses that are precipitated or exacerbated by cannabis use, or which simply occur in individuals who happen to have used cannabis (Thornicroft, 1990).

Chronic Psychosis

If cannabis can produce an acute organic psychosis the possibility must be considered that chronic cannabis use may produce a chronic psychosis (Ghodse, 1986). Although this is a possibility, there is no good evidence that chronic cannabis use causes a psychotic illness that persists beyond abstinence from cannabis (Thomas, 1993). This hypothesis is difficult to study because of the problem of distinguishing a chronic cannabis psychosis from a functional psychosis, such as schizophrenia, in which there is concurrent cannabis use (Negrete, 1983). Follow-up studies of patients with acute cannabis psychoses, if they could be reliably identified, would be the best way of throwing some light on this issue. The possibility that chronic cannabis use could perpetuate a chronic schizophrenic illness is considered below.

Other Psychiatric Disorders

An Amotivational Syndrome

Anecdotal reports that chronic heavy cannabis use impairs motivation and social performance have been described in societies with a long history of cannabis use, such as Egypt, the Caribbean and elsewhere (e.g., Brill & Nahas, 1984). Among young adults who were heavy cannabis users in the United States in the early 1970s, there were clinical reports (e.g., Kolansky & Moore, 1971; Millman & Sbriglio, 1986; Tennant & Groesbeck, 1972) of individuals who became apathetic, withdrawn, lethargic and unmotivated, apparently as a result of chronic heavy cannabis use (Brill & Nahas, 1984; McGlothlin & West, 1968). This constellation of symptoms was described as an "amotivational syndrome" (McGlothlin & West, 1968; Smith, 1968). All these reports were uncontrolled so that it has not been possible to disentangle the effects of chronic cannabis use from those of pre-existing personality and other psychiatric disorders (Edwards, 1976; Institute of Medicine, 1982; Millman & Sbriglio, 1986; Negrete, 1983).

It has proved difficult in controlled studies to obtain evidence to form a consensus on whether or not there is an amotivational syndrome. Field studies of chronic heavy cannabis users in societies with a tradition of such use, for example, Costa Rica (Carter, Coggins & Doughty, 1980) and Jamaica (Rubin & Comitas, 1975), have produced evidence that has usually been interpreted as failing to demonstrate the existence of the amotivational syndrome (e.g., Dornbush, 1974; Hollister, 1986; Negrete, 1988). Critics have argued, however, that these studies are unconvincing because the chronic users studied have come from socially marginal groups so that the cognitive and motivational demands of their everyday lives were insufficient to detect any impairment caused by chronic cannabis use (Cohen, 1982).

Other evidence suggests that an amotivational syndrome is likely to be rare, if it exists. Halikas et al. (1982), for example, followed up 100 regular cannabis users over six to eight years and inquired about symptoms of an amotivational syndrome. They found only three individuals who had ever experienced such a cluster of symptoms, and they did not differ in their patterns of use from cannabis users who did not show these symptoms.

The status of the amotivational syndrome remains contentious. Many clinicians find the cases of amotivational syndrome compelling, whereas many researchers are more impressed by the largely unsupportive findings of the field and epidemiological studies. The possibility has been kept alive by reports that regular cannabis users experience a loss of ambition and impaired school and occupational performance as adverse effects of their use (e.g., Hendin, Haas et al., 1987) and that some ex-cannabis users give impaired occupational performance as a reason for stopping (Jones, 1984). Although heavy users who request assistance to stop their use report impaired motivation as a *symptom* of cannabis use, a well-defined amotivational *syndrome* has not been documented. Instead of inventing a new psychiatric syndrome, it may be more parsimonious to regard impaired motivation as a symptom of chronic cannabis intoxication.

Other Psychiatric Disorders

There are a number of other rarer psychiatric symptoms and disorders that have been attributed to cannabis use. Because of their rarity, their existence is supported by only a small number of case histories in which individuals report unusual experiences and symptoms after using cannabis. These disorders include residual and late onset disorders, such as "flashbacks" — experiencing symptoms of cannabis intoxication days or weeks after the individual last used cannabis (Edwards, 1983); symptoms of depersonalization following cannabis intoxication (Moran, 1986; Thomas, 1993); and reports of amnestic disorders in chronic heavy cannabis users (Kolansky & Moore, 1971).

As noted in chapter 1, it is often difficult to decide whether these are: rare events that are coincidental with cannabis use; the effects of other drugs that are often taken together with cannabis; rare consequences of cannabis use occurring at doses much higher than those used recreationally or requiring unusual forms of personal vulnerability; or the results of interactions between the cannabis and other drugs. The effects of chronic cannabis use on memory are explored in chapter 6.

Comorbidity: Cannabis Use and Schizophrenia

A clinical association between heavy, chronic cannabis use and schizophrenia (e.g., Tennant & Groesbeck, 1972) has received some support from case-control studies of cannabis and other psychoactive drug use among schizophrenic patients (Schneier & Siris, 1987; Smith & Hucker, 1994). These studies have found that schizophrenic patients are more likely to have used psychotomimetic drugs such as amphetamines, cocaine and hallucinogens than other psychiatric patients (Dixon, Haas et al., 1990; Schneier & Siris, 1987; Weller, Ang et al., 1988) or normal controls (Breakey, Goodell et al., 1974; Rolfe, Tang et al., 1993). The results for cannabis use have been more mixed, with some finding a higher prevalence of use or abuse (e.g., Mathers, Ghodse et al., 1991) while others have not done so (Dixon, Haas et al., 1990; Mueser, Yarnold et al., 1990; Schneier & Siris, 1987). The ECA study also found an association between schizophrenia and drug abuse and dependence (Anthony & Helzer, 1991; Cuffel,

Heithoff & Lawson, 1993), which was replicated in a population survey of psychiatric disorder in Edmonton, Alberta, using the same ECA interview schedule and diagnostic criteria (Bland, Norman & Orn, 1987).

Precipitation

Many researchers have favored a causal interpretation of the association between cannabis use and schizophrenia, arguing that cannabis use precipitates schizophrenic disorders in persons who are vulnerable to developing the disorder, and possibly in persons who may not otherwise have developed the disorder. In support of this hypothesis, they cite reports that drug-abusing schizophrenic patients have an earlier age of onset of psychotic symptoms (with their drug use typically preceding the onset of symptoms), a better premorbid adjustment, fewer negative symptoms (e.g., withdrawal, anhedonia, lethargy), and a better response to treatment and outcome than schizophrenic patients who do not use drugs (Allebeck, Adamsson et al., 1993; Dixon, Haas et al., 1990; Hambrecht & Hafner, 1996; Schneier & Siris, 1987).

Other hypotheses have been advanced. Arndt et al. (1992), for example, have suggested that the association between cannabis use and an early onset of schizophrenia in persons with a good premorbid personality and outcome is spurious. On their hypothesis, schizophrenics with a better premorbid personality were simply more likely to be exposed to illicit drug use among peers than those who are socially withdrawn. Because of this prior exposure to drugs, these individuals are also more likely to use these drugs to cope with the symptoms of an emerging psychosis. Other investigators have failed to replicate the associations between cannabis use and clinical history and symptoms (e.g., Cuffel, Heithoff & Lawson, 1993; Kovasznay, Bromet et al., 1993; Zisook, Heaton et al., 1992).

Another possibility is that cannabis use is a consequence of schizophrenia; that is, it is a form of self-medication used to deal with either the unpleasant symptoms of schizophrenia, such as depression, anxiety, the negative symptoms of lethargy, and anhedonia, or with the side effects of the neuroleptic drugs used to treat it (Dixon, Haas et al., 1990). There is some support for this hypothesis. Dixon et al. (1990) surveyed 83 patients with schizophrenia or schizophreniform psychoses about the effects of various illicit drugs on their mood and symptoms. Their patients reported that cannabis reduced anxiety and depression and increased a sense of calm, at the cost of some increase in suspiciousness, and with mixed effects on hallucinations and energy. Supportive findings have come from a controlled study of the effect of cannabis use on schizophrenic symptoms (Peralta & Cuesta, 1992).

The most convincing evidence of an association between cannabis use and the precipitation of schizophrenia has been provided by a 15-year prospective study of cannabis use and schizophrenia in 50,465 Swedish conscripts (Andreasson, Allebeck et al., 1987). These researchers investigated the relationship between self-reported cannabis use at age 18 and the risk of receiving a diagnosis of schizophrenia in the subsequent 15 years, as indicated by inclusion in the Swedish psychiatric case register. The relative risk of receiving a diagnosis of schizophrenia was 2.4 times higher for those who had ever tried cannabis compared to those who had not. There was also a dose-response relationship between the risk of a diagnosis of schizophrenia and the number of times that the conscript had tried cannabis by age 18. The crude relative risk of developing schizophrenia was 1.3 times higher for those who had used cannabis 1 to 10 times, 3.0 times higher for those who had used cannabis between 1 and 50 times, and 6.0 times higher for those who had used cannabis more than 50 times (compared in each case to those who had not used cannabis).

The size of the risk was substantially reduced by statistical adjustment for variables that were independently related to the risk of developing schizophrenia (namely, having a psychiatric diagnosis at conscription and having parents who had divorced). Nevertheless, the relationship remained statistically significant and still showed a dose-response relationship. The risk of a diagnosis of schizophrenia for those who had smoked cannabis from 1 to 10 times was 1.5 times that of those who had never used, and the relative risk for those who had used 10 or more times was 2.3 times that of those who had never used.

Andreasson et al. (1987) and Allebeck (1991) argued that these data show that cannabis use can precipitate schizophrenia in vulnerable individuals. They rejected the hypothesis that cannabis consumption was a consequence of emerging schizophrenia since the cannabis users who developed schizophrenia had better premorbid personalities, a more abrupt onset and more positive symptoms than the non-users who developed schizophrenia (Andreasson, Allebeck & Rydberg, 1989). Moreover, there was still a dose-response relationship between cannabis use and schizophrenia among those conscripts who did not have a psychiatric history at age 18. They stressed that cannabis use "only accounts for a minority of all cases" since most of the 274 conscripts who developed schizophrenia had not used cannabis, and only 21 of them were heavy cannabis users.

A number of alternative explanations have been offered of the association. First, there was a large temporal gap between self-reported cannabis use at age 18 to 20 years and the development of schizophrenia over the next 15 years or so (Johnson, Smith & Taylor, 1988; Negrete, 1989). Because the diagnosis of schizophrenia was based on a case register, there was usually no information on whether the individuals continued to use cannabis up until the time that their schizophrenia was diagnosed. Andreasson et al. (1987) argued that it was most likely that cannabis use did persist since self-reported cannabis use at age 18 was also strongly related to the likelihood of attracting a diagnosis of drug abuse, and the more frequently cannabis had been used by age 18, the more likely the person was to receive such a diagnosis.

A second possibility was that the excess rate of "schizophrenia" among the heavy cannabis users included cannabis-induced toxic psychoses

that were mistakenly diagnosed as schizophrenia (Johnson, Smith & Taylor, 1988; Negrete, 1989). Andreasson et al. (1989) addressed this criticism by a study of the validity of the schizophrenia diagnoses in 21 conscripts in the case register (8 of whom had used cannabis and 13 of whom had not). This study indicated that 80 per cent of these cases met the *DSM-III* requirement that the symptoms had been present for at least six months, an observation that tends to exclude transient psychotic symptoms as the cause. This sample size (21 cases) was small, however, and the confidence interval around a 20 per cent rate of misdiagnosis of schizophrenia is between 3 per cent and 37 per cent.

Third, the relationship between cannabis use and schizophrenia may be a consequence of the use of other illicit psychoactive drugs. Longitudinal studies of illicit drug use indicate that intensity of cannabis use in late adolescence predicts the subsequent use of other illicit drugs. These include amphetamine (Johnson, 1988; Kandel & Faust, 1975), which can produce an acute paranoid psychosis (Angrist, 1983; Bell, 1973; Connell, 1959; Gawin & Ellinwood, 1988; Grinspoon & Hedblom, 1975) and which was the major illicit drug of abuse in Sweden during the study period (Inghe, 1969; Goldberg, 1968a; 1968b). Therefore, intervening amphetamine use may have produced a spurious association between cannabis use and schizophrenia.

A fourth possibility is that cannabis use at age 18 was a symptom of emerging schizophrenia. Andreasson et al. (1987) argued that this hypothesis was implausible because the dose-response relationship between cannabis use and the risk of a schizophrenia diagnosis held up among those who did not have a psychiatric history. The persuasiveness of this argument depends on how confident we can be that a *failure* to identify a psychiatric disorder at conscription means that no disorder was present.

The fifth criticism relates to the validity of self-reported cannabis use at conscription. Andreasson et al. (1987) acknowledged that there was likely to be underreporting of cannabis use because this information was not collected anonymously but they argued that this was most likely to lead to an underestimation of the relationship between cannabis use and the risk of schizophrenia. This will only be true, however, if the schizophrenic and non-schizophrenic conscripts were equally likely to underreport. If, for example, preschizophrenic subjects were more candid about their drug use the apparent relationship between cannabis use and schizophrenia would be due to response bias (Negrete, 1989). Although a possibility, this seems unlikely in view of the strong dose-response relationship with frequency of cannabis use, and the large size of the unadjusted relative risk of schizophrenia among heavy users.

When all these criticisms are considered, the Andreasson et al. (1987) study still provides strong evidence of an association between cannabis use and schizophrenia. Uncertainty remains about the causal significance of the association because it is unclear to what extent the relationship is a result of drug-induced psychoses being mistaken for schizophrenia and to what extent it is attributable to amphetamine rather than cannabis use.

If the relationship is causal, its public health significance needs to be kept in perspective. An estimate of the attributable risk based on the relative risk adjusted for psychiatric disorder (Feinstein, 1985) indicates that, at most, 7 per cent of cases of schizophrenia would be attributable to cannabis use. Even this small potential contribution to an increased incidence of schizophrenia seems difficult to accept since there is good independent evidence that the incidence of schizophrenia, and particularly of early-onset acute cases, declined during the 1970s, the period when the prevalence of cannabis use increased among young adults in Western Europe and North America (Der, Gupta & Murray, 1990).

Exacerbation

There is clinical evidence that schizophrenic patients who continue to use cannabis experience more psychotic symptoms (Weil, 1970) and have a worse clinical course than those who do not (Knudsen & Vilmar, 1984; Perkins, Simpson

& Tsuang, 1986; Turner & Tsuang, 1990). These observations have recently been supported by a number of controlled studies of the relationship between cannabis use and the clinical outcome of schizophrenia.

Negrete et al. (1986) conducted a retrospective study using clinical records of symptoms and treatment seeking among 137 schizophrenic patients with a disorder of at least six months' duration and three visits to their psychiatric service during the previous six months. Negrete et al. compared the prevalence of hallucinations, delusions and hospitalizations among the active users, the past users and those who had never used cannabis. There were higher rates of continuous hallucinations and delusions and of hospitalizations among active users which persisted after statistical control for differences in age and sex among the three user groups.

Negrete et al. argued that cannabis use exacerbated schizophrenic symptoms. They rejected the alternative hypothesis that patients with a poorer prognosis were more likely to use cannabis because they found that past cannabis users experienced fewer symptoms, and reported a high rate of adverse effects when using (91 per cent). They also discounted the possibility that these were toxic psychoses because in all cases the minimum duration of symptoms had been six months. They suggested three possible mechanisms by which cannabis use exacerbated schizophrenic symptoms: that cannabis disorganizes psychological functioning; that it causes a toxic psychosis that accentuates schizophrenic symptomatology; or that it interferes with the therapeutic action of antipsychotic medication.

Cleghorn et al. (1991), Jablensky et al. (1991) and Martinez-Arevalo et al. (1994) have provided supportive evidence for the hypothesis of Negrete et al. Cleghorn et al. compared the symptom profiles of schizophrenic patients with histories of substance abuse of varying severity, among whom cannabis was the most heavily used drug. Comparisons within a subset of the patients who were maintained on neuroleptic drugs revealed that the drug abusers had a higher prevalence of hallucinations, delusions and positive symptoms. Jablensky et al. reported in their two-year follow-up of 1,202 new schizophrenic patients in 10 countries that the use of "street drugs," including cannabis, during the follow-up period predicted a poorer outcome. Martinez-Arevalo et al. reported that continued use of cannabis during a one-year follow-up of 62 *DSM*-diagnosed schizophrenic patients predicted a higher rate of relapse and poorer compliance with treatment.

Linszen et al. (1994) recently reported a prospective study of outcome in 93 psychotic patients whose symptoms were assessed monthly over a year. Twenty-four of their patients were cannabis abusers (11 were less than daily users and 13 were daily cannabis users). Despite the small sample sizes, they found that the cannabis users relapsed to psychotic symptoms sooner and had more frequent relapses in the year of follow-up than patients who had not used cannabis. There was also a dose-response relationship, with the daily users relapsing earlier and more often than the less than daily users who, in turn, relapsed sooner and more often than the patients who did not use cannabis. These relationships persisted after multivariate adjustment for pre-morbid adjustment and alcohol and other drug use during the follow-up period.

Most but not all studies (e.g., Zisook, Heaton et al., 1992) have reported an association between continued cannabis use and exacerbation of psychotic symptoms in patients with schizophrenia. The major uncertainty about this relationship is the role of confounding factors, such as differences in premorbid personality, family history and other characteristics (Kavanagh, 1995). These factors are unlikely to have affected the WHO schizophrenia study (Jablensky, Sartorius et al., 1991) and the recent study of Linszen et al. (1994), both of which used multivariate statistical methods to adjust for many of these confounders.

Another difficulty is separating the contributions of cannabis from those of alcohol and other drugs to exacerbations of schizophrenic symptoms. It is rare for a schizophrenic patient to use cannabis *only* (Mueser, Bellack &

Blanchard, 1992). The concurrent use of alcohol is common, and the heavier their cannabis use, the more likely it is that patients also use psychostimulants and hallucinogens. Only the Linszen et al. (1994) study statistically adjusted for the effects of concurrent alcohol and drug use and found that the relationship persisted. Our confidence that the effect is attributable to cannabis would be increased by replications of the Linszen et al. finding.

Conclusion

Clinical and epidemiological research has clarified the status of the cannabis dependence syndrome. A reduced emphasis on tolerance and withdrawal in diagnostic criteria for drug dependence has removed a major reason for skepticism about the existence of a cannabis dependence syndrome. More positively, clinical and epidemiological research using standardized diagnostic criteria has produced good evidence for a cannabis dependence syndrome that affects a substantial minority of cannabis users. As with other drugs, the risk of developing dependence is highest among those with a history of daily cannabis use. About half of those who use cannabis daily for weeks and months, and between 1 in 10 and 1 in 5 of those who ever use cannabis, may become dependent on it.

The state of the evidence on an amotivational syndrome and cannabis-induced psychoses has not substantively changed since the 1981 WHO report. In both cases, the existence of these putative disorders still depends on clinical observations. Although there is reasonable self-report evidence that heavy cannabis use can impair motivation, an amotivational syndrome has not been clearly defined nor have its central features been clearly distinguished from the effects of chronic intoxication in chronic heavy cannabis users.

The existence of "cannabis psychoses" also depends on clinical observations of individuals developing acute psychotic disorders (both with and without organic features) following heavy cannabis use. The attribution of these disorders to cannabis use is based on the facts that a substantial minority of these individuals have no prior history of psychiatric disorder, and their disorders remit within days to weeks of abstinence from cannabis. There are also a limited number of case-control studies comparing the clinical symptoms and course of psychotic disorders in individuals who do and do not have cannabinoids in their urine. These studies have not, however, clearly defined the phenomenology of cannabis psychoses, nor have these disorders been distinguished from schizophrenia and other psychotic disorders that occur among cannabis users.

In addition to these major disorders, a number of other psychiatric disorders have been linked with cannabis use, including persistent depersonalization, "flashbacks," and amnestic disorders. These disorders are supported by only a small number of case histories. In the case of flashbacks, there is considerable uncertainty as to whether these effects were attributable to cannabis or other drug use.

Epidemiological research has produced clear evidence from case-control, cross-sectional and prospective studies of an association between cannabis use and schizophrenia. The prospective study of Andreasson et al. (1987) has shown a dose-response relationship between the frequency with which cannabis had been used by age 18 and the risks over the subsequent 15 years of being diagnosed as schizophrenic. The association is not in doubt, but its significance is still debated because it is unclear whether it reflects the precipitation of schizophrenia by cannabis use, the use of cannabis as a form of "self-medication" by schizophrenic individuals or a spurious association attributable to the use of other psychoactive drugs, such as amphetamines. It is much clearer that cannabis use can exacerbate the symptoms of schizophrenia in affected individuals.

There are two major research priorities for cannabis-induced psychiatric and behavioral disorders. These are the better delineation of the clinical features of cannabis dependence, including its responsiveness to interventions to assist users to stop and the design of intervention studies with psychotic individuals who use cannabis to see whether cessation of cannabis use improves their outcome.

References

Allebeck, P. (1991). Cannabis and schizophrenia: Is there a causal association? In G.G. Nahas & C. Latour (Eds.), *Physiopathology of Illicit Drugs: Cannabis, Cocaine, Opiates* (pp. 23–31). Oxford: Pergamon Press.

Allebeck, P., Adamsson, C., Engstrom, A. & Rydberg, U. (1993). Cannabis and schizophrenia: A longitudinal study of cases treated in Stockholm county. *Acta Psychiatrica Scandinavica, 88,* 21–24.

American Psychiatric Association. (1980). *Diagnostic and Statistical Manual of Mental Disorders* (3rd ed.). Washington, DC: American Psychiatric Association.

American Psychiatric Association. (1987). *Diagnostic and Statistical Manual of Mental Disorders* (3rd ed., rev.). Washington, DC: American Psychiatric Association.

American Psychiatric Association. (1994). *Diagnostic and Statistical Manual of Mental Disorders* (4th ed.). Washington, DC: American Psychiatric Association.

Andreasson, S., Allebeck, P., Engstrom, A. & Rydberg, U. (1987). Cannabis and schizophrenia: A longitudinal study of Swedish conscripts. *Lancet, 2,* 1483–1486.

Andreasson, S., Allebeck, P., & Rydberg, U. (1989). Schizophrenia in users and nonusers of cannabis. *Acta Psychiatrica Scandinavica, 79,* 505–510.

Angrist, B. (1983). Psychoses induced by central nervous system stimulants and related drugs. In I. Creese (Ed.), *Stimulants: Neurochemical, Behavioral and Clinical Perspectives* (pp. 1–30). New York: Raven Press.

Anthony, J.C. & Helzer, J.E. (1991). Syndromes of drug abuse and dependence. In L.N. Robins & D.A. Regier (Eds.), *Psychiatric Disorders in America* (pp. 116–154). New York: Free Press.

Anthony, J.C., Warner, L.A. & Kessler, R.C. (1994). Comparative epidemiology of dependence on tobacco, alcohol, controlled substances and inhalants: Basic findings from the National Comorbidity Study. *Clinical and Experimental Psychopharmacology, 2,* 244–268.

Arndt, S., Tyrrell, G., Flaum, M. & Andreasen, N.C. (1992). Comorbidity of substance abuse and schizophrenia: The role of premorbid adjustment. *Psychological Medicine, 22,* 379–388.

Bell, D. (1973). The experimental reproduction of amphetamine psychosis. *Archives of General Psychiatry, 29,* 35–40.

Bernardson, G. & Gunne, L.M. (1972). Forty-six cases of psychosis in cannabis abusers. *International Journal of Addictions, 7,* 9–16.

Bland, R.C., Newman, S.C. & Orn, H. (1987). Schizophrenia: Lifetime co-morbidity in a community sample. *Acta Psychiatrica Scandinavica, 75,* 383–391.

Breakey, W.R., Goodell, H., Lorenz, P.C. & McHugh, P.R. (1974). Hallucinogenic drugs as precipitants of schizophrenia. *Psychological Medicine, 4,* 255–261.

Brill, H. & Nahas, G.G. (1984). Cannabis intoxication and mental illness. In G.G. Nahas (Ed.), *Marihuana in Science and Medicine* (pp. 96–111). New York: Raven Press.

Carney, M.W.P., Bacelle, L. & Robinson, B. (1984). Psychosis after cannabis use. *British Medical Journal, 288,* 1047.

Carter, W.E., Coggins, W. & Doughty, P.L. (1980). *Cannabis in Costa Rica: A study of chronic marihuana use.* Philadelphia: Institute for the Study of Human Issues.

Chaudry, H.R., Moss, H.B., Bashir, A. & Suliman, T. (1991). Cannabis psychosis following bhang ingestion. *British Journal of Addiction, 86,* 1075–1081.

Chopra, G.S. & Smith, J.W. (1974). Psychotic reactions following cannabis use in East Indians. *Archives of General Psychiatry, 30,* 24–27.

Cleghorn, J.M., Kaplan, R.D., Szechtman, B., Szechtman, H., Brown, G.M. & Franco, S. (1991). Substance abuse and schizophrenia: Effect on symptoms but not on neurocognitive function. *Journal of Clinical Psychiatry, 52,* 26–30.

Cohen, S. (1982). Cannabis effects upon adolescent motivation. In *Marijuana and Youth: Clinical Observations on Motivation and Learning* (pp. 2–10). Rockville, MD: National Institute on Drug Abuse.

Cohen, S. & Johnson, K. (1988). Psychosis from alcohol or drug abuse. *British Medical Journal, 297,* 1270–1271.

Compton, D.R., Dewey, W.L. & Martin, B.R. (1990). Cannabis dependence and tolerance production. *Advances in Alcohol and Substance Abuse, 9,* 128–147.

Connell, P.H. (1959). *Amphetamine Psychosis* (Maudlsey Monograph No. 5, Institute of Psychiatry). London: Oxford University Press.

Cuffel, B.J., Heithoff, K.A. & Lawson, W. (1993). Correlates of patterns of substance abuse among patients with schizophrenia. *Hospital and Community Psychiatry, 44,* 247–251.

Der, G., Gupta, S. & Murray, R.M. (1990). Is schizophrenia disappearing? *Lancet, 1,* 513–516.

Didcott, P., Reilly, D., Swift, W. & Hall, W. (1997). *Long Term Cannabis Users on the New South Wales North Coast* (National Drug and Alcohol Research Centre Monograph No. 30). Sydney: National Drug and Alcohol Research Centre.

Dixon, L., Haas, G., Weiden, P.J., Sweeney, J. & Frances, A.J. (1990). Acute effects of drug abuse in schizophrenic patients: Clinical observations and patients' self-reports. *Schizophrenia Bulletin, 16*, 69–79.

Dornbush, R.L. (1974). The long-term effects of cannabis use. In L.L. Miller (Ed.), *Marijuana: Effects on Behavior* (pp.221–231). New York: Academic Press.

Drummond, L. (1986). Cannabis psychosis: A case report. *British Journal of Addiction, 81,* 139–140.

Edwards, G. (1976). Cannabis and the psychiatric position. In J.D.P. Graham (Ed.), *Cannabis and Health* (pp. 321–342). London: Academic Press.

Edwards, G. (1983). Psychopathology of a drug experience. *British Journal of Psychiatry, 143,* 509–512.

Edwards, G. & Gross, M.M. (1976). Alcohol dependence: Provisional description of a clinical syndrome. *British Medical Journal, 1,* 1058–1061.

Engstrom, A., Allebeck, P., Rodwall, Y. & Rydberg, U. (1985). Adverse psychic effects of cannabis — with special focus on Sweden. In D.J. Harvey, W. Paton & G. Nahas (Eds.), *Marihuana '84: Proceedings of the Oxford Symposium on Cannabis.* (pp. 593–604). Oxford: IRL Press.

European Monitoring Centre for Drugs and Drug Addiction. (1996). *1995 Annual Report on the State of the Drugs Problem in the European Union.* Lisbon: European Monitoring Centre for Drugs and Drug Addiction.

Fehr, K.O. & Kalant, H. (Eds.). (1983). *Cannabis and Health Hazards.* Toronto: Addiction Research Foundation.

Feinstein, A.R. (1985). *Clinical Epidemiology.* Philadelphia: W.B. Saunders.

Gawin, F.H. & Ellinwood, E.H. (1988). Cocaine and other stimulants: Actions, abuse and treatment. *New England Journal of Medicine, 318,* 1173–1182.

Georgotas, A. & Zeidenberg, P. (1979). Observations on the effects of four weeks of heavy marijuana smoking on group interaction and individual behavior. *Comprehensive Psychiatry, 20,* 427–432.

Ghodse, A.H. (1986). Cannabis psychosis. *British Journal of Addiction, 81,* 473–478.

Goldberg, L. (1968a). Drug abuse in Sweden. Part I. *Bulletin on Narcotics, 20* (1), 1–31.

Goldberg, L. (1968b). Drug abuse in Sweden. Part II. *Bulletin on Narcotics, 20* (2), 9–36.

Grinspoon, L. & Hedblom, P. (1975). *The Speed Culture: Amphetamine Abuse in America.* Cambridge, MA: Harvard University Press.

Gruber, A.J. & Pope, H.G. (1994). Cannabis psychotic disorder. Does it exist? *American Journal of the Addictions, 3*, 72–83.

Halikas, J.A., Goodwin, D.W. & Guze, S.B. (1971). Marihuana effects: A survey of regular users. *Journal of the American Medical Association, 217*, 692–694.

Halikas, J.A., Weller, R.A., Morse, C. & Shapiro, T. (1982). Incidence and characteristics of amotivational syndrome, including associated findings, among chronic marijuana users. In *Marijuana and Youth: Clinical Observations on Motivation and Learning* (pp. 11–26). Rockville, MD: National Institute on Drug Abuse.

Hambrecht, M. & Hafner, H. (1996). Substance abuse and the onset of schizophrenia. *Biological Psychiatry, 40*, 1155–1163.

Hendin, H., Haas, A.P., Singer, P., Eller, M. & Ulman, R. (1987). *Living High: Daily Marijuana Use Among Adults.* New York: Human Sciences Press.

Hollister, L.E. (1986). Health aspects of cannabis. *Pharmacological Reviews, 38*, 1–20.

Imade, A.G.T. & Ebie, J.C. (1991). A retrospective study of symptom patterns of cannabis-induced psychosis. *Acta Psychiatrica Scandinavica, 83*, 134–136.

Inghe, G. (1969). The present state of abuse and addiction to stimulant drugs in Sweden. In F. Sjoqvist & M. Tottie (Eds.), *Abuse of Central Stimulants* (pp. 187–214). New York: Raven Press.

Institute of Medicine. (1982). *Marijuana and Health.* Washington, DC: National Academy Press.

Jablensky, A., Sartorius, N., Ernberg, G., Anker, M., Korten, A., Cooper, J.E., Day, R. & Bertelsen, A. (1991). *Schizophrenia: Manifestations, Incidence and Course in Different Cultures. A World Health Organization Ten-Country Study* (Psychological Medicine Monograph Supplement No. 20). Geneva: World Health Organization.

Johnson, B.A., Smith, B.L. & Taylor, P. (1988). Cannabis and schizophrenia. *Lancet, 1*, 592–593.

Johnson, V. (1988). A longitudinal assessment of predominant patterns of drug use among adolescents and young adults. In G. Chesher, P. Consroe & R. Musty (Eds.), *Marijuana: An International Research Report* (pp. 173–182). Canberra: Australian Government Publishing Service.

Jones, R.T. (1984). Marijuana: Health and treatment issues. *Psychiatric Clinics of North America, 7*, 703–712.

Jones, R.T. & Benowitz, N. (1976). The 30-day trip — Clinical studies of cannabis tolerance and dependence. In M.C. Braude & S. Szara (Eds.), *Pharmacology of Marijuana* (Vol. 2, pp. 627–642). New York: Academic Press.

Jones, R.T., Benowitz, N. & Herning, R.I. (1981). The clinical relevance of cannabis tolerance and dependence. *Journal of Clinical Pharmacology, 21,* 143S–152S.

Kandel, D.B. & Davies, M. (1992). Progression to regular marijuana involvement: Phenomenology and risk factors for near daily use. In M. Glantz & R. Pickens (Eds.), *Vulnerability to Drug Abuse* (pp. 211–253). Washington, DC: American Psychological Association.

Kandel, D. & Faust, R. (1975). Sequence and stages in patterns of adolescent drug use. *Archives of General Psychiatry, 32,* 923–932.

Kavanagh, D.J. (1995). An intervention for substance abuse in schizophrenia. *Behaviour Change, 12,* 20–30.

Kessler, R.C., McGonagh, K.A., Zhao, S., Nelson, C.B., Hughes, M., Eshleman, S., Wittchen, U. & Kendler, K.S. (1994). Lifetime and 12-month prevalence of DSM-II-R psychiatric disorders in the United States. *Archives of General Psychiatry, 51,* 8–19.

Kolansky, H. & Moore, R.T. (1971). Effects of marihuana on adolescents and young adults. *Journal of the American Medical Association, 216,* 486–492.

Kosten, T.R., Rounsaville, B.J., Babor, T.F., Spitzer, R.L. & Williams, J.B.W. (1987). Substance-use disorders in DSM-III-R. *British Journal of Psychiatry, 151,* 834–843.

Kovasznay, B., Bromet, E., Schwartz, J.E., Ram, R., Lavelle, J. & Brandon, L. (1993). Substance abuse and onset of psychotic illness. *Hospital and Community Psychiatry, 44,* 567–571.

Knudsen, P. & Vilmar, T. (1984). Cannabis and neuroleptic agents in schizophrenia. *Acta Psychiatrica Scandinavica, 69,* 162–174.

Lewis, A. (1968). A review of the international clinical literature. In *Report of the Advisory Committee on Drug Dependence: Cannabis* (pp. 40–63). London: Her Majesty's Stationary Office.

Linszen, D.H., Dingemans, P.M. & Lenior, M.E. (1994). Cannabis abuse and the course of recent-onset schizophrenic disorders. *Archives of General Psychiatry, 51,* 273–279.

Machado, T. (1994). *Culture and Drug Use in Asian Settings: Research for Action.* Bangalore: St. John's Medical College.

Martinez-Arevalo, M.J., Calcedo-Ordonez, A. & Varo-Prieto, J.R. (1994). Cannabis consumption as a prognostic factor in schizophrenia. *British Journal of Psychiatry, 164,* 679–681.

Mathers, D.C., Ghodse, A.H., Caan, A.W. & Scott, S.A. (1991). Cannabis use in a large sample of acute psychiatric admissions. *British Journal of Addiction, 86,* 779–784.

McGlothin, W.H. & West, L.J. (1968). The marijuana problem: An overview. *American Journal of Psychiatry, 125,* 370–378.

McGuire, P., Jones, R., Harvey, I., Bebbington, P., Toone, B., Lewis, S. & Murray, R. (1994). Cannabis and acute psychosis. *Schizophrenia Research, 13,* 161–168.

McGuire, P., Jones, R., Harvey, I., Williams, M., McGuffin, P. & Murray, R. (1995). Morbid risk of schizophrenia for relatives of patients with cannabis associated psychosis. *Schizophrenia Research, 15,* 277–281.

Millman, R.B. & Sbriglio, R. (1986). Patterns of use and psychopathology in chronic marijuana users. *Psychiatric Clinics of North America, 9,* 533–545.

Moran, C. (1986). Depersonalisation and agoraphobia associated with marijuana use. *British Journal of Medical Psychology, 59,* 187–196.

Mueser, K.T., Bellack, A.S. & Blanchard, J.J. (1992). Comorbidity and substance abuse: Implications for treatment. *Journal of Consulting and Clinical Psychology, 60,* 845–856.

Mueser, K.T., Yarnold, P.R., Levinson, D.F., Singh, H., Bellack, A.S., Kee, K., Morrison, R.L. & Yadalam, K.G. (1990). Prevalence of substance abuse in schizophrenia: Demographic and clinical correlates. *Schizophrenia Bulletin, 16,* 31–56.

Negrete, J.C. (1983). Psychiatric aspects of cannabis use. In K.O. Fehr & H. Kalant (Eds.), *Cannabis and Health Hazards* (pp. 577–616). Toronto: Addiction Research Foundation.

Negrete, J.C. (1988). What's happened to the cannabis debate? *British Journal of Addiction, 83,* 359–372.

Negrete, J.C. (1989). Cannabis and schizophrenia. *British Journal of Addiction, 84,* 349–351.

Negrete, J.C., Knapp, W.P., Douglas, D. & Smith, W.B. (1986). Cannabis affects the severity of schizophrenic symptoms: Results of a clinical survey. *Psychological Medicine, 16,* 515–520.

Newcombe, M.D. (1992). Understanding the multidimensional nature of drug use and abuse: The role of consumption, risk factors and protective factors. In M. Glantz & R. Pickens (Eds.), *Vulnerability to Drug Abuse* (pp. 255–297). Washington, DC: American Psychological Association.

Onyango, R.S. (1986). Cannabis psychosis in young psychiatric inpatients. *British Journal of Addiction, 81,* 419–423.

Paes, M. (1986). Cannabis et psychopathologie. *Psychologie Médicale, 18,* 219–220.

Peralta, V. & Cuesta, M.J. (1992). Influence of cannabis abuse on schizophrenic psychopathology. *Acta Psychiatrica Scandinavica, 85,* 127–130.

Perkins, K.A., Simpson, J.C. & Tsuang, M.T. (1986). Ten-year follow-up of drug abusers with acute or chronic psychosis. *Hospital and Community Psychiatry, 37,* 481–484.

Poole, R. & Brabbins, C. (1996). Drug induced psychosis. *British Journal of Psychiatry, 168,* 135–138.

Robins, L.N. & Regier, D.A. (Eds.). (1991). *Psychiatric Disorders in America.* New York: Free Press.

Roffman, R.A., Stephens, R.S., Simpson, E.E. & Whitaker, D.L. (1988). Treatment of marijuana dependence: Preliminary results. *Journal of Psychoactive Drugs, 20,* 129–137.

Rolfe, M., Tang, C.M., Sabally, S., Todd, J.E., Sam, E.B. & Hatib N'Jie, A.B. (1993). Psychosis and cannabis abuse in Gambia: A case-control study. *British Journal of Psychiatry, 163,* 789–801.

Rottanburg, D., Robins, A.H., Ben-Arie, O., Teggin, A. & Elk, R. (1982). Cannabis-associated psychosis with hypomanic features. *Lancet, 2,* 1364–1366.

Rounsaville, B.J., Bryant, K., Babor, T., Kranzler, H. & Kadden, R. (1993). Cross-system agreement for substance use disorders. *Addiction, 88,* 337–348.

Rubin, V. & Comitas, L. (1975). *Ganja in Jamaica: A Medical Anthropological Study of Chronic Marihuana Use.* The Hague: Mouton.

Schneier, F.R. & Siris, S.G. (1987). A review of psychoactive substance use and abuse in schizophrenia: Patterns of drug choice. *Journal of Nervous and Mental Disorders, 175,* 641–652.

Smith, D.E. (1968). Acute and chronic toxicity of marijuana. *Journal of Psychedelic Drugs, 2,* 37–47.

Smith, J. & Hucker, S. (1994). Schizophrenia and substance abuse. *British Journal of Psychiatry, 165,* 13–21.

Stephens, R.S. & Roffman, R.A. (1993). Adult marijuana dependence. In J.S. Baer, G.A. Marlatt & R.J. MacMahon (Eds.), *Addictive Behaviors Across the Lifespan: Prevention, Treatment and Policy Issues* (pp. 202–218). Newbury Park, CA: Sage.

Swift, W., Hall, W. & Copeland, J. (1997). *Cannabis Dependence Among Long-term Users in Sydney, Australia* (NDARC Technical Report No. 47). Sydney: National Drug and Alcohol Research Centre.

Tennant, F.S. & Groesbeck, C.J. (1972). Psychiatric effects of hashish. *Archives of General Psychiatry, 27,* 133–136.

Thacore, V.R. & Shukla, S.R.P. (1976). Cannabis psychosis and paranoid schizophrenia. *Archives of General Psychiatry, 33,* 383–386.

Thomas, H. (1993). Psychiatric symptoms in cannabis users. *British Journal of Psychiatry, 163,* 141–149.

Thornicroft, G. (1990). Cannabis and psychosis: Is there epidemiological evidence for association. *British Journal of Psychiatry, 157,* 25–33.

Thornicroft, G., Meadows, G. & Politi, P. (1992). Is "cannabis psychosis" a distinct category? *European Psychiatry, 7,* 277–282.

Tien, A.Y. & Anthony, J.C. (1990). Epidemiological analysis of alcohol and drug use as risk factors for psychotic experiences. *Journal of Nervous and Mental Disease, 178,* 473–480.

Torres, M.L., Mattick, R.P., Chen, R. & Baillie, A. (1995). *Clients of Treatment Service Agencies: March 1995 Census Findings.* Canberra: Commonwealth Department of Human Services and Health.

Turner, W.M. & Tsuang, M.T. (1990). Impact of substance abuse on the course and outcome of schizophrenia. *Schizophrenia Bulletin, 16,* 87–95.

United States Office of National Drug Control Policy. (1994). *Pulse Check: National Trends in Drug Abuse, December 1994.* Washington, DC: Office of National Drug Control Policy.

United States Office of National Drug Control Policy. (1996). *Pulse Check: National Trends in Drug Abuse, December 1996.* Washington, DC: Office of National Drug Control Policy.

Weil, A. (1970). Adverse reactions to marihuana. *New England Journal of Medicine, 282,* 997–1000.

Weller, M.P.I., Ang, P.C., Latimer-Sayer, D.T. & Zachary, A. (1988). Drug abuse and mental illness. *Lancet, 1,* 977.

Weller, R.A. & Halikas, J. (1980). Objective criteria for the diagnosis of marijuana abuse. *Journal of Nervous and Mental Disease, 168,* 98–103.

Weller, R.A., Halikas, J. & Morse, C. (1984). Alcohol and marijuana: Comparison of use and abuse in regular marijuana users. *Journal of Clinical Psychiatry, 45,* 377–379.

Wells, J.E., Bushnell, J.A., Joyce, P.R., Oakley-Browne, M.A. & Hornblow, A.R. (1992). Problems with alcohol, drugs and gambling in Christchurch, New Zealand. In M. Abbot & K. Evans (Eds.), *Alcohol and Drug Dependence and Disorders of Impulse Control.* Auckland: Alcohol Liquor Advisory Council.

World Health Organization (WHO) (1992). *ICD-10 Classification of Mental and Behavioral Disorders: Clinical Descriptions and Diagnostic Guidelines.* Geneva: World Health Organization.

Woody, G.E., Cottler, L.B. & Caciola, J. (1993). Severity of dependence: Data from the DSM-IV field trials. *Addiction, 88,* 1573–1579.

Zisook, S., Heaton, R., Moranville, J., Kuck, J., Jernigan, T. & Braff, D. (1992). Past substance abuse and clinical course of schizophrenia. *American Journal of Psychiatry, 149,* 552–553.

Effects of Marijuana on Cell Nuclei: A Review of the Literature Relating to the Genotoxicity of Cannabis

Effects of Marijuana on Cell Nuclei: A Review of the Literature Relating to the Genotoxicity of Cannabis

DONALD G. MacPHEE

Cannabis and the cannabinoids are often said to have mutagenic and carcinogenic effects and to impair the biosynthesis of nucleic acids and proteins (see, for example, Jones, 1983). In displaying some or all of these toxicological properties, they do, however, resemble a great many innocuous plants, plant extracts and plant constituents, as well as a great many other natural compounds to which humans are regularly exposed. This latter point does not appear to be widely appreciated, perhaps because of the mistaken belief that chemicals or mixtures of chemicals with mutagenic and/or carcinogenic properties are rare among the vast numbers of chemicals in our natural environment. That such properties are not at all rare should be evident from the growing literature on the naturally occurring mutagens, carcinogens and otherwise harmful chemical substances that can be found in abundance in plants and other human and animal foods (Ames, 1983). This relatively recent knowledge should be borne in mind when making judgments about the older literature on the potentially harmful effects of cannabis and the cannabinoids in humans.

The term *cannabis* is usually applied to a crude material obtained from the plant *Cannabis sativa,* a plant that may well contain more than 400 chemicals, most of which are common to many plants. Only some 61 of the so-called cannabinoids appear to be specific to cannabis (see Dewey, 1986; Martin, 1986). Observations that cannabis and the cannabinoids possess some obvious harmful properties, including mutagenicity and potential carcinogenicity, are not unique, since other plant materials are known to share some of these properties.

Most drug use of cannabis involves smoking, and the inhaled constituents share many of the characteristics (and in many cases probably also the identity) of the constituents of tobacco smoke. Given the large numbers of constituents of both cigarette and marijuana smoke (both raw and arising from pyrolysis) that may have to be considered when assessing their final biological and toxicological effectiveness, it would be unwise to focus too much attention on the *in vitro* or *in vivo* toxicological properties of those few native constituents that possess other significant pharmacological activities (e.g., psychoactivity). Even if the principal psychoactive ingredient in marijuana ($\emptyset$-tetrahydrocannabinol or THC) eventually proves to be a potent mutagen and carcinogen — and most of the available evidence suggests that this is probably not the case — it may still be a mistake to focus too much attention upon quantifying the contribution which this particular chemical species could make to the adverse biological effects which can be associated with the regular inhalation of cannabis smoke as such.

A great deal of evidence collected over the years indicates that cannabis — and perhaps also one or more of the 61 or so of the cannabis-specific ingredients or "cannabinoids" that it contains — is capable of exerting significant effects on cellular organisms, most probably by interacting with the cell nucleus. The information obtained in many of these studies has been reviewed on several previous occasions and is dealt with under the following headings: effects on macromolecular synthesis, chromosomal aberrations, mutagenicity and carcinogenicity.

Effects on Macromolecular Synthesis

Most reviews of the potentially harmful effects of marijuana point out (1) that cannabinoids can interfere with the normal cell cycle (as shown, for example, in experiments in which the protozoan *Tetrahymena* was exposed to increasing doses of THC by Zimmerman & McClean in 1973); and (2) that cannabinoids can decrease synthesis of DNA, RNA and protein (as shown by Blevins & Regan in 1976). Such effects may be tissue-specific. For example, Paria et al. (1994) reported that injection of THC into ovariectomized or hypophysectomized mice at a dose of 5 or 10 mg/kg daily for seven days caused an increase in uterine wet weight and in incorporation of ^{3}H-thymidine into the nuclei of the total uterus. In contrast, Morgan et al. (1988) found that daily administration of THC to pregnant rats in a dose of 50 mg/kg (by gavage) from day 2 to day 22 of gestation did not affect DNA or RNA in the brains of the offspring, but reduced brain protein levels at postnatal days 7 and 14; the effect had disappeared by day 21. It will be of

interest to see how such differences between tissues correlate with the differences in cannabinoid receptor types and densities in the various tissues.

Hollister (1986) neatly summarized the significance of these and comparable findings when he commented that "on the one hand, exposure to smoke from cannabis may be carcinogenic. On the other, the changes in nucleic acid synthesis, were they to be specific for rapidly dividing cells, such as malignancies, might be useful therapeutically in their treatment" (p. 5). More recently, Tahir and Zimmerman (1992) have shown that THC (and to a lesser extent cannabidiol and cannabinol) can disrupt the formation of microtubules and microfilaments in rat cells in culture and hence may interfere with such diverse cellular processes as cell division, cell migration and neuron differentiation. It is possible that such properties may be of just as much value in treatment as they are usually assumed to be in pathology.

Effects on Gene Expression

Many compounds that have mutagenic and carcinogenic effects do so because they (or in some cases their metabolites) react directly with DNA in the cells in which they exert their effects. Other compounds may influence the processes leading to carcinogenesis (and probably also to mutagenesis) in other ways; some may do so without having any direct effect on DNA molecules. These include some compounds that are frequently referred to as *cancer promoters* (or perhaps tumor promoters), as well as some that are better termed *co-carcinogens,* and still others that may be termed *anti-carcinogens.* Although there may well be just as many mechanisms as there are compounds displaying pro- or anticancer activities, one mechanism by which some of them at least might be expected to operate is that often referred to simply as "modulation of gene expression."

Modulation of gene expression can be expected to result in a wide variety of cellular effects — some beneficial, others quite detrimental — in addition to those mentioned above as influencing mutation and cancer rates. Accordingly, evidence that a compound is capable of switching genes on and off (or up and down) is of considerable interest, not only to the general toxicologist, but also to the genetic toxicologist. Indeed, modulation of gene expression is a research field that is likely to be of growing interest to genetic toxicologists as more and more evidence becomes available in support of the view that epimutagenesis —involving non-mutational but heritable changes in methylation patterns, for example — may have an important part to play in the causation of certain forms of cancer.

One interesting recent study that appears to indicate a role for THC in regulating gene expression is that of Mailleux et al. (1994), in which a macroscopic quantitative *in situ* hybridization method was used to demonstrate that there was a significant increase in expression of the gene coding for the growth factor pleiotropin in cells of the adult rat forebrain after a single intraperitoneal injection of THC (5 mg/kg). The particular gene involved in this study is of interest, given that THC is primarily known for its psychoactive properties and since the authors' claim that theirs is the first report of THC regulation of growth factor gene expression in the brain must be taken seriously. It is hoped that further studies of the mechanisms underlying enhanced expression of other genes in the presence of THC will eventually provide useful information about the non-psychoactive effects of this particular compound on both cellular and organismal biology.

Chromosomal Aberrations

The results discussed in the previous section relate mainly to studies in which the investigators were primarily motivated by an interest in modes of action of drugs or druglike compounds, or else of effects on general physiological mechanisms of one sort or another. The test agents were usually therefore pure or near-pure cannabinoid compounds. In the experiments discussed in the next two sections, by contrast,

there is no such consistency of findings. This is to be expected since most human exposure to cannabis occurs by smoke inhalation; we need to know the outcomes of real-life exposure situations to assess the nature and extent of the health risks involved in marijuana use.

Direct analogies with the health risks of cigarette smoking are frequently used in discussions of the marijuana issue. In these discussions, the most important similarities are those that arise when we conduct toxicological assessments of substances to which people are primarily exposed by the inhalation route. Cigarette tobacco smoke, cigarette smoke condensates and cigarette tobacco extracts, and their marijuana equivalents, are all very complex and highly variable mixtures consisting of many hundreds of compounds (some identified, many not); such ill-defined mixtures give different results at different times and in different hands. This problem is apparent when test materials are prepared in different ways with different batches of material from different sources in which the THC or nicotine content may differ by quite substantial amounts (for example, from 1 to 8 per cent for THC). Given that there is such variability in levels of known ingredients and that there are so many unquantified *known* ingredients (let alone unquantified *unknown* ingredients), the results of even the simplest biological assays will sometimes appear positive and sometimes negative. Moreover, biological assays of complex mixtures may occasionally give negative results, not because there is too little of a particular substance in the mixture, but because there is too much. To take an extreme example, batches of cigarette tobacco that are heavily contaminated with a toxic metal, mercury or cadmium for example, or some other highly cytotoxic but not genotoxic chemical can be virtually guaranteed to give negative results in assays for genetic damage of any kind (primarily because there may be too few viable cells remaining to manifest the symptoms of genetic toxicity).

The results of genotoxicity tests conducted with individual components of complex mixtures should not be affected by as many variables as are tests with the mixtures as a whole. Even so, there may be difficulties in interpretation if some key principles relating to dose-response relationships are overlooked. For example, some chromosome-damaging effects can only ever be detected at very high dose levels of the test compound, and may not therefore predict heritable genetic effects with any certainty — if only because their effects are normally accompanied by cell death. In the context of more general genotoxicology testing, this key reservation reflects the fact that dead cells simply don't transmit their chromosome defects to *any* kind of progeny, mutant or otherwise.

Thus, not all clastogens (i.e., agents capable of breaking or otherwise seriously damaging chromosomes) are also mutagenic, since this by definition requires them to be capable of also causing heritable genetic changes to the exposed cells at doses that are fully compatible with cell survival. Therefore, even if a test chemical is already known to cause chromosome breaks and/or aberrations at high doses, it is still necessary to acquire reproducible data on its ability or lack of ability to cause heritable mutations (usually point mutations) before determining its genotoxicity profile. With this background, it is interesting to note that most reports that refer to the potential adverse biological effects of marijuana and its constituents do so on the basis of results obtained in chromosome studies. Although such studies have to be taken seriously, they might have contributed more confusion than enlightenment about the *genetic* hazards of cannabis smoking.

For example, in one much-cited paper, Henrich et al. (1980) described some attempts to assess the effects of cannabinoids on chromosome numbers in cultured human lymphocytes as a way of evaluating their supposed ability to produce chromosomal segregation errors. THC caused a statistically significant increase in chromosomal segregation errors, whereas cannabinol and cannabidiol did not. Among the wide range of chromosome changes observed, only anaphase lags and unequal segregations in bipolar divisions reached statistical significance. It was concluded that THC affects the formation of microtubules

and spindles and, hence, could be considered a mitotic poison. Thus, Henrich et al.'s results were said to complement the earlier findings of cells with increased or decreased DNA contents in experiments involving exposure of human lung explants to marijuana smoke (Leuchtenberger, Leuchtenberger et al., 1973a). Henrich and colleagues did observe intrachromosomal abnormalities (anaphase and telophase bridge formations) in the course of their own study, but these failed to reach statistical significance and so did not add greatly to earlier literature reports. Their own equivocal results were not inconsistent with an earlier ambivalent literature in which some workers (e.g., Gilmour, Bloom et al., 1971 and Stenchever, Kunysz & Allen, 1974) had observed increased incidences of chromosomal breaks in the lymphocytes of marijuana smokers, whereas others had not (Matsuyama, Yen et al., 1977; Morishima, Henrich et al., 1979; Nichols, Miller et al., 1974). Negative results were also obtained following *in vitro* exposure of cells to cannabis resin, crude cannabis extract and THC (Martin, Thorburn & Bryant, 1973; Neu, Powers et al., 1970; Stenchever, Parks & Stenchever, 1976).

By about 1990, Zimmerman and Zimmerman were able to conclude that the cannabinoids induced chromosome aberrations in both *in vivo* and *in vitro* studies, and that the aberrations involved included chromosomal breaks, deletions, translocations, errors in chromosomal separation and hyperploidy. They also pointed out that the lesions involved could be due to the clastogenic action of cannabinoids or to cannabinoid-induced disruption of mitotic events, or to both. On the basis of these later reports, Zimmerman and Zimmerman (1990–91) concluded that the conflicting reports in the earlier literature could probably be attributed to differences in experimental protocols, cell types or animals used.

Chiesara et al. (1983) appear to have been the first to report a significant clastogenic effect of cannabis in humans. They noted increased chromosome aberration levels in both heroin and marijuana addicts. However, a more recent comprehensive study by Piatti et al. (1989) failed to find increases in either chromosome aberrations or micronuclei in a group of young soldiers whose only form of drug abuse appeared to involve marijuana.

In the meantime, studies of sister chromatid exchanges (SCE) have also yielded positive results with marijuana. Vassiliades et al. (1986) studied the SCE levels in a group of 14 cannabis users and 14 controls, and found that the mean number of SCEs per cell was significantly higher in users (11.99, *sic*) than in controls (9.31, *sic*). Noting that Chiesara et al. (1983) had previously found an increased risk of chromosome damage in marijuana users, Vassiliades et al. suggested that their combined results indicated that the cells of cannabis and heroin users had a reduced capacity for repair of DNA damaged by various environmental factors. They hypothesized that this reduced capacity for repair might allow the fixation or retention of a greater fraction of lesions caused by normal environmental exposures, in which case the observed effects of cannabis usage on SCE formation would be attributable to indirect damage to DNA repair systems rather than direct damage to DNA molecules.

More recently, however, Jorgensen et al. (1991) described the results of a study of sister-chromatid exchanges in 22 tobacco smokers and 22 tobacco-plus-cannabis smokers. They found that while tobacco smokers had enhanced SCE levels by comparison with non-smokers, those who smoked cannabis and tobacco did not have SCE levels that were higher than those of tobacco smokers only. Their conclusion was that cannabis smoking *per se* was not genotoxic. More recently still, Behnke and Eyler (1993) briefly reviewed the literature on prenatal exposure of animals to marijuana. While conceding that "reports in the literature still seem controversial," they concluded that cannabinoids produce mitotic disruption in rodents and are weakly clastogenic as well. They were nevertheless uncertain as to whether or not these "changes can produce stable alterations in chromosomes that can be passed on to offspring" (p. 1354). Their overall conclusion was, however: "Although study designs have varied widely, the preponderance of

data on prenatal marijuana use supports an increased risk of chromosome abnormalities, poor pregnancy outcome, and long-term effects on exposed offspring" (p. 1355). It is not easy to reconcile these conclusions of Behnke and Eyler with one another, let alone with the fundamentally negative conclusions reached by Jorgensen et al. following their assessment of what must have been essentially the same literature.

Mutagenicity

In this section, heritable changes associated with marijuana usage are of primary interest, so that the available data on point mutations (whose transmissibility is seldom in doubt) will be of particular significance.

Complex Mixtures

Following a thorough review of the literature on the genetic effects of marijuana, Zimmerman and Zimmerman (1990–91) concluded: "In general these studies show that the cannabinoids are detrimental to the health of an individual" (p. 19).

In commenting to this effect, they noted that although there was broad agreement in the literature that cannabinoids can indeed cause chromosome abnormalities (which they described as "mutagenicity in the broad sense"), there was no consensus as to whether or not cannabinoids could induce heritable point mutations (a property which they termed "mutagenicity in a narrow sense"). It would appear from their (presumably careful) choice of words that the Zimmermans were not convinced by the evidence then available that the use or abuse of materials containing cannabinoids represented a convincing threat to the health of the offspring of users (as opposed to the health of individual users themselves).

Certainly the quality and consistency of the evidence relating to the potential effects of cannabinoids on the genetic material of living organisms was difficult to assess at the time the

Zimmermans were writing (1990–91), and indeed it is not much easier at the present time. The headings for the Zimmermans' review — mutagenic studies, cytogenetic analysis of germinal cells, and cytogenetic analysis of somatic cells — were clearly chosen for convenience in dealing with the available marijuana literature rather than to reflect a particular classification system for environmental genotoxins that was then in use.

More conventional classifications assume that the most important end-point to assess is the one referred to by geneticists simply as mutagenicity. Analysis of this property of mutagenicity *(sensu stricto)* requires an assessment of the potential of a test compound or compounds to cause heritable genetic damage in the organism of interest. A secondary but important consideration might involve assessing the potential of the same test material(s) to initiate tumors in appropriate tissues and in appropriate circumstances. Evidence that a test compound can inflict cytogenetic damage on somatic or germinal cells alike would be regarded primarily as providing supporting evidence for that compound to have mutagenic potential, *but would not in itself be regarded as conclusive.* As noted above, this is because not all of the cellular damage that is reflected in a cytogenetically demonstrable outcome will end up being inherited by progeny cells or organisms. Many of the grossest lesions — and those that are among the most immediately obvious — will terminate along with the cells in which they were first observed. Thus, evidence that a compound can produce chromosome damage in a given cell type is usually taken simply as evidence that the compound can reach and interact with the genetic material of cells of that type; it does not provide *prima facie* evidence of a capacity to generate heritable mutations, or of a potential to cause cancers by a mutation-driven mechanism.

Having made this point, there can be little doubt that both cannabis use (as judged by findings in cannabis users or animals exposed to marijuana smoke) and exposures to certain constituents of whole cannabis preparations (or in some cases cannabis smoke condensates) can produce genuinely mutagenic effects when judged by the more reliable end-points for assessing this important property. These exposures probably also have the potential to be carcinogenic as well as clastogenic, and therefore ought to be capable of causing visible cytogenetic effects in a wide range of experimental organisms. It should be emphasized that a similar claim cannot be made for "pure" cannabis or the cannabinoids *per se,* at the present time.

The results that lead to this conclusion, although individually somewhat variable in quality, are nevertheless quite convincing when taken as a whole. For example, Busch et al. (1979), Seid and Wei (1979), Wehner et al. (1980) and Sparacino et al. (1990) have all reported obtaining positive results with either cannabis extracts or smoke condensates in the Ames assay for mutagenicity. In passing, it should be noted that the Ames assay for mutagenicity, often described as "only" a bacterial assay, is widely acknowledged by practising genetic toxicologists as one of the most reliable and cost-effective ways of distinguishing truly genetically active chemicals (mutagens) from their genetically inactive counterparts (i.e., non-mutagens, a class that includes some well-known toxic compounds that are often wrongly assumed to be mutagenic).

In addition, Leuchtenberger et al. (1973b) found that cultured human lung cells exposed to marijuana smoke showed alterations in DNA content and aneuploidy (changes in chromosome number), while Morishima et al. (1979) reported finding cells with reduced chromosome numbers among cultured lymphocytes from both heavy and light marijuana smokers. Errors in chromosome segregation were also observed under a controlled marijuana treatment regime devised by Morishima et al. (1979). Moreover, the papers by Gilmour et al. (1971), Stenchever et al. (1974) and Chiesara et al. (1983) were concerned with the increased frequencies of chromosome abnormalities that can be shown to occur in cultured lymphocytes obtained from marijuana users.

Given the many resemblances between these mutagen-containing, marijuana-derived materials and comparable tobacco preparations, it is no surprise that cannabis and cannabis extracts have been shown to be carcinogenic to rodents in both skin-painting and inhalation studies (Hoffmann, Brunnemann et al., 1975; Rosenkrantz & Fleischman, 1979). To what extent do the results obtained with the cannabis preparations reflect their similarity to tobacco products, and to what extent are they a manifestation of cannabinoid pharmacology and toxicology? The literature to date presents very few results of carcinogenicity tests on individual cannabinoids such as THC (studies on the individual constituents of marijuana smoke such as the aromatic amines and polycyclic aromatic hydrocarbons are available, however — for details see Maskarinec, Alexander & Novotny, 1976; Merli, Wiester et al., 1981; Novotny, Kump et al., 1980). This point is discussed further below.

Studies with THC, Cannabis or Cannabinoids

In contrast to the findings for crude extracts of cannabis or cannabis smoke condensates, pure THC as such has given entirely negative results in well-conducted Ames-type Salmonella assays (Legator, Weber et al., 1976; Zimmerman, Stich & San, 1978). In view of this, it is interesting that a great many studies of the effects of cannabis preparations on chromosomes in intact animals, including some of the positive ones, have involved pure or relatively pure THC or other cannabinoids. The results of such studies should be viewed with considerable caution, and few observers who are familiar with the cytogenetic analysis of potentially hazardous chemicals will be surprised to find that they are far from uniform. As argued above, this is to be expected given the variety of test materials, test animals and application conditions and the difficulties of interpreting the results of many different types of test protocols.

Among the more recent findings in this area are the results of testing THC and certain other cannabinoids for their capacity to produce micronuclei (positive: Zimmerman & Raj, 1980; negative: Legator, Weber et al., 1976), chromosome

aberrations (positive: Zimmerman & Raj, 1980), sperm chromosome abnormalities (positive: Dalterio, Badr et al., 1982; negative: Zimmerman, Murer-Orlando & Richer, 1986, in a study that included C-banding), or dominant lethal mutations as judged by relative numbers of non-viable embryonic implants following treatment of male mice (positive: Dalterio, Badr et al., 1982; negative: Berryman, Anderson et al., 1992; Generoso, Cain et al., 1985; Legator, Weber et al., 1976).

The investigators who reported positive findings in the mouse dominant lethal assay (Dalterio, Badr et al., 1982) also reported finding a significantly increased frequency of heritable translocations among the offspring they were studying. Their study was a very small one, however, involving cytogenetic analysis of only eight progeny, and the original data were not presented in sufficient detail to allow an independent re-evaluation to be carried out. Very little significance should be attached to the findings of this study. A follow-up study conducted by Generoso et al. (1985), in which some 498 male progeny were examined, failed to find any evidence of heritable translocations. This is clearly the definitive study to date, the subsequent and largely confirmatory findings by Berryman et al. (1992) notwithstanding.

THC has also been administered to human subjects under controlled conditions and tested for its ability to induce chromosome abnormalities in cultured lymphocytes (Nichols, Miller et al., 1974). The results were entirely negative, but the study design has been criticized by Legator and Au (1987) and by Zimmerman and Zimmerman (1990–91) on a number of grounds. Among these was the important one that the lymphocytes that were collected before, during and after the study might well all have been exposed to appreciable amounts of the relevant drugs, in which case it would have been unrealistic to expect to see significant differences in their aberration frequencies. In addition, administration of marijuana or hashish extracts (by Nichols et al. in the 1974 study), or of marijuana by inhalation for 28 days by Matsuyama et al. (1977), also failed to produce abnormalities in the cultured human lymphocytes of volunteers. This means that very little significance can be attached to the findings reported in similarly designed studies with (presumably pure) THC. In a short note, Piatti et al. (1989) reported that they too were unable to detect increases in either chromosome aberrations or micronuclei in a study of young soldiers who abused marijuana, although they were able to detect such increases in soldiers who abused either heroin or heroin-plus-marijuana.

One other recent study that contains useful information about the potential mutagenicity of THC was conducted by Berryman et al. (1992). This study primarily measured co-mutagenicity, using either ethanol or THC in combination with the well-studied alkylating mutagen Trenimon™. It necessarily involved studying the rate of induction of dominant lethal mutations in mice by THC alone. These data indicated that THC alone had no effect on either pre-implantation loss or fetal mortality, or on the resulting mutation index. It was also established that THC was most unlikely to act in a co-mutagenic manner with either ethanol or Trenimon. The authors themselves seemed reluctant to conclude that their negative findings in well-conducted mouse dominant lethal assays ruled out possible mutagenic effects of cannabinoid exposure, even though they were able to demonstrate the mutagenicity of both controls (ethanol and Trenimon) under precisely the same experimental conditions. Their (negative) data was of a substantially higher quality than the earlier (positive) data that had been thoroughly overinterpreted by Dalterio et al. (1982). Inexplicably, however, Berryman et al. (1992) omitted to mention two other studies that had recorded negative findings with cannabinoids in mouse dominant lethal assays, namely, those by Legator et al. (1976) and Generoso et al. (1985). Given the variable quality of the four studies conducted to date, it is the negative one conducted by Generoso et al. that appears to be the most comprehensive — and therefore reliable — study of the *in vivo* mutagenicity of cannabinoids currently available for assessment.

Systematic Study of the Chemistry and Mutagenicity of Marijuana Smoke Condensate

Sparacino et al. (1990) have reported finding significant mutagenic activity in fractions prepared by extracting marijuana smoke condensates. Their study appears to differ from the others in that it was part of a systematic attempt to analyse the biologically active fractions of marijuana smoke condensates in some considerable depth. The findings released in their 1990 paper all appear to have been preliminary. They used bioassays (Ames-type Salmonella assays for mutagenicity) to determine which of several fractionation procedures led to a selective enrichment of mutagenic activity in their test materials. They commented, for example, that "the marijuana high-doses base fraction was sevenfold more mutagenic than either the tobacco or low-dose marijuana base-fraction," while "the more polar subfractions of the base fraction were more mutagenic than the less polar subfractions" (p. 138). In addition, they identified approximately 200 compounds by mass spectrometry, of which about half were amines and half of these again were aromatic amines; some alkylated pyrazoles and pyrazines were detected in very large amounts, as was an alkylated benzimidazole. (Some THC derivatives were also detected.) In concluding, they pointed out that the majority of the compounds that they identified had not yet been tested for mutagenicity. Data derived from testing these additional compounds may prove to be of great value in assessing the hazards of both tobacco and marijuana smoke.

Carcinogenicity

The fact that so many studies of the potential mutagenicity of cannabis and THC have been carried out may reflect the long-established and now widely accepted relationship between mutagenicity and carcinogenicity. Although some have downplayed the significance of this relationship in recent years, there is now no doubt that cancer is usually a mutational phenomenon. Indeed, in many cases, the precise base-pair changes involved in activating oncogenes or inactivating tumor suppressor genes have been identified in the DNA sequences of the genes concerned. The repeated findings of mutagenic activity in cannabis extracts and condensates (findings that almost certainly do not relate directly to their THC content) may well have important implications for human cancer and human mutagenicity.

The mutagenic compounds so far identified in marijuana smoke are most unlikely to contribute to respiratory cancer without also contributing in some way to various other forms of cancer. These mutagens appear to resemble closely those associated with tobacco smoke, in general properties and in amounts. It is reasonable to assume that they will be distributed via the bloodstream to many other organs (but see below). Thus we may eventually find associations between marijuana and cancers of the bladder, esophagus, mouth and tongue, and perhaps of the blood-forming cells in the bone marrow, but these will only become apparent if sufficient care is taken in the design of future studies.

As with cigarette tobacco smoking, our greatest concerns about the carcinogenicity of marijuana smoking have focused on the respiratory system, because the epithelial cells lining the organs of this system are assumed to be most exposed to the constituent chemicals of the smoke ingredients/smoke condensates. It should be remembered, however, that many of the most potentially troublesome chemicals present in tobacco and marijuana smoke are not themselves mutagenic or carcinogenic, but rather are pro-mutagens (or pro-carcinogens) requiring activation by mammalian metabolic enzymes to convert them to their biologically active forms. Since the metabolic processes involved in these particular transformations are usually functions of the liver, questions about which cell types are maximally exposed to the "ultimate" chemical mutagens are not as straightforward as they might first seem. However, drug-metabolizing enzymes of the cytochrome P450 family are also present in substantial amounts in pulmonary macrophages and are believed to play an important role in the activation of pulmonary carcinogens (Rauno, Pasanen et al., 1995; Wheeler & Guenthner, 1991).

One further point to be made is that marijuana smoke, like other combustion products (including tobacco smoke), is a lung irritant. In addition to containing mutagenic carcinogens, therefore, marijuana smoke may play a second and important role in the pathogenesis of human cancer, as a promoter. Several authors have suggested that cigarette smoking contributes to lung cancer by being both an initiator and a promoter because it has an irritant effect and therefore a mitogenic effect. Cigarette smokers who give up smoking reduce their risk of subsequently contracting lung cancer, in part at least because they are no longer exposed to the same degree of potentially mitogenic irritation. It is reasonable to assume that marijuana smoking may have a similar natural history. One possible implication of this suggestion is that former smokers of tobacco cigarettes who nevertheless continue to smoke marijuana may not enjoy the benefit of the reduced lung cancer risk. It will not be easy to mount an epidemiological study to test this suggestion, however.

Cancer Studies: Smoke and Other Complex Mixtures

In recent years, three case-control studies involving cancer patients have been undertaken, and all three have suggested at an association between prenatal cannabis use by mothers-to-be and certain rare cancers in their children. There are also many reports in the cannabis literature of drug-induced cellular changes in the respiratory systems of both humans and animals, of a sort that may be related to the onset or enhancement of tumors. Often these are referred to as precancerous alterations, or sometimes precancerous lesions (for example, see reports by Rosenkrantz & Fleischman, 1979; Tennant, 1980; and especially the summary in Table 2 of Leuchtenberger's 1982 review). Nevertheless, there are no confirmed reports of cancer induction in animals or positive epidemiological findings in humans.

Several physicians have reported on case-series of oropharyngeal cancers; the impact of these reports will largely depend on one's own assessment of the evidential value of some generally very sketchy reports (see "Cancers of the Respiratory System" for further discussion). However, there is at least one report in the early literature (Hoffmann, Brunnemann et al., 1975) of tumor formation in animals following skin-painting with cannabis smoke condensate, which desperately needs to be confirmed and then followed up by tests with extracts and fractions.

CHILDHOOD CANCERS

The first of the three case-control studies referred to above was that conducted by Robison et al. in 1988. This study involved telephone interviews with the parents of cases and appropriately selected control children, and it led the authors to suggest that there was an elevenfold increase in the risk of childhood non-lymphoblastic leukemia following maternal use of "mind-altering drugs" just prior to or during an index pregnancy. However, the actual percentages of drug-exposed mothers in this case-control study were only 5.0 per cent for leukemia cases and 0.5 per cent for the controls; these figures stand in marked contrast to those obtained in an earlier study of marijuana use during pregnancy in which it was noted that some 10 per cent of new mothers were prepared to admit to marijuana use during pregnancy if they were interviewed in person shortly after they had given birth (Linn, Schoenbaum et al., 1983).

In 1990, Kuijten et al. described findings in a case-control study of astrocytoma that included the observation that there was non-significant association between marijuana use during pregnancy and risk of this rare tumor in children (OR = 2.8, p = 0.07). More recently still, Grufferman et al. (1993) reported that there seemed to be an increased risk of the rare and highly malignant tumor of mesenchymal origin known as rhabdomyosarcoma in children whose parents used cocaine and marijuana. This was also a case-control study that depended on telephone interviews, and the key findings for "marijuana use" involved a threefold increase in risk with maternal use and a twofold increase with paternal use. However, no dose-response data was sought for any drug, and it proved impossible to determine whether marijuana and cocaine had independent effects since use of these two drugs was correlated. (This finding makes the complete absence of any record of cocaine use in the two earlier studies somewhat puzzling.) It may be worth noting that Kuijten et al. recorded a "strong, *but non-significant,* association with allergy shots" with an OR of 7.1 (p. 220, Grufferman, Schwartz et al., 1993).

More importantly, though, the possibility that many of the parents of cases (but not controls) might have had to undergo face-to-face interviews (which almost certainly would have included questions about their drug habits) at or around the time of their child's cancer diagnosis does not appear to have been taken into account in any of the case-control studies, even though such interviews could have had a profound influence on the telephone interviews of these parents. Future studies might well be designed to take such potential bias into account. Parents who have already answered "yes" to questions about drug use in face-to-face interviews may be less likely to give false-negative answers in later telephone interviews than parents who have never been confronted with such questions about their pregnancies. Parents of cases could not have known what records of earlier interviews might have been available to their telephone interviewers, for example.

It is also worth noting that none of the above studies was supported by the data on the changing incidences of the childhood cancers under investigation. If marijuana use is a significant factor in the etiology of some rare childhood cancers, one would expect to see the growing use of marijuana by young people in certain communities in the late 20th century reflected in the incidences of the relevant tumors among their children. Data on this point should not be difficult to obtain and should be relatively easy to analyse since many of the tumor types in question were formerly rather rare.

Chapter 8

CANCERS OF THE RESPIRATORY SYSTEM

In addition to these three studies of childhood cancer, there are a number of case reports in the medical literature to suggest that marijuana may be causal in cancers of the respiratory tract in exposed humans. For example, Taylor (1988) reported on 10 cases of respiratory tract carcinoma appearing before the age of 40 years, in contrast to the usual age of 60 to 70 years for such cancers; 5 of the 10 were heavy smokers of marijuana and 2 others were regular smokers. Similarly, Sridhar et al. (1994) compared 13 cases of lung cancer appearing before the age of 45 years with 97 cases in which the cancer appeared after the age of 45. Only 6 per cent of the older group had ever smoked cannabis, whereas all of the younger cases had, and all but one were current users of tobacco as well as marijuana. Both Taylor and Sridhar et al. suggested that cannabis use, especially in conjunction with tobacco, might be responsible for the early appearance of these cancers. In 1993 aWengen reported that some 34 young patients with squamous cell carcinomas of the oral cavity, tongue and pharynx, all of whom were chronic marijuana smokers, had been treated at the University of California Davis Medical Center, Sacramento, in the preceding seven years; aWengen suggested that these cancers were rapidly increasing among 20- to 40-year-olds. Several other case studies involving smaller numbers of patients were cited by Nahas and Latour (1992) in support of their claim that cancers of the mouth, jaw, tongue and lung due to marijuana smoking were "now being reported" in 19- to 30-year-olds. Nahas and Latour's use of the data from these case studies was heavily criticized by Christie and Chesher (1994) in a follow-up letter to the *Medical Journal of Australia.* Although there appears to be some limited (but suggestive) evidence that marijuana smoking may be important in the etiology of some forms of cancer, full-scale epidemiological studies in which great care is taken to deal with confounding variables have not been conducted, despite the fact that there are probably tens (perhaps hundreds) of millions of marijuana users around the world.

One experimental study that may have relevance to the potential carcinogenicity of smoking marijuana was recently conducted by Talaska et al. (1992). This study involved the measurement of carcinogen-DNA adducts in the lungs of monkeys exposed chronically to marijuana smoke. To obtain the necessary data, rhesus monkeys were exposed to marijuana smoke for either two days or seven days per week, or to ethanol-extracted marijuana smoke for seven days per week, or to a sham treatment for one year and then sacrificed seven months after the last exposure. The levels of carcinogen-DNA adducts in the lungs of the animals were then determined. Although the daily exposures in the study resulted in serum THC levels equivalent to those seen in human volunteers who smoke four to five marijuana cigarettes per day, the levels of aromatic carcinogen-DNA adducts in the lungs of animals exposed to marijuana smoke appeared to be no higher than those observed in untreated animals.

There were some indications in the data that the smoke from ethanol-extracted marijuana (which is essentially devoid of THC) may have had an effect that was somewhat greater than that of marijuana itself. Animals exposed daily to the ethanol-extracted material had the highest DNA-carcinogen levels in 14 of 21 adduct measures recorded using the nuclease P1 procedure (a procedure that appears to enhance the recovery of adducts resulting from exposures to polycyclic aromatic hydrocarbons). The authors concluded that the smoke from ethanol-extracted marijuana was not innocuous, and, although the supporting data did not reach statistical significance, it may actually have been more toxic than marijuana itself. In addition, they pointed out that their data were at variance with earlier work by others (Sparacino, Hyldburg & Hughes, 1990) that indicated that fractionated marijuana smoke could be highly genotoxic. They explained the apparent discrepancy by suggesting that extrapolation of findings from the bacterial assays employed by Sparacino et al., which had involved the use of "fixed" metabolic activation systems, to whole animal or human exposures was likely to be flawed, especially perhaps with respect to complex exposures. As they said, "these simpler systems may be unable to model the subtle perturbations that mixtures might cause in the metabolism of the whole animal" (p. 329). Clearly, the suggestions made by Talaska et al. (1992) are controversial and must be confirmed, as well as tested.

Cancer Studies with THC and Related Compounds

Perhaps more interesting than the many results that are available is the absence of data on skin-painting assays with THC and other cannabinoids. Even allowing for the difficulties of publishing negative results, it is hard to believe that such studies have not been conducted, yet they are not cited in the large volume of cannabis literature. Many will find it equally difficult to believe that full-scale carcinogenicity bioassays of THC have not been conducted, but this does seem to be the case according to the conventional literature. Whether the fault lies in failure to test or failure to publish negative results is not known. If such studies have not already been conducted, they should surely be carried out as a matter of urgency and their results should be published in full.

cancers of the respiratory tract and also certain other sites (including the bladder, esophagus, mouth and tongue) following distribution of individual pyrolysis products via the bloodstream to all parts of the body. Research priorities identified in this review include a need for skin-painting bioassays with THC and certain other constituents of marijuana smoke, together with a definite need for claims of an association between parental cannabis use and rare childhood cancers to be backed up with a clear demonstration that the same rare cancers have been increasing in incidence with increasing drug use over the last two or three decades. It also needs to be shown that any such increases are confined to the children of drug users.

Conclusion

A review of the literature indicates that cannabis smoke contains several mutagenic substances and may also therefore be carcinogenic in humans. Direct evidence on the latter point is still unavailable, however. Pure THC seems to lack either mutagenic or carcinogenic activity, and, surprisingly, there appears to be little information about the behavior of this compound in even the simplest of animal pre-screens for carcinogenicity (e.g., skin-painting tests). From the evidence to date, the most likely long-term consequences of prolonged heavy cannabis use would appear to be not too different from the risks associated with long-term (cigarette) tobacco use, namely,

Acknowledgments

I am most grateful to Pam Royle, Anetta Miller and Craig Lighton for their help in assembling the literature upon which this review was based. I also thank Dr. Wayne Hall for his most helpful and incisive comments on an earlier draft of this manuscript.

References

Ames, B.N. (1983). Dietary carcinogens and anticarcinogens. *Science, 221*, 1256–1263.

aWengen, D.F. (1993). Marijuana and malignant tumors of the upper aerodigestive tract in young patients: On the risk assessment of marijuana. *Laryngorhinootologie, 72*, 264–267.

Behnke, M. & Eyler, F.D. (1993). The consequences of prenatal substance use for the developing fetus, newborn and young child. *International Journal of the Addictions, 28*, 1341–1391.

Berryman, S.H., Anderson, R.A., Weis, J. & Bartke, A. (1992). Evaluation of the co-mutagenicity of ethanol and $\varnothing$-tetrahydrocannabinol with Trenimon. *Mutation Research, 278*, 47–60.

Blevins, R.D. & Regan, J.D. (1976). Delta-9-tetrahydrocannabinol: Effect on macromolecular synthesis in human and other mammalian cells. *Archives of Toxicology, 34*, 127–135.

Busch, F.W., Seid, D.A. & Wei, E.T. (1979). Mutagenic effects of marihuana smoke condensates. *Cancer Letters, 6*, 319–324.

Chiesara, E., Cutrufello, R. & Rizzi, R. (1983). Chromosome damage in heroin-marijuana and marijuana addicts. *Archives of Toxicology* (Suppl. 6), 128–130.

Christie, M.J. & Chesher, G.B. (1994). The human toxicity of marijuana. *Medical Journal of Australia, 161*, 338–339.

Dalterio, S., Badr, F., Bartke, A. & Mayfield, D. (1982). Cannabinoids in male mice: Effects on fertility and spermatogenesis. *Science, 216*, 315–316.

Dewey, W.L. (1986). Cannabinoid pharmacology. *Pharmacological Reviews, 38*, 151–178.

Generoso, W.M., Cain, K.T., Cornett, C.V. & Shelby, M.D. (1985). Tests for induction of dominant-lethal mutations and heritable translocations with Ø-tetrahydrocannabinol in male mice. *Mutation Research, 143*, 51–53.

Gilmour, D.G., Bloom, A.D., Lele, K.P., Robbins, E.S. & Maximillian, C. (1971). Chromosomal aberrations in users of psychoactive drugs. *Archives of General Psychiatry, 24*, 268–272.

Grufferman, S., Schwartz, A.G., Ruymann, F.B. & Maurer, H.M. (1993). Parents' use of cocaine and marijuana and increased risk of rhabdomyosarcoma in their children. *Cancer Causes and Control, 4*, 217–224.

Henrich, R.T., Nogawa, T. & Morishima, A. (1980). In vitro induction of segregational errors of chromosomes by natural cannabinoids in normal human lymphocytes. *Environmental Mutagenesis, 2*, 139–147.

Hoffmann, D., Brunnemann, K.D., Gori G.B. & Wynder, E.L. (1975). On the carcinogenicity of marijuana smoke. In V.C. Runeckles (Ed.), *Recent Advances in Phytochemistry* (pp. 63–81). New York: Plenum Press.

Hollister, L.E. (1986). Health aspects of cannabis. *Pharmacological Reviews, 38*, 1–20.

Jones, R.T. (1983). Cannabis and health. *Annual Reviews of Medicine, 32*, 247–258.

Jorgensen, K., Wulf, H.C., Husum, B. & Niebuhr, E. (1991). Sister-chromatid exchange in cannabis smokers. *Mutation Research, 261*, 193–195.

Kuijten, R.R., Bunin, G.R., Nass, C.C. & Meadows, A.T. (1990). Gestational and familial risk factors for childhood astrocytoma: Results of a case-control study. *Cancer Research, 50*, 2608–2612.

Legator, M.S. & Au, W.W. (1987). Need to reassess the genetic toxicology of drugs of abuse. In M.C. Braude & A.M. Zimmerman (Eds.), *Genetic and Perinatal Effects of Abused Substances* (pp. 3–26). Orlando, FL: Academic Press.

Legator, M.S., Weber, E., Connor, T. & Stockel, M. (1976). Failure to detect mutagenic effects of Ø-tetrahydrocannabinol in the dominant lethal test, host-mediated assay, blood urine studies and cytogenetic evaluation with mice. In C. Braude & S. Szara (Eds.), *Pharmacology of Marihuana* (pp. 699–709). New York: Raven Press.

Leuchtenberger, C. (1982). Effects of marihuana (cannabis) smoke on cellular biochemistry, utilizing in vitro test systems. In K.O. Fehr & H. Kalant (Eds.), *Adverse Health and Behavioural Consequences of Cannabis Use: Working Papers for the ARF/WHO Scientific Meeting, Toronto, 1981* (pp. 177–223). Toronto: Addiction Research Foundation.

Leuchtenberger, C., Leuchtenberger, R., Rutter, U. & Inui, H. (1973a). Effects of marihuana and tobacco smoke on DNA and chromosomal complement in human lung explants. *Nature, 242*, 403–404.

Leuchtenberger, C., Leuchtenberger, R. & Schneider, A. (1973b). Effects of marihuana and tobacco smoke on human lung physiology. *Nature, 241,* 137–139.

Linn, S., Schoenbaum, S.C., Monson, R.R., Rosner, R., Stubblefield, P.C. & Ryan, K.J. (1983). The association of marijuana use with outcome of pregnancy. *American Journal of Public Health, 73,* 1161–1164.

Mailleux, P., Preud'homme, X., Albala, N., Vanderwinden, J.M. & Vanderhaeghen, J.J. (1994). Delta-9-tetrahydrocannabinol regulaietes gene expression of the growth factor pleiotrophin in the forebrain. *Neuroscience Letters, 175,* 25–27.

Martin, B.R. (1986). Cellular effects of cannabinoids. *Pharmacological Reviews, 38,* 45–74.

Martin, P.A., Thorburn, M.J. & Bryant, S.A. (1973). In vivo and in vitro studies of the cytogenetic effects of *Cannabis sativa* in rats and men. *Teratology, 9,* 82–86.

Maskarinec, M., Alexander, G. & Novotny, M. (1976). Analysis of the acidic fraction of marijuana smoke condensate by capillary gas chromatography/mass spectrometry. *Journal of Chromatography, 126,* 559–568.

Matsuyama, S.S., Yen, F.S., Jarvik, L.F., Sparkes, R.S., Fu, T.K., Fisher, H., Reccius, N. & Frank, J.M. (1977). Marihuana exposure *in vivo* and human lymphocyte chromosomes. *Mutation Research, 48,* 255–262.

Merli, F., Wiester, D., Maskarinec, M., Novotny, M., Vassilanos, D. & Lee, M. (1981). Characterisation of the basic fraction of marijuana smoke condensate by capillary gas chromatography/mass spectrometry. *Analytical Chemistry, 53,* 1929–1935.

Morgan, B., Brake, S.C., Hutchings, D.E., Miller, N. & Gamagaris, Z. (1988). Delta-9-tetra-hydrocannabinol during pregnancy in the rat: Effects on development of RNA, DNA, and protein in offspring brain. *Pharmacology, Biochemistry and Behavior, 31,* 365–369.

Morishima, A., Henrich, R.T., Jayaraman, J. & Nahas, G.G. (1979). Hypoploid metaphases in cultured lymphocytes of marihuana smokers. In G.G. Nahas & W.D.M. Paton (Eds.), *Marihuana: Biological Effects: Analysis, Metabolism, Cellular Responses, Reproduction and Brain, Advances in the Biosciences* (pp. 371–376). Oxford: Pergamon Press.

Nahas, G. & Latour, C. (1992). The human toxicity of marijuana. *Medical Journal of Australia, 156,* 495–497.

Neu, R.L., Powers, H.O., King, S. & Gardner, L.I. (1970). Delta-8-tetrahydrocannabinol and Ø⁹-tetrahydrocannabinol: Effects on cultured human lymphocytes. *Journal of Clinical Pharmacology, 10,* 228–230.

Nichols, W.W., Miller, R.C., Heneen, W., Bradt, C., Hollister, L.E. & Kanter, S. (1974). Cytogenetic studies on human subjects receiving marihuana and Ø⁹-tetrahydro-cannabinol. *Mutation Research, 26,* 413–417.

Novotny, M., Kump, R., Merli, F. & Todd, L. (1980). Capillary gas chromatography/mass spectrometric determination of nitrogen aromatic compounds in complex mixtures. *Chemistry*, *52*, 401–406.

Paria, B.C., Wang, X.N. & Dey, S.K. (1994). Effects of chronic treatment with delta-9-tetrahydrocannabinol on uterine growth in the mouse. *Life Sciences*, *55*, 729–734.

Piatti, E., Rizzi, R., Re, F. & Chiesara, E. (1989). Genotoxicity of heroin and cannabis in humans. *Pharmacological Research*, *21* (Suppl. 1), 59–60.

Rauno, H., Pasanen, M., Mäenpää, J., Hakkola, J. & Pelkonen, O. (1995). Expression of extrahepatic cytochrome P450 in humans. In G.M. Pacifici & G.N. Fracchia (Eds.), *Advances in Drug Metabolism in Man* (pp. 233–287). Brussels: European Commission.

Robison, L.L., Buckley, J.D., Daigle, A.E., Wells, R., Benjamin, D., Arthur, D.C. & Hammond, G.D. (1988). Maternal drug use and risk of childhood nonlymphoblastic leukaemia among offspring: An epidemiologic investigation implicating marijuana. *Cancer*, *63*, 1904–1911.

Rosenkrantz, H. & Fleischman, R.W. (1979). Effects of cannabis on the lungs. In G.G. Nahas & W.D.M. Paton (Eds.), *Marihuana: Biological Effects: Analysis, Metabolism, Cellular Responses, Reproduction and Brain, Advances in the Biosciences* (pp. 279–299). Oxford: Pergamon Press.

Seid, D.A. & Wei, E.T. (1979). Mutagenic activity of marihuana smoke condensates. *Pharmacologist*, *21*, 204.

Sparacino, C.M., Hyldburg, P.A. & Hughes, T.J. (1990). *Chemical and biological analysis of marijuana smoke condensate* (NIDA Research Monograph No. 99, pp. 121–140). Washington, DC: U.S. Government Printing Office.

Sridhar, K.S., Raub, W.A., Jr., Weatherby, N.L., Metsch, L.R., Surratt, H.L., Inciardi, J.A., Duncan, R.C., Anwyl, R.S. & McCoy, C.B. (1994). Possible role of marijuana smoking as a carcinogen in the development of lung cancer at a young age. *Journal of Psychoactive Drugs*, *26*, 285–288.

Stenchever, M.A., Kunysz, J.J. & Allen, M.A. (1974). Chromosome breakage in users of marijuana. *American Journal of Obstetrics and Gynecology*, *118*, 106–113.

Stenchever, M.A., Parks, K.J. & Stenchever, M.R. (1976). Effects of delta-8-tetrahydrocannabinol and Ø-tetrahydrocannabinol, and crude marihuana on human cells in tissue culture. In G.G. Nahas, W.D.M. Paton & J.E. Idänpään-Heikkila (Eds.), *Marihuana: Chemistry, Biochemistry, and Cellular Effects* (pp. 257–263). New York: Springer-Verlag.

Tahir, S.K. & Zimmerman, A.M. (1992). Cytoskeletal organization following cannabinoid treatment in undifferentiated and differentiated PC12 cells. *Biochemical Cell Biology*, *70*, 1159–1173.

Talaska, G., Schamer, M., Bailey, J.R., Ali, S.F., Scallet, A.C., Slikker, W., Jr. & Paule, M.G. (1992). No increase in carcinogen-DNA adducts in the lungs of monkeys exposed chronically to marijuana smoke. *Toxicology Letters*, *63*, 321–332.

Taylor, F.M. (1988). Marijuana as a potential respiratory tract carcinogen: A retrospective analysis of a community hospital population. *Southern Medical Journal*, *81*, 1213–1216.

Tennant, F.S. (1980). Histopathologic and clinical abnormalities of the respiratory system in chronic hashish smokers. In L.S. Harris (Ed.), *Problems of Drug Dependence, 1979* (NIDA Research Monograph No. 27, pp. 309–315). Washington, DC: U.S. Government Printing Office.

Vassiliades, N., Mourelatos, D., Dozi-Vassiliades, J., Epivatianos, P. & Hatzitheodoridou, P. (1986). Induction of sister-chromatid exchanges in heroin-cannabis, heroin and cannabis addicts. *Mutation Research*, *170*, 125–127.

Wehner, F.C., Van Rensburg, S.J. & Thiel, P.G. (1980). Mutagenicity of marijuana and Transkei tobacco smoke condensates in the Salmonella/microsome assay. *Mutation Research*, *77*, 135–142.

Wheeler, C.W. & Guenthner, T.M. (1991). Cytochrome P-450-dependent metabolism of xenobiotics in human lung. *Journal of Biochemical Toxicology*, *6*, 163–169.

Zimmerman, A.M. & McClean, D.K. (1973). Action of narcotic and hallucinogenic agents on the cell cycle. In A.M. Zimmerman, G.M. Padilla & I.L. Cameron (Eds.), *Drugs and the Cell Cycle* (p. 67). New York: Academic Press.

Zimmerman, A.M., Murer-Orlando, M.L. & Richer, C.L. (1986). Effects of cannabinoids on spermatogenesis *in vivo*. *Cytobios*, *45*, 7–15.

Zimmerman, A.M. & Raj, A.Y. (1980). Influence of cannabinoids on somatic cells *in vivo*. *Pharmacology*, *21*, 277–287.

Zimmerman, A.M., Stich, H. & San, R. (1978). Nonmutagenic action of cannabinoids *in vitro*. *Pharmacology*, *16*, 333–343.

Zimmerman, S. & Zimmerman, S. (1990–91). Genetic effects of marijuana. *International Journal of the Addictions*, *25*, 19–33.

CHAPTER 9

Cannabis Effects on the Respiratory System

Cannabis Effects on the Respiratory System

DONALD P. TASHKIN

Abundant epidemiologic, physiologic and clinical evidence has implicated regular tobacco smoking as the most important cause of lung cancer and chronic obstructive pulmonary disease (COPD), which consists of chronic obstructive bronchitis and emphysema. Tobacco smoking has also been found to predispose to the development of respiratory tract infection. These respiratory consequences of tobacco are probably mediated by a number of different mechanisms, including respiratory tract irritation and injury, mutagenic and carcinogenic effects and impairment in pulmonary host defences. Next to tobacco, cannabis is one of the most widely smoked substances worldwide. Cannabis yields many of the same smoke contents as tobacco, including respiratory tract irritants and carcinogens, with the major exceptions of nicotine in tobacco and over 60 cannabinoid compounds in cannabis (Hoffmann, Brunnemann et al., 1975; Novotny, Lee & Bartle, 1976; Sparacino, Hyldburg & Hughes, 1990). Given the fact that cannabis is generally smoked far less frequently than tobacco, however, it remains unclear whether habitual smoking of cannabis can result in pulmonary disorders similar to those caused by tobacco. This question has been addressed, either directly or indirectly, by a number of studies carried out both in experimental animals and in humans within the last two decades. This chapter provides an in-depth review of the published reports of these studies, with a primary focus on those studies reported since 1982.

Older Studies (Prior to 1982)

Animal Studies

EFFECTS OF CANNABIS ON AIRWAY AND LUNG PARENCHYMAL HISTOPATHOLOGY

A few animal studies were conducted in the 1970s to examine possible effects of cannabis on pulmonary histopathology. Results of these studies suggested that habitual exposure to marijuana smoke can cause airway and parenchymal lung injury. For example, in tracheotomized dogs, severe inflammation of the smaller airways and destruction of the ciliated epithelial cells of the trachea with replacement by squamous epithelium occurred after 30 months of exposure to the smoke of four marijuana cigarettes a day (Roy, Magnan-Lapointe et al., 1976). Although these experimental canine exposures to cannabis were greater than the usual recreational human exposures, it is noteworthy that the observed changes were more marked than those noted after exposure of a parallel group of dogs to the same amount of tobacco smoke over a similar span of time. In rats, after 87 days of exposure to doses of cannabis smoke comparable to those used recreationally by humans, dose-related acute alveolitis and pneumonitis localized in the proximity of respiratory bronchioles or alveolar ducts were noted and these progressed to chronic focal pneumonia after one year of exposure (Fleischman, Baker & Rosenkrantz, 1979; Fleischman, Hayden et al., 1975; Rosenkrantz & Fleischman, 1979). These pulmonary lesions contained an admixture of granulomatous, chronic and acute inflammation, and some areas also showed early fibrosis and alveolar cell hyperplasia. In both of the above animal models, qualitatively similar morphologic abnormalities were observed in the experimental and control groups, but the alterations in the marijuana-exposed animals were of greater severity and frequency of occurrence. Moreover, in the marijuana-exposed animals, the severity and extent of the lesions were related to the duration and intensity of exposure to marijuana smoke. Another important finding was that, with the exception of tracheal squamous metaplasia in the canine model that might have been attributed to the chronic tracheostomy (Roy, Magnan-Lapointe et al., 1976), the histopathologic alterations mostly affected the small-airway region of the lung.

Although the results of the few animal studies cited above suggest that the long-term effects of chronic exposure to marijuana smoke can be injurious to the lung, these results may not be extrapolatable to humans because of differences in smoking topography, effective dose to the respiratory tract, duration of exposure and coincident exposures, as well as species differences.

EFFECTS OF CANNABIS ON ALVEOLAR MACROPHAGE STRUCTURE, NUMBER AND FUNCTION

The alveolar macrophage is the key cell in the lung's defence against infection and toxic injury. It is also principally responsible for mediating inflammatory responses in the lung through release of toxic oxygen species and a variety of cytokines that are capable of causing lung injury and parenchymal destruction. Huber (Drath, Shorey et al., 1979) reported that marijuana exposure can induce metabolic and structural alterations in rat alveolar macrophages, including the intracellular accumulation of lipolysosomes containing tissue-damaging enzymes with the potential for mediating lung inflammation and destruction. Huber et al. (1975) also found that the bactericidal activity of rat alveolar macrophages was depressed *in vitro* by water-soluble cytotoxic components of the gas phase of fresh marijuana smoke. Based on data obtained using an *in vitro* model with wetted surfaces simulating the moist mucosa of the upper and lower respiratory tract, Huber and colleagues (1991) subsequently determined that the most likely gas-phase cytotoxins (acrolein and acetaldehyde) were nearly completely absorbed by only a small fraction of the wetted surface, thus eliminating their potential for *in vivo* alveolar macrophage cytotoxicity. Exposure of rats to marijuana or tobacco smoke for 30 consecutive days failed to alter the number of alveolar macrophages subsequently obtained by bronchopulmonary lavage or the ability of these cells to phagocytose *Staphylococcus aureus,* compared to macrophages obtained from control, unexposed animals (Drath, Shorey et al., 1979). On the contrary, however, the same laboratory observed that *in vivo* inactivation of pathogenic bacteria aerosolized into the lungs was impaired in a dose-dependent manner in rats exposed to increasing amounts of whole fresh marijuana smoke, including smoke from THC-extracted marijuana smoke (Huber, Pochay et al., 1980). Taken together, these findings suggest that cannabis smoking can impair the host defences of the lung against infection and other noxious insults due to non-cannabinoid toxic components within the smoke other than highly water-soluble gas-phase cytotoxins.

Human Studies

SHORT-TERM PHYSIOLOGIC EFFECTS OF CANNABIS

Several early laboratory-controlled studies examined the short-term effects of smoked marijuana, as well as oral $\varnothing$-tetrahydrocannabinol (THC), on airway dynamics. These are reviewed in greater detail elsewhere (Tashkin, 1991). Briefly, Vachon et al. (1973) and Tashkin et al. (1973) observed significant decreases in airway resistance (R_{aw}) and increases in specific airway conductance (SG_{aw}) in healthy regular smokers of marijuana within minutes of smoking marijuana containing 1.0 to 2.6 per cent THC (3.23 to 7 mg/kg bodyweight), indicating an acute bronchodilator response. These changes were noted immediately after completion of smoking, peaked at 15 to 20 minutes and persisted for at least 60 minutes. A placebo marijuana preparation (from which the cannabinoids had been extracted) elicited no changes in R_{aw} or SG_{aw}, while the bronchodilator response was restored by another placebo preparation that had been "spiked" with synthetic THC. These results suggested, therefore, that the bronchodilator effect was due mainly to THC and not to other ingredients in marijuana. This conclusion is supported by other studies demonstrating a dose-dependent bronchodilator response to oral administration of 10 to 20 mg of synthetic THC (Tashkin, Shapiro & Frank, 1973). Interestingly, the bronchodilator response to smoked marijuana in healthy volunteers was greater than that to a therapeutic dose of a nebulized beta-adrenergic agonist (isoproterenol, 1250 mcg), indicating that THC is a potent bronchodilator. Moreover, in marked contrast to the bronchodilator effect of smoked marijuana, smoking a single tobacco cigarette caused mild, but statistically significant, bronchoconstriction, probably due to an irritant effect of tobacco smoke on the airway epithelium causing vagally mediated reflex bronchospasm.

The acute bronchodilator response to both smoked marijuana and oral THC noted in healthy volunteers was also observed in asthmatic subjects with mild to moderate airways obstruction (mean FEV_1 67.4 per cent predicted), although the asthmatics, in contrast to the normal subjects, showed a proportionately greater response to isoproterenol than to marijuana (Tashkin, Shapiro & Frank, 1974), as well as a less marked bronchodilator response to oral THC. In addition to dilating the airways of stable asthmatics, smoked marijuana has also been shown to cause rapid reversal of bronchoconstriction induced experimentally by methacholine inhalation or exercise in asthmatic subjects (Tashkin, Shapiro et al., 1975). These findings suggested that THC, the physiologically active bronchodilator compound in marijuana, might have therapeutic potential in asthma. However, smoking is not a satisfactory route of administration of THC for therapeutic bronchodilation because of the numerous other ingredients in the smoke, including noxious gases and particulates that are capable of causing chronic bronchial irritation and/or malignant change after long-term use (see below). Oral THC is also not suitable for therapeutic use in asthma because of its unwanted non-bronchodilator effects, including central nervous system intoxication and tachycardia in relation to its only modest bronchodilator properties. Furthermore, tolerance to the bronchodilator effect of THC has been demonstrated after several weeks of use (Tashkin, Shapiro et al., 1976).

A few studies have attempted to exploit the therapeutic potential of THC in asthma by administering pure THC in aerosol form, thereby obviating harmful effects of other smoke components and minimizing the psychotropic effects of THC due to relatively limited systemic absorption of the nebulized THC from the tracheobronchial tree, as opposed to the alveolar surface. In one study, however, bronchoconstriction was induced by 5 to 20 mg THC that was delivered as an aerosol from a metered-dose inhaler (MDI) to asthmatic subjects (Tashkin, Reiss et al., 1977). This paradoxical response was presumably due to an irritating effect of relatively high concentrations of aerosolized THC (a phenolic compound) at localized sites in the airway leading to reflex bronchospasm in individuals with sensitive airways. On the other hand, others have succeeded in producing significant bronchodilation (without any instances of bronchospasm) in asthmatics administered a smaller dose of nebulized THC (0.2 mg) from an MDI (Williams, Hartley & Graham, 1976), although the time to peak bronchodilation was relatively slow, thus limiting therapeutic utility. Systemic effects of THC were not observed with these low doses delivered topically to the airways. Nevertheless, an MDI delivering low doses of THC for use as a bronchodilator in asthma would have the potential for abuse, since higher doses capable of producing psychotomimetic effects could be achieved simply by increasing the number of inhalations. It appears, therefore, that THC itself, whether in the form of smoked marijuana or as a pure synthetic compound administered orally or as an aerosol, is not suitable for therapeutic use in asthma. An alternative approach to promoting the therapeutic potential of cannabis in asthma would be to synthesize an analogue of THC that retained its bronchodilator properties but was devoid of undesirable systemic effects. Thus far, such efforts have not been successful (Tashkin, 1991).

SHORT-TERM EFFECTS OF CANNABIS ON GAS EXCHANGE AT REST AND DURING EXERCISE

Shapiro and colleagues (1976) examined the effects of smoking active versus placebo marijuana on gas exchange at rest and during progressively increasing exercise. At rest, compared to placebo, active marijuana (approximately 900 mg, 2 per cent THC) produced no change in breathing rate or depth, minute ventilation, oxygen production, CO_2 production,

respiratory exchange ratio (R), arterial blood gases or blood lactate concentration, despite a modest increase in dead space (15 ± 6 mL) and a substantial increase in heart rate (25.8 ± 6.1 min^{-1}). At each level of cycloergometer exercise after smoking active marijuana, changes in arterial blood gases, blood lactate, minute ventilation, oxygen consumption, CO_2 production and R were similar to the changes at the same exercise level after placebo marijuana, although the absolute heart rate at comparable levels of exercise was greater after active marijuana. On the other hand, the maximal level of exercise tolerance after marijuana smoking was diminished by a mean of 300 kg-m/min compared to the average maximal level achieved after placebo (1500 kg-m/min). The decrease in maximal exercise tolerance after active marijuana was felt to be due to an additive effect of THC-induced tachycardia and exercise-related tachycardia, so that peak heart rate with exercise was achieved at a lower work rate after marijuana than placebo.

CLINICAL-PHYSIOLOGIC EFFECTS OF CANNABIS USE

Only a few older (before 1982) studies have addressed the question whether regular cannabis smoking can cause clinically significant damage to the human respiratory system, and the results of these studies are conflicting. Older reports of bronchitis after heavy or chronic smoking of cannabis are either anecdotal or based on uncontrolled clinical observations. For example, in India, Chopra (1973) observed an apparently high prevalence of asthma, bronchitis and nose and throat irritation among 124 selected cannabis users and, in Jamaica, Hall (1975) noted that an emphysematous configuration of the chest was particularly common among frequent, heavy users of cannabis. Neither of these authors, however, systematically compared their observations in cannabis smokers with findings in a control group of subjects. Nor did they control for the important confounding variable of concomitant tobacco smoking. In contrast to the above observations, a Greek study failed to find a higher prevalence of "bronchitis" among 44 chronic hashish users (who also smoked tobacco) compared to tobacco-smoking controls, although cough and throat irritation were common complaints among the hashish smokers (Boulougouris, Panayiotopoulos et al., 1976). This study may be criticized, however, since subject selection forced exclusion of those with incapacitating illness and the frequent finding of cough among the hashish users raises doubts as to the validity of the authors' definition of "bronchitis."

In a cross-sectional Jamaican study of lung function, mean values of forced vital capacity (FVC), forced expiratory volume in one second (FEV_1) and arterial PO_2 were all found to be lower in 30 cannabis (ganja) users (who smoked an average of seven cannabis cigarettes per day for a mean of 17 years) than in 30 control non-cannabis users, but the differences were not statistically significant (Cruickshank, 1976). Moreover, the cannabis users did not differ from the control subjects with respect to clinical evidence of respiratory disease. This study was flawed, however, by the failure to control for the variable of tobacco smoking, since both the cannabis smokers and their controls smoked tobacco, the effects of which could have masked any effect of marijuana. In a Costa Rican study, no significant differences were noted in FEV_1 or maximal mid-expiratory flow rate ($FEF_{25-75 \text{ per cent}}$), a sensitive measure of small airways dysfunction, between 40 cannabis smokers (average of 9.6 joints per day for 10 years) and 40 age- and tobacco-matched controls (Hernandez-Bolanos, Swenson & Coggins, 1976). The results of the latter two studies are difficult to interpret, however, because the samples of cannabis users examined were small and apparently not randomly selected, thereby raising the possibility of selection bias. Moreover, both studies were cross-sectional, raising the possibility that the samples of cannabis users examined represented a "survivor population" and that potentially damaging effects of cannabis were underestimated if those harmed by long-term heavy cannabis use were too sick to participate in the study.

To evaluate the impact of cannabis smoking on lung function over time, Tashkin et al. (1976) performed extensive lung function tests on 28 young healthy experienced cannabis smokers at different times before, during and after a several week period of daily smoking of greater than their usual quantities of cannabis. In this prospective study, baseline spirometric tests (FVC, FEV_1 and $FEF_{25-75 \text{ per cent}}$), as well as closing volume and $\oslash N_2/L$ (sensitive tests of peripheral airways function), were all within statistically normal limits. However, daily smoking of 1 to 20 (average of 5) marijuana joints (20 mg THC per joint) a day over 47 to 59 days caused mild but statistically significant decreases in several tests of lung function, some of which were correlated with the daily average number of joints smoked per individual. Although the observed absolute decreases in lung function were not large, if these changes were annualized, the extrapolated rates of decline in lung function would be several-fold higher than those observed in healthy non-smokers. Consequently, if lung function continued to deteriorate at the same rate observed during the course of the study, individuals who continued to smoke an average of five joints per day would become disabled by respiratory insufficiency in a few years. Since the latter consequence of heavy, habitual cannabis use is not clinically obvious, it is more likely that heavy cannabis smoking over several weeks causes a subacute impairment in lung function that subsequently stabilizes or progresses at a much slower rate. Whether or not these physiologic changes in habitual cannabis users will progress to clinically significant airways obstruction after years or decades of continued regular use of cannabis is not known at present (see "Newer Studies" below).

EFFECTS OF CANNABIS USE ON AIRWAY HISTOPATHOLOGY AND ALVEOLAR MACROPHAGE STRUCTURE

Among young U.S. servicemen in West Germany who smoked more than 50 grams of hashish per month and sought medical attention for respiratory symptoms, Tennant et al. (1971) and Henderson et al. (1972) found frequent evidence of upper airway inflammation (rhinitis, pharyngitis, sinusitis), as well as clinical and functional evidence of bronchitis and asthma. Several of the patients with chronic cough underwent bronchoscopy and biopsy of the tracheal epithelium. Microscopically, extensive cellular abnormalities were noted, including loss of cilia, proliferation of basal epithelial cells and atypical cells — changes that are felt to be precursors to the subsequent development of bronchogenic carcinoma in regular tobacco smokers. Although most of these men also smoked tobacco along with hashish, they were in an age group in which such extensive microscopic abnormalities involving the central airways have not generally been noted in smokers of tobacco alone. In a follow-up study, Tennant (1980) performed bronchoscopy in an additional group of 30 heavy hashish smokers (25 to 150 g/month for 3 to 24 months), of whom seven did not smoke tobacco. Three non-smoking control subjects and three smokers of tobacco alone (mean of 1.6 packs per day for 11.3 years) also underwent bronchoscopy. All of the smokers of both hashish and tobacco showed extensive microscopic abnormalities in their tracheal biopsies similar to those previously observed, whereas similar abnormalities were found in only two of seven smokers of hashish alone, in one of three smokers of tobacco alone and in none of the non-smokers. These findings suggest that combined use of cannabis and tobacco may cause more respiratory tract damage than use of either substance alone.

Alveolar macrophages harvested by lung washings from habitual cannabis users have shown electron dense and lucent inclusions on electron microscopy similar to those found in macrophages from regular tobacco smokers (Mann, Cohen et al., 1971). Whether these ultrastructural abnormalities are associated with clinically relevant defects in alveolar macrophage function remains to be determined (see "Newer Studies" below).

EFFECTS OF CANNABIS ON RESPIRATORY CARCINOGENESIS

The following older evidence (briefly summarized) suggests that habitual smoking of marijuana may predispose to the development of respiratory tract cancer, independent of the effect of tobacco smoking.

- The tar phase of the smoke from marijuana contains approximately 50 per cent more of some carcinogenic hydrocarbons than the smoke from a comparable quantity of unfiltered tobacco (Hoffmann, Brunnemann et al., 1975), thus increasing the burden of carcinogens delivered to the respiratory tract of smokers of marijuana, particularly in comparison with smokers of filtered tobacco, for a given quantity of plant material smoked.

- Hamster lung explants exposed to marijuana smoke over a period of two years led to accelerated malignant transformation within three to six months of marijuana exposure compared to control explants (Leuchtenberger & Leuchtenberger, 1976).

- In the Ames Salmonella/microsome test, marijuana smoke condensate induced numbers of mutations comparable to those produced by an equivalent amount of tobacco tar, suggesting the ability to cause genetic mutations that could predispose to malignancy (Busch, Seid & Wei, 1979; Wehner, Van Rensburg & Thiel, 1980).

- The extensive metaplastic and dysplastic changes that were noted in the bronchial epithelium of heavy, habitual smokers of hashish (Henderson, Tennant & Guerry, 1972; Tennant, 1980) are similar to those noted in heavy smokers of tobacco who subsequently develop bronchogenic carcinoma and may thus be considered precursors of lung cancer (Auerbach, Gere et al., 1957; Auerbach, Stout et al., 1961).

Newer Studies
(After 1982)

Animal Studies

EFFECTS OF CANNABIS EXPOSURE ON LUNG PHYSIOLOGY AND MORPHOLOGY IN RATS

To study the comparative effects of tobacco and marijuana on the lung, Huber and Mahajan (1988) exposed pathogen-free rats to marijuana and tobacco smoke both acutely in progressively increasing doses and chronically for six months. After sacrifice of the animals, physiologic measurements of lung elasticity were obtained as indicators of parenchymal destruction (as seen in pulmonary emphysema). In addition, fixed inflated lung sections were examined microscopically using morphometric and stereologic techniques to quantify surface areas and lung tissue densities for morphologic assessment of emphysematous changes. Tobacco smoke exposure induced morphologic and physiologic changes that reflected a loss of lung parenchyma and a decrease in lung elasticity, consistent with emphysema. In contrast, exposure to a similar quantity of marijuana smoke for the same duration resulted in no detectable morphologic or physiologic abnormalities. These findings suggest that chronic exposure to the smoke of tobacco, but not marijuana, leads to emphysematous changes in the lungs of experimental animals.

EFFECTS OF CANNABIS EXPOSURE ON LUNG HISTOPATHOLOGY IN MONKEYS

Fligiel et al. (1991) examined formalin-inflated, sectioned lungs from four groups of periadolescent male rhesus monkeys (six animals per group) that were sacrificed seven months after a one-year period of daily marijuana, placebo or sham smoke inhalation. Each group was exposed to either:

1. high-dose marijuana (one marijuana cigarette daily);
2. low-dose marijuana (one marijuana cigarette two days per week and sham smoke five days per week);
3. placebo (one extracted marijuana cigarette daily); or
4. sham (sham smoke daily).

The peak plasma THC levels attained in these monkeys were equivalent to those predicted for humans after smoking four to five medium-potency marijuana cigarettes. The authors considered, therefore, that the inhalation by their monkeys of one marijuana cigarette per day for one year was equivalent to heavy chronic marijuana use in the human. Light microscopic examination of the lung sections after sacrifice revealed a greater frequency of several histopathologic abnormalities (alveolitis and granulomatous inflammation) in all smoking groups compared to the non-smoking sham group. A higher frequency of other microscopic abnormalities (bronchiolitis, bronchiolar squamous metaplasia and interstitial fibrosis) was noted in the marijuana-smoking groups compared to the placebo-smoking and non-smoking sham groups. The severity of many of the changes, including respiratory bronchiolitis, bronchiolar squamous metaplasia and peribronchiolar/interstitial fibrosis, as well as the frequency with which these changes were observed, was related to the amount of marijuana the animals inhaled. These small airways abnormalities are similar to those observed in human tobacco smokers and are considered precursors to the development of chronic obstructive bronchitis and emphysema (Niewoehner, Kleinerman & Rice, 1974). Moreover, interstitial alveolitis similar to that observed in the lungs of these monkeys has also been considered an early precursor to emphysema in humans (Anderson & Foraker, 1961). The findings from this prospective study, therefore, indicate that exposure of primates to marijuana smoke results in distinctive histopathologic alterations that may represent precursor lesions to more severe changes that are characteristic of chronic obstructive bronchitis and emphysema. In addition, one particular abnormality — alveolar cell hyperplasia with focal atypia — was found only in the marijuana-smoking monkeys. Since atypical alveolar cell hyperplasia has been found in humans with adenocarcinoma, the latter observation suggests a possible relationship to invasive malignant neoplasm. Further studies in larger numbers of primates with a longer follow-up period are needed to better define the morbid consequences of these morphologic alterations.

EFFECTS OF CANNABIS EXPOSURE ON ALVEOLAR MACROPHAGE STRUCTURE AND FUNCTION IN PRIMATES

Cabral and colleagues (1991) examined alveolar macrophages obtained at sacrifice from the same four groups of rhesus monkeys exposed to the smoke from low- and high-dose marijuana, the smoke from ethanol-extracted marijuana (placebo) or sham smoking conditions for one year, followed by a seven-month period of no smoke exposure. Macrophages from all the animals exposed to high- or low-dose marijuana or placebo marijuana contained numerous intracytoplasmic particulate inclusions. Since the mean half-life of alveolar macrophages is only approximately 27 days and a seven-month interval separated the cessation of experimental exposure to marijuana and sacrifice of the animals, these observations indicate that marijuana smoke-derived particulates recycle from macrophage to macrophage during macrophage turnover within the lung. This recycling process provides a mechanism whereby alveolar macrophages may be persistently exposed to THC within the intracytoplasmic inclusions, even after cessation of marijuana smoking. Macrophages exposed to low- and high-dose marijuana smoke contained an increased number and size of cytoplasmic vacuoles, irregularity in cell surface outline and "blebs" extending from the cell surface, consistent with earlier observations in the alveolar macrophages of human marijuana smokers (Davis, Brody & Adler, 1979). Moreover, most of the macrophages from the monkeys exposed to high-dose marijuana exhibited a spherical conformation after adherence to plastic. The expression of cell surface blebs and the assumption of a spherical shape by alveolar macrophages are consistent with toxic injury to cell surface membranes with alterations in membrane permeability. These morphologic changes might reflect impairment in macrophage function, such as phagocytosis, as demonstrated for murine peritoneal macrophages exposed *in vitro* to THC (Lopez-Cepero, Friedman et al., 1986). Alveolar macrophages of monkeys exposed to marijuana smoke also exhibited inhibition of protein synthesis in response to stimulation by lipopolysaccharide, suggesting a diminished capacity of the macrophages to respond to external stimuli. Since newly expressed proteins are associated with the varied activities of activated macrophages, these findings imply that chronic exposure to marijuana may impair the antimicrobial and immunoregulatory function of alveolar macrophages.

Human Studies

CLINICAL-PHYSIOLOGIC EFFECTS OF CANNABIS USE

To evaluate possible pulmonary effects of habitual smoking of marijuana with or without tobacco, Tashkin et al. (1987) administered a detailed respiratory questionnaire and an extensive battery of lung function tests to a convenience sample of young habitual smokers of marijuana alone (MS; n = 144) or with tobacco (MTS; n = 135) and age-matched control subjects who smoked tobacco alone (TS; n = 70) or were non-smokers (NS; n = 97), who resided in the Los Angeles area. MS and MTS smoked an average of 49 to 57 joint-years (mean daily number of joints times number of years smoked) and MTS and TS smoked a mean of 16 to 22 pack-years of tobacco cigarettes. In all smoking groups, including the marijuana-only group, prevalence of chronic cough (18 to 24 per cent), sputum production (20 to 26 per cent), wheeze (25 to 37 per cent) and > 1 prolonged episode of acute bronchitis during the previous three years (10 to 14 per cent) was significantly higher than in the non-smokers ($p < 0.05$; chi square). No difference in prevalence of chronic respiratory symptoms was noted between MS and TS, nor were additive effects of marijuana and tobacco on symptom prevalence observed. These findings indicate that heavy, habitual smoking of marijuana with or without concomitant tobacco is associated with a higher prevalence of symptoms of chronic bronchitis and a higher incidence of acute bronchitis than is observed among non-smokers, although additive effects of combined marijuana and tobacco smoking on the prevalence of chronic or acute respiratory symptoms could not be demonstrated.

Lung function test results from the same study (Tashkin, Coulson et al., 1987) indicated an association between the smoking of marijuana, but not tobacco, and an obstructive abnormality in the large, central airways, as indicated by abnormal increases in airway resistance and decreases in specific airway conductance. In contrast, tobacco, but not marijuana, smoking was associated with abnormalities in several tests reflecting small airways obstruction, including closing volume and slope of phase III of the single-breath oxygen test, as well as abnormalities in carbon monoxide diffusing capacity (or gas transfer). Since small airways dysfunction and impairment in diffusing capacity are early physiologic indicators of chronic obstructive airways disease (which primarily affects the small, peripheral airways) and pulmonary emphysema (which is characterized by destruction of alveolar walls with resultant impairment in gas transfer), these findings do not support the concept that heavy, habitual smoking of marijuana predisposes to the development of chronic *obstructive* pulmonary disease (COPD) or emphysema. These results are also consistent with the experimental findings of Huber and Mahajan (1988) in rats.

COPD may be defined as "chronic *obstructive* bronchitis" and/or emphysema. An essential component of COPD is air flow *obstruction* (American Thoracic Society, 1962). "Chronic bronchitis" is characterized by chronic cough and sputum production on most days for at least three months a year and for at least two years. The symptoms of chronic bronchitis are believed to be due to mucus hypersecretion that results from structural alterations in the airways induced by cigarette smoking: i.e., hyperplasia of mucus-secreting surface epithelial cells (goblet cells) and hypertrophy of submucosal bronchial mucus glands leading to increased production of mucus, and loss of ciliated epithelial cells resulting in diminished ability of the airways to transport mucus up the tracheobronchial tree in the absence of cough. Chronic bronchitis, i.e., mucus hypersecretion, can occur *with* or *without* airways *obstruction* and is therefore not necessarily equated with COPD. The findings from the above-cited study suggest that habitual marijuana smoking leads to symptoms of chronic bronchitis, but probably does not predispose to the development of COPD, i.e., to chronic *obstructive* bronchitis or emphysema.

In comparison with the latter study, data from the Tucson epidemiological study of airways obstructive disease provided both confirmatory and contradictory results (Bloom, Kaltenborn et al., 1987). In the Tucson study, 2,251 Caucasian, non-Hispanic subjects were recruited from a random stratified cluster of households in the general community. In 1981–83, these subjects underwent forced expiratory spirometry and answered a questionnaire including questions about respiratory symptoms and the duration and intensity of smoking tobacco and non-tobacco (mainly marijuana) cigarettes. Since few subjects over age 40 years admitted to smoking non-tobacco cigarettes, analysis was restricted to the respondents 15 to 40 years of age, including 56 smokers of non-tobacco (marijuana) plus tobacco cigarettes, 54 smokers of non-tobacco cigarettes alone, 209 smokers of tobacco alone and 502 non-smokers. Average lifetime cumulative non-tobacco cigarette use was 58.2 cigarette years (number of non-tobacco cigarettes per week times number of years smoked), while mean tobacco cigarette use among current smokers was 8.7 pack-years. Findings from this population-based study revealed a significantly greater frequency of symptoms of chronic bronchitis (cough and sputum production), as well as wheezing, in smokers of non-tobacco (mostly marijuana) cigarettes alone (26 to 40 per cent) compared to the prevalence of the same symptoms in non-smokers (13 to 23 per cent), in agreement with the findings from the Los Angeles study (Tashkin, Coulson et al., 1987). In contrast to the Los Angeles study, however, findings from the Tucson survey also suggested *additive* effects of tobacco and non-tobacco (mostly marijuana) cigarettes on the frequency of abnormal respiratory symptoms that were reported by a significantly higher percentage of combined smokers (63 to 68 per cent), compared to smokers of either substance alone (26 to 54 per cent).

Spirometric results of the Tucson study also documented a significant relationship in men between airways obstruction and the smoking of non-tobacco (marijuana) cigarettes in comparison with non-smokers of non-tobacco products, as indicated by significantly lower values for forced expiratory flow rates at low lung volumes (an index of small airways obstruction) and for FEV_1/FVC ratio in the marijuana smokers than the non-smokers. Moreover, the severity of the airways obstruction was even greater in the non-tobacco-only smokers than in the tobacco-only smokers and was greatest in the combined smokers of both types of cigarettes, implying an additive effect of marijuana and tobacco. These findings, which are in disagreement with the results of the Los Angeles study, suggest that marijuana smoking may be an important determinant of the development of obstructive airways disease in young men. Possible reasons for the discrepancy between the results of these two studies include differences in the study design (convenience sample vs. random sample derived from the general community), failure in the Tucson study to control for possible use of other smoked substances besides cannabis and tobacco, differences in intensity and cumulative lifetime amount of cannabis smoke exposure, and possible confounding effects of differing exposures to atmospheric pollutants in the two communities.

Follow-up data from four consecutive surveys of the Tucson longitudinal study conducted between 1981–83 and 1985–88 provided information on non-tobacco (mostly marijuana) smoking, respiratory symptoms and lung function in 856 subjects who participated in at least two of the surveys (Sherrill, Krzyzanowski et al., 1991). Findings from this longitudinal study indicated an increased risk of respiratory symptoms in current non-tobacco smokers, after adjustment for age, tobacco smoking and occurrence of the symptom on the previous survey: estimated odds ratio (OR) 1.73 for chronic cough, 1.53 for chronic phlegm, and 2.01 for wheeze. The risk of these symptoms increased with the duration of non-tobacco smoking and persisted several years after quitting non-tobacco cigarettes. Moreover, the risk of these symptoms increased with the amount of non-tobacco cigarettes smoked weekly, suggesting a dose-response relationship between chronic respiratory symptoms and the level of marijuana usage. In addition, a significant reduction in ventilatory function (FEV_1, FEV_1/FVC ratio and maximal expiratory flow at 50 per cent of the FVC) was found $\geq$ 1 year after the first report of current non-tobacco smoking. The estimated decrement in FEV_1 due to continuing non-tobacco cigarette smoking was 142 mL (or approximately 5 per cent of the average FEV_1 level in non-smokers), which was twice as large as the estimated decrement due to current tobacco smoking (68 mL). The effects of smoking non-tobacco and tobacco cigarettes were not additive. These findings in a community sample suggest that marijuana smoking, particularly if continued over several years, has a significant deleterious effect on chronic respiratory symptoms and ventilatory function that is at least as great as, or greater in magnitude than, the effect of regular cigarette smoking. It is also noteworthy that significant detrimental effects on respiratory symptoms and lung function were evident even though the average consumption of marijuana cigarettes was less than one per day.

The possible role of daily smoking of marijuana in the development of chronic obstructive pulmonary disease was also assessed by Tashkin and colleagues (1997), who evaluated the effect of habitual use of marijuana with or without tobacco on the age-related change in lung function (measured as FEV_1) in comparison with the effect of non-smoking and regular tobacco smoking. A convenience sample of 394 healthy young Caucasian adults (68 per cent males; mean age 33 ± 6 [SD] years), including, at study entry, 131 heavy, habitual smokers of marijuana alone, 112 smokers of marijuana plus tobacco, 65 regular smokers of tobacco alone and 86 non-smokers of either substance, were recruited from the greater Los Angeles community. FEV_1 was measured at study entry in all participants and in 255 of the 394 subjects (65 per cent) on up to six additional occasions at intervals of ± 1 year (mean 1.7 ± 1.1 [SD] year) over a period of eight years; the mean interval from first to last visit was 4.9 ± 2.0 years. Random effects models were used to estimate mean rates of decline in FEV_1 and to compare these rates between smoking groups. Males showed a significant effect of tobacco, but not marijuana, on FEV_1 decline ($p < 0.05$). Among women, marijuana smoking was not associated with greater declines in FEV_1 than non-smoking. In neither men nor women was there an additive effect of marijuana and tobacco or a significant relationship between the number of marijuana joints smoked per day and the rate of decline in FEV_1. These authors concluded that regular tobacco, but not marijuana, smoking is associated with greater annual rates of decline in lung function than non-smoking. These findings do not support an association between regular marijuana smoking and chronic obstructive pulmonary disease, but do not exclude the possibility of other adverse respiratory effects.

The reason for the discrepancy between the results of the two longitudinal studies, one conducted in Los Angeles (Matthias, Tashkin et al., 1997) and the other in Tucson (Sherrill, Krzyzanowski et al., 1991), is unclear. One reason might be due to sampling differences, since the randomly selected Tucson sample was more likely to be representative of the marijuana-smoking population as a whole than the Los Angeles

convenience sample which may have selectively underrecruited "sicker" smokers. Other possible reasons for these discrepant findings include differences in environmental or occupational exposures, concomitant substance abuse (aside from tobacco — such as crack cocaine, phencyclidine or heroin), intensity and continuity of marijuana smoking and other host characteristics, such as allergy and concomitant illness. With regard to possible confounding by differences in intensity and/or continuity of marijuana use, it is noteworthy that the marijuana smokers in the Los Angeles study were particularly heavy current users (mean of over three joints per day); they reported heavy lifetime cumulative use (mean of 45 to 56 joint-years, defined as the number of joints *per day* times the number of years smoked); and most (82 per cent of MTS and 73 per cent of MS) continued to smoke marijuana during the entire follow-up period (Matthias, Tashkin et al., 1997). In contrast, the marijuana smokers in the Tucson cohort were much lighter smokers (< 1 joint per day, on the average) and reported a much lower lifetime intensity of use (mean of 8.3 marijuana joint-years, when calculated as the number of joints *per day* times the number of years smoked) (Sherrill, Krzyzanowski et al., 1991). Although the authors do not specify the continuity of marijuana use in their cohort of marijuana users, continuing or quitting marijuana smoking did not influence the decrements in lung function estimated from their model. Thus, differences in current and lifetime amount of marijuana use or in continuity of use during the course of follow-up do not appear to account for the discrepant results of the two studies. One would not expect the more intense and prolonged use among the Los Angeles marijuana smokers to have resulted in the much *lower* rate of decline in FEV_1 relative to non-smoking (and even tobacco smoking) than that which was observed in the Tucson study.

As part of a larger study examining the effects of cannabis on female reproductive function, 15 healthy women who smoked an average of 1.7 ($\pm$ 1.4 SD) marijuana cigarettes per day for a mean of 10.5 ± 3.7 years underwent pulmonary function testing, including measurement of the single-breath diffusing capacity of the lung (D_LCO) in 12 of the 15 subjects (Tilles, Goldenheim et al., 1986). Nine of the total group of 15 marijuana smokers also smoked tobacco, whereas only six were smokers of marijuana only. Results were compared with those obtained in 27 non-smoking and 26 tobacco-smoking women. No abnormalities in forced expiratory flow rates or lung volumes were observed in this small group of marijuana smokers, irrespective of concomitant tobacco smoking. D_LCO in the marijuana-only smokers (n = 5) was similar (87 ± 18 per cent predicted) to that in the non-smoking controls (92 ± 11 per cent predicted), whereas the D_LCO of the tobacco-only smokers was reduced (80 ± 7 per cent predicted). The D_LCO of the combined smokers of marijuana plus tobacco (n = 7) was significantly reduced (65 ± 17 per cent predicted) in comparison not only with the non-smoking control group but also with the tobacco-only smoking group. The authors indicated that these results suggest that heavy marijuana smoking may have an additive effect to that of tobacco smoking on the gas exchange surface of the lung. However, caution is required in interpreting the results of this study because of the very small number of smokers of both marijuana and tobacco who were examined (n = 5). Moreover, in the much larger sample of marijuana plus tobacco smokers (n = 135) studied by Tashkin et al. (1987), no such additive effect of marijuana and tobacco smoking on D_LCO was observed.

Previous data suggest that regular tobacco smoking may lead to non-specific airways hyper-responsiveness (AHR) independent of effects on airways obstruction, possibly due to tobacco-related bronchial inflammation. AHR is felt to be a risk factor predisposing some smokers to develop COPD. Since marijuana smoke contains respiratory irritants that elicit cough and produce histopathologic alterations (including inflammation) in bronchial mucosa, Tashkin et al. (1993) examined the effect of habitual smoking of marijuana and/or other smoked substances (tobacco and cocaine) on AHR in 113 marijuana-only smokers, 61 tobacco-only smokers, 76 smokers of marijuana plus tobacco and 102 non-smokers participating in an on-going cohort study of the pulmonary effects of smoking illicit substances. Subjects underwent methacholine inhalation challenge testing; positive responses were defined by declines in FEV_1 of ≥ 20 per cent or ≥ 10 per cent from postdiluent control values after five inhalations of each concentration of methacholine (1 to 25 mg/mL). Although no significant differences were found in prevalence of positive responses to methacholine between non-smokers and smokers of marijuana alone (chi square), logistic regression revealed statistically significant associations between marijuana smoking and positive responses to some concentrations of methacholine (≤ 10 mg/mL). However, no dose-response relationship was found between AHR (defined by the slope of the methacholine dose-response curve) and either the current intensity or cumulative lifetime amount of marijuana smoking. In addition, no evidence of an additive or potentiating influence of marijuana on the association between tobacco and AHR was demonstrated. These findings suggest that heavy, habitual marijuana smoking has an inconsistent effect on AHR that does not add to or potentiate the effect of tobacco on AHR.

Tashkin et al. (1997) attempted to evaluate the impact of continuing or changing smoking status for regular use of marijuana and/or tobacco on chronic respiratory symptoms in their cohort of 446 non-smokers (NS) and habitual smokers (S) of marijuana (M) and/or tobacco (T). For this purpose, they invited participants in this longitudinal study to undergo repeated administration of a detailed drug use and respiratory questionnaire at intervals of ≥ 1 year over a mean total span of 9.8 years. Follow-up questionnaires were administered to 68 per cent of the study sample at least once. Comparisons between responses to the first and last questionnaire were averaged across subjects within each smoking category as defined at study entry (1) for those whose smoking status did not change (MS, n = 73; MTS, n = 41; TS, n = 40; and NS, n = 77) and (2) for those whose smoking status changed (MS → NS, n = 28; MTS → MS, n = 12; MTS → NS, n = 8; MTS → TS, n = 12; TS → NS, n = 10). Although, in general, prevalence of symptoms declined slightly from first to last visit among those whose smoking status did not change, these differences were not statistically significant (McNemar's; p > 0.05). In contrast, substantial declines in symptom prevalence were noted among MS, MTS and TS whose smoking status changed to NS, but not among MTS whose status changed to MS or TS. These findings indicate that continuing smoking of marijuana and/or tobacco is associated with persistence of symptoms of chronic bronchitis, while complete cessation of smoking is accompanied by substantial declines in symptoms.

EFFECTS OF CANNABIS ON CARBON MONOXIDE ABSORPTION IN THE LUNG

Pulmonary absorption of carbon monoxide (CO) from inhaled tobacco or marijuana smoke causes an elevation in blood carboxyhemoglobin (COHb) levels. Elevated blood levels of COHb have important adverse health effects due to the associated impairment in tissue oxidation. Wu et al. (1988) observed that the boost in blood COHb saturation within two minutes of completion of smoking a single marijuana cigarette (840 mg, 0.004 per cent THC) was more than four times greater than the boost in blood COHb measured within two minutes of smoking a single tobacco cigarette (1,010 mg) ($p < 0.01$). Tashkin et al. (1991) subsequently determined that the major factor responsible for the greater COHb boost immediately after smoking marijuana compared to tobacco was the approximately fourfold longer duration of breath holding associated with marijuana, compared to tobacco, cigarette smoking. The physiological consequences of the marked boost in COHb after a single marijuana cigarette include interference with diffusion of oxygen into pulmonary capillary blood, a reduction in the oxygen-carrying capacity of the blood and impairment in release of oxygen from hemoglobin in the tissues. Because THC causes acute dose-related increases

in heart rate and, therefore, in myocardial oxygen requirements, the marked boost in COHb immediately after smoking marijuana could lead to a critical imbalance between reduced myocardial oxygen supply and increased oxygen demand, especially in individuals with underlying coronary artery disease.

In contrast to the considerably greater *acute* effect of smoking marijuana compared to tobacco on pulmonary CO absorption, the *chronic* impact of even heavy habitual marijuana smoking on blood COHb levels appears to be relatively modest compared to the effect of regular tobacco smoking. Mean blood COHb levels of habitual smokers of marijuana measured > 7 hours after marijuana was last smoked (in 78 per cent of the subjects) (1.71 ± 0.07 [SEM] per cent) were only 36.4 per cent of the mean COHb levels of regular smokers of tobacco alone (4.69 ± 0.26 per cent) and only 40 per cent higher than the COHb levels of non-smokers (1.22 ± 0.06 per cent), compared to 3.8-fold higher levels in the tobacco smokers (Tashkin, Wu & Djahed, 1988). Since the half-life of CO clearance from the body is only four hours, the latter results are probably due to the markedly lower frequency of marijuana smoking than tobacco smoking and the resultant longer average time interval since marijuana (as compared to tobacco) was last smoked prior to blood sampling for COHb. Thus, in comparison with the relatively short average interval between the smoking of consecutive tobacco cigarettes during the waking hours (approximately 1.0 to 1.5 hours), more time is generally available for CO generated by marijuana smoking to be cleared from the circulating blood in the much longer interval between the smoking of consecutive marijuana cigarettes. The significantly lower baseline (presmoking) COHb levels in the blood of habitual smokers of marijuana-only compared to smokers of tobacco implies a lower *chronic* cardiovascular risk than is incurred by regular tobacco smokers. However, because baseline levels of COHb are still moderately elevated in marijuana-only smokers compared to non-smokers, some chronically increased risk of marijuana smoking due to carbon monoxide-related interference with tissue oxygenation might still be present. Furthermore, there may also be long-term adverse effects due to repeated, relatively large boosts in COHb immediately after smoking each marijuana cigarette.

EFFECTS OF CANNABIS ON CONTROL OF BREATHING

Because THC has potent psychophysiologic properties, several investigators have studied its effects on central ventilatory drive with conflicting results. Ventilatory responses to rebreathing carbon dioxide (CO_2) have been shown by different workers to decrease (Bellville, Swanson & Aqleh, 1975), increase (Zwillich, Doekel et al., 1978) or not change (Vachon, Fitzgerald et al., 1973) acutely after smoking marijuana, and one study demonstrated a stimulant effect of marijuana on metabolism. A recent, more detailed study of control of breathing responses to smoking marijuana of varying potency (0 to 27 mg THC) has failed to reveal any acute effect of marijuana on central or peripheral ventilatory drive or on metabolic rate in habitual marijuana smokers (Wu, Wright et al., 1992).

EFFECTS OF CANNABIS USE ON LUNG HISTOPATHOLOGY

Morris (1985) reported histopathological changes in the lungs of 13 known marijuana smokers, 15 to 40 years of age, all of whom died suddenly and, with one exception, violently and were free of cardiac disease, pulmonary infection or malignancy. Unfortunately, no information was available concerning the extent of use of marijuana, tobacco or other drugs. The major findings included focal or diffuse, light to heavy infiltrations of heavily pigmented alveolar macrophages within the alveolar spaces. Focal areas of fibrosis were also noted within alveolar walls and around small bronchi in areas of heavy infiltration with alveolar macrophages. In nearly all cases, there was also evidence of ulceration of the mucosal epithelium of small bronchi and bronchioles. Although the contribution of tobacco smoking to these histological alterations could not be ascertained, it is noteworthy that one of

the cases, a 15-year-old boy who had smoked marijuana for two years, did not smoke tobacco. This case showed extensive focal infiltration of heavily pigmented macrophages within and around bronchioles and focal early fibrosis, despite a relatively short duration of smoking marijuana alone. Clearly, additional autopsy studies of known smokers of cannabis alone and with other substances are needed to define the effects of cannabis on lung pathology better.

EFFECTS OF CANNABIS USE ON MICROSCOPIC AND VISUAL EVIDENCE OF AIRWAY INJURY

Studies conducted at UCLA as part of an ongoing project to evaluate the pulmonary effects of habitual use of marijuana (Tashkin, Coulson et al., 1987) used flexible fibre optic bronchoscopy (FFB) to systematically evaluate the gross and histopathologic features of the lower respiratory tract in study participants who volunteered to undergo FFB. Subjects in whom FFB was performed included habitual, heavy smokers of marijuana alone (MS; n = 30) and with tobacco (MTS; n = 17), smokers of tobacco only (TS; n = 15) and non-smokers (NS; n = 11); most of these subjects did not report significant respiratory symptoms (Tashkin, Fligiel et al., 1990). During FFB, mucosa from the primary carina and randomly selected secondary and tertiary carinae of the right middle or lower lobe was biopsied and processed for light microscopy (Gong, Fligiel et al., 1987). The following histopathologic features of the bronchial epithelial biopsies were assessed by a single pathologist (who was unaware of the subject's smoking category) using the criteria of Auerbach and colleagues (1957; 1961): basal cell hyperplasia; stratification; squamous metaplasia; goblet cell hyperplasia; cellular disorganization; nuclear variation; mitotic figures; increased nuclear-to-cytoplasmic ratio; inflammation; and basement membrane thickening. Biopsies revealed that habitual smoking of marijuana alone (an average of 3 to 4 joints per day) caused a greater frequency and severity of abnormalities for most of the epithelial features examined compared to the changes noted in the non-smokers and at least as extensive abnormalities as those observed in the smokers of tobacco alone (22 cigarettes per day), despite the marked disparity between the daily number of marijuana vs. tobacco cigarettes consumed. These histopathological abnormalities included basal cell hyperplasia, stratification, goblet cell metaplasia, increased nuclear-to-cytoplasmic ratio and basement membrane thickening. In a larger sample of marijuana and/or tobacco smokers (40 MS, 44 MTS, 31 TS and 53 NS) from the same study (Fligiel, Roth et al., 1997), all of the above histopathologic abnormalities were more frequently observed in the marijuana-only smokers than in the non-smokers. Moreover, for nearly all histologic features examined, abnormalities were noted more frequently in the combined smokers of marijuana plus tobacco than in smokers of either substance alone, suggesting additive effects of marijuana and tobacco on bronchial epithelial histopathology.

To further assess possible cannabis-induced airway inflammation, Roth et al. (1998) performed videobronchoscopy and bronchial mucosal biopsies in 40 healthy subjects, aged 20 to 49 years, of whom 10 were non-smokers, 10 habitually smoked marijuana alone, 10 regularly smoked tobacco alone and 10 smoked both marijuana and tobacco on a regular basis. Videotapes were scored in a blinded manner for central airway erythema, edema and secretions using a modified bronchitis index. Scores for these visual features of bronchitis were significantly higher in MS, TS and MTS than in NS. Mucosal biopsies from the same subjects were examined for the presence of vascular hyperplasia, submucosal edema, inflammatory cell infiltrates and goblet cell hyperplasia as pathologic correlates of the visual endoscopic findings. Biopsies from 97 per cent of smokers, but from none of the non-smokers, were positive for at least two of these features. These findings suggest that regular smoking of marijuana by young adults is associated with significant airway injury that is similar in frequency, type and magnitude to that noted in the lungs of tobacco smokers.

The above findings are important for several reasons. First, all the marijuana smokers were young adults, most of whom had no respiratory symptoms or significant lung function abnormality. These observations suggest that habitual marijuana can cause potentially serious airway pathology at a relatively early age despite the absence of any clinical or physiologic evidence of disease. Second, the prevalence and extent of the histopathologic abnormalities noted in the marijuana-only and tobacco-only smokers were comparable, suggesting that habitual marijuana smoking may be at least as damaging to the epithelium of the central airways as the smoking of tobacco. This observation is somewhat surprising because of the far smaller daily number of marijuana joints smoked by the marijuana-only smokers (three to four joints) than the daily number of tobacco cigarettes smoked by the tobacco-only smokers (> 20), suggesting a more damaging effect of marijuana than tobacco per cigarette smoked. Third, the more frequent abnormalities noted in the combined smokers of marijuana and tobacco suggests an additive effect of the two substances on airway injury, consistent with earlier observations of Tennant (1980) in heavy smokers of hashish and/or tobacco. It is of interest, however, that the heavy hashish smokers examined by Tennant were generally symptomatic and many had lung function abnormality, in contrast to the smokers of Tashkin et al. (1990), most of whom were asymptomatic with normal lung function. Finally, some of the changes that were noted in the bronchial epithelium of smokers of marijuana with or without tobacco, particularly squamous metaplasia, cellular disorganization, nuclear variation, mitotic figures and increased nuclear-to-cytoplasmic ratio, may be considered to be precursors of subsequent bronchogenic carcinoma. These findings support the concept that habitual smoking of marijuana may be an important risk factor for the subsequent development of respiratory tract malignancy.

It is also of interest that the studies of marijuana-induced pulmonary histopathologic abnormalities in humans yielded results somewhat different from those of animal studies. The principal changes noted in human subjects consisted of evidence of epithelial injury in the central airways (trachea and major bronchi) (Gong, Fligiel et al., 1987; Fligiel, Roth et al., 1997; Tennant, 1980), whereas the animal studies (Fleischman, Baker & Rosenkrantz, 1979; Fleischman, Hayden et al., 1975; Roy, Magnan-Lapointe et al., 1976) showed mainly small-airway alterations with less extensive changes in the larger airways than noted in humans. These differences could be due, at least in part, to the technical limitations of fibre optic bronchoscopy, which make it difficult to sample tissue from the peripheral airways of human volunteers.

EFFECTS OF CANNABIS USE ON ALVEOLAR CYTOLOGY, ALVEOLAR MACROPHAGE STRUCTURE AND ALVEOLAR CELL FUNCTION

Pulmonary alveolar macrophages (PAMs) are the principal cells in the peripheral air spaces of the lung and key elements in the lung's immune defence system. Examination of the cells recovered from the distal air spaces of the lung by bronchial alveolar lavage (BAL) at the time of bronchoscopy in smokers of marijuana and/or tobacco and non-smokers revealed an increase in the number of PAMs from all smoking groups compared with non-smokers (Barbers, Gong et al., 1987). The increased numbers of PAMs from the marijuana smokers were independent of concomitant tobacco smoking, although an additive effect of marijuana and tobacco was suggested. Subsequent studies in which the replication of PAMs was determined by measuring the incorporation of [^{3}]thymidine into the DNA of dividing cells suggested that the major mechanism of the accumulation of PAMs in the alveoli of smokers of marijuana and/or tobacco was *in situ* replication rather than recruitment from the circulation (Barbers, Evans et al., 1991). The observed increases in PAMs probably represent an inflammatory response to smoking-induced lung injury, implying an adverse effect of marijuana on the peripheral air spaces of the lung that is independent of and additive to that of tobacco.

Examination of PAMs obtained from the same subjects by transmission electron microscopy has revealed dramatic ultrastructural abnormalities in the PAMs of smokers of marijuana and/or tobacco, consisting of larger and more complex cytoplasmic inclusions than in the PAMs of non-smokers (Beals, Fligiel et al., 1989; abstract). In addition, definite ultrastructural differences were noted between the PAMs of marijuana-only and tobacco-only smokers, implying that exposure to marijuana or tobacco could lead to differences in the functional activity of these important cells.

Sherman and co-workers (Sherman, Campbell et al., 1991) assessed the effect of marijuana smoking on the antimicrobial activity of PAMs by measuring the ability of PAMs obtained from non-smokers and smokers of marijuana and/or tobacco to phagocytose (ingest) and destroy *Candida albicans* and to produce superoxide anion (O_2^-) under both basal and stimulated conditions. O_2^- production (a measure of the cellular respiratory burst) was studied because of its possible role in microbial killing. Findings from these studies indicated that marijuana smoking did not alter the phagocytic behavior or respiratory burst of human PAMs, but that it did impair the ability of these cells to destroy ingested *Candida albicans*. These results contrasted with the effects of tobacco smoking that also impaired the fungicidal activity of PAMs but increased their respiratory burst. The mechanism(s) for smoking-induced defect in microbial killing may differ between marijuana and tobacco smokers and requires further study. The clinical implications of these findings are that habitual marijuana smoking, like regular tobacco smoking, diminishes the capacity of the lungs to kill invading micro-organisms, thus decreasing resistance to pulmonary infection. Furthermore, since oxidants, including O_2^-, released from PAMs are capable of causing lung damage, the observation that the PAMs of marijuana-only smokers did not produce increased amounts of O_2^- when compared to PAMs of non-smokers, in contrast to the substantially higher levels of O_2^- released by the PAMs of tobacco smokers, may account for the absence of abnormalities in small airway function and alveolar diffusing capacity in marijuana-only smokers, in contrast to the presence of such findings in smokers of tobacco, with or without marijuana (Sherman, Campbell et al., 1991; Sherman, Roth et al., 1991).

Baldwin et al. (1997) recently studied the function of alveolar macrophages obtained by bronchoalveolar lavage from the lungs of healthy non-smokers (n = 22) and habitual smokers of marijuana alone (n = 10) or tobacco alone (n = 11). Alveolar macrophages recovered from marijuana-only, but not tobacco-only, smokers were deficient in their ability both to phagocytose and to kill *Staphylococcus aureus,* as well as in their ability to kill tumor target cells. Studies using N^G-monomethyl-L-arginine monoacetate, an inhibitor of nitric oxide synthase, suggested that alveolar macrophages from marijuana smokers, unlike those from non-smokers and tobacco smokers, were unable to use nitric oxide as an antibacterial effector molecule. Moreover, alveolar macrophages from marijuana smokers, but not tobacco smokers, when stimulated with lipopolysaccharide, produced subnormal amounts of certain pro-inflammatory cytokines (tumor necrosis factor-α, granulocyte-macrophage colony stimulating factor and interleukin-6), which may play a role in the inflammatory response to bacterial infection.

The above-cited findings indicate that frequent marijuana smoking can cause airway injury, lung inflammation and impaired pulmonary defences against infection that may predispose to clinically important lung disease. This possibility is supported by an epidemiologic study that systematically reviewed medical records to assess the real health consequences of marijuana, controlling for the effects of tobacco, alcohol and sociodemographic factors (Polen, Sidney et al., 1993). The medical experience of daily or near-daily marijuana smokers who never smoked tobacco (n = 452) was compared with that of a demographically similar group of non-smokers of either substance (n = 450). After adjustment for sex, age, race, education, marital status and alcohol consumption, frequent marijuana smokers had small increased risks of outpatient visits for respiratory illness (relative risk [RR] = 1.19; 95 per cent confidence interval [CI] = 1.01, 1.41), injuries (RR = 1.32; CI = 1.10, 1.57), and other types of illnesses (RR = 1.09; CI = 1.02, 1.16) compared with non-smokers. Thus, these findings demonstrate that frequent marijuana smoking is a significant independent risk factor for the development of respiratory illness, as well as injuries and other medical problems.

The impairment in host defences suggested by the findings that alveolar macrophages from the lungs of healthy, habitual marijuana smokers were suppressed in their ability to kill fungal and bacterial organisms and to release pro-inflammatory cytokines raises the possibility of potentially serious health consequences in patients with pre-existing immune deficits due to AIDS, organ transplantation (receiving immunosuppressive therapy to prevent rejection of the transplant) or cancer (receiving immunosuppressive chemotherapy). The latter possibility is supported by reports of fungal and bacterial pneumonias in patients with AIDS or organ transplantation who used marijuana (Caiaffa, Vlahov et al., 1994; Denning, Follansbee et al., 1991). Moreover, among HIV-positive individuals, active marijuana use has been found to be a significant risk factor for rapid progression from HIV infection to AIDS and acquisition of opportunistic infections and/or Kaposi's sarcoma (Newell, Mansell et al., 1985; Tindall, Philpot et al., 1988).

EFFECTS OF CANNABIS ON SUBPOPULATIONS OF LYMPHOCYTES OBTAINED BY BRONCHOALVEOLAR LAVAGE

Wallace et al. (1994) examined the effect of heavy, habitual use of marijuana and/or tobacco on lymphocyte subpopulation profiles in bronchoalveolar lavage (BAL) fluid obtained from 19 heavy, habitual marijuana smokers (MS), 9 marijuana and tobacco smokers (MTS), 14 tobacco-only smokers (TS) and 14 non-smokers (NS). Marijuana use was associated with increased numbers of alveolar macrophages but no differences in the total numbers of lymphocytes or neutrophils in BAL fluid, whereas tobacco use was associated with increases in the numbers of all three types of inflammatory cells. Moreover, the bronchoalveolar T-lymphocyte phenotypic profiles of marijuana users differed from the profiles of tobacco smokers: in marijuana smokers, the concentration of CD4 cells was similar to that of non-smokers, while CD8 cell numbers were decreased, whereas, in tobacco smokers, lower percentages of CD4 lymphocytes and higher concentrations of CD8 cells with reduced CD4/CD8 cell ratios were found. The latter immunoregulatory abnormalities may disturb pulmonary defence mechanisms and thereby predispose to malignancy and infection. On the other hand, the lymphocyte subpopulation alterations exhibited by the tobacco smokers were not apparent in the marijuana users or were too small to be detected in the small sample of subjects examined. In peripheral blood, marijuana, but not tobacco, use was associated with significantly higher percentages of CD4 cells, lower percentages of CD8 cells and higher CD4/CD8 ratios. In a previous study (Wallace, Tashkin et al., 1988), the same authors found a suppressive effect of tobacco, but not marijuana, on mitogen responsiveness of peripheral blood lymphocytes. Taken together, these findings suggest that marijuana and tobacco have different effects on lower respiratory tract and circulating immunoregulatory T-lymphocyte subpopulations, as well as peripheral blood lymphocyte function.

EFFECTS OF CANNABIS ON BRONCHIAL CYTOLOGY

Roby and colleagues (1991) investigated the cytologic effects of marijuana smoking on the bronchial airways from three-day pooled expectorated sputum processed using conventional cytopathologic techniques and analysed microscopically using quantitative methodology, as well as qualitative interpretation. Subjects consisted of 25 habitual smokers of marijuana only for at least two years and age-matched (mean age 28 years) non-marijuana controls, including 25 regular smokers of tobacco only and 25 non-smokers. In quantitative comparisons, marijuana smokers had significantly higher levels of macrophages, neutrophils, columnar epithelial cells, metaplastic cells and mucous spirals than non-smokers ($p < 0.0001$). Marijuana smokers scored slightly lower on all cytomorphic components than tobacco smokers. In qualitative comparisons, marijuana smokers had significantly elevated levels of eosinophils, reactive columnar cells, benign bronchial hyperplasia and purse cells. Purse cells are large, flat squamous epithelial cells with a large cytoplasmic vacuole; Canti (1988) believes that these cells are usually associated with malignancy but can occur in inflammatory conditions. On the average, more marijuana smokers exhibited increased levels of all these cells than did either tobacco smokers or non-smokers. On the other hand, dysplastic cells, which are considered to be a premalignant transformation of the normal bronchial mucosa, were found in only one of the marijuana smokers (4 per cent) and three of the tobacco smokers (12 per cent), and all four of these cases exhibited only mild dysplasia. These cytomorphic findings in expectorated sputum are consistent with qualitatively and quantitatively similar reactive changes in the tracheobronchial mucosa to chronic irritation from inhaled marijuana or tobacco smoke. As well, they complement the results of the histopathologic studies of tracheobronchial epithelium of non-smokers and smokers of marijuana or tobacco cited above (Fligiel, Roth, 1997; Gong, Fligiel et al., 1987). Previous data suggest that about 15 per cent of tobacco cigarette smokers with moderate dysplasia show progression to lung cancer (Greenberg, Hunter et al., 1986). The relatively low frequency and mild severity of dysplasia in this small sample of young smokers of either marijuana or tobacco neither support nor negate a causal relationship between marijuana smoking and lung cancer. More data are needed to determine the rates of progression or reversibility of bronchial dysplasia in relation to marijuana use.

EFFECTS OF CANNABIS ON RESPIRATORY CARCINOGENESIS

The following newer evidence (since 1982) supplements older data in support of the concept that habitual smoking of marijuana may be an important risk factor for the development of respiratory tract malignancy.

- The above-cited studies demonstrating a high prevalence of extensive histopathologic abnormalities in the bronchial epithelium of young, heavy habitual smokers of marijuana (with or without tobacco) (Fligiel, Roth et al., 1997; Gong, Fligiel et al., 1987) supplement findings from earlier studies of extensive metaplastic and dysplastic changes in the tracheal mucosa of heavy smokers of hashish (Henderson, Tennant & Guerry, 1972; Tennant, 1980) that may be precursors of bronchogenic carcinoma. Moreover, these changes appear to be additive to those induced by concomitant tobacco smoking, thereby potentially magnifying the risk of respiratory tract malignancy.

- The tar phase of marijuana smoke, as already noted, contains many of the same carcinogenic compounds contained in tobacco smoke, including nitrosamines, reactive aldehydes and up to a 50 per cent higher concentration of carcinogenic polycyclic hydrocarbons (PAHs), including benz[α]pyrene (Hoffmann, Brunnemann et al., 1975). Benz[α]pyrene, which has recently been shown to promote mutations in the p53 oncogene (Dinissenko, Pao et al., 1996), is believed to play an important role in human cancer.

- Smoking of one marijuana cigarette led to the deposition in the lower respiratory tract of a fourfold greater quantity of insoluble smoke particulates (tar) than did smoking a filtered tobacco cigarette of comparable weight (Wu, Tashkin et al., 1988). The higher content of carcinogenic PAHs in marijuana tar and the relatively greater deposition of marijuana tar

in the lung act together to amplify exposure of the marijuana smoker to the carcinogens in the tar phase, thus potentially increasing the risk of respiratory tract carcinogenesis. The markedly increased respiratory deposition of tar during marijuana, compared to tobacco, smoking was due partly to the reduced filtering capacity of the marijuana cigarette (producing a relatively greater tar yield) and partly to differences in smoking topography for the two types of cigarettes, especially the fourfold greater breath holding time after inhaling marijuana than tobacco smoke (Tashkin, Gliederer et al., 1991). These differences in cigarette filtration and smoking topography, leading to the delivery of more particulates and gaseous irritants to the respiratory tract in the smoke from marijuana than the smoke from tobacco, may account for the previously noted observations that smokers of only three to four marijuana joints a day have a frequency of chronic respiratory symptoms and tracheobronchial histopathology similar to that of smokers of ≥ 20 tobacco cigarettes a day.

- Preliminary findings suggest that marijuana smoke activates cytochrome P4501A1 (CYP1A1), the enzyme primarily responsible for converting PAHs, such as benz[α]pyrene, into active carcinogens (Marques-Magallanes, Taskin et al., 1997). PAHs in tar are known to be capable themselves of inducing the CYP1A1 enzyme through a pathway that involves binding to an aryl hydrocarbon receptor in the cell which then becomes complexed to a nuclear transporter protein. This complex is translocated into the cell nucleus where promoter sequences on DNA are activated and the gene that codes for the CYP1A1 enzyme is transcribed. Recent studies have shown that bronchial epithelial cells in biopsies from marijuana smokers stain strongly for the antibody to the CYP1A1 enzyme, while staining is absent or only weak in biopsies from non-smokers, implying that regular exposure to marijuana smoke induces the CYP1A1 enzyme *in vivo* (Marques-Magallanes,

Tashkin et al., 1997). Incubation of liver cells *in vitro* with tar from marijuana smoke is also capable of activating the CYP1A1 enzyme.

- Bronchial immunohistology revealed overexpression of molecular markers of lung tumor progression in smokers of marijuana (Barsky, Roth et al., 1998).

- Alveolar macrophages from marijuana-only smokers have reduced ability to kill tumor cell targets (Baldwin, Tashkin et al., 1997).

- THC inhibits the development of anti-tumor immunity both *in vitro* and *in vivo*. Anti-tumor immunity depends on the ability of antigen-presenting dendritic cells to stimulate the proliferation of T lymphocytes that selectively recognize and destroy tumor cells, but not normal cells. In *in vitro* studies in which dendritic cells and T cells were incubated in the presence or absence of THC, THC suppressed T cell proliferation in a dose-dependent manner (Roth, Zhu et al., 1997). At the same time, THC inhibited the release of protective pro-inflammatory cytokines (interferon-γ) that may help mediate the T-cell proliferative response.

- Pretreatment of mice with THC for two weeks prior to implanting Lewis lung cancer cells (a non-small-cell immunogenic carcinoma) into the animals caused larger, faster-growing tumors. THC-stimulated enhanced growth of these tumors was correlated with the production by cells associated with the tumor of decreased amounts of pro-inflammatory cytokines (e.g., interferon-γ) and increased amounts of immunosuppressive cytokines (e.g., transforming growth factor-b and interleukin-10) (Zhu, Stolina et al., 1998). These results suggest that THC impairs the development of anti-tumor immunity *in vivo* and parallels the findings of THC-related inhibition of anti-tumor immunity in the *in vitro* studies cited above.

- Several cases have been reported of respiratory tract malignancy (tongue, tonsil, lip, pyriform sinus, paranasal sinus, larynx, lung) in relatively young (age < 40 years) habitual marijuana smokers (Donald, 1991; Ferguson, Hasson & Walker, 1989; Taylor, 1988). Of particular interest is the finding by Taylor that of the 10 patients < 40 years of age who were identified from a total pool of 887 patients of all ages with upper or lower respiratory tract cancer, 7 were heavy or regular users of marijuana and 1 probably used marijuana. Ferguson and colleagues reported the development of metastatic epidermoid carcinoma of the lung in a 27-year-old Jamaican who had smoked 20 joints of marijuana per day for longer than 16 years; this patient also admitted to occasional cocaine use and tobacco smoking, but his total tobacco exposure was equivalent to ≤ 10 pack-years. Although these reports implicate marijuana smoking as a possible cause of cancer of the upper aerodigestive tract, as well as of the lower respiratory tract, most of the patients were exposed to other risk factors, namely tobacco and/or alcohol. On the other hand, 1 of the 6 patients reported by Donald and 2 of the 10 reported by Taylor did not use tobacco or alcohol. Moreover, the development of respiratory tract cancers in young individuals is rare, even in the presence of other etiologic factors, such as regular tobacco smoking and alcohol consumption, thus pointing to marijuana as a potentially important cause of respiratory tract cancer, especially in younger individuals. In further support of this view is the report of two additional cases of squamous cell carcinoma of the tongue in men (ages 37 and 52 years) who chronically smoked marijuana but had no other identifiable risk factors (Caplan & Brigham, 1990). It is also possible that when other risk factors, such as tobacco, are present, an effect of marijuana on respiratory tract carcinogenesis may be additive to that of the other factor(s). These case-series reports suggest that marijuana may play a role in the development of human respiratory cancer. Without a control group, however, the effect of marijuana use on cancer risk cannot be estimated, nor can the potentially confounding effect of tobacco and other risk factors be controlled.

- The only epidemiologic study that examined an association between marijuana and cancer was recently published by Sidney et al. (1997). These investigators at Kaiser Permanente in Northern California followed a cohort of 65,000 health plan members who were 15 to 49 years of age in 1979–85, at which time they completed self-administered questionnaires about marijuana use and other health-related factors. This cohort was followed for detection of the development of new cancers until 1993. Over this period of time, 182 tobacco-related cancers were detected, of which 97 were lung malignancies. No effects of lifetime or current marijuana use on the risk of these cancers was found. The major limitation of this study is that those subjects who are likely to have been heavy or long-term users of marijuana were probably not followed long enough to detect an effect on cancer risk since the peak incidence of respiratory cancer occurs in later life. Furthermore, despite the large cohort size, there may not have been a sufficient number of heavy and/or long-term marijuana smokers to observe an effect. In addition, the following points need to be made with respect to the Sidney et al. study: (1) the average age at follow-up was only 43 years, much too young to expect an increased rate of cancers; (2) deaths may have been missed among cohort members who left the state; and (3) cigarette smoking and alcohol use were only modestly associated with premature mortality in the cohort, a fact probably related to the relatively young age of the cohort.

Despite the lack of compelling epidemiologic evidence to date, findings from the biochemical, cellular, immunologic, genetic, tissue and animal studies cited above provide a biologically plausible basis for the hypothesis that marijuana is a risk factor for human cancer. What is required to address this hypothesis more convincingly is a population-based case-control study of sufficiently large numbers of lung cancer cases and cases of upper aerodigestive tumors (cancers of the oral cavity and pharynx, larynx and esophagus), as well as non-cancer controls, to demonstrate a statistically significant association, if one exists. Because of the long period of time required for induction of human carcinomas (latency period) and the infrequent use of marijuana in the general U.S. population prior to 1966, no adequately powered epidemiologic studies have as yet examined the association between marijuana and cancer. However, at the present time, epidemiologic investigation of this association may have become more feasible. Approximately 30 years have elapsed since the start of widespread marijuana use in the United States among teenagers and young adults, who are currently reaching an age when respiratory cancers are more common. Any epidemiologic assessment of the risk of marijuana smokers for respiratory cancer must take into account the confounding influence of concomitant use of other substances, including tobacco and alcohol. An important obstacle to efforts to study the health effects of marijuana smoking using medical records searches for documentation of cannabis use is the nearly universal failure of physicians to query their patients concerning the use of marijuana (Polen, Sidney et al., 1993; Tashkin, 1993).

One mechanism by which malignancy is believed to be initiated is through formation of covalent adducts between carcinogens and DNA which, in turn, can lead to oncogene activation through point mutations and chromosome alterations (reviewed by Talaska, Schamer et al., 1992). Carcinogen-DNA adducts in human lung tissue have been associated with tobacco smoking (Phillips, Hewer et al., 1988). In a recently reported study, Talaska et al. (1992) failed to find any statistically significant increase in aromatic carcinogen-DNA adducts in the lungs of rhesus monkeys sacrificed seven months after exposure two to seven days per week to marijuana smoke for one year. It is of interest, however, that 15 of 22 adduct measures were highest in the monkeys exposed to ethanol-extracted marijuana and 12 of 22 measures were lowest in the sham-exposed animals, suggesting an abnormal trend at least in the animals treated with modified marijuana. Although this study failed to find that smoking unmodified marijuana increased lung tissue levels of carcinogen-DNA adducts, it is possible that exposures, while relatively intense (equivalent to human consumption of four to five marijuana cigarettes per day), were not of sufficiently long duration to initiate carcinogenesis. Longer-term studies involving exposures to marijuana smoke and its components in a suitable animal model are warranted.

OTHER PULMONARY COMPLICATIONS OF CANNABIS

Marijuana use has been associated with spontaneous pneumothorax and/or pneumomediastinum (Feldman, Sullivan et al., 1993; Mattox, 1976; Miller, Spiekerman & Hepper, 1972), presumably due to the frequent performance of Valsalva manoeuvres during breath holding after deep inhalation of marijuana smoke, leading to rupture of subpleural blebs or alveoli with dissection of air along the vessels and bronchi to the pleural space or mediastinum. An association between tobacco smoking and increased risk of spontaneous pneumothorax has also been noted, presumably due to tobacco-induced lung damage (Bense, Eklung et al., 1987). Contamination of marijuana with *Aspergillus fumigatus* can cause lung disease, as illustrated by case reports of bronchopulmonary aspergillosis (Llamas, Hart & Schneider, 1978) and invasive aspergillosis in immunocompromised smokers (Chusid, Gelfland et al., 1975; Denning, Follansbee et al., 1991; Hamadeh, Ardehali et al., 1988). With regard to the latter complication, it is noteworthy that most illegally obtained marijuana is contaminated with *Aspergillus* species, a ubiquitous fungus (Kagen, Kurup et al., 1983). Such contamination has been shown to cause serious,

invasive fungal infection in marijuana smokers with impaired immunity, particularly individuals with AIDS (Denning, Follansbee et al., 1991). In a report from Puerto Rico, four policemen developed acute pulmonary histoplasmosis in temporal association with the search and destruction of a marijuana patch (Ramirez, 1990). This report raises the possibility that acute pulmonary histoplasmosis may be a hitherto unrecognized hazard of marijuana plant destruction by drug enforcement personnel.

Conclusion

Although further study of the impact of regular marijuana smoking on the lung is certainly warranted, enough evidence has already accumulated to justify counselling by physicians against the smoking of marijuana as a potential risk factor for the development of lung disease. The available evidence also suggests the possibility of a particularly increased risk of infectious pulmonary complications of marijuana smoking in individuals with impaired immunity due to malignancy, cancer chemotherapy, AIDS or other conditions. Additional studies are needed to investigate this possibility, in view of the current interest in medicinal marijuana for the treatment of the wasting syndrome of AIDS and of nausea and vomiting due to cancer chemotherapy (Voth & Schwartz, 1997).

Summary

Worldwide, after tobacco, cannabis is probably the most commonly smoked substance. With the exception of nicotine in tobacco and over 60 cannabinoids in cannabis, the smoke from these two compounds share many of the same respiratory irritants and carcinogens. In fact the tar phase of the smoke of marijuana has about 50 per cent more of some of the carcinogens than a comparable quantity of unfiltered tobacco.

Histopathology

Early animal studies indicated that prolonged high-dose exposure to marijuana smoke could result in parenchymal lung injury. The findings of later experimental studies suggest that high-dose cannabis exposure is associated with the development of bronchiolitis and carries the risk of invasive malignancy such as that produced by tobacco smoke. The histopathological changes occurred mainly in the distal airways and air spaces and included acute and chronic inflammation, fibrosis and alveolar cell hyperplasia. Later prospective investigations undertaken on primates found changes such as bronchiolar squamous metaplasia and peribronchiolar/interstitial fibrosis. The severity of these small airway changes was related to the dose and duration of cannabis exposure. Atypical cell hyperplasia with focal atypia was also found.

In human studies, on the other hand, the principal respiratory damage caused by long-term cannabis smoking is an epithelial injury of the trachea and major bronchi. The difference between the findings in animal and human studies is probably due to the fact that observations in humans are limited to those that can be made by bronchoscopy. Human bronchoscopic studies undertaken on young adults who had few respiratory symptoms found evidence of histological changes in the central airways among heavy cannabis smokers. These changes included basal cell hyperplasia, stratification, goblet cell metaplasia, and basement membrane thickening. The studies were also suggestive of an additive effect of cannabis and tobacco smoking. Further, the histological abnormalities resulting from cannabis consumption were more severe per marijuana cigarette smoked than for tobacco.

Autopsies undertaken on cannabis smokers who had no respiratory symptomatology at time of death also found changes in the form of focal infiltration by pigmented macrophages around bronchioles and within alveolar spaces, and focal fibrosis within alveolar walls. In this study, the relative contribution of tobacco to these changes could not be ascertained with certainty except in one case who had not smoked tobacco.

Immune Defence

The function of alveolar macrophages, key cells in the lung's defence against infection, has been shown to be impaired by cannabis smoke in both animal and human studies. Although animal studies failed to demonstrate a change in macrophage numbers following cannabis smoke exposure, subsequent investigations in humans, comparing non-smokers to cannabis and tobacco smokers, suggested an increase in habitual cannabis smokers. This probably reflects an immunological response to any lung injury induced by cannabis smoke. The effect is independent of tobacco consumption.

Macrophage cells harvested in these human studies have alterations in their morphology, possibly reflecting an impairment in cell function. Residual particles from cannabis smoke in the form of intracytoplasmic inclusions have been found to be cycled between subsequent generations of macrophages as part of the process of cellular turnover. While there is a suggestion in human studies that cannabis smoking did not alter phagocytosis of *Candida albicans* or respiratory burst, it did impair phagocytosis of *Staphylococcus aureus* and destruction of ingested fungi and bacteria. The mechanism of macrophage impairment in fungicidal and bactericidal activity has not been fully elucidated and requires further investigation, although preliminary data suggest that marijuana-related impairment in macrophage production of reactive oxygen species, reactive oxygen intermediates and pro-inflammatory cytokines may be playing a role. The above studies suggest that regular cannabis consumption reduces the respiratory immune response to invading organisms. Further, serious invasive fungal infections as a result of cannabis contamination have been reported among individuals who are immuno-compromised, including a series of patients who were affected by AIDS.

These findings suggest that frequent heavy cannabis consumption over prolonged periods can cause airway injury, lung inflammation and impaired pulmonary defence against infection. Epidemiological studies that have adjusted for sex, age, race, education and alcohol consumption suggest that daily marijuana smokers have a slightly elevated risk of respiratory illness compared to non-smokers. Other epidemiologic studies in HIV-positive individuals have identified marijuana use as a significant risk factor for acquisition of opportunistic infections and/or Kaposi's scarcoma.

Lung Physiology

Several studies on humans have demonstrated an acute bronchodilator effect of both smoked cannabis and oral THC. These findings have been replicated in both healthy and asthmatic populations. However, the potential therapeutic use of cannabis and synthetic cannabinoids has been largely discounted for a variety of reasons.

Two studies in relatively young populations compared respiratory symptoms and lung function in non-smokers and long-term smokers of both cannabis and tobacco (Bloom, Kaltenborn et al., 1987; Tashkin, Coulson et al., 1987). In both studies, heavy habitual cannabis consumption, with or without tobacco, was associated with a higher prevalence of symptoms of chronic bronchitis and a higher incidence of acute bronchitis than in the non-smoking group.

However, the studies disagreed about effects on peripheral airway function. One longitudinal study indicated that cannabis consumption was associated with increased large airway resistance but not with the development of small airways dysfunction or diffusion impairment that are characteristic of chronic obstructive bronchopulmonary disease or emphysema. The other study found a significant deleterious effect on ventilatory function of small airways among habitual cannabis smokers. The effect was at least as great as the effect of tobacco consumption. Recent studies have also failed to agree on whether any impairment in pulmonary function is additive to the effects of tobacco consumption. Both the site of impairment and potential interaction between cannabis and tobacco require further investigation.

While the pulmonary absorption of carbon monoxide from cannabis smoke is relatively high compared to that from tobacco smoke, the impact of this on heavy habitual consumers is modest. This probably reflects the short half life for clearance of carbon monoxide, and the relatively longer times between occasions of cannabis use. However, the carboxyhemoglobin levels in cannabis smokers are higher than in non-smokers; this may result in a slight interference with tissue oxygenation.

Recent more detailed studies have failed to demonstrate any acute effect of cannabis on central or peripheral ventilatory drive or any chronic effect on non-specific airways hyper-responsiveness.

Carcinogenesis

Biochemical, cellular, immunologic, genetic, tissue and animal studies provide a biologically plausible basis for the concern that marijuana may play a role in the development of respiratory cancer. While this concern is reinforced by reports of cancer of the upper aerodigestive tract in young adults with a history of heavy cannabis use, the lack of a control group in these case-series does not permit a true estimate of the impact of marijuana on cancer risk. In the only epidemiological study that has thus far assessed the association between marijuana and cancer, no effect of marijuana use on respiratory cancer risk was found. However, this study was limited by the fact that marijuana users were not followed long enough to detect an effect. Well-designed and adequately powered epidemiological studies of the association of marijuana and cancer should be a high priority for research on the possible adverse health effects of chronic cannabis use.

References

American Thoracic Society. (1962). Definitions and classification of chronic bronchitis, asthma and pulmonary emphysema. *American Review of Respiratory Disease, 85,* 762–767.

Anderson, A.E. & Foraker, A.G. (1961). Pathogenic implications of alveolitis in pulmonary emphysema. *Archives of Pathology, 72,* 44–58.

Auerbach, O., Gere, J.B., Forman, J.B., Petrick, T.G., Smokin, H.J., Muehsam, G.E., Kassourny, D. & Stout, A.P. (1957). Changes in the bronchial epithelium in relation to smoking and cancer of the lung. *New England Journal of Medicine, 256,* 97–104.

Auerbach, O., Stout, A.P., Hammond, E.D. & Garfinkel, L. (1961). Changes in bronchial epithleium in relation to cigarette smoking and its relation to lung cancer. *New England Journal of Medicine, 265,* 253–267.

Baldwin, G.C., Tashkin, D.P., Buckley, D.M., Park, A.N., Dubinett, S.M. & Roth, M.D. (1997). Habitual smoking of marijuana and cocaine impairs alveolar macrophage function and cytokine production. *American Journal of Respiratory and Critical Care Medicine, 156,* 1606–1613.

Barbers, R.G., Evans, M.J., Gong, H., Jr. & Tashkin, D.P. (1991). Enhanced alveolar monocytic phagocyte (macrophage) proliferation in tobacco and marijuana smokers. *American Review of Respiratory Disease, 143,* 1092–1095.

Barbers, R.G., Gong, H., Jr., Tashkin, D.P., Oishi, J. & Wallace, J.M. (1987). Differential examination of bronchoalveolar lavage cells in tobacco cigarette and marijuana smokers. *American Review of Respiratory Disease, 135,* 1271–1275.

Barsky, S.H., Roth, M.D., Kleerup, E.C., Simmons, M. & Tashkin, D.P. (1998, in press). Molecular alterations in bronchial epithelium in habitual smokers of marijuana, cocaine and/or tobacco. *Journal of the National Cancer Institute.*

Beals, T.F., Fligiel, S.E.G., Stuth, S. & Tashkin, D.P. (1989, May). *Morphological alterations of alveolar macrophages from marijuana smokers.* Paper presented at the annual meeting of the American Thoracic Society, Cincinnati, OH. *American Review of Respiratory Disease, 139* (Part 2), A336.

Bellville, J.W., Swanson, G.D. & Aqleh, K.A. (1975). Respiratory effect of delta-9-tetrahydrocannabinol. *Clinical Pharmacology and Therapeutics, 17,* 541–548.

Bense, L., Eklung, G., Odont, D. & Wiman, L-G. (1987). Smoking and increased risk of contracting spontaneous pneumothorax. *Chest, 92,* 1009–1012.

Bloom, J.W., Kaltenborn, W.T., Paoletti, P., Camilli, A. & Lebowitz, M.D. (1987). Respiratory effects of non-tobacco cigarettes. *British Medical Journal, 295,* 1516–1518.

Boulougouris, J.C., Panayiotopoulos, C.P., Antypas, E., Liakos, A. & Stefanis, C. (1976). Effects of chronic hashish use on medical status in 44 users compared with 38 controls. *Annals of the New York Academy of Sciences, 282*, 168–172.

Busch, F.W., Seid, D.A. & Wei, E.T. (1979). Mutagenic activity of marihuana smoke condensates. *Cancer Letters, 6*, 319–324.

Cabral, G.A., Stinnett, A.L., Bailey, J., Ali, S.F., Paule, M.G., Scallet, A.C. & Slikker, W., Jr. (1991). Chronic marijuana smoke alters alveolar macrophage morphology and protein expression. *Pharmacology, Biochemistry and Behavior, 40*, 643–649.

Caiaffa, W.T., Vlahov, D., Graham, N.M., Astemborski, J., Solomon, L., Nelson, K.E. & Muñoz, A. (1994). Drug smoking, *Pneumocystis carinii* pneumonia, and immuno-suppression increase risk of bacterial pneumonia in human immunodeficiency virus-seropositive infection drug users. *American Journal of Respiratory and Critical Care Medicine,150*, 1493–1498.

Canti, G. (1988). *A Colour Atlas of Sputum Cytology: The Early Diagnosis of Lung Cancer.* London: Wolfe Medical Publications.

Caplan, G.A. & Brigham, B.A. (1990). Marijuana smoking and carcinoma of the tongue: Is there an association? *Cancer, 66*, 1005–1006.

Chopra, G.S. (1973). Studies on psycho-clinical aspects of long-term marihuana use in 124 cases. *International Journal of the Addictions, 8*, 1015–1026.

Chusid, M.J., Gelfland, J.A., Nutter, C. & Fauci, A.S. (1975). Pulmonary aspergillosis, inhalation of contaminated marijuana smoke, chronic granulomatous disease (letter). *Annals of Internal Medicine, 82*, 682–683.

Cruickshank, E.K. (1976). Physical assessment of 30 chronic cannabis users and 30 matched controls. *Annals of the New York Academy of Sciences, 282*, 162–167.

Davis, G.S., Brody, A.R. & Adler, K.B. (1979). Functional and physiologic correlates of human alveolar macrophage cell shape and surface morphology. *Chest, 75*, 280–282.

Denning, D.W., Follansbee, S.E., Scolaro, M., Norris, S., Edelstein, H. & Stevens, D.A. (1991). Pulmonary aspergillosis in the acquired immunodeficiency syndrome. *New England Journal of Medicine, 324*, 654–662.

Dinissenko, M.F., Pao, A., Tang, M.-S. & Pfeifer, G.P. (1996). Preferential formation of benz[α]pyrene adducts at lung cancer mutational hotspots in P53. *Science, 274*, 430–432.

Donald, P.J. (1991). Advanced malignancy in the young marijuana smoker. *Advances in Experimental Medicine and Biology, 288*, 33–56.

Drath, D.B., Shorey, J.M., Price, L. & Huber, G.L. (1979). Metabolic and functional characteristics of alveolar macrophages recovered from rats exposed to marijuana smoke. *Infection and Immunity, 25,* 268–272.

Endicott, J.N., Skipper, P. & Hernandez, L. (1993). Marijuana and head and neck cancer. In H. Friedman, S. Specter & T.W. Klein (Eds.), *Drug of Abuse, Immunity, and Immunodeficiency* (pp. 107–112). New York: Plenum Press.

Feldman, A.L., Sullivan, J.T., Passero, M.A. & Lewis, D.C. (1993). Pneumothorax in polysubstance abusing marijuana and tobacco smokers: 3 cases. *Journal of Substance Abuse, 5,* 183–186.

Ferguson, R.P., Hasson, J. & Walker, S. (1989). Metastatic lung cancer in a young marijuana smoker (letter). *Journal of the American Medical Association, 261,* 41–42.

Fleischman, R.W., Baker, J.R. & Rosenkrantz, H. (1979). Pulmonary pathologic changes in rats exposed to marijuana smoke for one year. *Toxicology and Applied Pharmacology, 47,* 557–566.

Fleischman, R.W., Hayden, D.W., Braude, M.C. & Rosenkrantz, H. (1975). Chronic marijuana inhalation toxicity in rats. *Toxicology and Applied Pharmacology, 34,* 467–478.

Fligiel, S.E.G., Beals, T.F., Tashkin, D.P., Paule, M.G., Scallet, A.C., Ali, S.F., Bailey, J.R. & Slikker, W., Jr. (1991). Marijuana exposure and pulmonary alterations in primates. *Pharmacology, Biochemistry and Behavior, 40,* 637–642.

Fligiel, S.E.G., Roth, M.D., Kleerup, E.C., Barsky, S.H., Simmons, M.S. & Tashkin, D.P. (1997). Tracheobronchial histopathology in habitual smokers of cocaine, marijuana and/or tobacco. *Chest, 112,* 319–326.

Gong, H., Jr., Fligiel, S., Tashkin, D.P. & Barbers, R.G. (1987). Tracheobronchial changes in habitual, heavy smokers of marijuana with and without tobacco. *American Review of Respiratory Disease, 136,* 142–149.

Greenberg, S.D., Hunter, N.R., Taylor, G.R., Swank, P.R., Winkler, D.G., Spjut, H.J., Estrada, R.G., Grenia, C., Clark, M. & Herson, J. (1986). Application of cell-image analysis to the diagnosis of cellular atypia in sputum: A review. *Diagnostic Cytopathology, 2,* 168–174.

Hall, J.A.S. (1975). *Testimony in marijuana-hashish epidemic and its impact on United States security: Hearings of the Committee on the Judiciary, United States Senate* (pp. 147–154). Washington, DC: Government Printing Office.

Hamadeh, R., Ardehali, A., Locksley, R.M. & York, M.K. (1988). Fatal aspergillosis associated with smoking contaminated marijuana, in a marrow transplant recipient. *Chest, 94,* 432–433.

Henderson, R.L., Tennant, F.S., Jr. & Guerry, R. (1972). Respiratory manifestations of hashish smoking. *Archives of Otolaryngology, 95*, 248–251.

Hernandez-Bolanos, J., Swenson, E.W. & Coggins, W.J. (1976). Preservation of pulmonary function in regular, heavy, long-term marijuana smokers. *American Review of Respiratory Disease, 113* (Suppl.), 100 (Abstract).

Hoffmann, D., Brunnemann, K.D., Gori, G.B. & Wynder, E.L. (1975). On the carcinogenicity of marijuana smoke. In V.C. Runeckles (Ed.), *Recent Advances in Phytochemistry* (pp. 63–81). New York: Plenum Press.

Huber, G.L., First, M.W. & Grubner, O. (1991). Marijuana and tobacco smoke gas-phase cytotoxins. *Pharmacology, Biochemistry and Behavior, 40*, 629–636.

Huber, G.L. & Mahajan, V.K. (1988). The comparative response of the lung to marihuana or tobacco smoke inhalation. In G. Chesher, P. Consroe & R. Musty (Eds.), *Marijuana: An International Research Report. Proceedings of Melbourne Symposium on Cannabis 2–4 September, 1987* (National Campaign Against Drug Abuse Monograph Series No. 7, pp. 19–24). Canberra: Australian Government Publishing Service.

Huber, G.L., Pochay, V.E., Pereira, W., Shea, J.W., Hinds, W.C., First, M.W. & Sornberger, G.C. (1980). Marijuana, tetrahydrocannabinol, and pulmonary antibacterial defenses. *Chest, 77*, 403–410.

Huber, G.L., Simmons, G.A., McCarthy, C.R., Cutting, M.B., Laguarda, R. & Pereira, W. (1975). Depressant effect of marihuana smoke on antibactericidal activity of pulmonary alveolar macrophages. *Chest, 68*, 769–773.

Kagen, S.L., Kurup V.P., Sohnle, P.G. & Fink, J.N. (1983). Marijuana smoking and fungal sensitization. *Journal of Allergy and Clinical Immunology, 71*, 389–393.

Leuchtenberger, C. & Leuchtenberger, R. (1976). Cytological and cytochemical studies of the effects of fresh marihuana cigarette smoke on growth and DNA metabolism of animal and human lung cultures. In M.C. Braude & S. Szara (Eds.), *The Pharmacology of Marijuana* (pp. 595–612). New York: Raven Press.

Llamas, R., Hart, D.R. & Schneider, N.S. (1978). Allergic bronchopulmonary aspergillosis associated with smoking moldy marijuana. *Chest, 73*, 871–872.

Lopez-Cepero, M., Friedman, M., Klein, T. & Friedman, H. (1986). Tetrahydrocannabinol-induced suppression of macrophage spreading and phagocytic activity in vitro. *Journal of Leukocyte Biology, 39*, 679–686.

Mann, P.E.G., Cohen, A.B., Finley, T.N. & Ladman, A.J. (1971). Alveolar macrophages: Structural and functional differences between non-smokers and smokers of marihuana and tobacco. *Laboratory Investigation, 25*, 111–120.

Marques-Magallanes, J.A., Tashkin, D.P., Serafian, T., Stegeman, J. & Roth, M.D. (1997, June). In vivo *and* in vitro *activation of cytochrome P4501A1 by marijuana smoke*. Paper presented by D.P. Tashkin at the 1997 Symposium on the Cannabinoids of the International Cannabinoid Research Society, Stone Mountain, GA.

Matthias, P., Tashkin, D.P., Marques-Magallanes, J.A., Wilkins, J.N. & Simmons, M.S. (1997). Effects of varying marijuana potency on deposition of tar and delta-9-THC in the lung during smoking. *Pharmacology, Biochemistry and Behavior, 58*, 1145–1150.

Mattox, K.L. (1976). Pneumomediastinum in heroin and marijuana users. *JACEP, 5*, 26–28.

Miller, W.E., Spiekerman, R.E. & Hepper, N.G. (1972). Pneumomediastinum resulting from performing Valsalva maneuvers during marijuana smoking. *Chest, 62*, 233–234.

Morris, R.R. (1985). Human pulmonary histopathological changes from marijuana smoking. *Journal of Forensic Sciences, 30*, 345–349.

Newell, G.R., Mansell, P.W., Wilson, M.B., Lynch, H.K., Spitz, M.R. & Hersh, E. (1985). Risk factor analysis among men referred for possible acquired immune deficiency syndrome. *Preventive Medicine, 14*, 81–91.

Newton, C.A., Klein, T.W. & Friedman, H. (1994). Secondary immunity to *Legionella pneumophilia* and Th1 activity are suppressed by $\varnothing^9$-tetrahydrocannabinol injection. *Infection and Immunity, 62*, 4015–4020.

Niewoehner, D.E., Kleinerman, J. & Rice, D.B. (1974). Pathologic changes in the peripheral airways of young cigarette smokers. *New England Journal of Medicine, 291*, 755–758.

Novotny, M., Lee, M.L. & Bartle, K.D. (1976). A possible chemical basis for the higher mutagenicity of marijuana smoke as compared to tobacco smoke. *Experientia, 32*, 280–282.

Phillips, D.H., Hewer, A., Martin, C.N., Garner, R.C. & King, M.M. (1988). Correlation of DNA adduct levels in human lung with cigarette smoking. *Nature, 336*, 790–792.

Polen, M.R., Sidney, S., Tekawa, I.S., Sadler, M. & Friedman, G.D. (1993). Health care use by frequent marijuana smokers who do not smoke tobacco. *Western Journal of Medicine, 158*, 596–601.

Ramirez, J. (1990). Acute pulmonary histoplasmosis: newly recognized hazard of marijuana plant hunters. *American Journal of Medicine, 88* (Suppl. 5), 60N–62N.

Roby, T.J., Hubbard, G.A. & Swan, G.E. (1991). Cytomorphologic features in the tracheo-bronchial airways of marijuana smokers. *Diagnostic Cytopathology, 7*, 229–234.

Rosenkrantz, H. & Fleischman, R.W. (1979). Effects of cannabis on the lungs. In G.G. Nahas & W.D.M. Paton (Eds.), *Marihuana: Biological Effects: Analysis, Metabolism, Cellular Responses, Reproduction and Brain, Advances in the Biosciences* (pp. 279–299). Oxford: Pergamon Press.

Roth, M.D., Kleerup, E.C., Arora, A., Barsky, S. & Tashkin, D.P. (1998). Airway inflammation in young marijuana and tobacco smokers. *American Journal of Respiratory and Critical Care Medicine, 157*, 928–937.

Roth, M.D., Zhu, L., Sharma, S., Stolina, M., Park, A.N., Chen, K., Tashkin, D.P. & Dubinett, S.M. (1997, June). $\varnothing^9$-tetrahydrocannabinol inhibits antigen-presentation *in vitro* and anti-tumor immunity *in vivo*. Paper presented at the 1997 Symposium on the Cannabinoids of the International Cannabinoid Research Society, Stone Mountain, GA.

Roy, P.E., Magnan-Lapointe, F., Huy, N.D. & Boutet, M. (1976). Chronic inhalation of marijuana and tobacco in dogs: Pulmonary pathology. *Research Communications in Chemical Pathology and Pharmacology, 14*, 305–317.

Rubin, V. & Comitas, L. (1975). Respiratory function and hematology. In V. Rubin & L. Comitas (Eds.), *Ganja in Jamaica: A Medical Anthropological Study of Chronic Marihuana Use* (pp. 87–102). The Hague: Mouton.

Shapiro, B.J., Reiss, S., Sullivan, S.F., Tashkin, D.P., Simmons, M.S. & Smith, R.T. (1976). *Cardiopulmonary effects of marijuana smoking during exercise*. Paper presented at the annual meeting of the American College of Chest Physicians, Atlanta, GA. *Chest, 70*, 441.

Sherman, M.P., Campbell, L.A., Gong, H., Jr., Roth, M.D. & Tashkin, D.P. (1991). Antimicrobial and respiratory burst characteristics of pulmonary alveolar macrophages recovered from smokers of marijuana alone, smokers of tobacco alone, smokers of marijuana and tobacco, and nonsmokers. *American Review of Respiratory Disease, 144*, 1351–1356.

Sherman, M.P., Roth, M.D., Gong, H., Jr. & Tashkin, D.P. (1991). Marijuana smoking, pulmonary function and lung macrophage oxidant release. *Pharmacology, Biochemistry and Behavior, 40*, 663–669.

Sherrill, D.L., Krzyzanowski, M., Bloom, J.W. & Lebowitz, M.D. (1991). Respiratory effects of non-tobacco cigarettes: A longitudinal study in general population. *International Journal of Epidemiology, 20*, 132–137.

Sidney, S., Beck, J.E., Tekawa, I.S., Quesenberry, C.P. & Friedman, G.D. (1997). Marijuana use and mortality. *American Journal of Public Health, 87*, 585–590.

Sparacino, C.M., Hyldburg, P.A. & Hughes, T.J. (1990). *Chemical and biological analysis of marijuana smoke condensate* (NIDA Research Monograph No. 9, pp. 121–140). Washington, DC: U.S. Government Printing Office.

Sridhar, K.S., Raub, W.A., Jr., Weatherby, N.L., Metsch, L.R., Surratt, H.L., Inciardi, J.A., Duncan, R.C., Anwyl, R.S. & McCoy, C.B. (1994). Possible role of marijuana smoking as a carcinogen in the development of lung cancer at a young age. *Journal of Psychoactive Drugs*, *26*, 285–288.

Talaska, G., Schamer, M., Bailey, J.R., Ali, S.F., Scallet, A.C., Slikker, W., Jr. & Paule, M.G. (1992). No increase in carcinogen-DNA adducts in the lungs of monkeys exposed chronically to marijuana smoke. *Toxicology Letters*, *63*, 321–332.

Tashkin, D.P. (1991). Marijuana and lung function. In R.R. Watson (Ed.), *Biochemistry and Physiology of Substance Abuse III* (pp. 41–69). Boca Raton, FL: CRC Press.

Tashkin, D.P. (1993). Is frequent marijuana smoking harmful to health? *Western Journal of Medicine*, *158*, 635–637.

Tashkin, D.P., Coulson, A.H., Clark, V.A., Simmons, M., Bourque, L.B., Duann, S., Spivey, G.H. & Gong, H. (1987). Respiratory symptoms and lung function in habitual, heavy smokers of marijuana alone, smokers of marijuana and tobacco, smokers of tobacco alone, and nonsmokers. *American Review of Respiratory Disease*, *135*, 209–216.

Tashkin, D.P., Fligiel, S., Wu, T.-C., Gong, H., Jr., Barbers, R.G., Coulson, A.H., Simmons, M.S. & Beals, F. (1990). Effects of habitual use of marijuana and/or cocaine on the lung. In C.N. Chiang & R.L. Hawks (Eds.), *Research Findings on Smoking of Abused Substances* (NIDA Research Monograph No. 99, pp. 63–87) (DHHS Publication No. ADM 90-1690). Washington, DC: U.S. Government Printing Office.

Tashkin, D.P., Gliederer, F., Rose, J., Chang, P., Hui, K.K., Yu, J.L. & Wu, T.-C. (1991). Effects of varying marijuana smoking profile on deposition of tar and absorption of CO and delta-9-THC. *Pharmacology, Biochemistry and Behavior*, *40*, 651–656.

Tashkin, D.P., Reiss, S., Shapiro, B.J., Calvarese, B., Olsen, J.L. & Lodge, J.W. (1977). Bronchial effects of aerosolized $\varnothing$-tetrahydrocannabinol in healthy and asthmatic subjects. *American Review of Respiratory Disease*, *115*, 57–65.

Tashkin, D.P., Shapiro, B.J. & Frank, I.M. (1973). Acute pulmonary physiologic effects of smoked marijuana and oral $\varnothing$-tetrahydrocannabinol in healthy young men. *New England Journal of Medicine*, *289*, 336–341.

Tashkin, D.P., Shapiro, B.J. & Frank, I.M. (1974). Acute effects of smoked marijuana and oral $\varnothing$-tetrahydrocannabinol on specific airway conductance in asthmatic subjects. *American Review of Respiratory Disease*, *109*, 420–428.

Tashkin, D.P., Shapiro, B.J., Lee, Y.E. & Harper, C.E. (1975). Effects of smoked marijuana in experimentally induced asthma. *American Review of Respiratory Disease*, *112*, 377–386.

Tashkin, D.P., Shapiro, B.J., Lee, Y.E. & Harper, C.E. (1976). Subacute effects of heavy marihuana smoking on pulmonary function in healthy men. *New England Journal of Medicine*, *294*, 125–129.

Tashkin, D.P., Simmons, M.S., Chang, P., Liu, H. & Coulson, A.H. (1993). Effect of smoked substance abuse on airways hyperresponsiveness. *American Review of Respiratory Disease, 147*, 97–103.

Tashkin, D.P., Simmons, M.S., Clark, V.A. & Coulson, A.H. (1988). Longitudinal changes in respiratory symptoms and lung function in nonsmokers, tobacco smokers and heavy, habitual smokers of marijuana with and without tobacco. In G. Chesher, P. Consroe & R. Musty (Eds.), *Marijuana: An International Research Report. Proceedings of Melbourne Symposium on Cannabis 2–4 September, 1987* (National Campaign Against Drug Abuse, Monograph Series No. 7, pp. 25–30). Canberra: Australian Government Publishing Service.

Tashkin, D.P., Simmons, M.S., Sherrill, D.L. & Coulson, A.H. (1997). Heavy habitual marijuana smoking does not cause an accelerated decline in FEV_1 with age: A longitudinal study. *American Journal of Respiratory and Critical Care Medicine, 155*, 141–148.

Tashkin, D.P., Wu, T.-C. & Djahed, B. (1988). Acute and chronic effects of marijuana vs. tobacco smoking on blood carboxyhemoglobin levels. *Journal of Psychoactive Drugs, 20*, 27–31.

Taylor, F.M. (1988). Marijuana as a potential respiratory tract carcinogen: A retrospective analysis of a community hospital population. *Southern Medical Journal, 81*, 1213–1216.

Tennant, F.S., Jr. (1980). Histopathologic and clinical abnormalities of the respiratory system in chronic hashish smokers. *Substance and Alcohol Actions/Misuse, 1*, 93–100.

Tennant, F.S., Preble, M., Prendergast, T.J. & Ventry, P. (1971). Medical manifestations associated with hashish. *Journal of the American Medical Association, 216*, 1965–1969.

Tilles, D.S., Goldenheim, P.D., Johnson, D.C., Mendelson, J.A., Mellow, N.K. & Hales, C.A. (1986). Marijuana smoking as cause of reduction in single-breath carbon monoxide diffusing capacity. *American Journal of Medicine, 80*, 601–606.

Tindall, B., Philpot, C.R., Cooper, D.A., Gold, J., Donovan, B., Penny, R. & Barnes, T. (1988). The Sydney AIDS project: Development of acquired immunodeficiency syndrome in a group of HIV seropositive homosexual men. *Australian and New Zealand Journal of Medicine, 18*, 8–15.

Vachon, L., Fitzgerald, M.X., Solliday, N.H.F., Gould, I.A. & Gaensler, E.A. (1973). Single-dose effect of marihuana smoke: Bronchial dynamics and respiratory center sensitivity in normal subjects. *New England Journal of Medicine, 288*, 985–989.

Voth, E.A. & Schwartz, H. (1997). Medicinal applications of delta-9-tetrahydrocannabinol and marijuana. *Annals of Internal Medicine, 126*, 792–798.

Wallace, J.M., Oishi, J.S., Barbers, R.G., Simmons, M.S. & Tashkin, D.P. (1994). Cellular and lymphocytic subpopulation profiles in bronchoalveolar lavage fluid from tobacco and marijuana smokers. *Chest, 105*, 847–852.

Wallace, J.M., Tashkin, D.P., Oishi, J.S. & Barbers, R.G. (1988). Peripheral blood lymphocyte subpopulations and mitogen responsiveness in tobacco and marijuana smokers. *Journal of Psychoactive Drugs, 20*, 9–14.

Wehner, F.C., Van Rensburg, S.J. & Thiel, P.G. (1980). Mutagenicity of marijuana and Transkei tobacco smoke condensates in the Salmonella/microsome assay. *Mutation Research, 77*, 135–142.

Williams, S.J., Hartley, J.P.R. & Graham, J.D.P. (1976). Bronchodilator effect of $\varnothing$-tetra-hydrocannabinol administered by aerosol to asthmatic patients. *Thorax, 31*, 720.

Wu, D.-H., Wright, R.S., Sassoon, C.S.H. & Tashkin, D.P. (1992). Acute effects of smoked marijuana of varying potency on ventilatory drive and metabolic rate in habitual marijuana smokers. *American Review of Respiratory Disease, 146*, 716–721.

Wu, T.-C., Tashkin, D.P., Djahed, B. & Rose, J.E. (1988). Pulmonary hazards of smoking marijuana as compared with tobacco. *New England Journal of Medicine, 318*, 347–351.

Zhu, L., Stolina, M., Sharma, S., Roth, M., Tashkin, D.P. & Dubinett, S.M. (1998). THC suppresses anti-tumor immunity and promotes growth in murine lung cancer. *American Journal of Respiratory and Critical Care Medicine, 157*, A319.

Zwillich, C.W., Doekel, R., Hammill, S. & Weil, J.V. (1978). The effects of smoked marijuana on metabolism and respiratory control. *American Review of Respiratory Disease, 118*, 885–891.

Cannabis and Immunity

Cannabis and Immunity

THOMAS W. KLEIN

An explosion in the numer of cannabis and immunity papers has occurred over the last 10 to 15 years. Whole animal and tissue culture systems have now established that cannabinoids, especially $\varnothing$-tetrahydrocannabinol (THC), either increase or decrease the function of a variety of immune cells. This variation in drug effects depends upon experimental factors such as drug concentration, timing of drug delivery, and the type of cell function analysed. Because of this ability to either increase or decrease immune function, cannabinoids should now be considered immunomodulators capable of perturbing immune homeostasis upon either injection or addition to tissue culture. Although cannabinoids modulate immunity, it is also clear that the immune system is relatively resistant to these drugs in that many effects appear to be relatively small and totally reversible, occur at concentrations higher than needed to induce psychoactivity (> 10 µM or > 5 mg/kg), and are not always linked to psychoactivity. This would suggest that cannabinoid effects on immune cells are not due to mechanisms involving the newly described cannabinoid receptor in spite of the fact that receptor activity has been detected in these cells. It must be proposed at this time, therefore, that cannabinoids modulate immune cell function through both cannabinoid receptor and non-receptor mechanisms. Regarding the public health impact of smoking marijuana, unfortunately, this issue is still unclear. Although many studies have established THC as an immunomodulator, few have employed animal or human subject paradigms designed to test the effects of drug exposure on host resistance to microbes and tumors. These types of studies are needed and will require the cooperation of immunologists, infectious disease specialists, oncologists and pharmacologists.

Human, Monkey and Rodent Macrophages *in vivo*

Reports in the 1970s suggested that marijuana smoke or THC induced various changes in cultured macrophages such as suppression of bactericidal capacity or alterations in morphology (see Tables 1 and 3; Arif & Archibald, 1981; Friedman, Klein & Specter, 1991; Friedman, Shivers & Klein, 1994; Hollister, 1988; Klein &

Friedman, 1990; Specter, Lancz & Hazelden, 1990). However, extension of these studies to whole animals suggested that rat alveolar macrophages were only moderately affected following 30 consecutive days of "smoking." Changes were noted in morphology (Davies, Sornberger & Huber, 1979), cellular oxygen consumption and superoxide generation following phagocytosis (Drath, Shorey et al., 1979). Phagocytosis of bacteria was not significantly affected by marijuana smoke (Drath, Shorey et al., 1979) but was by tobacco smoke. More recently, similar studies have been done in humans (Sherman, Roth et al., 1991) and monkeys (Cabral, Stinnett et al., 1991). Pulmonary alveolar macrophages were obtained by lavage from patient groups including non-smokers, marijuana smokers, tobacco smokers and tobacco and marijuana smokers, and these cells were studied along with lung function. It was observed that tobacco smoking rather than marijuana smoking resulted in lung changes and suppression of macrophage superoxide production (Sherman, Roth et al., 1991). In the monkey studies, however, changes were noted in alveolar macrophages obtained from animals exposed for one year to daily marijuana smoking followed by a seven-month rest period (Cabral, Stinnett et al., 1991). Here, the cells from drug-treated animals displayed changes in morphology as well as altered expression of certain cellular proteins suggestive of altered cellular function.

Human and Rodent Macrophages *in vitro*

As with many studies on marijuana and immunity, *in vitro* effects of THC on macrophage function have been consistently and repeatedly shown (see Tables 2 and 4). Most work has been done using rodent peritoneal macrophages and drug concentrations ranging from 1 µM to 100 µM. Lopez-Cepero et al. (1986) demonstrated mouse peritoneal cell cultures were suppressed in terms of surface contact-induced spreading and phagocytosis of yeast by THC concentrations ranging from 1 to 50 µM. The drug effect was fully reversible and had no effect on cell viability. Similar results were obtained using human, mononuclear phagocyte cultures with drug effects starting at 5 µM (Specter, Lancz & Goodfellow, 1991).

Regarding drug effects on macrophage cytokine production, Klein and Friedman reported in 1990 that THC in the range of 10 to 30 µM increased the IL1 bioactivity in the supernatant of cultured, mouse peritoneal macrophages. IL1 is an inflammatory and immunomodulatory protein produced by macrophages and other cells in response to tissue injury and infection. The increase in bioactivity was surprising in that THC had been shown to suppress immune function of cultured splenocytes and it was therefore expected to decrease production of immune cytokines such as IL1. Further studies showed THC increased the processing and release of IL1, rather than increasing the cellular production of the protein (Zhu, Newton et al., 1994). The molecular mechanisms responsible for this are not clear but could involve effects on either apoptosis or the cellular production of prostaglandins and cAMP. Indeed, THC activation of the cannabinoid receptor decreases the cellular production of cAMP and drug treatment of macrophages has been shown to increase the cellular release of arachidonic acid and prostaglandins (Burstein, 1991).

In contrast to the above results, THC treatment of other types of macrophage cultures has been reported to suppress the production of another pro-inflammatory cytokine, TNF. An initial report suggested THC treatment (0.1 to 10 µM) of macrophage cell lines such as RAW264.7 and J774A.1 suppressed the release of antiviral factors suggestive of a suppression in cytokine production (Cabral & Vasquez, 1992). Subsequently, supernatant TNF was directly shown to be suppressed by THC treatment (10 to 32 µM) in a macrophage culture system employing IFN co-treatment and low fetal calf serum culture conditions (Zheng, Specter & Friedman, 1992). Further studies showed THC treatment of RAW264.7 cell cultures suppressed the cellular processing of the precursor TNF molecule to the active secreted form of the protein (Fisher-Stenger, Pettit & Cabral, 1993). The suppression of TNF, however, is culture-system-specific because the supernatant level of TNF is increased in cultures of THP-1 cells previously differentiated by phorbol myristate acetate treatment (Shivers, Newton et al., 1994). From these studies, it would appear best to characterize the drug effect on cytokine levels as a modulation rather than suppression or increase. As with other THC effects, the drug is most effective in concentrations above 10 µM.

Macrophage function can also be studied in terms of antimicrobial capacity. Arata et al. (1991) reported THC treatment (around 10 µM) suppressed both the endogenous and endotoxin-activated, antimicrobial activity of mouse peritoneal macrophages against the facultative intracellular bacterial pathogen, *Legionella pneumophila.* Although the mechanism for this effect was not described, it was suggested that alterations in prostaglandin levels of cAMP might be involved (Arata, Klein et al., 1991). Another study, employing THC injections into mice prior to removing activated peritoneal macrophages, revealed the drug treatment (multiple injections of 25 to 100 mg/kg) suppressed the antimicrobial activity of the macrophages when tested against target cells infected with either *Naeglaria fowleri* amoeba or herpes simplex virus (HSV) (Burnette-Curley, Marciano-Cabral et al., 1993). Again, the mechanism of the drug effect was not reported but was suggested to be related to suppression of macrophage effector molecules.

Human and Monkey Lymphocytes *in vivo*

T and B lymphocytes are now known to be major regulatory and effector cells participating in all aspects of immunity including both cell-mediated and humoral immunity. It was reasoned, therefore, that if marijuana or cannabinoids modulated immune function, this should be reflected in changes in the number and function of lymphocytes. Studies in the 1970s were conflicting in that leukocyte numbers and functions were either suppressed (see Table 1; Cushman & Khurana, 1976; Gupta, Grieco, & Cushman, 1974; Nahas, Suciu-Foca et al., 1974; Petersen, Graham & Lemberger, 1976) or unaffected (Lau, Tubergen et al., 1976; Rachelefsky, Opelz et al., 1976; Silverstein & Lessin, 1974; White, Brin & Janicki, 1975) by marijuana smoking. These studies were done using various patient groups including either habitual outpatient marijuana abusers or abusers institutionalized and given marijuana for the duration of the study. No strict association was observed between the method of drug intake and immune suppression; however, suppression was frequently observed among non-institutionalized, outpatient abusers suggesting lifestyle factors other than marijuana abuse may have contributed to the immunosuppression. To control for variations attributable to lifestyle, several studies were done using monkeys. Daul and Heath (1975) studied immunoglobulin levels and the mitogen response of peripheral blood lymphocytes in rhesus monkeys exposed to daily marijuana smoke for a period of six months. High, medium and low doses of smoke were tested. They observed that monkeys exposed to high doses of smoke had a significant reduction in blood cell mitogen responses as well as a reduction in serum IgG and IgM levels. In other studies, rhesus monkeys injected with THC (2.5 mg/kg) for three weeks had significantly elevated blood neutrophil levels; however, these returned to normal within several weeks after treatment (Silverman, Darnell et al., 1982). Lymphocyte numbers were not affected by drug treatment in these studies.

More recently, human studies have appeared each employing quite different designs. In 1988, Wallace et al. reported on findings employing an outpatient group of marijuana abusers and tobacco abusers. Although no information was provided on the extent of marijuana and tobacco use, the tobacco group showed a significant decrease in

TABLE 1.

Cannabinoid Effects on Immunity: Human and Monkey Studies *in vivo*

Cell type	Function	Drug effect	Reference
Macrophages	Superoxide release	No effect	Sherman, Roth et al., 1991[1]
	Morphology	↑ Vacuoles	Cabral, Stinnett et al., 1991[2]
	Protein expression	↑	Cabral, Stinnett et al., 1991[2]
Lymphocytes	Antibody production	↑ or ↓	Nahas & Osserman, 1991[1]
		↑	Daul & Heath, 1975[2,3]
		No effect	Rachelefsky, Opelz et al., 1976[1]
	Lymphoproliferation	Mitogen response	Nahas, Suciu-Foca et al., 1974[1]
		↓	Petersen, Graham & Lemberger, 1976[1]
			Daul & Heath, 1975[2,3]
		No effect	Lau, Tubergen et al., 1976[1]
			Rachelefsky, Opelz et al., 1976[1]
			White, Brin & Janicki, 1975[1]
			Wallace, Tashkin et al., 1988[1]
			Dax, Pilotte et al., 1989[1]
		Alloantigen response	Petersen, Graham & Lemberger, 1976[1]
		No effect	Rachelefsky, Opelz et al., 1976[1]
	T cell rosettes	↓	Petersen, Graham & Lemberger, 1976[1]
			Gupta, Grieco & Cushman, 1974[1]
			Cushman & Khurana, 1976[1]
	B cell rosettes	No effect	Gupta, Grieco & Cushman, 1974[1]
	Lymphocyte profiles	↑ CD4/CD8 ratio	Wallace, Tashkin et al., 1988[1]
		No effect	Dax, Pilotte et al., 1989[1]
	Delayed skin test	No effect	Silverstein & Lessin, 1974[1]
Killer cells	NK activity	No effect	Dax, Pilotte et al., 1989[1]
	ADCC	No effect	Dax, Pilotte et al., 1989[1]

Note: ↑ increase; ↓ decrease; [1] humans, lifestyles vary; [2] monkeys; [3] dose-dependent

peripheral blood lymphoproliferative response to mitogens, while the marijuana group showed an increase in the T cell CD4/CD8 ratio. A subsequent study (Dax, Pilotte et al., 1989) reported findings with institutionalized subjects given a relatively small amount of marijuana (up to three cigarettes per day) for only four days. White blood cell and lymphocyte subset counts were unaffected by marijuana exposure; furthermore, killer cell function of the blood lymphocytes was also not affected. In a more recent study (Nahas & Osserman, 1991), institutionalized subjects allowed marijuana *ad libitum* for four weeks were used. As a group, the subjects averaged 12.5 cigarettes per day (range 5.3 to 16.3) with each cigarette containing 20 mg THC. Their results showed a significant drop in the serum concentration of IgG which persisted for two weeks following the cessation of smoking. In contrast to the drop in IgG, the serum level of IgD significantly increased during and after smoking. IgA and IgM levels were not significantly affected in this study. From these studies, it appears that marijuana smoking/exposure is associated with moderate disturbances in lymphocyte number and function; however, the contribution of these disturbances to the long-term health of the host is still not known.

Human Lymphocytes *in vitro*

Cannabinoid suppression of the function of cultured, human lymphoid cells has also been reported (see Table 2). In the 1970s, several reports documented the suppressive effect of THC on the function of peripheral blood lymphocytes including suppression of leukocyte migration (Schwartzfarb, Needle & Chavez-Chase, 1974) and suppression of lymphoproliferation (Nahas, Morishima & Desoize, 1977). As with all *in vitro* culture systems, significant suppression was observed at 10 μM and higher drug concentrations. It is also of interest to note

---

TABLE 2.

Cannabinoid Effects on Immunity: Human Studies *in vitro*

Cell type	Function	Drug effect	Reference
Macrophages	Spreading and phagocytosis	↓	Specter, Lancz & Goodfellow, 1991[1]
	TNFα release	↓ ↑	Zheng, Specter & Friedman, 1992[1] Shivers, Newton et al., 1994[1,2]
	IL1 bioactivity	↑	Shivers, Newton et al., 1994[1,2]
	IL6 release	↓	Shivers, Newton et al., 1994[1,2]
Lymphocytes	Lymphoproliferation	↓ ↓ ↑ or ↓	Specter 1990[1] Nahas, Morishima & Desoize, 1977[3] Luo, Patel et al., 1992[1,4]
	Intracellular cAMP	↓	Diaz, Specter & Coffey, 1993[1]
	Cytokines	↑ or ↓	Watzl, Scuderi & Watson, 1991[1,4]
	Leukocyte migration	↓	Schwartzfarb, Needle & Chavez-Chase, 1974[1]
Killer cells	NK activity	↓ ↓	Specter, Klein et al., 1986[1] Specter & Lancz, 1991[1]
Neutrophils	Antifungal activity	↓	Djeu, Wand & Friedman, 1991[1]

Note: ↑ increase; ↓ decrease; [1] treatment with THC; [2] human macrophage cell line; [3] treatment with various cannabinoids; [4] dose-dependent

---

that regarding drug structure/activity considerations, non-psychoactive cannabinoids were demonstrated to be marginally more potent than THC (Nahas, Morishima & Desoize, 1977). Taken together, these results suggest that cannabinoids suppress the function of cultured cells by mechanisms other than those involving the cannabinoid receptor.

In the 1980s, a few reports confirmed and extended these findings. For example, it was reported (Specter, Klein et al., 1986) that THC at a concentration of around 30 µM suppressed natural killer (NK) cell activity when added to cultures of peripheral blood mononuclear cells. This effect was totally reversible suggesting suppression was not due to drug toxicity. Related studies (Specter & Lancz, 1991) showed 11-OH-THC also suppressed NK activity at concentrations between 10 and 100 µM and that the suppression could be reversed by adding the lymphocyte growth factor IL2 to the cultures. Suppression of lymphoproliferation in response to T cell mitogens was also observed under similar conditions (Specter, Lancz & Hazelden, 1990). The mechanism of these drug effects may be at least partially related to cellular adenylate cyclase activity because recently THC has been shown to suppress agonist-induced cAMP in lymphocyte cultures via a mechanism involving a pertussis toxin-sensitive G protein (Diaz, Specter & Coffey, 1993).

Cannabinoid treatment of human lymphoid cultures has also been reported to modulate cytokine production (Watzl, Scuderi & Watson, 1991). The drug treatment led to both increases and decreases in the supernatant level of cytokines such as IL2, IFNγ, and TNF. Lower THC concentrations (e.g., 3 µM) caused an increase in cytokines while higher concentrations (30 µM) caused a decrease.

Human Neutrophils
in vitro

The antimicrobial capacity of human polymorphonuclear leukocytes (PMNs) has also been shown to be suppressed *in vitro* following THC treatment (Djeu, Wand & Friedman, 1991). Here, drug concentrations from 3 to 6 µM were effective in suppressing not only antimicrobial activity against *Candida albicans* but also superoxide production. However, it must be noted that the culture conditions in this study employed serum concentrations of only 2 per cent, which might have contributed to the apparent increased potency of the drug.

Rodent Lymphocytes
in vivo

Many studies have reported cannabinoid effects on the immune system of rodents (see Table 3). Rodent studies are important complements to human studies because many immune paradigms are readily available in rodent systems, and the lifestyle confounds encountered in human studies are eliminated. Animal studies are also an important way to test directly the effect of cannabinoid treatment on resistance to challenges with tumors and microbes.

Antibody Production

Studies in the 1970s suggested that THC, as well as other cannabinoids, injected into mice suppressed the development of the primary antibody response (Smith, Harris et al., 1978; Zimmerman, Zimmerman et al., 1977). The greatest suppression occurred at doses of 10 mg/kg or higher and following treatment with both psychoactive and non-psychoactive cannabinoids. These results were subsequently extended to drug effects on the secondary antibody response (Baczynsky & Zimmerman, 1983). Here, THC doses of 10 to 15 mg/kg significantly suppressed the secondary antibody response to SRBC (sheep red blood cells) in addition to the primary response. Cannabinol and cannabidiol at these doses had no effect. Drug effects on T cell dependent and T cell independent antibody responses have also been reported (Schatz, Koh

TABLE 3.

Cannabinoid Effects on Immunity: Rodent Studies *in vivo*

Cell type	Function	Drug effect	Reference
Macrophages	Morphology	↑ lipid inclusions ↓ cytoplasmic volume	Davies, Sornberger et al., 1979[1]
	Phagocytosis	No effect	Drath, Shorey et al., 1979[1]
	Superoxide release	↓	Drath, Shorey et al., 1979[1]
	Antimicrobial activity	↓	Burnette-Curley, Marciano-Cabral et al., 1993[2,5]
Lymphocytes	Antibody production	↓ or no effect	Zimmerman, Zimmerman et al., 1977[2] Baczynsky & Zimmerman, 1983[2] Smith, Harris et al., 1978[2] Titishov, Mechoulam & Zimmerman, 1989[3] Schatz, Koh & Kaminski, 1993[2]
	IFN	↓ or no effect	Cabral, Lockmuller & Mishkin, 1986[2] Blanchard, Newton et al., 1986[2]
	Delayed skin test	↓	Smith, Harris et al., 1978[2]
Killer cells	NK activity	↓	Patel, Borysenko et al., 1985[4] Klein, Newton & Friedman, 1987[2]
	CTL activity	↓	Klein, Kawakami et al., 1991[2] Fisher-Stenger, Updegrove et al., 1992[2]
Other	Tumor growth	↓	Watson 1989[1]
	Resistance to infection	↓ antibacterial	Bradley, Munson et al., 1977[2,6] Morahan, Klykken et al., 1979[2,7] Ashfaq, Watson & ElSohly, 1987[1,8]
		↓ antiviral	Morahan, Klykken et al., 1979[2,9] Miskin & Cabral, 1985[2,9] Cabral, Mishkin et al., 1986[4,9] Specter, Lancz & Goodfellow, 1991[2,9,10]
		↑ serum cytokines	Klein, Newton et al., 1993[2]
		↓ secondary immunity	Klein, Newton & Friedman, 1994[2,11]
	Autoimmunity	↓	Lyman, Sonett et al., 1989[4]

Note: ↑ increase; ↓ decrease; [1] "smoking" rats or mice; [2] mice injected with THC; [3] mice treated with HU-210; [4] rats or guinea pigs injected with THC; [5] resistance to protozoa; [6] resistance to Gram-negative bacteria; [7] resistance to *Legionella monocytogenes*; [8] resistance to *Staphylococcus aureus*; [9] resistance to herpes simplex; [10] resistance to Friend leukemia virus; [11] resistance to *Legionella pneumophila*

& Kaminski, 1993). Here, oral administration of THC (50 to 200 mg/kg for seven consecutive days prior to antigen injection) was shown to suppress the T dependent response to SRBC but not the T independent response to DNP-ficoll (dinitrophenyl coupled to ficoll). Similar results were obtained *in vitro* using normal splenocytes and THC concentrations in the range of 3 to 30 μM. From these and other studies the authors concluded THC was primarily affecting the function of T lymphocytes (Schatz, Koh & Kaminski, 1993). Recently, the effect of the synthetic cannabinoids HU-210 and HU-211 on the anti-SRBC antibody response has been reported (Titishov, Mechoulam & Zimmerman, 1989). Anti-SRBC activity was measured by both serum hemagglutination titers as well as the number of splenocyte, plaque-forming cells (PFC). THC (> 5 mg/kg) and HU-210 (> 0.05 mg/kg) were shown to significantly suppress both measures of antibody production when given as a daily injection with and after antigen injection. The non-psychoactive enantiomer HU-211 suppressed only the PFC response. If injection of the drugs was delayed until two days following antigen injection, serum titers and PFCs were suppressed only by HU-210 (0.1 mg/kg) and not HU-211. These studies are remarkable for the relatively low doses of cannabinoid needed to produce an immunomodulatory effect. Also, because HU-210 has a much higher cannabimimetic effect than HU-211 it is possible that the cellular and molecular mechanisms involved in the induction of the antibody response are susceptible to both cannabinoid receptor and non-receptor mechanisms whereas the later stages of the response are susceptible to only receptor-mediated drug effects (see "Cannabinoid Receptors and Immunity").

Killer Cells

The recognition of natural killer (NK) cells as important in host defences against tumors and microbes suggested these cells as targets of cannabinoid effects. Accordingly, Patel et al.

(1985) were the first to show THC injection into rats decreased the splenic NK activity. Animals were treated daily for 25 days with a single injection of THC (3 mg/kg) and the NK activity was decreased between 25 and 50 per cent. Attenuation of the THC effect was observed following a co-injection of naloxone suggesting that the drug might be suppressing NK cell activity by an indirect mechanism. A similar suppression of NK activity was reported in mice following one or two daily injections of 50 mg/kg THC (Klein, Newton & Friedman, 1987), and the lytic activity of splenic, cytotoxic T lymphocytes (CTLs) was also suppressed by a single injection of the same dose (Klein, Kawakami et al., 1991). These results suggest that killer cell activity is negatively influenced by either repeated injections of relatively low THC doses or the bolus injection of a high drug dose.

Interferon

Cytokines mediate intercellular communication and therefore regulate immunity and inflammation during host defence against foreign antigens. The production of these substances could also be targets of cannabinoid effects on host defence. By the mid-1980s, the cytokine actions of interferons (IFN) were widely known and a few reports demonstrated that THC injection altered their production. Cabral and colleagues (Cabral, Lockmuller & Mishkin, 1986) reported that four daily injections of THC (> 5 mg/kg) suppressed the increase in serum IFN titers in response to cytokine inducers such as poly I:C (polyinosinic:polycytidylic acid) and herpes simplex virus (HSV). Non-psychoactive cannabidiol had no suppressive effect. Another report showed a similar effect of THC injection in a paradigm involving chronic drug treatment (Blanchard, Newton et al., 1986). Mice were injected every five days with 50 mg/kg THC for up to eight weeks and the spleens were removed and stimulated *in vitro* for IFN production. Under these conditions, IFN production was shown to be deficient in animals as early as two weeks following drug injection.

Other *in vivo* Studies in Rodents

Several other reports have appeared describing cannabinoid exposure and animal responses involving immune function (see Table 3). In one report (Watson, 1989), rats were exposed to long-term marijuana or placebo cigarette smoke and then implanted with sarcoma 180 tumor cells. Surprisingly, smoke exposure increased rather than decreased host resistance to the tumor challenge. Because placebo cigarettes also increased resistance and because injection of THC had no effect, it was concluded that marijuana smoke stimulates immunity by factors other than cannabinoids. Another report described the effect of THC injection on the laboratory model of multiple sclerosis, experimental allergic encephalomyelitis (Lyman, Sonett et al., 1989). Rats were given THC (5 mg/kg per day) on 1, 3, 5, 7 and 9 days postsensitization and evaluated for disease and the development of central nervous system (CNS) symptoms and mortality. The drug-treated rats had significantly fewer symptoms and mortality than controls, suggesting that the drug inhibited the development of the autoimmune response or immune-mediated inflammatory mechanisms causing the neurological symptoms.

Rodent Lymphocytes *in vitro*

Antibody Formation

It has become possible to study factors affecting antibody production using *in vitro* culture techniques (see Table 4). In one report (Baczynsky & Zimmerman, 1983b) splenocyte cultures were treated with varying concentrations of THC, cannabinol or cannabidiol and immunized by the addition of SRBC antigen. The splenocytes were from mice previously immune-primed to SRBC. The results showed both THC

(1 to 5 μM) and cannabidiol (5 μM) suppressed the antibody-producing capacity of the cultures. THC (32 μM) and 11-hydroxy-THC (32 μM) were also reported to suppress antibody formation in splenocyte cultures obtained from unprimed mice (Klein & Friedman, 1990). Neither study provided any clues as to the cellular or molecular mechanisms responsible for the cannabinoid effect. These *in vitro* studies support results obtained *in vivo* showing cannabinoid injection is associated with antibody suppression (see above).

Killer Cells

Animal studies in rodents suggested cannabinoid injection suppressed lymphocyte-mediated cytolytic activity. To learn more about the cellular basis for these *in vivo* observations, subsequent studies were performed *in vitro*. One of the first reports described cannabinoid effects on mouse splenic NK activity (Klein, Newton & Friedman, 1987). THC and 11-OH-THC were reported to suppress the cytolytic activity of semi-purified NK cells by about 60 per cent in a concentration-dependent manner using drug concentrations in the range of 10 to 32 μM. In addition, cell viability was not affected, and 11-OH-THC was more potent in suppressing NK activity. THC concentrations below 10 μM were subsequently shown to be without effect (Lu & Ou, 1989). Regarding mechanisms, the drug effect was shown to be independent of cellular calcium mobilization and to suppress at a stage following target cell binding and during the programming for lysis. The failure of NK cells to become activated in the presence of the drug was at least partially explained by studies showing suppression of responsiveness to IL2 (Kawakami, Klein et al., 1988a; 1988b). This cytokine, binding to IL2 receptors on NK cells, induces cellular proliferation and activation to become so-called lymphokine-activated killer (LAK) cells. THC and 11-OH-THC in the concentration range of 10 to 32 μM suppressed the proliferation and LAK cell activity of both splenic NK cells and a cloned, NK-like cell line (Kawakami,

TABLE 4.

Cannabinoid Effects on Immunity: Rodent Studies *in vitro*

Cell type	Function	Drug effect	Reference
Macrophages	Spreading and phagocytosis	↓	Lopez-Cepero, Friedman et al., 1986[1,2]
	IL1 bioactivity	↑	Klein & Friedman, 1990[1,2] Shivers, Newton et al., 1994[1,2]
	IL1 release	↑	Zhu, Newton et al., 1994[1,2]
	TNFα release	↓	Zheng, Specter & Friedman, 1992[1] Fischer-Stenger, Pettit et al., 1993[1]
	Antiviral factors	↓	Cabral & Vasquez, 1992[1]
	Antibacterial activity	↓	Arata, Keline et al., 1991[1,3]
	Arachidonic acid metabolism	↑	Burstein, 1991[1,2]
Lymphocytes	Lymphoproliferation	Mitogen response ↓ ↓ ↑ or ↓ ↑ or ↓	Klein, Newton et al., 1985[1,4] Pross, Klein et al., 1990[1,5] Pross, Nakano et al., 1992[1,6] Luo, Patel et al. 1992[1,2]
	Antibody production	↓ or no effect ↓	Baczynsky & Zimmerman, 1983[7] Klein & Friedman, 1990[7]
	IFN	↓	Blanchard, Newton et al., 1986[1]
	Calcium mobilization	↓	Yebra, Klein & Friedman, 1992[1]
Killer cells	NK activity	↓ ↓ No effect	Kawakami, Klein et al., 1988b[1] Klein, Newton & Friedman, 1987[1] Lu & Ou, 1989[1,2]
	CTL activity	↓ No effect	Klein, Kawakami et al., 1991[1] Lu & Ou, 1989[1,2]
	LAK activity	↓ ↓	Kawakami, Klein et al., 1988a[1] Kawakami, Klein et al., 1988b[1]
	IL2 binding	↓	Zhu, Igarashi et al., 1993[1]

Note: ↑ increase; ↓ decrease; [1] treatment with THC; [2] dose-dependent; [3] resistance to *Legionella pneumophila*; [4] T cell and B cell activation; [5] CD4 and CD8 activation; [6] mitogen-dependent; [7] treatment with various cannabinoids

Klein et al., 1988b). Subsequent studies in the cell line showed that THC treatment suppressed IL2 bioactivity by decreasing the number of high and intermediate affinity IL2 receptors on the NK cell surface (Zhu, Igarashi et al., 1993) by mechanisms involving the decreased cellular production of the IL2 receptor γ protein rather than production of the α and β chains (Zhu, Igarashi et al., 1995). The cellular production of the latter two chains was actually increased by drug treatment. These results, although obtained with relatively high concentrations of cannabinoids, strongly suggest that these drugs can simultaneously increase the cellular production of some immunologically relevant proteins while decreasing the production of others.

Killer cells other than NK cells are also suppressed by cannabinoids. The cytolytic activity of murine splenocyte, cytotoxic T lymphocytes (CTL) was shown to be depressed by about 60 per cent following incubation with THC or 11-OH-THC in the concentration range of 10 to 50 μM (Klein, Kawakami et al., 1991). The type of targets used were allogeneic and TNP (trinitrophenyl)-modified syngeneic targets. *In vivo*-induced CTLs appeared to be more sensitive to drug effects than *in vitro*-induced ones, and as with NK cells, the drug did not affect the viability of the CTLs, was suppressing a step in the lytic process at some point following target cell binding, and was suppressing the proliferative response of the killer cells (Klein, Kawakami et al., 1991). It is likely that cannabinoids are suppressing CTL activity similar to NK activity, by mechanisms involving IL2 biology.

Lymphocyte Proliferation

A necessary and fundamental consequence of immune activation is the proliferation of various lymphocyte antigen reactive clones. The antigen-induced proliferation can be mimicked using lectin proteins and certain microbial products that are lymphocyte mitogens. For decades, it has been common practice to measure mitogen-induced lymphoproliferation when assessing the immunomodulating potential of all types of

agents. The marijuana and immunity literature is no exception; indeed, human and animal studies have shown *in vivo* and *in vitro* drug effects on this testing parameter. In this regard, *in vitro* studies using rodent cell cultures have extended our perspective on cannabinoid influence on immunity and lymphocytes. For example, this type of study showed B lymphocytes were somewhat more sensitive to cannabinoid suppression than T lymphocytes (Klein, Newton et al., 1985). The proliferation of cultured, murine splenocytes in response to lipopolysaccharide (B cell mitogen) were suppressed by lower concentrations (i.e., 6 μM) of THC and 11-OH-THC than was the response to T cell mitogens, suggesting that B cell immunity (i.e., antibody production) might be more sensitive to cannabinoid suppression. In this regard, it is interesting to note that drug-induced suppression of antibody production is the most consistently reported finding in the marijuana literature.

Other studies have reported drug-induced changes in T lymphocyte proliferation. For example, it has been reported (Pross, Klein et al., 1990) that suppressor/cytotoxic T cells of the CD8[+] phenotype were suppressed to a greater degree than CD4[+], T helper cells in mitogen-stimulated cultures. This group also showed (Pross, Nakano et al., 1992) that if splenocyte cultures were treated with a different mitogen (e.g., antibody to CD3) THC increased rather than decreased lymphoproliferation. This increase was THC dose-dependent (i.e., 16 μM increased while 32 μM decreased proliferation) and was again observed mainly in CD8[+] cells. This report, along with another showing that low-dose THC (e.g., 1 μM) enhances lectin-induced proliferation (Luo, Patel et al., 1992), suggests that treatment of lymphocytes does not always lead to suppression of function and therefore the drug might be considered as a modulator of immune function.

It has already been suggested (see above) that at least one of the molecular mechanisms contributing to drug effects on lymphoproliferation is a deficiency in the functioning of the IL2/IL2 receptor system. A recent report suggests that a drug-induced suppression in intracellular calcium mobilization might also be involved (Yebra, Klein & Friedman, 1992). This event is an essential component of receptor/ligand signal transduction during lymphocyte activation. The normal rise in cytosolic calcium in mouse thymocyte cultures stimulated with mitogen was suppressed by THC (13 μM) after only a 10-minute drug exposure. The drug effect was further shown to be suppressing both calcium influx from the extracellular pool as well as intracellular release (Yebra, Klein & Friedman, 1992). Because calcium mobilization is dependent upon membrane phospholipid metabolism, it was speculated that cannabinoids might be interfering with the substrates or enzymes controlling inositol phosphate production.

Resistance to Infection: Animal Studies

A primary function of the immune system is to lessen the morbidity and mortality associated with infections. Indeed, the AIDS epidemic has painfully illustrated this point. It is reasonable, therefore, to conclude that cannabinoid-induced immunomodulation should be linked to modulation of host resistance to infection. Several reports in the 1970s suggested such a link. Macrophage antimicrobial activity is suppressed by cannabinoid exposure (see above, "Human and Rodent Macrophages *in vitro*"). Furthermore, host resistance to infection is diminished by drug treatment. Bradley et al. (1977) reported an enhanced susceptibility of mice to combination injections of THC and living or killed Gram-negative bacteria and endotoxin. Morahan et al. (1979) also reported enhanced mortality following drug treatment and infection with either *Listeria monocytogenes* or HSV. Drug doses having the greatest effect in these studies were in the 100 mg/kg range, therefore frustrating attempts to extrapolate these findings to

human drug abuse. More recently, bacterial infections have been examined in mice using THC doses in the 5 mg/kg range (Klein, Newton et al., 1993; Klein, Newton & Friedman, 1994). Two distinct drug effects on resistance to infection were observed that depended upon the dose and timing of drug injection. For example, mice given two THC injections (8 mg/kg), one day before and one day after a sublethal, primary infection with *Legionella pneumophila*, displayed mortality resembling septic shock within minutes following the second THC injection. Indeed, drug treatment appeared to be exacerbating the systemic mobilization of acute phase cytokines such as TNF (Klein, Newton et al., 1993), which are responsible for septic shock. On the other hand, if only one injection was given or doses below 5 mg/kg were used, all the mice survived the primary infection but failed to survive a subsequent challenge with a lethal dose of bacteria. In other words, these mice failed to develop immune memory in response to the primary, sublethal infection (Klein, Newton & Friedman, 1994). The cellular and molecular mechanisms responsible for this drug effect on immune memory are not clear at this time, nor is the role of psychoactive cannabinoids and cannabinoid receptors understood. However, the studies do suggest that THC injected into mice affects several different mechanisms of host resistance and occurs at drug doses in a range similar to that ingested during human abuse (Ashfaq, Watson & ElSohly, 1987; Mishkin & Cabral, 1985; Nahas, Morishima & Desoize, 1977).

Another study examining drug effects on bacterial infection employed a mouse, smoke-exposure model (Ashfaq, Watson & ElSohly, 1987). Mice were exposed to marijuana smoke or placebo for either 4 days or 60 days using a smoke-exposure machine. The cigarette dose-equivalent was 5 to 10 cigarettes per day. Following smoke exposure, the mice were given an intradermal injection of *Staphylococcus aureus* and the dermal necrotic index of the host response was monitored. The non-cannabinoid constituents of marijuana smoke decreased the severity of the necrotic lesions, suggesting to the authors that these substances might be immunostimulatory. However, it is also possible that these substances suppressed the inflammatory response in the skin resulting in reduced development of visible lesions. Whatever the mechanism, psychoactive components of the smoke did not appear to be involved since THC injection had no effect on lesion development.

THC effects on virus infection have also been reported. The resistance of mice to HSV infection was suppressed by four daily doses (15 or 100 mg/kg) of THC given around the time of intravaginal infection (Mishkin & Cabral, 1985). Frequency and severity of vaginal lesions, virus shedding, mortality, anti-herpes serum antibody and anti-herpes delayed hypersensitivity skin response were all measured and found to be adversely affected by drug treatment. This suggested the drug was suppressing the host response to infection by decreasing immune activation. Host resistance to HSV was also demonstrated in a guinea pig model wherein THC was injected at 0.2 to 25 mg/kg for a total of four daily injections per week for three weeks (Cabral, Mishkin et al., 1986). The animals were infected at the start of drug treatment. THC in the 5-mg/kg range increased the frequency and severity of infection similar to the mouse studies. The per-day dose was lower in the guinea pig studies, but the course of injection was longer than in the mouse studies. Subsequent mouse studies confirmed suppression of cell-mediated immunity following drug treatment in that anti-herpes splenocyte proliferation (Cabral, McNerney & Mishkin, 1987a) and cytotoxic T lymphocyte killing activity (Fischer-Stenger, Updegrove & Cabral, 1992) were suppressed in drug-treated animals.

Altered immunity to HSV infection might involve drug effects on virus target cells in addition to effects on immune cells. For example, treatment of HSV target cell cultures with THC (1 to 10 μM) caused an increase in virus release following infection but had no effect on cellular virus production (Cabral, McNerney & Mishkin, 1987b). Furthermore, much higher concentrations of drug suppressed herpes infectivity of cultured target cells (Lancz, Specter & Brown, 1991). Although the mechanisms for these effects were not elucidated, drug effects on target cell membranes or virus envelopes were suggested.

THC injection into mice has also been reported to increase susceptibility to co-infection with the murine retrovirus, Friend leukemia virus (FLV) and HSV (Specter, Lancz et al., 1991). Groups of mice were infected with FLV, followed seven days later by HSV infection. The injection of THC (80 mg/kg) two days before and two days after HSV infection significantly reduced the mean mortality time relative to groups injected with either virus alone. The mechanism responsible for this effect was not established although modulation of NK cell function and IFN production were proposed.

Resistance to Infections and Tumors: Human Studies

Reports of various infections and cancers associated with marijuana use have been reported over the past 10 years. Several of these deserve mention because of the possible effects on public health. Taylor et al. (1982) demonstrated that marijuana can serve as a source of transmission of bacterial pathogens. This study documented 85 cases of enteritis caused by *Salmonella muenchen* transmitted by contaminated marijuana. Disease outbreaks in several U.S. states were all traced to a similar *Salmonella muenchen* biotype that was found in high amounts in marijuana samples. Fungal infection and allergic bronchospasm to various species of *Aspergillus* also appear to be problems associated with marijuana use (Hamadeh, Ardehali et al., 1988; Kagen, Kurup et al., 1983; Levitz & Diamond, 1991). Patients with underlying immunodeficiency are particularly susceptible to serious infection following exposure to these fungi and recently it has been suggested that marijuana be sterilized by heat treatment prior to smoking (Levitz & Diamond, 1991).

Malignancies of the upper aerodigestive tract have also been associated with marijuana use. Donald (1986; 1991) reported nine patients with these types of cancers who presented at ages much younger than normal (mean age of 28.5 years). Five of the group reported little use of tobacco and alcohol but all used marijuana. A similar group of "young" patients (median age 36) was presented by Endicott et al. (1993) wherein 20 of 23 used marijuana. Smaller case reports of one or two patients with this type of cancer and a history of marijuana use have also been reported (Almadori, Paludetti et al., 1990; Caplan & Brigham, 1990). The cause and effect relationship between cancer and marijuana smoking is not established by these reports; however, they do indicate that there is an increased risk of this type of cancer associated with smoking marijuana, as there is with tobacco and alcohol consumption. In addition, these studies suggest that the cause of these cancers stems from localized effects of marijuana products on neoplastic transformation and immune function rather than on systemic immunity of the host.

Cannabinoid Receptors and Immunity

A major recent discovery in marijuana research is the cannabinoid receptor (CR). CRs were definitively demonstrated in rat brain membrane preparations by showing stereospecific binding of various cannabinoid agonists (Devane, Dysarz et al., 1988). Agonist binding studies also showed an inhibition of cAMP accumulation by means of a Gi protein (Howlett, Johnson et al., 1988). The cDNA encoding the binding activity was cloned in 1990 from a rat cerebral cortex cDNA library (Matsuda, Lolait et al., 1990) using a probe

derived from the sequence of bovine substance-K receptor. Although the CR protein has not been isolated and characterized to date, the translated sequence of the cDNA suggests a protein of 473 AA in length with several transmembrane regions, which is a member of the G-protein-coupled family of receptors (Matsuda, Lolait et al., 1990). The human counterpart of this gene activity has also been cloned from a human brain cDNA library using a probe based on conserved sequences in the G-protein-receptor family (Gérard, Mollereau et al., 1991). The deduced AA sequence suggested a protein of 472 residues that was 97 per cent identical to the rat brain protein and 100 per cent identical in the transmembrane regions (Gérard, Mollereau et al., 1991). Expression of the gene was detected in brain and testis but not in other peripheral tissues. Recently, a second gene has been cloned from a human leukemic cell line (HL60) cDNA library using a probe based on the G-protein-receptor family (Munro, Thomas & Abu-Shaar, 1993). The deduced amino acid sequence was only 44 per cent identical to the brain receptor and unlike the brain gene was not expressed in the brain but rather in macrophages in the spleen. This and the fact that the order of binding potency of various receptor agonists differed from the brain receptor suggests the possibility that at least two CRs exist and the distribution is tissue-specific. Multiple receptors are also suggested by the demonstration of a cannabinoid-regulated, N-type calcium channel that is coupled to a pertussis toxin-sensitive G-protein but is independent of intracellular cAMP (Mackie & Hille, 1992).

Cannabinoid effects on cells are also believed to occur by receptor-independent mechanisms. The high lipid solubility of cannabinoids, promoting the partition into cell membranes, may represent a way for these agents to disrupt the function of membrane proteins and therefore cell function (Makriyannis & Rapaka, 1990). These effects would be expected to occur at drug concentrations higher than those causing receptor-mediated changes and, indeed, this has recently been observed in CHO (Chinese hampster ovary) cells transfected with cannabinoid receptor cDNA (Felder, Veluz et al., 1992). Here, stereoselectivity was demonstrated for both cannabinoid binding and inhibition of cAMP accumulation, but not for the release of arachidonic acid and intracellular calcium. The IC50 doses for inhibition of cAMP accumulation were in the low nanomolar range, whereas the release of arachidonate and calcium occurred at doses higher than µM and also occurred in untransfected CHO cells (Felder, Veluz et al., 1992). Others have reported a role for CR coupled to phospholipases through a G-protein in the THC-induced release of arachidonic acid (Audette, Burstein et al., 1991).

The demonstration of cannabinoid binding sites and CR gene expression in lymphoid tissue raises important questions concerning the role of CR in immune cell function and immunomodulation by THC. Kaminski et al. (1992) were the first to report CR gene expression in lymphoid tissue. Specifically, mouse splenocytes were shown to display specific binding for the synthetic cannabinoid CP-55,940 characterized by a single binding site, a Kd of 910 pM, and a Bmax of 1,000 sites per cell. Supporting a role of the brain CR gene in splenocyte drug binding and immunomodulation, mRNA was demonstrated by reverse transcription–polymerase chain reaction (RT–PCR) in splenocyte preparations using primers and probes based on the brain CR cDNA, and in addition structure-activity studies showed a correlation between suppression of the *in vitro* antibody response and the potency of various cannabimimetic agents (Kaminski, Abood et al., 1992). As already stated above, this receptor appears to differ from the one reported by Munro not only in amino acid sequence, but also in tissue distribution and the order of affinity for various ligands.

Human leukocytes have also been reported to contain CR transcripts of the brain gene (Bouaboula, Rinaldi et al., 1993). Using RT–PCR with human CR primers, message was observed in human spleen, tonsils and blood leukocytes with B cells showing the highest mRNA level and CD4 T cells the lowest. Several leukocyte cell lines were also shown to express

the brain CR mRNA including Daudi, and THP1, but not Jurkat. We have also observed, in mouse splenocyte subsets, that the brain gene mRNA is highest in B cells, followed by T cells and macrophages, and that stimulated leukocytes express higher levels of CR mRNA than unstimulated cells (Daaka, Friedman & Klein, 1996). This suggests that the brain CR gene is differentially expressed in immune cell subpopulations and is regulated during leukocyte activation.

Conclusion

It is now clear that THC modulates the function of immune cells including lymphocytes, macrophages, and polymorphonuclear cells (PMNs). Virtually every function examined, from antibody production to phagocytosis, is affected in some way by the drug, especially when *in vitro* models are employed; however, for the most part, relatively high drug concentrations are required, immunomodulation is not related to psychoactivity, and the effects are reversible. Little is known at this time concerning the molecular mechanisms responsible for the drug effects, but it is likely that both cannabinoid receptor and non-receptor events are involved. Future studies should be aimed at establishing a relationship between cannabinoid-induced immunomodulation and altered host resistance to microbes and tumors. In addition, it will be of interest to establish the role of cannabinoid receptors in drug effects on host immunity as well as the role of these receptors in the regulation of the normal immune response.

Summary

Many research papers on cannabis and immune system functions in whole animals and tissue culture systems have been published in the past 10 to 15 years (Friedman, Shivers & Klein, 1994; Klein, Friedman & Specter, 1998).

Cannabinoids, especially THC, have been shown to modify the function of a variety of immune cells, increasing some responses and decreasing others. This variation in drug effects depends upon experimental factors such as drug concentration, timing of drug delivery and the type of cell function analysed. The range of cell types and functions studied is very broad, ranging from studies on the morphology of macrophages to the levels of transcription factors in lymphocytes. The results of these investigations indicate that cannabinoids are immunomodulators, i.e., capable of perturbing immune system homeostasis when administered to the whole animal or when added in cell culture. However, it is also clear that the immune system is relatively resistant to these drugs in that many of the effects appear to be relatively small, totally reversible after removal of the cannabinoid, and produced only at concentrations higher than those required for psychoactivity (> 10 μM *in vitro* and 5 mg/kg *in vivo*). Moreover, immunomodulatory effects can be produced by non-psychoactive cannabinoids. Thus, the immunomodulatory effects of cannabinoids may not be exclusively mediated by cannabinoid receptors, even though such receptors have been demonstrated in these cells. However, the demonstration of a cannabinoid receptor subtype (CB_2) in immune cells that is not expressed in brain suggests that these receptors may be involved in drug-induced immunomodulation.

The health impact of cannabis-induced immunomodulation is still unclear. Few studies exist employing animal paradigms or human trials assessing the effects of cannabis exposure on host resistance to bacteria, viruses and tumors. The studies that have been done in this area employed rather high cannabinoid doses and therefore have limited relation to the marijuana smoking experience. It is clear that additional studies are needed involving the cooperation of immunologists, infectious disease specialists, oncologists, pharmacologists and epidemiologists.

References

Almadori, G., Paludetti, G., Ottavaiani, F. & D'Alatri, L. (1990). Marijuana smoking as a possible cause of tongue carcinoma in young patients. *Journal of Laryngology and Otology, 104*, 896–899.

Arata, S., Klein, T.W., Newton, C. & Friedman, H. (1991). Tetrahydrocannabinol treatment suppresses growth restriction of *Legionella pneumophila* in murine macrophage cultures. *Life Sciences, 49*, 473–479.

Arif, A. & Archibald, H.D. (1981). *Report of an ARF/WHO Scientific Meeting of Adverse Health and Behavioral Consequences of Cannabis Use.* Toronto: Addiction Research Foundation.

Ashfaq, M.K., Watson, E.S. & ElSohly, H.N. (1987). The effect of subacute marijuana smoke inhalation on experimentally induced dermonecrosis by *S. aureus* infection. *Immunopharmacology and Immunotoxicology, 9*, 319–331.

Audette, C.A., Burstein, S.H., Doyle, S.A. & Hunter, S.A. (1991). G-protein mediation of cannabinoid-induced phospholipase activation. *Pharmacology, Biochemistry and Behavior, 40*, 559–563.

Baczynsky, W.O.T. & Zimmerman, A.M. (1983a). Effects of $\varnothing^9$-tetrahydrocannabinol, cannabinol, and cannabidiol on the immune system in mice: I. *In vivo* investigation of the primary and secondary immune response. *Pharmacology, 26*, 1–11.

Baczynsky, W.O.T. & Zimmerman, A.M. (1983b). Effects of $\varnothing^9$-tetrahydrocannabinol, cannabinol, and cannabidiol on the immune system in mice: II. *In vitro* investigation using cultured mouse splenocytes. *Pharmacology, 26*, 12–19.

Blanchard, D.K., Newton, C., Klein, T.W., Stewart, W.E., II & Friedman, H. (1986). *In vitro* and *in vivo* suppressive effects of delta-9-tetrahydrocannabinol on interferon production by murine spleen cells. *International Journal of Immunopharmacology, 8*, 819–824.

Bouaboula, M., Rinaldi, M., Carayon, P., Carillon, C., Delpech, B., Shire, D., Le Fur, G. & Casellas, P. (1993). Cannabinoid-receptor expression in human leukocytes. *European Journal of Biochemistry, 214*, 173–180.

Bradley, S.G., Munson, A.E., Dewey, W.L. & Harris, L.S. (1977). Enhanced susceptibility of mice to combinations of $\varnothing^9$-tetrahydrocannabinol and live or killed gram-negative bacteria. *Infection and Immunity, 17*, 325–329.

Burnette-Curley, D., Marciano-Cabral, F., Fischer-Stenger, K. & Cabral, G.A. (1993). Delta-9-tetrahydrocannabinol inhibits cell contact-dependent cytotoxicity of Bacillus Calmétte-Guérin-activated macrophages. *International Journal of Immunopharmacology, 15*, 371–382.

Burstein, S. (1991). Cannabinoid induced changes in eicosanoid synthesis by mouse peritoneal cells. In H. Friedman, S. Specter & T.W. Klein (Eds.), *Drug of Abuse, Immunity, and Immunodeficiency* (pp. 107–112). New York: Plenum Press.

Cabral, G.A., Lockmuller, J.C. & Mishkin, E.M. (1986). $\varnothing$-Tetrahydrocannabinol decreases alpha/beta interferon response to Herpes simplex virus type 2 in the B6C3F1 mouse. *Proceedings of the Society for Experimental Biology and Medicine, 181*, 305–311.

Cabral, G.A., McNerney, P.J. & Mishkin, E.M. (1987a). Delta-9-tetrahydrocannabinol inhibits the splenocyte proliferative response to Herpes simplex virus type 2. *Immunopharmacology and Immunotoxicology, 9*, 361–370.

Cabral, G.A., McNerney, P.J. & Mishkin, E.M. (1987b). Effect of micromolar concentrations of delta-9-tetrahydrocannabinol on Herpes simplex virus type 2 replication *in vitro*. *Journal of Toxicology and Environmental Health, 21*, 277–293.

Cabral, G.A., Mishkin, E.M., Marciano-Cabral, F., Coleman, P., Harris, L. & Munson, A.E. (1986). Effect of $\varnothing$-tetrahydrocannabinol on Herpes simplex virus type 2 vaginal infection in the guinea pig. *Proceedings of the Society for Experimental Biology and Medicine, 182*, 181–186.

Cabral, G.A., Stinnett, A.L., Bailey, J., Ali, S.F., Paule, M.G., Scallet, A.C. & Slikker, W., Jr. (1991). Chronic marijuana smoke alters alveolar macrophage morhpology and protein expression. *Pharmacology, Biochemistry and Behavior, 40*, 643–649.

Cabral, G.A. & Vasquez, R. (1992). $\varnothing$-Tetrahydrocannabinol suppresses macrophage extrinsic antiherpes virus activity. *Proceedings of the Society for Experimental Biology and Medicine, 199*, 255–263.

Caplan, G.A. & Brigham, B.A. (1990). Marijuana smoking and carcinoma of the tongue: Is there an association? *Cancer, 66*, 1005–1006.

Cushman, P. & Khurana, R. (1976). Marijuana and T lymphocyte rosettes. *Clinical Pharmacology and Therapeutics, 19*, 310–317.

Daaka, Y., Friedman, H. & Klein, T.W. (1996). Cannabinoid receptor proteins are increased in Jurkat, human T-cell line after mitogen activation. *Journal of Pharmacology and Experimental Therapeutics, 276*, 776–783.

Daul, C.B. & Heath, R.G. (1975). The effect of chronic marihuana usage on the immunological status of rhesus monkeys. *Life Sciences, 17*, 875–882.

Davies, P., Sornberger, G.C. & Huber, G.L. (1979). Effects of experimental marijuana and tobacco smoke inhalation on alveolar macrophages: A comparative stereologic study. *Laboratory Investigation, 41*, 220–223.

Dax, E.M., Pilotte, N.S., Adler, W.H., Nagel, J.E. & Lange, W.R. (1989). The effects of 9-ene-tetrahydrocannabinol on hormone release and immune function. *Journal of Steroid Biochemistry, 34,* 263–270.

Devane, W.A., Dysarz, F.A., III, Johnson, M.R., Melvin, L.S. & Howlett, A.C. (1988). Determination and characterization of a cannabinoid receptor in rat brain. *Molecular Pharmacology, 34,* 605–613.

Diaz, S., Specter, S. & Coffey, R.G. (1993). Suppression of lymphocyte andenosine 3':5'-cyclic monophosphate (cAMP) by delta-9-tetrahydrocannabinol. *International Journal of Immunopharmacology, 15,* 523–532.

Djeu, J.Y., Wand, M. & Friedman, H. (1991). Adverse effect of $\emptyset$-tetrahydrocannabinol on human neutophil function. In H. Friedman, S. Specter & T.W. Klein (Eds.), *Drug of Abuse, Immunity, and Immunodeficiency* (pp. 57–62). New York: Plenum Press.

Donald, P.J. (1986). Marijuana smoking — possible cause of head and neck carcinoma in young patients. *Otolaryngology — Head and Neck Surgery, 94,* 517–521.

Donald, P.J. (1991). Advanced malignancy in the young marijuana smoker. In H. Friedman, S. Specter & T.W. Klein (Eds.), *Drug of Abuse, Immunity, and Immunodeficiency* (pp. 33–46). New York: Plenum Press.

Drath, D.B., Shorey, J.M., Price, L. & Huber, G.L. (1979). Metabolic and functional characteristics of alveolar macrophages recovered from rats exposed to marijuana smoke. *Infection and Immunity, 25,* 268–272.

Endicott, J.N., Skipper, P. & Hernandez, L. (1993). Marijuana and head and neck cancer. In H. Friedman, S. Specter & T.W. Klein (Eds.), *Drug of Abuse, Immunity, and Immunodeficiency* (pp. 107–112). New York: Plenum Press.

Felder, C.C., Veluz, J.S., Williams, H.L., Briley, E.M. & Matsuda, L.A. (1992). Cannabinoid agonists stimulate both receptor- and nonreceptor-mediated signal transduction pathways in cells transfected with an expressing cannabinoid receptor clones. *Molecular Pharmacology, 42,* 838–845.

Fischer-Stenger, K., Pettit, D.A.D. & Cabral, G.A. (1993). $\emptyset$-Tetrahydrocannabinol inhibition of tumor necrosis factor-α: Suppression of post-translational events. *Journal of Pharmacology and Experimental Therapeutics, 267,* 1558–1565.

Fischer-Stenger, K., Updegrove, A.W. & Cabral, G.A. (1992). $\emptyset$-Tetrahydrocannabinol decreases cytotoxic T lymphocyte activity to Herpes simplex virus type 1-infected cells. *Proceedings of the Society for Experimental Biology and Medicine, 200,* 422–430.

Friedman, H., Klein, T. & Specter, S. (1991). Immunosuppression by marijuana and components. In R. Ader, D.L. Felten & N. Cohen (Eds.), *Psychoneuroimmunology* (pp. 931–953). New York: Academic Press.

Friedman, H., Shivers, S.C. & Klein, T.W. (1994). Drugs of abuse and the immune system. In J.H. Dean, M.I. Luster, A.E. Munson & I. Kimber (Eds.), *Immunotoxicology and Immunopharmacology* (pp. 303–322). New York: Raven Press.

Gérard, C.M., Mollereau, C., Vassart, G. & Parmentier, M. (1991). Molecular cloning of a human cannabinoid receptor. *Biochemical Journal, 279*, 129–134.

Gupta, S., Grieco, M.H. & Cushman, P., Jr. (1974). Impairment of rosette-forming T lymphocytes in chronic marihuana smokers. *New England Journal of Medicine, 291*, 874–876.

Hamadeh, R., Ardehali, A., Locksley, R.M. & York, M.K. (1988). Fatal aspergillosis associated with smoking contaminated marijuana, in a marrow transplant recipient. *Chest, 94*, 432–433.

Hollister, L.E. (1988). Marijuana and immunity. *Journal of Psychoactive Drugs, 20*, 3–8.

Howlett, A.C., Johnson, M.R., Melvin, L.S. & Milne, G.M. (1988). Nonclassical cannabinoid analgetics inhibit adenylate cyclase: Development of a cannabinoid receptor model. *Molecular Pharmacology, 33*, 297–302.

Kagen, S.L., Kurup, V.P., Sohnle, P.G. & Fink, J.N. (1983). Marijuana smoking and fungal sensitization. *Journal of Allergy and Clinical Immunology, 71*, 389–393.

Kaminski, N.E., Abood, M.E., Kessler, F.K., Martin, B.R. & Schatz, A.R. (1992). Identification of a functionally relevant cannabinoid receptor on mouse spleen cells that is involved in cannabinoid-mediated immune modulation. *Molecular Pharmacology, 42*, 736–742.

Kawakami, Y., Klein, T.W., Newton, C., Djeu, J., Dennert, G., Specter, S. & Friedman, H. (1988a). Suppression by cannabinoids of a cloned cell line with natural killer cell activity. *Proceedings of the Society for Experimental Biology and Medicine, 187*, 355–359.

Kawakami, Y., Klein, T.W., Newton, C., Djeu, J., Specter, S. & Friedman, H. (1988b). Suppression by delta-9-tetrahydrocannabinol of interleukin 2-induced lymphocyte proliferation and lymphokine-activated killer cell activity. *International Journal of Immunopharmacology, 10*, 485–488.

Klein, T.W. & Friedman, H. (1990). Modulation of murine immune cell function by marijuana components. In R.R. Watson (Ed.), *Drugs of Abuse and Immune Function* (pp. 87–111). Boca Raton, FL: CRC Press.

Klein, T.W., Friedman, H. & Specter, S. (1998). Marijuana, immunity and infection. *Journal of Neuroimmunology, 83*, 102–115.

Klein, T.W., Kawakami, Y., Newton, C. & Friedman, H. (1991). Marijuana components suppress induction and cytolytic function of murine cytotoxic T cells in vitro and in vivo. *Journal of Toxicology and Environmental Health, 32*, 465–477.

Klein, T.W., Newton, C. & Friedman, H. (1987). Inhibition of natural killer cell function by marijuana components. *Journal of Toxicology and Environmental Health, 20,* 321–332.

Klein, T.W., Newton, C. & Friedman, H. (1994). Resistance to *Legionella pneumophila* suppressed by the marijuana component, tetrahydrocannabinol. *Journal of Infectious Diseases, 169,* 1177–1179.

Klein, T.W., Newton, C., Widen, R. & Friedman, H. (1985). The effect of delta-9-tetrahydro-cannabinol and 11-hydroxy-delta-9-tetrahydrocannabinol on T-lymphocyte and B-lymphocyte mitogen responses. *Journal of Immunopharmacology, 7,* 451–466.

Klein, T.W., Newton, C., Widen, R. & Friedman, H. (1993). $\varnothing^9$-Tetrahydrocannabinol injection induces cytokine-mediated mortality of mice infected with *Legionella pneumophila. Journal of Pharmacology and Experimental Therapeutics, 267,* 635–640.

Lancz, G., Specter, S. & Brown, H.K. (1991). Suppressive effect of Δ-9-tetrahydrocannabinol on Herpes simplex virus infectivity *in vitro. Proceedings of the Society for Experimental Biology and Medicine, 196,* 401–404.

Lau, R.J., Tubergen, D.G., Barr, M., Jr. & Domino, E.F. (1976). Phytohemagglutinin-induced lymphocyte transformation in human receiving $\varnothing^9$-tetrahydrocannabinol. *Science, 192,* 805–807.

Levitz, S.M. & Diamond, R.D. (1991). Aspergillosis and marijuana. *Annals of Internal Medicine, 115,* 578–588.

Lopez-Cepero, M., Friedman, M., Klein, T. & Friedman, H. (1986). Tetrahydrocannabinol-induced suppression of macrophage spreading and phagocytic activity in vitro. *Journal of Leukocyte Biology, 39,* 679–686.

Lu, F. & Ou, D.W. (1989). Cocaine or $\varnothing^9$-tetrahydrocannabinol does not affect cellular cytotoxicity in vitro. *International Journal of Immunopharmacology, 11,* 849–852.

Luo, Y.D., Patel, M.K., Wiederhold, M.D. & Ou, D.W. (1992). Effects of cannabinoids and cocaine on the mitogen-induced transformations of lymphocytes of human and mouse origins. *International Journal of Immunopharmacology, 14,* 49–56.

Lyman, W.D., Sonett, J.R., Brosnan, C.F., Elkin, R. & Bornstein, M.B. (1989). $\varnothing^9$-Tetrahydrocannabinol: A novel treatment for experimental autoimmune encephalomylitis. *Journal of Neuroimmunology, 23,* 73–81.

Mackie, K. & Hille, B. (1992). Cannabinoids inhibit N-type calcium channels in neuroblastoma-glioma cells. *Proceedings of the National Academy of Sciences of the United States of America, 89,* 3825–3829.

Makriyannis, A. & Rapaka, R.S. (1990). The molecular basis of cannabinoid activity. *Life Sciences, 47,* 2173–2184.

Matsuda, L.A., Lolait, S.J., Brownstein, M.J., Young, A.C. & Bonner, T.I. (1990). Structure of a cannabinoid receptor and functional expression of the cloned cDNA. *Nature*, *346*, 561–564.

Mishkin, E.M. & Cabral, G.A. (1985). Delta-9-tetrahydrocannabinol decrease host resistance to Herpes simplex virus type 2 vaginal infection in the B6C3F1 mouse. *Journal of General Virology*, *66*, 2539–2549.

Morahan, P.S., Klykken, P.C., Smith, S.H., Harris, L.S. & Munson, A.E. (1979). Effects of cannabinoids on host resistance to *Listeria monocytogenes* and Herpes simplex virus. *Infection and Immunity*, *23*, 670–674.

Munro, S., Thomas, K.L. & Abu-Shaar, M. (1993). Molecular characterization of a peripheral receptor for cannabinoids. *Nature*, *365*, 61–65.

Nahas, G.G., Morishima, A. & Desoize, B. (1977). Effects of cannabinoids on macro-molecular synthesis and replication of cultured lymphocytes. *Federation Proceedings*, *36*, 1748–1752.

Nahas, G.G. & Osserman, E.F. (1991). Altered serum immunoglobulin concentration in chronic marijuana smokers. In H. Friedman, S. Specter & T.W. Klein (Eds.), *Drug of Abuse, Immunity, and Immunodeficiency* (pp. 25–32). New York: Plenum Press.

Nahas, G.G., Suciu-Foca, N., Armand, J-P. & Morishima, A. (1974). Inhibition of cellular mediated immunity in marihuana smokers. *Science*, *183*, 419–420.

Patel, V., Borysenko, M., Kumar, M.S.A. & Millard, W.J. (1985). Effects of acute and subchronic ∅-tetrahydrocannabinol administration on the plasma catecholamine, β-endorphin, and corticosterone levels and splenic natural killer cell activity in rats. *Proceedings of the Society for Experimental Biology and Medicine*, *180*, 400–404.

Petersen, B.H., Graham, J. & Lemberger, L. (1976). Marihuana, tetrahydrocannabinol, and T-cell function. *Life Sciences*, *19*, 395–400.

Pross, S.H., Klein, T.W., Newton, C.A., Smith, J., Widen, R. & Friedman, H. (1990). Differential suppression of T-cell subpopulations by THC (delta-9-tetrahydro-cannabinol). *International Journal of Immunopharmacology*, *12*, 539–544.

Pross, S.H., Nakano, Y., Widen, R., McHugh, S., Newton, C., Klein, T.W. & Friedman, H. (1992). Differing effects of delta-9-tetrahydrocannabinol (THC) on murine spleen cell populations dependent upon stimulators. *International Journal of Immunopharmacology*, *14*, 1019–1027.

Rachelefsky, G.S., Opelz, G., Mickey, M.R., Lessin, P., Kiuchi, M., Silverstein, M.J. & Stiehm, E.R. (1976). Intact humoral and cell-mediated immunity in chronic marijuana smoking. *Journal of Allergy and Clinical Immunology*, *58*, 483–490.

Schatz, A.R., Koh, W.S. & Kaminski, N.E. (1993). Δ^9-Tetrahydrocannabinol selectly inhibits T-cell dependent humoral immune responses through direct inhibition of accessory T-cell function. *Immunopharmacology, 26,* 129–137.

Schwartzfarb, L., Needle, M. & Chavez-Chase, M. (1974). Dose-related inhibition of leukocyte migration by marijuana and delta-9-tetrahydrocannabinol (THC) in vitro. *Journal of Clinical Pharmacololgy, 14,* 35–41.

Sherman, M.P., Roth, M.D., Gong, H., Jr. & Tashkin, D.P. (1991). Marijuana smoking, pulmonary function and lung macrophage oxidant release. *Pharmacology, Biochemistry and Behavior, 40,* 663–669.

Shivers, S.C., Newton, C., Friedman, H. & Klein, T.W. (1994). Δ^9-Tetrahydrocannabinol (THC) modulates IL-1 bioactivity in human monocyte/macrophage cell lines. *Life Sciences, 54,* 1281–1289.

Silverman, A.Y., Darnell, B.J., Montiel, M.M., Smith, C.G. & Asch, R.H. (1982). Response of rhesus monkey lymphocytes to short-term administration of THC. *Life Sciences, 30,* 107–115.

Silverstein, M.J. & Lessin, P. (1974). Normal skin test response in chronic marijuana users. *Science, 186,* 740–741.

Smith, S.H., Harris, L.S., Uwaydah, I.M. & Munson, A.E. (1978). Structure-activity relationships of natural and synthetic cannabinoids in suppression of humoral and cell-mediated immunity. *Journal of Pharmacology and Experimental Therapeutics, 207,* 165–170.

Specter, S. (1990). Marijuana and immunosuppression in man. In R.R. Watson (Ed.), *Drugs of Abuse and Immune Function* (pp. 73–85). Boca Raton, FL: CRC Press.

Specter, S., Klein, T.W., Newton, C., Mondragon, M., Widen, R. & Friedman, H. (1986). Marijuana effects of immunity: Suppression of human natural killer cell activity by delta-9-tetrahydrocannabinol. *International Journal of Immunopharmacology, 8,* 741–745.

Specter, S. & Lancz, G. (1991). Effects of marijuana on human natural killer cell activity. In H. Friedman, S. Specter & T.W. Klein (Eds.), *Drug of Abuse, Immunity, and Immunodeficiency* (pp. 47–56). New York: Plenum Press.

Specter, S., Lancz, G. & Goodfellow, D. (1991). Suppression of human macrophage function in vitro by Δ^9-tetrahydrocannabinol. *Journal of Leukocyte Biology, 50,* 423–426.

Specter, S., Lancz, G. & Hazelden, J. (1990). Marijuana and immunity: Tetrahydrocannabinol mediated inhibition of lymphocyte blastogenesis. *International Journal of Immunopharmacology, 12,* 261–267.

Specter, S., Lancz, G., Westrich, G. & Friedman, H. (1991). Delta-9-tetrahydrocannabinol augments murine retroviral induced immunosuppression and infection. *International Journal of Immunopharmacology, 13*, 411–417.

Taylor, D.N., Wachsmuth, I.K., Shangkuan, Y-H., Schmidt, E.V., Barrett, T.J., Schrader, J.S., Scherach, C.S., McGee, H.B., Feldman, R.A. & Brenner, D.J. (1982). Salmonellosis associated with marijuana: A multistate outbreak traced by plasmid fingerprinting. *New England Journal of Medicine, 306*, 1249–1253.

Titishov, N., Mechoulam, R. & Zimmerman, A.M. (1989). Stereospecific effects of (–)- and (+)-7-hydroxoy-delta-6-tetrahydrocannabinol-dimethylheptyl on the immune system of mice. *Pharmacology, 39*, 337–349.

Wallace, J.M., Tashkin, D.P., Oishi, J.S. & Barbers, R.G. (1988). Peripheral blood lymphocyte subpopulations and mitogen responsiveness in tobacco and marijuana smokers. *Journal of Psychoactive Drugs, 20*, 9–14.

Watson, E.S. (1989). The effect of marijuana smoke exposure on murine sarcoma 180 survival in Fisher rats. *Immunopharmacology and Immunotoxicology, 11*, 211–222.

Watzl, B., Scuderi, P. & Watson, R.R. (1991). Influence of marijuana components (THC and CBD) on human mononuclear cell cytokine secretion in vitro. In H. Friedman, S. Specter & T.W. Klein (Eds.), *Drug of Abuse, Immunity, and Immunodeficiency* (pp. 63–70). New York: Plenum Press.

White, S.C., Brin, S.C. & Janicki, B.W. (1975). Mitogen-induced blastogenic responses of lymphocytes from marihuana smokers. *Science, 188*, 71–72.

Yebra, M., Klein, T.W. & Friedman, H. (1992). $\varnothing$-Tetrahydrocannabinol suppressed concanavalin A induced increase in cytoplasmic free calcium in mouse thymocytes. *Life Sciences, 51*, 151–160.

Zheng, Z-M., Specter, S. & Friedman, H. (1992). Inhibition by delta-9-tetrahydrocannabinol of tumor necrosis factor alpha production by mouse and human macrophages. *International Journal of Immunopharmacology, 14*, 1445–1452.

Zhu, W., Igarashi, T., Friedman, H. & Klein, T.W. (1995). Delta-9-tetrahydrocannabinol (THC) causes the variable expression of IL2 receptor subunits. *Journal of Pharmacology and Experimental Therapeutics, 274*, 1001–1007.

Zhu, W., Igarashi, T., Qi, Z.T., Newton, C., Widen, R.E., Friedman, H. & Klein, T.W. (1993). Delta-9-tetrahydrocannabinol (THC) decreases the number of high and intermediate affinity IL-2 receptors of the IL-2 dependent cell line NKB61A2. *International Journal of Immunopharmacology, 15*, 401–408.

Zhu, W., Newton, C., Daaka, Y., Friedman, H. & Klein, T.W. (1994). $\varnothing$-Tetrahydro-cannabinol enhances the secretion of interleukin 1 from endotoxin-stimulated macrophages. *Journal of Pharmacology and Experimental Therapeutics, 270*, 1334–1339.

Zimmerman, S., Zimmerman, A.M., Cameron, I.L. & Laurence, H.L. (1977). $\varnothing$-Tetrahydro-cannabinol, cannabidiol and cannabinol effects on the immune response of mice. *Pharmacology, 15*, 10–23.

Cannabis Effects on Endocrine and Reproductive Function

Cannabis Effects on Endocrine and Reproductive Function

LAURA MURPHY

indings in the 1970s that cannabis exposure can affect endocrine and reproductive function in humans and experimental animals (for reviews see Abel, 1981; Bloch, 1983; Bloch, Thysen et al., 1978) resulted in a dramatic increase in research activity in these respective areas in subsequent years. The later studies continued to characterize the actions of cannabinoids on the endocrine and reproductive systems and began to examine potential sites and mechanisms of cannabis action. Progress has been significant, particularly in the area of cannabinoid effects on the reproductive endocrine system. Although much of the research has focused on the effects of cannabis in the male, interest in research with female animal models has escalated in the last several years. The plethora of new and important data from many different laboratories clearly indicate that the endocrine and reproductive systems in males and females are affected in a detrimental fashion by cannabis and its cannabinoid constituents. Furthermore, recent studies have demonstrated that specific cannabinoid receptors in the brain are responsible for mediating many of the endocrine and reproductive actions of cannabinoids. The function of cannabinoid receptors and endogenous cannabinoid compounds in the regulation of the endocrine and reproductive systems remains an important topic for future studies.

Female Reproductive Hormones

Experimental Animal Studies

Delta-9-tetrahydrocannabinol (THC), the principal psychoactive constituent of cannabis, alters anterior pituitary secretion of the gonadotropins, luteinizing hormone (LH) and follicle-stimulating hormone (FSH), and the lactogenic hormone, prolactin, when administered acutely or in repeated doses to intact and ovariectomized experimental animals. Acute administration of THC significantly reduced serum LH levels in ovariectomized rats (Johnson, Asch & Reiter, 1980; Marks, 1973; Steger, Silverman et al., 1980; 1981), mice (Dalterio, Mayfield & Bartke, 1983) and monkeys (Besch, Smith et al., 1977; Smith, Besch et al., 1979). The decrease in mean peripheral LH concentrations by THC most likely reflects an inhibition in pulsatile LH secretion, since doses of THC as low as 0.0625 mg/kg iv (intravenous) abolished the pulsatile fluctuations in serum LH typical of the ovariectomized rat (Tyrey, 1978; 1980). Although THC doses of 62.5 µg/kg suppressed LH secretion for less than 30 minutes, the duration of suppression increased with larger doses, continuing for 1 to 2 hours following a 4-mg/kg dose (Tyrey, 1978). In the ovariectomized rhesus monkey, THC doses of 0.6 to 5.0 mg/kg im (intramuscular), resulted in a prompt and significant decrease in both LH and FSH levels that lasted for 12 to 24 hours depending on the dose level of THC (Smith, Besch et al., 1979). Thus, these studies demonstrated that the duration of LH suppression, not the magnitude of suppression, was dose-dependent. Although THC-induced alterations in plasma levels of FSH have not been demonstrated in the ovariectomized rat (Steger, Silverman et al., 1981), acute THC treatment (50 mg/kg) has been shown to reduce plasma levels of both LH and FSH in the ovariectomized mouse (Dalterio, Mayfield & Bartke, 1983) and rhesus monkey (Smith, Besch et al., 1979).

In the intact cycling female rat, serum LH levels were reduced following acute or subchronic THC administration (Chakravarty, Shah et al., 1979; Chakravarty, Sheth & Ghosh, 1975). Oral THC administration reduced plasma levels of both LH and FSH in intact diestrous female mice (Dalterio, Mayfield & Bartke, 1983). In addition to suppressing basal LH levels in the female, THC also inhibited the preovulatory surges of LH and FSH and blocked ovulation in intact rats (Ayalon, Nir et al., 1977; Nir, Ayalon et al., 1973) and rabbits (Asch, Fernandez et al., 1979), and blocked the steroid-induced LH surge in estrogen-primed ovariectomized rats (Steger, Silverman et al., 1980). Moreover, the occurrence of the first ovulation in the maturing female rat was delayed following peripubertal administration of THC (Field & Tyrey, 1986). In the rhesus monkey, THC administration during the first 18 days of the follicular phase of the menstrual cycle blocked the preovulatory estrogen and LH surges and subsequent ovulation for several months after treatment (Asch, Smith et al., 1981). When administered during the luteal phase of the menstrual cycle, acute THC treatment lowered progesterone levels (Almirez, Smith et al., 1983), whereas daily THC administration had no effect on circulating progesterone levels but blocked ovulation during the following cycle (Asch, Smith et al., 1979b). Chronic THC

treatment completely suppressed LH and sex-steroid levels and blocked ovulation in the female rhesus monkey (Smith, Almirez et al., 1983).

Tonic prolactin levels were significantly decreased following acute or subchronic THC treatment in intact (Chakravarty, Shah et al., 1979; Chakravarty, Sheth & Ghosh, 1975) and ovariectomized female rats (Hughes, Everett & Tyrey, 1981; Johnson, Asch & Reiter, 1980). Furthermore, the rise in serum prolactin at the time of the preovulatory gonadotropin surge was blocked following intraperitoneal (Nir, Ayalon et al., 1973) or intravenous (Hughes, Everett & Tyrey, 1984) THC administration. In the estrogen-primed ovariectomized rat, THC suppressed tonic prolactin release and the surge of prolactin induced by a second injection of estrogen (Steger, DePaolo et al., 1983). Moreover, the nocturnal prolactin surge that occurs in pseudo-pregnant animals was temporally delayed or completely blocked by single or multiple injections of THC (Hughes & Tyrey, 1982). THC also blocked suckling-induced prolactin surges in lactating rats (Bromley, Rabii et al., 1978; Tyrey & Hughes, 1984). Although the effects of THC on prolactin release are primarily inhibitory, in ovariectomized rats in which frontal afferents to the medial hypothalamus were cut, THC produced a dose-related increase in serum prolactin suggesting that THC may also have prolactin-stimulating properties (Tyrey, 1986).

The effect of THC on serum prolactin levels was also examined in intact (Asch, Smith et al., 1979b; 1981) and ovariectomized female monkeys (Asch, Smith et al., 1979a). Administration of THC to ovariectomized monkeys reduced serum prolactin concentrations by 85 per cent within 30 to 90 minutes of drug administration (Asch, Smith et al., 1979a). In intact animals, short-term THC treatment during days 1 through 18 of the follicular phase of the menstrual cycle had no effect on serum prolactin levels, but animals were anovulatory during the subsequent posttreatment cycle, and prolactin levels were significantly elevated during the posttreatment period (Asch, Smith et al., 1981). Moreover, chronic

THC treatment disrupted menstrual cyclicity and produced significant decreases in average prolactin levels (Smith, Almirez et al., 1983). After two to four months of chronic THC treatment, tolerance to THC developed and prolactin levels were not different from untreated controls.

Human Studies

In an early study, women who reported using marijuana at least four times a week were studied over two menstrual cycles, and blood samples were obtained for analysis of gonadotropins and sex steroids (Bauman, 1980). When compared to a group of non-marijuana users, it was found that marijuana smokers had shorter menstrual cycles due to an inadequate luteal phase. Moreover, prolactin levels were significantly suppressed and testosterone levels were elevated in the group of marijuana smokers. In a different study, self-reported chronic marijuana users were not found to have any changes in circulating levels of LH, FSH and prolactin when compared to non-marijuana users (Block, Farinpour & Schlechte, 1991). However, the hormonal response to cannabis exposure may depend on the stage of the menstrual cycle. When the acute effects of marijuana smoking on plasma LH, prolactin and sex-steroid hormones were evaluated during the follicular and luteal phases of the menstrual cycle in groups of adult female volunteers, it was found that during the luteal phase of the menstrual cycle, plasma LH and prolactin levels were significantly suppressed at 60 to 120 minutes after the initiation of marijuana smoking (Mendelson, Mello & Ellingboe, 1985; Mendelson, Mello et al., 1986). There was no effect of cannabis exposure on LH or prolactin levels during the follicular phase or on the sex steroids during either the follicular or the luteal phases of the menstrual cycle. When the acute effects of marijuana smoking were examined in healthy adult women during the periovulatory phase of the menstrual cycle, there was a significant increase in plasma LH and prolactin levels but no change in circulating estradiol or progesterone levels after marijuana smoking (Mendelson, Mello et al., 1985).

In menopausal women, smoking a 1-gram marijuana cigarette containing 1.83 per cent THC did not significantly affect plasma LH levels at any time following marijuana smoking (Mendelson, Cristofaro et al., 1985). Together, these studies indicate that the hormone milieu at the time of exposure may dictate a woman's hormonal response to marijuana smoking.

Male Reproductive Hormones

Experimental Animal Studies

In the mature male rat, acute or chronic treatment with THC administered intramuscularly (Symons, Teale & Marks, 1976), subcutaneously (Chakravarty, Sheth et al., 1982), intraperitoneally (Puder, Nir et al., 1985) or orally (Fernández-Ruiz, Navarro et al., 1992; Murphy, Steger et al., 1990; Steger, Murphy et al., 1990) lowered plasma levels of LH. Although a single exposure to either cannabinol (CBN) or cannabidiol (CBD) did not alter LH secretion, co-administration with THC augmented the duration of the inhibitory action of THC on LH release (Murphy, Steger et al., 1990). Following intravenous administration, THC (1.0 mg/kg) significantly reduced LH levels within 10 minutes of its administration and blocked pulsatile LH secretion in castrate, testosterone-treated rats (Murphy, Chandrashekar & Bartke, 1994). The infusion of THC into the third ventricle of the brain of adult male rats resulted in decreased serum LH levels, but did not affect FSH secretion (Wenger, Rettori et al., 1987). In male mice, acute oral administration of THC (50 mg/kg) produced a significant decrease in plasma levels of LH and FSH (Dalterio, Bartke et al., 1978). Although oral administration of a single large dose of CBN or CBD failed to alter plasma LH or FSH levels in immature or adult male mice (Dalterio, Bartke et al., 1978), subchronic exposure to CBN reduced plasma levels of both gonadotropins (Dalterio, 1980). An acute dose of THC (5 mg/kg, im) suppressed LH levels in mature male rhesus monkeys (Smith, Moore et al., 1976). Moreover, THC administration reduced systemic testosterone concentrations in male mice (Dalterio, Bartke et al., 1978; Dalterio, Bartke & Mayfield, 1983), rats (Maskarinec, 1978; Steger, Murphy et al., 1990; Symons, Teale & Marks, 1976), and monkeys (Smith, Moore et al., 1976).

Studies suggest that multiple injections of THC either increased or had no effect on circulating prolactin levels, whereas acute THC exposure tended to inhibit prolactin secretion in male rodents. Subchronic administration of THC had no effect on serum or pituitary prolactin levels (Chakravarty, Sheth et al., 1982) or increased serum prolactin levels in male rats (Daley, Branda et al., 1974), while acute THC treatment significantly reduced serum prolactin levels 30 minutes after injection (Kramer & Ben-David, 1974; 1978). Daily intracerebroventricular infusions of THC (20 or 50 μg for one week) had no effect on plasma prolactin levels in prepubertal and young adult male rats (Collu, 1976), whereas a single infusion of THC (4 μg) suppressed prolactin levels (Rettori, Wenger et al., 1988). Furthermore, the increase in plasma prolactin that occurs in male rats exposed to sexually receptive female conspecifics has recently been shown to be blocked as a result of acute THC pretreatment (Murphy, Gher et al., 1994). Plasma prolactin levels were reduced in male mice after a single oral dose of THC (50 mg/kg) while chronic THC treatment was without effect (Dalterio, Michael et al., 1981). Moreover, acute CBN exposure reduced prolactin levels in stressed male mice (Dalterio, Michael et al., 1981). In the intact adult male rhesus monkey, a single injection of THC resulted in reduced serum prolactin concentrations by 74 per cent within 30 to 90 minutes of drug administration (Asch, Smith et al., 1979a).

Human Studies

Early studies reported that acute and chronic cannabis exposure produced a transient reduction in levels of both plasma gonadotropin and testosterone in human males (Cohen, 1976; Kolodny, Masters et al., 1974; 1976; Schaefer, Gunn & Dubowski, 1975) or had no effect on either pituitary LH or FSH secretion (Cushman, 1975) or systemic testosterone concentrations (Hembree, Zeidenberg & Nahas, 1976; Mendelson, Ellingboe et al., 1978; Mendelson, Kuehnle et al., 1974). Later studies demonstrated that plasma LH levels were significantly reduced while testosterone concentrations were unchanged after smoking one or two standardized marijuana cigarettes (Cone, Johnson et al., 1986). Daily exposure to either oral THC or standardized marijuana cigarettes was shown to have no affect on plasma levels of LH or testosterone in men who were prior marijuana users (Dax, Pilotte et al., 1989). Moreover, circulating levels of LH, FSH, prolactin and testosterone were not different in self-reported marijuana users versus non-users of the drug (Block, Farinpour & Schlechte, 1991).

No significant changes in prolactin levels were detected in male subjects who were marijuana smokers (Kolodny, Masters et al., 1974) or who were administered THC (Lemberger, Crabtree et al., 1975). Moreover, circulating prolactin concentrations were not significantly altered following acute oral administration of either THC (17.5 milligrams) or the synthetic cannabinoid, Nabilone (2 milligrams), or after smoking a marijuana cigarette containing 1.83 per cent THC (Mendelson, Ellingboe & Mello, 1984). Smoking one or two marijuana cigarettes containing 2.8 per cent THC also did not have a significant effect on plasma prolactin levels in men when compared to placebo-smoking control subjects (Cone, Johnson et al., 1986). However, long-term cannabis users who smoked a cigarette containing 1.5 grams of cannabis oil exhibited a slight increase in plasma prolactin levels 30 minutes after smoking and another rise in prolactin after four days of cannabis deprivation (Markianos & Stefanis, 1982). In another study, baseline plasma prolactin levels were significantly reduced in heavy marijuana smokers and were further reduced after oral THC administration (Dax, Pilotte et al., 1989).

Chapter 11

Although cannabinoids have a primarily inhibitory effect on reproductive hormones in male experimental animals, the effects of cannabinoids in the human male are not as straightforward. The conflicting results in these human studies could reflect differences in experimental procedures and the possible effects of previous cannabis exposure (i.e., tolerance), and of other drugs, in test subjects — effects that can be carefully controlled for in animal studies. However, the findings that chronic cannabis exposure does affect human reproductive function (Hembree, Nahas et al., 1979; Hembree, Zeidenberg & Nahas, 1976; Issidorides, 1979; Kolodny, Masters et al., 1974) suggests that cannabinoids do alter the reproductive hormones that control testicular function and/or have a direct effect on testicular parameters.

Other Hormones

In addition to effects on the reproductive endocrine system, there is considerable evidence that cannabinoid exposure can affect the hypothalamic-pituitary-adrenal axis. Early animal studies have demonstrated that THC is a potent stimulator of adrenocorticotropin (ACTH) release in male rats (Dewey, Peng & Harris, 1970; Kokka & Garcia, 1974). Acute THC administration also elevated plasma corticosterone levels in male (Kubena, Perhach & Barry, 1971; Puder, Weidenfeld et al., 1982) and female rats (Jackson & Murphy, 1997; Neto, Nunes & Carvalho, 1975) and male mice (Dalterio, Michael et al., 1981; Johnson, Dewey & Bloom, 1981). The intracerebroventricular infusion of either THC or anandamide, an endogenous ligand of the cannabinoid receptor, stimulated ACTH and corticosterone release in a dose-dependent manner and caused a pronounced depletion of corticotropin-releasing hormone (CRH) in the median eminence of the brain of male rats (Weidenfeld, Feldman & Mechoulam, 1994). It has been demonstrated that tolerance develops to the effect of THC on

ACTH release, but not on corticosterone secretion following chronic THC administration in male rats (Rodríguez de Fonseca, Murphy et al., 1992).

Interestingly, men who were heavy cannabis users did not exhibit alterations in cortisol (Block, Farinpour & Schlechte, 1991; Cruickshank, 1976) or impaired adrenocortical reactivity to ACTH (Perez-Reyes, Brine & Wall, 1976). However, one study has reported decreased plasma cortisol and growth hormone levels following insulin-induced hypoglycemia in THC-exposed men (Benowitz, Jones & Lerner, 1976).

In early studies, it was shown that THC was inhibitory to growth hormone secretion in male rats (Collu, Letarte et al., 1974; Kokka & Garcia, 1974) and mice (Dalterio, Michael et al., 1981). However, other studies have demonstrated either no change (Harclerode & Pennebacker, 1985) or an increase (Collu, 1976) in growth hormone in male rats treated with THC. More recently it has been shown that intracerebroventricular infusion of THC suppresses growth hormone secretion in adult male rats (Rettori, Wenger et al., 1988). Although differences in animal models and route and doses of THC administration may be sufficient to explain the variable growth hormone responses to THC reported above, certainly more studies are warranted to determine conclusively the effects of cannabis exposure on growth hormone in both males and females.

Few other endocrine systems have been studied. Circulating thyroxine levels have been shown to be reduced following acute (Hillard, Farber et al., 1984; Nazar, Kairys et al., 1977) or chronic (Rosenkrantz & Esber, 1980) THC administration in male rats. In adult rhesus monkeys, serum thyroxine concentrations were decreased by chronic THC but increased by CBD (Esber, Rosenkrantz & Bogden, 1976; Esber, Zavorskas et al., 1979). The finding that suckling-induced milk release was inhibited following THC treatment in lactating rats was one of the first studies to suggest that THC may also affect the release of the posterior pituitary hormone, oxytocin (Tyrey & Murphy, 1988).

Sites and Mechanisms of Cannabis Action

Site of Action

Many studies showing that cannabinoid exposure reduced testicular, seminal vesicle and prostate weights (Okey & Truant, 1975), decreased ovarian weight (Murphy, Rodríguez de Fonseca & Steger, 1991), increased pituitary and adrenal weights (Collu, 1976) and altered anterior and posterior pituitary hormone release and gonadal steroid secretion (Murphy, Steger & Bartke, 1990) suggested that cannabinoids may have direct effects on peripheral endocrine tissue. Indeed, cannabinoids have been demonstrated to directly inhibit steroidogenesis in cultured ovarian (Bloch, 1983; Reich, Laufer et al., 1982) and testicular cells (Dalterio, Bartke et al., 1978; Hembree, Zeidenberg & Nahas, 1976) and to alter multiple biochemical parameters in ovarian (Adashi, Jones & Hsueh, 1983; Murphy, Steger & Bartke, 1990) and testicular (Husain, 1985; Newton, Murphy & Bartke, 1993) tissues following in vitro incubation. Therefore, cannabinoids can directly affect endocrine organs and alter hormone synthesis and secretion which, in turn, may indirectly affect pituitary hormone release.

Increasing evidence suggests, however, that although chronic cannabis exposure may have pronounced effects on peripheral endocrine tissue, most of the physiological effects of occasional cannabis use can be attributed to its action within the central nervous system, which can then ultimately affect pituitary hormone release (Murphy & Bartke, 1992). Changes in the release of pituitary hormones may be the primary mode by which cannabinoids are able to affect peripheral endocrine function. Moreover, this action of cannabis does not appear to be exerted directly at the pituitary gland (Hughes, Everett & Tyrey, 1981; Murphy, Steger & Bartke, 1990; Rettori, Wenger et al., 1988; Wenger, Rettori et al., 1987), but is instead mediated by cannabinoid action within the brain. Studies using animals with CNS lesions have defined specific brain regions responsible for cannabinoid-induced effects on LH (Puder, Nir et al., 1985; Murphy & Tyrey, 1986a), prolactin (Hughes, Everett & Tyrey, 1984; Tyrey, 1986) and ACTH secretion (Puder, Weidenfeld et al., 1982). Subsequent investigations have determined that the direct infusion of THC into specific regions of the brain inhibited LH (Wenger, Rettori et al., 1987), ACTH (Weidenfeld, Feldman & Mechoulam, 1994), prolactin and growth hormone secretion (Rettori, Wenger et al., 1988) in experimental animals. Moreover, intracerebroventricular THC administration increased hypothalamic content of the neuropeptide, LH-releasing hormone or LHRH (Wenger, Rettori et al., 1987) and decreased CRH concentrations (Weidenfeld, Feldman & Mechoulam, 1994). Thus, cannabinoids appear to act in specific regions of the brain and alter the release of neuropeptides responsible for maintaining both tonic and cyclic pituitary hormone secretion.

Mechanism of Action

NEUROPEPTIDES AND NEUROTRANSMITTERS

The potential mechanisms by which cannabinoids act to alter neuroendocrine function have been widely studied for a number of years (for review see Murphy, Steger & Bartke, 1990), but in recent years significant progress has been achieved in this area. According to recent evidence, THC does not appear to directly inhibit LHRH secretion since it has been shown that the incubation of hypothalamic (Fienhold, 1993) or median eminence tissue (Rettori, Aguila et al., 1990) with THC in vitro does not inhibit basal LHRH release. Moreover, electrochemical stimulation of the medial preoptic area of the brain readily induced gonadotropin surges sufficient to elicit an ovulatory response in THC-blocked proestrous rats, suggesting that the LHRH neurons remain capable of responding to stimuli during THC exposure (Murphy & Tyrey, 1986b; Tyrey, 1992). Instead, cannabinoids appear to alter facilitative and/or inhibitory neurotransmitters and neuromodulators that regulate LHRH secretion. Indeed, THC has been shown to alter noradrenergic (Murphy, Steger et al., 1990; Patel, Borysenko & Kumar, 1985), dopaminergic (Rodríguez de Fonseca, Fernández-Ruiz et al., 1992), serotoninergic (Taylor & Fennessy, 1979), opioidergic (Corchero, Fuentes et al., 1997; Kumar & Chen, 1983) and GABAergic (Revuelta, Cheney et al., 1979) neuronal systems. Moreover, a correlation between THC-induced changes in the function of these neuromodulators and corresponding changes in LHRH and/or LH secretion has recently been elucidated. Several studies have demonstrated a concomitant reduction in norepinephrine activity and LHRH and/or LH secretion in ovariectomized, steroid-primed (Steger, DePaolo et al., 1983), and intact male rats (Murphy, Steger et al., 1990), which strongly suggests that THC may inhibit norepinephrine facilitation of LHRH and, thus, LH secretion. Furthermore, prostaglandin E_2, which mediates the stimulatory action of norepinephrine on LHRH release, may also be affected by THC exposure (Adrian & Murphy, 1992; Rettori, Aguila et al., 1990). Although THC does increase levels of hypothalamic opioids (Kumar & Chen, 1983), which have been shown to be inhibitory to LH release, opioid receptor antagonists were unable to block the effect of THC on pulsatile LH release in the ovariectomized rat (Keller, Kohli & Murphy, 1990). Several studies have shown that THC increased brain serotonin content *in vivo* (Taylor & Fennessy, 1979) and facilitated serotonin synthesis (Johnson & Dewey, 1978) and release (Johnson, Ho & Dewey, 1976) from brain synaptosomal preparations *in vitro*. Taken together, these data indicate that THC may influence serotonergic neuronal systems that are inhibitory to LHRH secretion. THC-induced LH suppression was rarely accompanied by alterations in hypothalamic dopamine neurotransmission (Murphy, Steger et al., 1990; Steger, DePaolo et al., 1983), which is primarily inhibitory to LHRH release. Interestingly, the

neurohormone CRH may also be involved in the ability of cannabinoids to suppress LHRH and LH release. Pretreatment with the CRH receptor antagonist, α-helical CRH, significantly reduced THC-induced LH suppression in female rats (Jackson & Murphy, 1997). Therefore, THC may elicit multiple modulatory actions on LHRH neurons by inhibiting the stimulatory role of norepinephrine on LHRH secretion and activating the inhibitory serotonergic and CRH neuronal systems.

Neurotransmitter and neuropeptide systems that may be involved in the ability of cannabinoids to alter prolactin and growth hormone secretion have also been investigated. In the male rat, THC increased hypothalamic dopamine content (Rodríguez de Fonseca, Fernández-Ruiz et al., 1992) and decreased circulating prolactin levels (Kramer & Ben-David, 1978; Rodríguez de Fonseca, Fernández-Ruiz et al., 1992). Furthermore, dopamine receptor antagonists have been shown to block the suppressive effect of THC on prolactin release in male rats (Kramer & Ben-David, 1978). Thus, inhibitory dopaminergic mechanisms may be involved in the ability of THC to alter prolactin secretion. It has also been demonstrated that serotonin receptor antagonists block THC-induced prolactin suppression (Kramer & Ben-David, 1978). Moreover, increasing evidence suggests that THC may have direct pituitary actions to prevent the ability of vasoactive intestinal peptide (VIP) (Murphy & Rodríguez de Fonseca, 1991) or estradiol (Murphy, Newton et al., 1991) to stimulate prolactin release from anterior pituitary cells *in vitro*.

Interestingly, THC has been shown to directly stimulate the release of somatostatin, a growth hormone inhibiting factor, from median eminence tissue *in vitro* (Rettori, Aguila et al., 1990), suggesting that the suppressive effect of THC on growth hormone release may be mediated in part by direct stimulation of somatostatin release. The effects of cannabinoid exposure on growth hormone releasing hormone are not known.

RECEPTOR-MEDIATED MECHANISMS OF ACTION

Whether cannabinoids alter neurotransmitter activity by inducing membrane perturbation and thus modifying neurotransmitter receptor functionality is not clear (Martin, 1986). Several studies have demonstrated that cannabinoids can alter binding characteristics of β-noradrenergic (Hillard & Bloom, 1982; 1984), dopaminergic (Bloom, 1984; Rodríguez de Fonseca, Fernández-Ruiz et al., 1992), and opioidergic (Vaysse, Gardner & Zukin, 1987) receptor systems. However, correlations between changes in receptor binding and affects on pituitary hormone secretion have not been forthcoming.

Because cannabinoids and steroids contain many similarities of chemical structure and physical property, the possibility that THC could exert action at steroid hormone target sites has been investigated for many years (Dewey, 1986; Martin, 1986). Indeed, experimental evidence suggests that cannabinoids can interact with estrogen (Martin, 1986), androgen (Purohit, Ahluwahlia & Vigersky, 1980) and glucocorticoid receptor systems (Eldridge, Murphy & Landfield, 1991). Several studies have demonstrated similarities between the reproductive actions of THC and estrogens in both females and males (Bloch, Thysen et al., 1978), suggesting that THC possessed estrogen-like activity. Although an early study reported that THC was a weak competitor for estrogen binding to rat uterine cytoplasmic receptors (Rawitch, Schultz & Kurt, 1977), subsequent studies found that THC was unable to compete with estradiol binding to cytosol preparations from rat (Okey & Bondy, 1978), rhesus monkey and human uteri (Smith, Besch & Besch, 1979). Furthermore, cannabinoids failed to directly activate estrogen receptors or antagonize the transcription and cell proliferative responses to estradiol (Ruh, Taylor et al., 1997). One study has demonstrated that THC and CBN modestly compete for dihydrotestosterone binding to androgen receptors in rat prostate cytosol (Purohit, Ahluwahlia & Vigersky, 1980). Furthermore, THC may exert both ago-nist and antagonistic effects in the glucocorticoid receptor system of the rat hippocampus (Eldridge, Murphy & Landfield, 1991). Therefore, cannabinoids may exert some action at steroid hormone target sites; however, it remains to be established whether these *in vitro* findings represent the actions of cannabinoids on the endocrine and reproductive systems *in vivo*.

A substantial amount of attention has recently focused on a membrane receptor for cannabinoids in the brain (for reviews see Howlett, Bidaut-Russell et al., 1990; Pertwee, 1993; 1997). Autoradiographic studies using synthetic ligands have demonstrated site-specific concentrations of cannabinoid receptors in the brain, including a diffuse concentration of cannabinoid receptors in the hypothalamus (Herkenham, Lynn et al., 1990). Moreover, it has recently been demonstrated that cannabinoid receptors are localized on neurons expressing the neuromodulatory peptides, substance P and enkephalin (Mailleux & Vanderhaeghen, 1994). The intracerebroventricular infusion of anandamide, an endogenous ligand of the cannabinoid receptor, stimulated ACTH and corticosterone release in a dose-dependent manner and caused a significant depletion of CRH in the median eminence of the brain of male rats (Weidenfeld, Feldman & Mechoulam, 1994). Systemic administration of anandamide and/or methanandamide has also been shown to inhibit prolactin and LH secretion in male and female rats (Fernández-Ruiz, Muñoz et al., 1997; Murphy, Muñoz et al., in press) and stimulate ACTH and corticosterone release in female rats (Murphy, Muñoz et al., in press). That specific cannabinoid receptors mediate the effects of natural and synthetic cannabinoid compounds on hormone release is supported by findings that specific and potent agonists for brain cannabinoid receptors stimulate ACTH and inhibit LH and prolactin release in rats (Murphy, Muñoz et al., in press), whereas pretreatment with the cannabinoid receptor antagonist SR14176A, blocks the effects of cannabinoid compounds on hormone secretion (Fernández-Ruiz, Muñoz et al., 1997; Murphy, Muñoz et al., in press). Furthermore, cannabinoid receptors in sea urchin sperm have been demonstrated to mediate the inhibitory effects of THC on the acrosome reaction (Chang, Berkery et al., 1993). Together, these findings indicate that cannabinoid receptors are involved in mediating the actions of cannabinoids on endocrine and reproductive parameters.

Reproduction and Development

Cannabinoid Effects on Sex Behavior and Fertility

Early experimental studies reported decreased sexual activity and an increased latency to mount in male rats exposed to THC (Merari, Barak & Plaves, 1973) or hashish (Corcoran, Amit et al., 1974). Subsequent studies have demonstrated that the increase in hypothalamic catecholamine activity and concomitant increase in plasma LH levels in male rats exposed to sexually receptive female rats is completely blocked by THC pre-treatment (Murphy, Gher et al., 1994). In this same study, THC treatment decreased the percentage of male rats exhibiting copulatory behavior and increased the latency periods to mount and intromit. In male mice, copulatory behavior parameters were significantly suppressed by high doses of acute (Dalterio, Bartke et al., 1978; Shrenker & Bartke, 1985) or chronic THC treatment (Dalterio, 1980). Moreover, perinatal THC exposure disrupted copulatory behavior in adult male mice (Dalterio, 1980) and rats. To date, controlled studies investigating the effects of cannabis exposure on copulatory behavior of the adult female have not been reported. However, a recent study has demonstrated that prenatal THC exposure reduced the ability of the adult female offspring to exhibit lordosis (Murphy, Gher & Szary, 1995).

There is very little literature concerning the effects of cannabis on fertility *per se* (Wright, Smith et al., 1976). However, the findings that cannabinoids interfere with normal hypothalamic-pituitary-gonadal function (Murphy, Steger & Bartke, 1990) and can disrupt ovulation (Murphy & Tyrey, 1986b; Smith, Almirez et al., 1983) and sperm production (Bloch, 1983) and sperm function (Chang, Berkery et al., 1993) give credence to the theory that fertility may be affected. Moreover, cannabinoids may interfere with the ability for successful implantation to occur (Chávez & Murphy, 1990; Das, Paria et al., 1995). Components of marijuana may affect the uterus directly (Bloch, Thysen et al., 1978) or indirectly via the hypothalamo-pituitary-gonadal axis (Murphy, Steger & Bartke, 1990), thus creating an intrauterine environment that is non-receptive to implantation-stage embryos or incompatible with continued growth and development of the embryo.

Developmental Effects of Early Cannabinoid Exposure

Chronic marijuana use by mothers before and during pregnancy was reportedly associated with neurobehavioral changes in their newborn, compared to the newborn of non-marijuana users (Fried, 1980; 1982). The offspring of women who chronically used marijuana during pregnancy, compared to those of non-users, had lower birthweights and were more likely to have abnormalities compatible with the fetal alcohol syndrome (Hingson, Alpert et al., 1982). Other studies have reported decreased birthweight and crown-rump length in offspring of mothers identified by urine assay as marijuana users (Zuckerman, Frank et al., 1989). As well, an increased frequency of premature births occurred among women who chronically used marijuana during pregnancy (Gibson, Baghurst & Colley, 1983). Animal evidence suggests that high doses of cannabis may cause birth malformations (Abel, 1985; Bloch, 1983); however, cannabis effects on fetal resorption and growth retardation are more consistently reported (Abel, 1985). Rhesus monkey infants whose mothers received daily oral THC prior to and during lactation, presented evidence of altered visual attention, which appeared to be characterized by sustained focus on a novel stimulus (Golub, Sassenrath & Chapman, 1981). Delayed reflex development has been observed in rat pups exposed to THC on days 10 to 12 of gestation (Borgen, Davis & Pace, 1973). Rat offspring exhibited delayed incisor eruption and retarded development of cliff avoidance and the visual placing reflex (Borgen, Davis & Pace, 1973). Pups also presented evidence of retarded weight gain and eye opening (Fried, 1976). Low doses of THC (1 µg/kg) given during the third week of gestation are associated with reduced litter size and decreased birthweight of offspring (Wenger, Croix et al., 1992). The offspring from pregnant rats exposed to high doses of THC (50 mg/kg) on gestation days (GD) 2 to 22, exhibited transitory changes in both somatic and brain growth (Morgan, Brake et al., 1988). Therefore, prenatal cannabinoid exposure affects the development of a number of maturational events.

The timing of cannabinoid exposure during the prenatal period appears to influence the hormonal response measured in the adult animal. Perinatal THC exposure on GD 20 (Dalterio, 1980) or postnatal treatment on day 1 postpartum (Dalterio, Steger et al., 1984b), resulted in a marked elevation in plasma LH levels or a significant decrease in plasma LH levels, respectively, in intact male mice. However, prenatal THC exposure on GD 18 had no apparent effect on plasma gonadotropin levels in intact adult male mice (Dalterio, Steger et al., 1984a). In adult male rats, prenatal THC exposure on GD 14 to 19 did not affect plasma levels of LH (Murphy, Gher & Szary, 1995).

Prenatal cannabinoid exposure can also alter the normal development of nigrostriatal, mesolimbic and tuberoinfundibular dopaminergic neurons, reflected by changes in several biochemical indices of their activity measured at perinatal ages (Rodríguez de Fonseca, Cebeira et al., 1990; 1991; Walters & Carr, 1986; 1988). Moreover, the male offspring exhibited enhanced hypothalamic dopaminergic activity and decreased serum prolactin levels (Rodríguez de Fonseca, Cebeira et al., 1991). Perinatal THC

exposure significantly inhibited male copulatory behavior parameters in mice (Dalterio, 1980) and rats (Murphy, Gher & Szary, 1995). Adult female rats exposed to THC on GD 14 to 19 (Murphy, Gher & Szary, 1995) or during the first five days after birth (Kumar, Solomon et al., 1986) exhibited irregular estrous cycles or constant diestrous smears compared to vehicle-administered controls. In addition, serum LH levels were significantly reduced when compared to control females (Kumar, Solomon et al., 1986). When the adult female rats exposed to THC on GD 14 to 19 were ovariectomized and primed with estrogen and progesterone, the number of animals exhibiting lordosis behavior was significantly reduced (Murphy, Gher & Szary, 1995).

Conclusion

Cannabinoids have been shown to have profound effects on the endocrine and reproductive systems of experimental animals. In animals, acute cannabinoid administration causes significant decreases in LH, prolactin, testosterone, growth hormone and thyroxine and produces increases in ACTH and corticoserone. Furthermore, cannabinoid exposure affects animal copulatory behavior and may affect fertility. Unfortunately, less is known on how and if cannabis affects hormone secretion and fertility in humans and the offspring of pregnant women who smoke marijuana. The identification of cannabinoid receptors in the brains of humans and animals supports a central nervous system site of cannabinoid action in the ability of cannabinoids alter hormone secretion. Furthermore, the ability of endogenous cannabinoid compounds to alter hormone release and reproductive function suggests a potential role for endogenous cannabinoids in the regulation of the endocrine and reproductive stystems.

Chapter 11

References

Abel, E.L. (1981). Marihuana and sex: A critical survey. *Drug and Alcohol Dependence, 8*, 1–22.

Abel, E.L. (1985). Effects of prenatal exposure to cannabinoids. In T.M. Pinkert (Ed.), *Current Research on the Consequences of Maternal Drug Abuse* (NIDA Research Monograph No. 59, pp. 20–35)(DHHS Publication No. 85-1400). Washington, DC: U.S. Government Printing Office.

Adashi, E.Y., Jones, P.B.C. & Hsueh, A.J.W. (1983). Direct antigonadal activity of cannabinoids: Suppression of rat granulosa cell functions. *American Journal of Physiology, 244*, E177–E185.

Adrian, B.A. & Murphy, L.L. (1992). Inhibition of pulsatile luteinizing hormone secretion by delta-9-tetrahydrocannabinol is reversed by prostaglandin E2 infusion in the median eminence of the ovariectomized rat. *Endocrinology* (Suppl.), 101 (Abstract No. 198).

Almirez, R.G., Smith, C.G. & Asch, R.H. (1983). The effects of marijuana extract and delta-9-tetrahydrocannabinol on luteal function in the Rhesus monkey. *Fertility and Sterility, 39*, 212–215.

Asch, R.H., Fernandez, E.O., Smith, C.G. & Pauerstein, C.J. (1979). Precoital single doses of ∅-tetrahydrocannabinol block ovulation in the rabbit. *Fertility and Sterility, 31*, 331–334.

Asch, R.H., Smith, C.G., Siler-Khodr, T.M. & Pauerstein, C.J. (1979b). Acute decreases in serum prolactin concentrations caused by ∅-tetrahydrocannabinol in nonhuman primates. *Fertility and Sterility, 32*, 571–575.

Asch, R.H., Smith, C.G., Siler-Khodr, T.M. & Pauerstein, C.J. (1981). Effects of ∅-tetrahydrocannabinol during the follicular phase of the Rhesus monkey (Macaca mulatta). *Journal of Clinical Endocrinology and Metabolism, 52*, 50–55.

Asch, R.H., Smith, C.G., Siler-Khodr, T.M. & Pauerstein, C.J. (1979a). Effects of delta-9-tetrahydrocannabinol on gonadal steroidogenic activity in vivo. *Fertility and Sterility, 32*, 576–582.

Ayalon, D., Nir, I., Cordova, T., Bauminger, S., Puder, M., Naor, Z., Kashi, R., Zor, U., Harell, A. & Lindner, H.R. (1977). Acute effect of ∅-tetrahydrocannabinol on the hypothalamo-pituitary-ovarian axis in the rat. *Neuroendocrinology, 23*, 31–42.

Bauman, J. (1980). Marijuana and the female reproductive system (Testimony Before the Subcommittee on Criminal Justice of the Committee on the Judiciary, U.S. Senate). In *Health Consequences of Marijuana Use* (pp. 85–97). Washington, DC: U.S. Government Printing Office.

Benowitz, N.L., Jones, R.T. & Lerner, C.B. (1976). Depression of growth hormone and cortisol response to insulin-induced hypoglycemia after prolonged oral delta-9-tetrahydrocannabinol administration in man. *Journal of Clinical Endocrinology and Metabolism, 42,* 938–941.

Besch, N.F., Smith, C.G., Besch, P.K. & Kaufmann R.H. (1977). The effect of marihuana (delta-9-tetrahydrocannabinol) on the secretion of luteinizing hormone in the ovariectomized rhesus monkey. *American Journal of Obstetrics and Gynecology, 128,* 635–642.

Bloch, E. (1983). Effects of marijuana and cannabinoids on reproduction, endocrine function, development and chromosomes. In K.O. Fehr & H. Kalant (Eds.), *Cannabis and Health Hazards* (pp. 355–432). Toronto: Addiction Research Foundation.

Bloch, E., Thysen, B., Morrill, G.A., Gardner, E. & Fujimoto, G. (1978). Effects of cannabinoids on reproduction and development. *Vitamins and Hormones, 36,* 203–258.

Block, R.I., Farinpour, R. & Schlechte, J.A. (1991). Effects of chronic marijuana use on testosterone, luteinizing hormone, follicle stimulating hormone, prolactin and cortisol in men and women. *Drug and Alcohol Dependence, 28,* 121–128.

Bloom, A.S. (1984). Effects of cannabinoids on neurotransmitter receptors in the brain. In S. Agurell, W.L. Dewey & R.E. Willette (Eds.), *The Cannabinoids: Chemical, Pharmacologic and Therapeutic Aspects* (pp. 575–589). New York: Academic Press.

Borgen, L.A., Davis, W.M. & Pace, H.B. (1973). Effects of prenatal $\varnothing$-tetrahydrocannabinol on the development of rat offspring. *Pharmacology, Biochemistry and Behavior, 1,* 203–206.

Bromley, B.L., Rabii, J., Gordon, J.H. & Zimmerman, E. (1978). Delta-9-tetrahydrocannabinol inhibition of suckling-induced prolactin release in the lactating rat. *Endocrine Research Communications, 5,* 271–278.

Chakravarty, I., Shah, P.G., Sheth, A.R. & Ghosh, J.J. (1979). Mode of action of delta-9-tetrahydrocannabinol on hypothalamo-pituitary function in adult female rats. *Journal of Reproductive Fertility, 57,* 113–115.

Chakravarty, I., Sheth, A.R. & Ghosh, J.J. (1975). Effect of acute $\varnothing$-tetrahydrocannabinol treatment on serum LH and prolactin levels in adult female rats. *Fertility and Sterility, 26,* 947–948.

Chakravarty, I., Sheth, P.R., Sheth, A.R. & Ghosh, J.J. (1982). Delta-9-tetrahydrocannabinol: Its effect on hypothalamo-pituitary system in male rats. *Archives of Andrology, 8,* 25–27.

Chang, M.C., Berkery, D., Schuel, R., Laychock, S.G., Zimmerman, A.M., Zimmerman, S. & Schuel, H. (1993). Evidence for a cannabinoid receptor in sea urchin sperm and its role in blockade of the acrosome reaction. *Molecular Reproduction and Development, 36,* 507–516.

Chávez, D.J. & Murphy, L.L. (1990). Deleterious effects of delta-9-tetrahydrocannabinol (THC) on periimplantation mouse embryos *in vitro*. *Journal of Cell Biology, 111* (5), 483a (Part 2, Abstract No. 2708).

Cohen, S. (1976). The 94-day cannabis study. *Annals of the New York Academy of Sciences, 282,* 211–220.

Collu, R. (1976). Endocrine effects of chronic intraventricular administration of ∅-tetrahydrocannabinol to prepubertal and adult male rats. *Life Sciences, 18,* 223–230.

Collu, R., Letarte, J., Leboeuf, G. & Ducharme, J.R. (1974). Endocrine effects of chronic administration of psychoactive drugs. *Life Sciences, 16,* 533–542.

Cone, E.J., Johnson, R.E., Moore, J.D. & Roache, J.D. (1986). Acute effects of smoking marijuana on hormones, subjective effects and performance in male human subjects. *Pharmacology, Biochemistry and Behavior, 24,* 1749–1754.

Corchero, J., Fuentes, J.A. & Manzanares, J. (1997). ∅-Tetrahydrocannabinol increases proopiomelanocortin gene expression in the arcuate nucleus of the rat hypothalamus. *European Journal of Pharmacology, 323,* 193–195.

Corcoran, M.E., Amit, Z., Malsbury, C.W. & Daykin, S. (1974). Reduction in copulatory behavior of male rats following hashish injections. *Research Communications in Chemical Pathology and Pharmacology, 7,* 779–782.

Cruickshank, E.K. (1976). Physical assessment of 30 chronic cannabis users and 30 matched controls. *Annals of the New York Academy of Sciences, 282,* 162–167.

Cushman, P. (1975). Plasma testosterone levels in healthy male marijuana smokers. *American Journal of Drug and Alcohol Abuse, 2,* 269–275.

Daley, Y.D., Branda, L.A., Rosenfeld, Y. & Younglai, E.V. (1974). Increase of serum prolactin in male rats by (–)-trans-delta-9-tetrahydrocannabinol. *Endocrinology, 63,* 415–416.

Dalterio, S.L. (1980). Perinatal or adult exposure to cannabinoids alters male reproductive functions in mice. *Pharmacology, Biochemistry and Behavior, 12,* 143–153.

Dalterio, S., Bartke, A. & Mayfield, D. (1983). Cannabinoids stimulate and inhibit testosterone production in vitro and in vivo. *Life Sciences, 32,* 605–612.

Dalterio, S., Bartke, A., Roberson, C., Watson, D. & Burstein, S. (1978). Direct and pituitary-mediated effects of ∅-THC and cannabinol on the testis. *Pharmacology, Biochemistry and Behavior, 8,* 673–678.

Dalterio, S.L., Mayfield, D.L. & Bartke, A. (1983). Effects of ∅-THC on plasma hormone levels in female mice. *Substance and Alcohol Actions/Misuse, 4,* 339–345.

Dalterio, S.L., Michael, S.D., Macmillan, B.T. & Bartke, A. (1981). Differential effects of cannabinoid exposure and stress on plasma prolactin, growth hormone and corticosterone levels in male mice. *Life Sciences, 28*, 761–766.

Dalterio, S.L., Steger, R., Mayfield, D. & Bartke, A. (1984a). Early cannabinoid exposure influences neuroendocrine and reproductive functions in male mice. I. Prenatal effects. *Pharmacology, Biochemistry and Behavior, 20*, 107–113.

Dalterio, S.L., Steger, R., Mayfield, D. & Bartke, A. (1984b). Early cannabinoid exposure influences neuroendocrine and reproductive functions in mice: II. Postnatal effects. *Pharmacology, Biochemistry and Behavior, 20*, 115–123.

Das, S.K., Paria, B.C., Chakraborty, I. & Dey, S.K. (1995). Cannabinoid ligand-receptor signaling in the mouse uterus. *Proceedings of the National Academy of Sciences of the United States of America, 92*, 4332–4336.

Dax, E.M., Pilotte, N.S., Adler, W.H., Nagel, J.E. & Lange, W.R. (1989). The effects of 9-ene-tetrahydrocannabinol on hormone release and immune function. *Journal of Steroid Biochemistry and Molecular Biology, 34*, 263–270.

Dewey, W.L. (1986). Cannabinoid pharmacology. *Pharmacological Reviews, 38*, 151–178.

Dewey, W.L., Peng, T-C. & Harris, L.S. (1970). The effect of 1-trans-$\varnothing$-tetrahydrocannabinol on the hypothalamo-hypophyseal-adrenal axis of rats. *European Journal of Pharmacology, 12*, 382–384.

Eldridge, J.C., Murphy, L.L. & Landfield, P.W. (1991). Cannabinoids and the hippocampal glucocorticoid receptor: Recent findings and possible significance. *Steroids, 56*, 226–231.

Esber, H.J., Rosenkrantz, H. & Bogden, A.E. (1976). Assessment of the effect of $\varnothing$-tetrahydrocannabinol on testicular and thyroid hormone levels in rats. *Federation Proceedings, 35*, 727.

Esber, H.J., Zavorskas, P.A., Bogden, A.E. & Rosenkrantz, H. (1979). Effect of cannabidiol on serum thyroxine levels in adult rhesus monkeys. *Federation Proceedings, 38*, 1030.

Fernández-Ruiz, J.J., Muñoz, R.M., Romero, J., Villanua, M.A., Makriyannis, A. & Ramos, J.A. (1997). Time course of the effects of different cannabimimetics on prolactin and gonadotrophin secretion: Evidence for the presence of CB1 receptors in hypothalamic structures and their involvement in the effects of cannabimimetics. *Biochemical Pharmacology, 53*, 1919–1927.

Fernández-Ruiz, J.J., Navarro, M., Hernández, M.L., Vaticón, D. & Ramos, J.A. (1992). Neuroendocrine effects of an acute dose of $\varnothing$-tetrahydrocannabinol: Changes in hypothalamic biogenic amines and anterior pituitary hormone secretion. *Neuroendocrinology Letters, 14*, 349–355.

Field, E. & Tyrey, L. (1986). Blockade of first ovulation in pubertal rats by delta-9-tetrahydro-cannabinol: Requirement for advanced treatment due to early initiation of the critical period. *Biology of Reproduction, 34,* 512–517.

Fienhold, J.W. (1993). The effect of delta-9-tetrahydrocannabinol on luteinizing hormone-releasing hormone secretion from male and female hypothalami in vitro. Master's thesis, Southern Illinois University, Carbondale.

Fried, P.A. (1976). Short and long-term effects of pre-natal cannabis inhalation upon rat offspring. *Psychopharmacology (Berl), 50,* 285–291.

Fried, P.A. (1980). Marijuana use by pregnant women: Neurobehavioral effects in neonates. *Drug and Alcohol Dependence, 6,* 415–424.

Fried, P.A. (1982). Marijuana use by pregnant women and effects on offspring: An update. *Neurobehavioral Toxicology and Teratology, 4,* 451–454.

Gibson, G.T., Baghurst, P.A. & Colley, D.P. (1983). Maternal alcohol, tobacco and cannabis consumption and the outcome of pregnancy. *Australian and New Zealand Journal of Obstetrics and Gynaecology, 23,* 15–19.

Golub, M.S., Sassenrath, E.N. & Chapman, L.F. (1981). Regulation of visual attention in offspring of female monkeys treated chronically with $\varnothing$-tetrahydrocannabinol. *Developmental Psychobiology, 14,* 507–512.

Harclerode, J.E. & Pennebacker, P.K. (1985). The effect of delta-9-tetrahydrocannabinol on rat serum and pituitary growth hormone levels. In D.J. Harvey (Ed.), *Marihuana '84: Proceedings of the Oxford Symposium on Cannabis* (pp. 529–536). Oxford: IRL Press.

Hembree, W.C., III, Nahas, G.G., Zeidenberg, P. & Huang, H.F.S. (1979). Changes in human spermatozoa associated with high dose marihuana smoking. In G.G. Nahas & W.D.M. Paton (Eds.), *Marihuana: Biological Effects: Analysis, Metabolism, Cellular Responses, Reproduction and Brain, Advances in the Biosciences* (pp. 429–439) (Vols. 22 & 23). Oxford: Pergamon Press.

Hembree, W.C., III, Zeidenberg, P. & Nahas, G.G. (1976). Marihuana's effect on human gonadal function. In G.G. Nahas (Ed.), *Marihuana: Chemistry, Biochemistry, and Cellular Effects* (pp. 521–532). New York: Springer-Verlag.

Herkenham, M., Lynn, A.B., Little, M.D., Johnson, M.R., Melvin, L.S., De Costa, B.R. & Rice, K.C. (1990). Cannabinoid receptor localization in brain. *Proceedings of the National Academy of Sciences of the United States of America, 87,* 1932–1936.

Hillard, C.J. & Bloom, A.S. (1982). $\varnothing$-Tetrahydrocannabinol-induced changes in beta-adrenergic receptor binding in mouse cerebral cortex. *Brain Research, 235,* 370–377.

Hillard, C.J. & Bloom, A.S. (1984). Further studies of the interaction of delta-9-tetrahydro-cannabinol with the beta-adrenergic receptor. In S. Agurell, W.L. Dewey & R.E. Willette (Eds.), *The Cannabinoids: Chemical, Pharmacologic and Therapeutic Aspects* (pp. 591–602). New York: Academic Press.

Hillard, C.J., Farber, N.E., Hagen, T. & Bloom, A.S. (1984). The effects of THC on serum thyrotropin levels in the rat. *Pharmacology, Biochemistry and Behavior, 20,* 547–550.

Hingson, R., Alpert, J., Day, N., Dooling, E., Kayne, H., Morelock, S., Oppenheimer, E. & Zuckerman, B. (1982). Effects of maternal drinking and marijuana use on fetal growth and development. *Pediatrics, 70,* 539–546.

Howlett, A.C., Bidaut-Russell, M., Devane, W.A., Melvin, L.S., Johnson, M.R. & Herkenham, M. (1990). The cannabinoid receptor: Biochemical, anatomical and behavioral characterization. *Trends in Neuroscience, 13,* 420–423.

Hughes, C.L., Jr., Everett, J.W. & Tyrey, L. (1981). $\varnothing$-Tetrahydrocannabinol suppression of prolactin secretion in the rat: Lack of direct pituitary effect. *Endocrinology, 109,* 876–880.

Hughes, C.L., Jr., Everett, J.W. & Tyrey, L. (1984). Effects of delta-9-tetrahydrocannabinol on serum prolactin in female rats bearing CNS lesions: Implications for site of drug action. In S. Agurell, W.L. Dewey & R.E. Willette (Eds.), *The Cannabinoids: Chemical, Pharmacologic and Therapeutic* Aspects (pp. 497–519). Orlando, FL: Academic Press.

Hughes, C.L., Jr. & Tyrey, L. (1982). Effects of (–)-trans-$\varnothing$-tetrahydrocannabinol on serum prolactin in the pseudopregnant rat. *Endocrine Research Communications, 9,* 25–36.

Husain, S. (1985). Involvement of cellular energetics in the gonadal effects of delta-9-tetrahydrocannabinol (THC). In D.J. Harvey (Ed.), *Marihuana '84: Proceedings of the Oxford Symposium on Cannabis* (pp. 391–398). Oxford: IRL Press.

Issidorides, M.R. (1979). Observations in chronic hashish users: Nuclear aberrations in blood and sperm and abnormal acrosomes in spermatozoa. In G.G. Nahas & W.D.M. Paton (Eds.), *Marihuana: Biological Effects: Analysis, Metabolism, Cellular Responses, Reproduction and Brain, Advances in the Biosciences* (pp. 377–387) (Vols. 22 & 23). Oxford: Pergamon Press.

Jackson, A.L. & Murphy, L.L. (1997). Role of the hypothalamo-pituitary-adrenal axis in the suppression of luteinizing hormone release by delta-9-tetrahydrocannabinol. *Neuroendocrinology, 65,* 446–452.

Johnson, K.M. & Dewey, W.L. (1978). The effect of $\varnothing$-tetrahydrocannabinol on the conversion of [³H]tryptophan to 5-[³H]hydroxytryptamine in the mouse brain. *Journal of Pharmacology and Experimental Therapeutics, 207,* 140–150.

Johnson, K.M., Dewey, W.L. & Bloom, A.S. (1981). Adrenalectomy reverses the effects of delta-9-THC on mouse brain 5-hydroxytryptamine turnover. *Pharmacology, 23,* 223–229.

Johnson, K.M., Ho, B.T. & Dewey, W.L. (1976). Effects of ∅-tetrahydrocannabinol on neurotransmitter accumulation and release mechanism in rat forebrain synaptosomes. *Life Sciences, 19*, 347–356.

Johnson, L.Y., Asch, R.H. & Reiter, R.J. (1980). Failure of pinealectomy to affect acute changes in plasma levels of luteinizing hormone and prolactin in ovariectomized rats following ∅-tetrahydrocannabinol administration. *Substance and Alcohol Actions/Misuse, 1*, 355–359.

Keller, P., Kohli, M. & Murphy, L.L. (1990). Naloxone reverses but does not prevent delta-9-tetrahydrocannabinol-induced inhibition of pulsatile LH secretion in ovariectomized rats. *Society for Neuroscience Abstracts, 16*, 1101.

Kokka, N. & Garcia, J.F. (1974). Effects of ∅-THC on growth hormone and ACTH secretion in rats. *Life Sciences, 15*, 329–338.

Kolodny, R.C., Lessin, R.C., Toro, G., Masters, W.H. & Cohen, S. (1976). Depression of plasma testosterone with acute marihuana administration. In M.C. Braude & S. Szara (Eds.), *The Pharmacology of Marihuana* (pp. 217–225). New York: Raven Press.

Kolodny, R.C., Masters, W.H., Kolodny, R.M. & Toro, G. (1974). Depression of plasma testosterone levels after chronic intensive marijuana use. *New England Journal of Medicine, 290*, 872–874.

Kramer, J. & Ben-David, M. (1974). Suppression of prolactin secretion by acute administration of ∅-THC in rats. *Proceedings of the Society for Experimental Biology and Medicine, 147*, 482–484.

Kramer, J. & Ben-David, M. (1978). Prolactin suppression by (–)∅9-tetrahydrocannabinol (THC): Involvement of serotonergic and dopaminergic pathways. *Endocrinology, 103*, 452–457.

Kubena, R.K., Perhach, J.L., Jr. & Barry H., III. (1971). Corticosterone elevation mediated centrally by ∅-tetrahydrocannabinol in rats. *European Journal of Pharmacology, 14*, 89–92.

Kumar, A.M., Solomon, J., Patel, V., Kream, R.M., Drieze, J.M. & Millard, W.J. (1986). Early exposure to ∅-tetrahydrocannabinol influences neuroendocrine and reproductive functions in female rats. *Neuroendocrinology, 44*, 260–264.

Kumar, M.S.A. & Chen, C.L. (1983). Effect of an acute dose of ∅-THC on hypothalamic luteinizing hormone releasing hormone and met-enkephalin content and serum levels of testosterone and corticosterone in rats. *Substance and Alcohol Actions/Misuse, 4*, 37–43.

Lemberger, L., Crabtree, R., Rowe, H. & Clemons, J. (1975). Tetrahydrocannabinoids and serum prolactin levels in man. *Life Sciences, 16*, 1339–1343.

Mailleux, P. & Vanderhaeghen, J.J. (1994). Delta-9-Tetrahydrocannabinol regulates substance P and enkephalin mRNA levels in the caudate-putamen. *European Journal of Pharmacology, 267,* R1–R3.

Markianos, M. & Stefanis, C. (1982). Effects of acute cannabis use and short-term deprivation on plasma prolactin and dopamine-β-hydroxylase in long-term users. *Drug and Alcohol Dependence, 9,* 251–255.

Marks, B.H. (1973). Ø-Tetrahydrocannabinol and LH secretion. *Progress in Brain Research, 39,* 331–338.

Martin, B.R. (1986). Cellular effects of cannabinoids. *Pharmacological Reviews, 38,* 45–74.

Maskarinec, M.P. (1978). Endocrine effects of cannabis in male rats. *Toxicology and Applied Pharmacology, 45,* 615–628.

Mendelson, J.H., Cristofaro, P., Ellingboe, J., Benedikt, R. & Mello, N.K. (1985). Acute effects of marihuana on luteinizing hormone in menopausal women. *Pharmacology, Biochemistry and Behavior, 23,* 765–768.

Mendelson, J.H., Ellingboe, J., Kuehnle, J.C. & Mello, N.K. (1978). Effects of chronic marihuana use on integrated plasma testosterone and luteinizing hormone levels. *Journal of Pharmacology and Experimental Therapeutics, 207,* 611–617.

Mendelson, J.H., Ellingboe, J. & Mello, N.K. (1984). Acute effects of natural and synthetic cannabis compounds on prolactin levels in human males. *Pharmacology, Biochemistry and Behavior, 20,* 103–106.

Mendelson, J.H., Kuehnle, J., Ellingboe, J. & Babor, T.F. (1974). Plasma testosterone levels before, during and after chronic marihuana smoking. *New England Journal of Medicine, 291,* 1051–1055.

Mendelson, J.H., Mello, N.K., Cristofaro, P., Ellingboe, J. & Benedikt, R. (1985). Acute effects of marihuana on pituitary and gonadal hormones during the periovulatory phase of the menstrual cycle. In L.S. Harris (Ed.), *Problems of Drug Dependence: 1984* (pp. 24–31). Washington, DC: U.S. Government Printing Office.

Mendelson, J.H., Mello, N.K. & Ellingboe, J. (1985). Acute effects of marihuana smoking on prolactin levels in human females. *Journal of Pharmacology and Experimental Therapeutics, 232,* 220–222.

Mendelson, J.H., Mello, N.K., Ellingboe, J., Skupny, A.S.T., Lex, B.W. & Griffin, M. (1986). Marihuana smoking suppresses luteinizing hormone in women. *Journal of Pharmacology and Experimental Therapeutics, 237,* 862–866.

Merari, A., Barak, A. & Plaves, M. (1973). Effects of Ø$^{(2)}$-tetrahydrocannabinol on copulation in the male rat. *Psychopharmacologia, 28,* 243–246.

Morgan, B., Brake, S.C., Hutchings, D.E., Miller, N. & Gamagaris, Z. (1988). Delta-9-tetrahydrocannabinol during pregnancy in the rat: Effects on development of RNA, DNA, and protein in offspring brain. *Pharmacology, Biochemistry and Behavior, 31*, 365–369.

Murphy, L.L. & Bartke, A. (Eds.) (1992). *Marijuana/Cannabinoids: Neurobiology and Neurophysiology.* Boca Raton, FL: CRC Press.

Murphy, L.L., Chandrashekar, V. & Bartke, A. (1994). Delta-9-tetrahydrocannabinol inhibits pulsatile luteinizing hormone secretion in the male rat: Effect of intracerebroventricular norepinephrine infusion. *Neuroendocrinology Letters, 16*, 1–7.

Murphy, L.L., Gher, J., Steger, R.W. & Bartke, A. (1994). Effects of ∅-tetrahydrocannabinol on copulatory behavior and neuroendocrine responses of male rats to female conspecifics. *Pharmacology, Biochemistry and Behavior, 49*, 1–7.

Murphy, L.L., Gher, J. & Szary, A. (1994). Prenatal cannabinoid exposure and effects on reproductive and immune parameters of the male and female offspring. *International Cannabis Research Society Annual Meeting, Montreal* (Abstract).

Murphy, L.L., Gher, J. & Szary, A. (1995). Effects of prenatal exposure to delta-9-tetrahydrocannabinol on reproductive, endocrine and immune parameters of male and female rat offspring. *Endocrine, 3*, 875–879.

Murphy, L.L., Muñoz, R.M., Adrian, B.A. & Villanua, M.A. (in press). Function of cannabinoid receptors in the neuroendocrine regulation of hormone secretion. *Seminars in the Neurosciences.*

Murphy, L.L., Newton, S.C., Dhali, J. & Chávez, D. (1991). Evidence for a direct anterior pituitary site of delta-9-tetrahydrocannabinol action. *Pharmacology, Biochemistry and Behavior, 40*, 603–607.

Murphy, L.L. & Rodríguez de Fonseca, F. (1991). Acute effects of delta-9-tetrahydrocannabinol on VIP-induced cAMP accumulation and prolactin release by rat anterior pituitary cells. *Journal of Cell Biology, 115* (3), 78a (Part 2, Abstract No. 454).

Murphy, L.L., Rodríguez de Fonseca, F. & Steger, R.W. (1991). ∅-Tetrahydrocannabinol antagonism of the anterior pituitary response to estradiol in immature female rats. *Steroids, 56*, 97–102.

Murphy, L.L., Steger, R.W. & Bartke, A. (1990). Psychoactive and nonpsychoactive cannabinoids and their effects on reproductive neuroendocrine parameters. In R.R. Watson (Ed.), *Biochemistry and Physiology of Substance Abuse* (Vol. 2) (pp. 73–93). Boca Raton, FL: CRC Press.

Murphy, L.L., Steger, R.W., Smith, M.S. & Bartke, A. (1990). Effects of delta-9-tetrahydrocannabinol, cannabinol and cannabidiol, alone and in combinations, on luteinizing hormone and prolactin release and on hypothalamic neurotransmitters in the male rat. *Neuroendocrinology, 52*, 316–321.

Murphy, L.L. & Tyrey, L. (1986a). Inhibition of LH and PRL by ⌀-tetrahydrocannabinol in medial basal hypothalamic-deafferentated ovariectomized rats. *First International Congress of Neuroendocrinology, Abstract No. 30* (p. 30). Basel: S. Karger.

Murphy, L.L. & Tyrey, L. (1986b). Induction of LH release by electrochemical stimulation of the medial preoptic area in delta-9-tetrahydrocannabinol-blocked proestrous rats. *Neuroendocrinology, 43*, 471–475.

Nazar, B., Kairys, D.J., Fowler, R. & Harclerode, J. (1977). Effects of ⌀-tetrahydrocannabinol on serum thyroxine concentrations in the rat. *Journal of Pharmacy and Pharmacology, 29*, 778–779.

Neto, J.P., Nunes, J.F. & Carvalho, F.V. (1975). The effects of chronic cannabis treatment upon brain 5-hydroxytryptamine, plasma corticosterone and aggressive behavior in female rats with different hormonal status. *Psychopharmacology, 42*, 195–200.

Newton, S.C., Murphy, L.L. & Bartke, A. (1993). In vitro effects of psychoactive and non-psychoactive cannabinoids on immature rat sertoli cell function. *Life Sciences, 53*, 1429–1437.

Nir, I., Ayalon, D., Tsafriri, A., Cordova, T. & Lindner, H.R. (1973). Suppression of the cyclic surge of luteinizing hormone secretion and of ovulation in the rat by Δ^1-tetrahydrocannabinol. *Nature (London), 243*, 470–471.

Okey, A.B. & Bondy, G.P. (1978). Δ^9-Tetrahydrocannabinol and 17β-estradiol bind to different macromolecules in estrogen target tissues. *Science, 200*, 312–314.

Okey, A.B. & Truant, G.S. (1975). Cannabis demasculinizes but is not estrogenic. *Life Sciences, 17*, 1113–1118.

Patel, V., Borysenko, M. & Kumar, M.S.A. (1985). Effect of ⌀-THC on brain and plasma catecholamine levels as measured by HPLC. *Brain Research Bulletin, 14*, 85–90.

Perez, R.M., Cerezo, A., Sanz, N. & Hernandez, R. (1996). Prenatal and adult treatments with THC: Effects on hormone levels and sexual behavior in male rats. *Neuroscience Research Communications, 19*, 179–188.

Perez-Reyes, M., Brine, D. & Wall, M.E. (1976). Clinical study of frequent marijuana use: Adrenal cortical reserve metabolism of a contraceptive agent and development of tolerance. *Annals of the New York Academy of Sciences, 282*, 173–179.

Pertwee, R. (1993). The evidence for the existence of cannabinoid receptors. *General Pharmacology, 24*, 811–824.

Pertwee, R.G. (1997). Pharmacology of cannabinoid CB_1 and CB_2 receptors. *Pharmacology and Therapeutics, 74*, 129–180.

Puder, M., Nir, I., Siegel, R.A., Weidenfeld, J. & Ayalon, D. (1985). The effect of ∅-tetra-hydrocannabinol on luteinizing hormone release in castrated and hypothalamic deafferentated male rats. *Experimental Brain Research*, *59*, 213–216.

Puder, M., Weidenfeld, J., Chowers, I., Nir, I., Conforti, N. & Siegel, R.A. (1982). Corticotrophin and corticosterone secretion following ∅-tetrahydrocannabinol, in intact and in hypothalamic deafferentated male rats. *Experimental Brain Research*, *46*, 85–88.

Purohit, V., Ahluwahlia, B.S. & Vigersky, R.A. (1980). Marihuana inhibits dihydrotestosterone binding to the androgen receptor. *Endocrinology*, *107*, 848–850.

Rawitch, A.B., Schultz, G.S. & Kurt, E.E. (1977). Competition of ∅-tetrahydrocannabinol with estrogen in rat uterine estrogen receptor binding. *Science*, *197*, 1189–1191.

Reich, R., Laufer, N., Lewysohn, O., Cordova, T., Avalon, D. & Tsafriri, A. (1982). In vitro effects of cannabinoids on follicular function in the rat. *Biology of Reproduction*, *27*, 223–231.

Rettori, V., Aguila, M.C., Gimeno, M.F., Franchi, A.M. & McCann, S.M. (1990). In vitro effect of delta-9-tetrahydrocannabinol to stimulate somatostatin release and block that of luteinizing hormone-releasing hormone by suppression of the release of prostaglandin E_2. *Proceedings of the National Academy of Sciences of the United States of America*, *87*, 10063–10066.

Rettori, V., Wenger, T., Snyder, G., Dalterio, S. & McCann, S.M. (1988). Hypothalamic action of delta-9-tetrahydrocannabinol to inhibit the release of prolactin and growth hormone in the rat. *Neuroendocrinology*, *47*, 498–503.

Revuelta, A.V., Cheney, D.L., Wood, P.L. & Costa, E. (1979). GABAergic mediation in the inhibition of hippocampal acetylcholine turnover rate elicited by ∅-tetrahydro-cannabinol. *Neuropharmacology*, *18*, 523–530.

Rodríguez de Fonseca, F., Cebeira, M., Fernández-Ruiz, J.J., Navarro, M. & Ramos, J.A. (1991). Effects of pre- and perinatal exposure to hashish extracts on the ontogeny of brain dopaminergic neurons. *Neuorscience*, *43*, 713–723.

Rodríguez de Fonseca, F., Cebeira, M., Hernández, M.L., Ramos, J.A. & Fernández-Ruiz, J.J. (1990). Changes in brain dopaminergic indices induced by perinatal exposure to cannabinoids in rats. *Developmental Brain Research*, *51*, 237–240.

Rodríguez de Fonseca, F., Fernández-Ruiz, J.J., Murphy, L.L., Cebeira, M., Steger, R.W., Bartke, A. & Ramos, J.A. (1992). Acute effects of Δ9-tetrahydrocannabinol on dopaminergic activity in several rat brain areas. *Pharmacology, Biochemistry and Behavior*, *42*, 269–275.

Rodríguez de Fonseca, F., Murphy, L.L., Bonnin, A., Eldridge, J.C., Bartke, A. & Fernández-Ruiz, J.J. (1992). $\emptyset$-tetrahydrocannabinol administration affects anterior pituitary, corticoadrenal and adrenomedullary functons in male rats. *Neuroendocrinology (Life Science Advances)*, *11*, 147–156.

Rosenkrantz, H. & Esber, H.J. (1980). Cannabinoid-induced hormone changes in monkeys and rats. *Journal of Toxicology and Environmental Health*, *6*, 297–313.

Ruh, M.F., Taylor, J.A., Howlett, A.C. & Welshons, W.V. (1997). Failure of cannabinoid compounds to stimulate estrogen receptors. *Biochemical Pharmacology*, *53*, 35–41.

Schaefer, C.F., Gunn, C.G. & Dubowski, K.M. (1975). Normal plasma testosterone concentrations after marihuana smoking. *New England Journal of Medicine*, *292*, 867–868.

Shrenker, P. & Bartke, A. (1985). Suppression of male copulatory behavior by $\emptyset$-THC is not dependent on changes in plasma testosterone or hypothalamic dopamine or serotonin content. *Pharmacology, Biochemistry and Behavior*, *22*, 415–420.

Smith, C.G., Almirez, R.G., Berenberg, J. & Asch, R.H. (1983). Tolerance develops to the disruptive effects of $\emptyset$-tetrahydrocannabinol on primate menstrual cycle. *Science*, *219*, 1453–1455.

Smith, C.G., Besch, N.F., Smith, R.G. & Besch, P.K. (1979). Effect of tetrahydrocannabinol on the hypothalamic-pituitary axis in the ovariectomized rhesus monkey. *Fertility and Sterility*, *31*, 335–339.

Smith, C.G., Moore, C.E., Besch, N.F. & Besch, P.K. (1976). The effect of marihuana (delta-9-tetrahydrocannabinol) on the secretion of sex hormones in the mature male Rhesus monkey. *Clinical Chemistry*, *22*, 1184–1186.

Smith, R.G., Besch, N.F. & Besch, P.K. (1979). Inhibition of gonadotropin by $\emptyset$-tetrahydrocannabinol: Mediation by steroid receptors? *Science*, *204*, 325–327.

Steger, R.W., DePaolo, L., Asch, R.H. & Silverman, A.Y. (1983). Interactions of $\emptyset$-tetrahydrocannabinol (THC) with hypothalamic neurotransmitters controlling luteinizing hormone and prolactin release. *Neuroendocrinology*, *37*, 361–370.

Steger, R.W., Murphy, L.L., Bartke, A. & Smith, M.S. (1990). Effects of psychoactive and nonpsychoactive cannabinoids on the hypothalamic-pituitary axis of the adult male rat. *Pharmacology, Biochemistry and Behavior*, *37*, 299–302.

Steger, R.W., Silverman, A.Y., Johns, A. & Asch, R.H. (1981). Interactions of cocaine and $\emptyset$-tetrahydrocannabinol with the hypothalamo-hypophyseal axis of the female rat. *Fertility and Sterility*, *35*, 567–572.

Steger, R.W., Silverman, A.Y., Siler-Khodr, T.M. & Asch, R.H. (1980). The effect of $\emptyset$-tetrahydrocannabinol on the positive and negative feedback control of luteinizing hormone release. *Life Sciences*, *27*, 1911–1916.

Symons, A.M., Teale, J.D. & Marks, V. (1976). Effects of $\varnothing$-tetrahydrocannabinol on the hypothalamic-pituitary-gonadal system in the maturing male rat. *Journal of Endocrinology, 68*, 43P.

Taylor, D.A. & Fennessy, M.R. (1979). The effect of (–)-trans-$\varnothing$-tetrahydrocannabinol on regional brain levels and subcellular distribution of monoamines in the rat. *Clinical and Experimental Pharmacology and Physiology, 6*, 541–548.

Tyrey, L. (1978). Delta-9-tetrahydrocannabinol suppression of episodic luteinizing hormone secretion in the ovariectomized rat. *Endocrinology, 102*, 1808–1814.

Tyrey, L. (1980). Delta-9-tetrahydrocannabinol: A potent inhibitor of episodic luteinizing hormone secretion. *Journal of Pharmacology and Experimental Therapeutics, 213*, 306–308.

Tyrey, L. (1986). Reversal of the delta-9-tetrahydrocannabinol inhibitory effect on prolactin secretion by rostral deafferentation of the medial basal hypothalamus. *Neuroendocrinology, 44*, 204–210.

Tyrey, L. (1992). Delta-9-tetrahydrocannabinol attenuates luteinizing hormone release induced by electrochemical stimulation of the medial preoptic area. *Biology of Reproduction, 47*, 262–267.

Tyrey, L. & Hughes, C.L., Jr. (1984). Inhibition of suckling-induced prolactin secretion by $\varnothing$-tetrahydrocannabinol. In S. Agurell, W.L. Dewey & R.W. Willette (Eds.), *The Cannabinoids: Chemical, Pharmacologic and Therapeutic Aspects* (pp. 487–495). Orlando, FL: Academic Press.

Tyrey, L. & Murphy, L.L. (1988). Inhibition of suckling-induced milk ejections in the lactating rat by delta-9-tetrahydrocannabinol. *Endocrinology, 123*, 469–472.

Vaysse, P.J.-J., Gardner, E.L. & Zukin, R.S. (1987). Modulation of rat brain opioid receptors by cannabinoids. *Journal of Pharmacology and Experimental Therapeutics, 241*, 534–539.

Walters, D.E. & Carr, L.A. (1986). Changes in brain catecholamine mechanisms following perinatal exposure to marihuana. *Pharmacology, Biochemistry and Behavior, 25*, 763–768.

Walters, D.E. & Carr, L.A. (1988). Perinatal exposure to cannabinoids alters neurochemical development in rat brain. *Pharmacology, Biochemistry and Behavior, 29*, 213–216.

Weidenfeld, J., Feldman, S. & Mechoulam, R. (1994). Effect of the brain constituent anandamide, a cannabinoid receptor agonist, on the hypothalamo-pituitary-adrenal axis in the rat. *Neuroendocrinology, 59*, 110–112.

Wenger, T., Croix, D., Tramu, G. & Leonardelli, J. (1992). Effects of $\varnothing$-tetrahydrocannabinol on pregnancy, puberty, and the neuroendocrine system. In L.L. Murphy & A. Bartke (Eds.), *Marijuana/Cannabinoids: Neurobiology and Neurophysiology* (pp. 539–560). Boca Raton, FL: CRC Press.

Wenger, T., Rettori, V., Snyder, G.D., Dalterio, S. & McCann, S.M. (1987). Effects of delta-9-tetrahydrocannabinol on the hypothalamic-pituitary control of luteinizing hormone and follicle-stimulating hormone secretion in adult male rats. *Neuroendocrinology, 46*, 488–493.

Wright, P.L., Smith, S.H., Keplinger, M.L., Calandra, J.C. & Braude, M.C. (1976). Reproductive and teratologic studies with $\varnothing^9$-tetrahydrocannabinol and crude marijuana extract. *Toxicology and Applied Pharmacology, 38*, 223–235.

Zuckerman, B., Frank, D., Hingson, R., Amaro, H., Levenson, S., Kayne, H., Parker, S., Vinci, R., Aboagye, K., Fried, L., Cabral, H., Timperi, R. & Bauchner, H. (1989). Effects of maternal marijuana and cocaine use on fetal growth. *New England Journal of Medicine, 320*, 762–768.

Cannabis During Pregnancy: Neurobehavioral Effects in Animals and Humans

Cannabis During Pregnancy: Neurobehavioral Effects in Animals and Humans

DONALD E. HUTCHINGS AND PETER A. FRIED

A reader of the scientific literature on cannabis invariably encounters two unrelated pieces of information that appear in nearly every contemporary article — first, that cannabis or marijuana is the most widely used of all illicit drugs available in the United States and second, that $\varnothing^9$-tetrahydrocannabinol (THC) is the major psychoactive ingredient. The first of these — the popularity of marijuana — remains a guiding impetus to continue studies of its health-related effects. But it is the second fact — the role of THC — that requires some additional comment.

Indeed, THC is the principal active ingredient in marijuana, producing almost all of the characteristic pharmacological effects. But the term has become so inextricably associated with marijuana that it is viewed by some, erroneously, as nearly synonymous with marijuana or misperceived as meaning "synthetic" marijuana. Given the complexity of marijuana botany, chemistry and pharmacology, the confusion is understandable. Prerequisite to a meaningful discussion is some familiarity with basic terms and definitions of marijuana-related products and discussion of a few interpretive problems related to human and animal studies of its developmental toxicity.

First, here is a brief list of commonly used terms in the cannabis literature:

- cannabis is the crude material from the plant *Cannabis sativa;*
- marijuana is usually a mixture of crushed leaves, twigs, seeds and sometimes flowers;
- *Sinsemilla* is a seedless variety of high-potency marijuana originally grown in Northern California;
- hashish is a resin obtained by pressing, scraping and shaking the plant, and hash oil is a very potent solvent extract (Marijuana and Health, 1982).

PLANT CHEMISTRY

Cannabis contains more than 400 chemicals, many common to all plants. Sixty-one of these are unique to cannabis and are collectively referred to as cannabinoids. Because of its potent pharmacological activity, THC has been the most extensively studied. It is important to appreciate, however, that other cannabinoids, for example, cannabidiol (CBD) and cannabinol (CBN), though exerting little or no psychoactive effects, do have biological activity. CBD is an anticonvulsant and appears, at least under some conditions, to attenuate the effects of THC, whereas CBN appears to exert weak cannabinoid activity (for review, see Dewey, 1986; Martin, 1986).

TABLE 1.

Marijuana and Tobacco Reference Cigarette Analysis of Mainstream Smoke (abbreviated list*)

Mainstream smoke		Marijuana cigarette	Tobacco cigarette
I. Gas phase			
Carbon monoxide	(vol. %)	3.99	4.58
	(mg)	17.60	20.20
Carbon dioxide	(vol. %)	8.27	9.38
	(mg)	57.30	65.00
Acetaldehyde	μg	1200.00	980.00
Acetone	μg	443.00	578.00
Benzene	μg	76.00	67.00
Toluene μ	μg	112.00	108.00
Vinyl chloride	ng**	5.40	12.40
II. Particulate phase			
Cannabidiol	μg	190.00	–
THC	μg	820.00	–
Cannabinol	μg	190.00	–
Nicotine	μg	–	2850.00
Benz(a)anthracene	ng**	75.00	43.00
Benzo(a)pyrene	ng**	31.00	21.00

* Some 150 compounds are identified in marijuana smoke.
** Known carcinogen

SMOKE CHEMISTRY

In the United States, most cannabis is consumed by smoking marijuana, a mode of administration that, by virtue of the products of pyrolysis, complicates an understanding of its pharmacology and toxicity. Marijuana smoke shares certain chemical characteristics with tobacco smoke; both contain hundreds of chemicals of known or potential biological activity in a mixture of very small particles and a gas-vapor phase. The amounts of a few constituents in tobacco and marijuana cigarette smoke are compared in Table 1.

How much active material is actually absorbed by the smoker depends on the manner in which the cigarette is smoked. The more "efficient" the technique, the higher the tissue concentrations of absorbed material. In the United States, a common marijuana smoking technique is to inhale deeply and hold the smoke for as long as possible.

Although the dose of THC can be accurately specified in human laboratory studies by the use of prepared experimental material, "street" marijuana shows extreme variation in the content of THC alone from 0 per cent or trace amounts to levels as potent as 18 per cent. Parenthetically, throughout the 1970s, THC concentrations of cannabis confiscated by the Drug Enforcement Agency in the United States averaged around 1 to 2 per cent. Subsequently, averages increased to 3 to 5 per cent and potency remains high (NIDA Marijuana Project, 1988). Moreover, cannabis from different sources also varies widely in the proportion of other chemicals including cannabinoids.

These considerations pose a number of dilemmas for both human and animal researchers interested in the developmental toxicity of cannabis. First, basic to an understanding of the pharmacology and toxicity of a compound is knowing how much active substance is delivered to biological tissues. A major advantage of animal studies is the ability to administer specified quantities of a compound in order to describe dose-response effects precisely. Nearly all of the developmental animal studies, because of practical advantages, have investigated THC — it is a biologically active, quantifiable chemical constituent of cannabis and clearly exerts some degree of dose-related embryotoxicity. It is important to emphasize, however, that THC represents only one ingredient of the natural material, and effects produced by other cannabinoids and cannabis-related products and their interactions may also prove significant. Though an obvious remedy would be to expose rats to marijuana smoke, the amount of THC delivered in smoke can only be approximated and only small amounts are actually absorbed (Fried, 1976).

Human reproductive studies, however, typically investigate the effects of smoked marijuana. In order to approximate dose response, experimental groups are usually defined with respect to usage pattern, for example, the number of marijuana "joints" smoked per day or week. But since the potency of the material being used by a particular study population is seldom reported — probably because it is unknown — specifying usage as "low," "moderate" or "high" yields a less-than-reliable estimate of actual potency. Thus, problems of interpretation arise, especially when findings between laboratories are in disagreement. If, for example, one research group finds evidence of dysmorphogenesis or neurobehavioral deficits and another does not, there is no way of knowing whether quantitative as well as qualitative difference in the smoked material may be contributing to different outcomes.

One could reasonably argue that a lack of complete information about the nature and potency of the maternally abused substance is certainly not unique to marijuana. But with the other major abuse compounds — alcohol, opioids, cocaine and phencyclidine — we have far more assurance in human studies that it is primarily these compounds, possibly along with some adulterants, that are being used and it is these compounds, without the adulterants, that are administered to laboratory animals.

These issues are raised, not to imply that marijuana research can only yield chaotic and uninterpretable results, but to show that we need to appreciate certain constraints in the interpretation, comparison and extrapolation of cannabis research data. Animal studies of THC, though of demonstrated value, are not studies of marijuana. By the same token, human studies would be greatly enhanced if more information were provided about the nature of the cannabis being used as well as the amount of cannabinoids actually entering the body.

THC During Pregnancy in the Rat

Following the identification of THC as the major psychoactive ingredient in marijuana in the 1970s and its availability for animal research, animal studies of its developmental toxicity began appearing. Many of these studies reported that cannabis, but chiefly THC, was not only teratogenic but also capable of producing neurobehavioral deficits in the offspring. Abel (for review, see Abel, 1985) was among the first researchers to point out serious methodological and interpretive flaws that characterized this early literature. A major problem shared by many of these studies, he argued, was that adverse effects observed in the offspring may not have been produced by direct drug effects on the embryo and fetus, but rather were secondary to THC-induced maternal toxicity. For example, one potent effect of THC administration in rats is a substantial inhibition of food and water intake with consequent maternal undernutrition and dehydration. Also, as revealed in later research, THC can disrupt normal maternal care at parturition, and through hormonal effects can inhibit milk production and let-down, all with possible adverse consequences for the neurobehavioral development of the offspring (for additional discussion of these issues, see Hutchings, 1985).

The remedy for these problems was clear. In order to obtain interpretable results from developmental animal studies of prenatally administered THC, all researchers would need to incorporate controls for the reduction in maternal food and water intake, as well as for effects that could result from being reared by a drug-impaired dam. While there may have been continued interest in the United States for studying the developmental effects of cannabis, the

National Institute on Drug Abuse (NIDA), in light of the criticisms of the earlier work, ceased funding new research on cannabis and reproduction if the proposed studies failed to include appropriate nutritional and fostering controls. Then, in the mid-1980s, a "crack" cocaine epidemic began sweeping the United States. The use of crack, particularly among pregnant addicts, overshadowed any lingering interest in cannabis. As developmental researchers shifted their focus to the effects of cocaine, there followed a dramatic reduction in the publication of developmental animal studies of cannabis and THC. In fact, the two neurobehavioral animal studies reported below were the only research of their kind to appear in the literature during this period, and a recent search of the animal literature has failed to locate any adequately controlled neurobehavioral studies since. There was, however, a continuing interest in cannabis research, but the major emphasis was on studies of the newly discovered cannabinoid receptor (for review, see Abood & Martin, 1992). Included in this effort and relevant to an understanding of how pre- and postnatal effects of THC are mediated, the ontogeny of cannabinoid receptor in rat brain from birth through late adulthood has recently been described (Belue, Howlett et al., 1995).

The studies reported here (Brake, Hutchings et al., 1987; Hutchings, Brake et al., 1987) used essentially the same design: two dose levels of THC, 15 or 50 mg/kg per day, were administered to pregnant rats. The compound was dissolved in sesame oil and administered by gastric intubation. To study potential effects on major developmental events, exposure was initiated on day 8 of gestation, the beginning of organogenesis, and continued through fetogenesis to term. To control for the effects of reduced food and water intake among THC-exposed dams, pair-fed (PF) controls were administered the vehicle alone and allowed to eat and drink only the amount consumed by the 50-mg/kg group on the same gestation days. A group of non-treated (NT) controls were left undisturbed, except for weighing, throughout pregnancy. In addition, to obviate possible postnatal effects of being reared by a drug-treated dam, all experimental and control litters were reared by surrogate dams. The results of these first studies were derived from a total of some 73 dams and their 940 offspring and are summarized as follows.

Maternal Nutrition and Embryotoxicity

Among the dams receiving 50 mg/kg of THC, food and water intake as shown in Figure 1 was initially reduced to 75 to 80 per cent of NT controls but then recovered over three to four days to

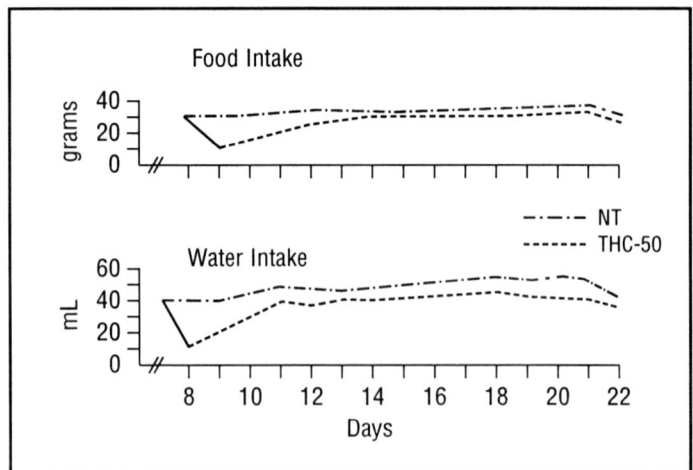

FIGURE 1.

Mean food and water intake for the non-treated controls and THC-treated dams from gestation days 7 through 22

approximately a 15 to 20 per cent reduction until term. Compared with the non-treated dams, both dose-level drug groups and PF controls gained significantly less bodyweight from conception to term. While offspring mortality did not differ between the NT and PF controls, significant dose-related increases in offspring mortality were observed among the THC groups.

Of particular interest was the observation of a dose-related increase in the sex ratio of live offspring. In many studies carried out in this laboratory over several years, a sex ratio of 50 per cent, ± 5 per cent, for both NT and PF controls is typically found. Among litters from dams receiving 50 mg/kg of THC, we consistently find

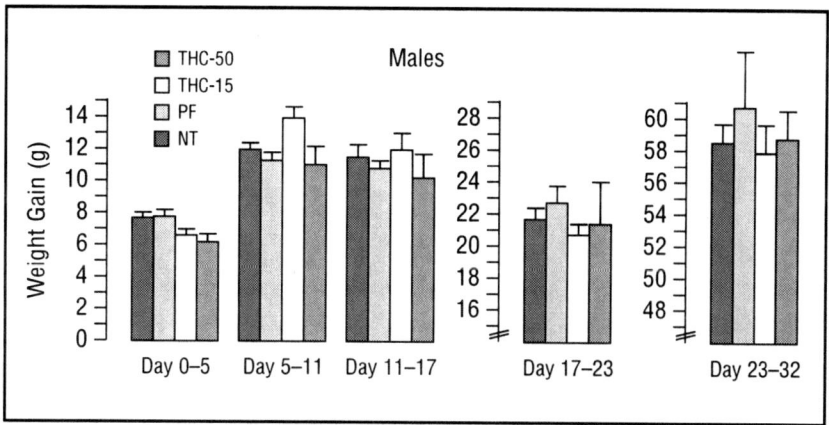

FIGURE 2.

Mean weight gained by THC-exposed and control male offspring from birth to 32 days of age

a significant dose-related increase in the proportion of male offspring ranging from 57 per cent (Hutchings, Brake et al., 1987) to 61 per cent (Morgan, Brake et al., 1988). The data further indicate that this results from a selective lethal effect on female embryos. Interestingly, Tennes et al. (1985) found in a study of women who smoked marijuana during pregnancy that heavy use was similarly associated with a significant increase in male over female births. However, because the women were recruited into the study well into their pregnancy, spontaneous abortion or early loss of female conceptuses cannot explain their sex-ratio effects.

Offspring Growth

Although birthweights were reduced among the drug-exposed offspring, this appeared to result largely from the reduced maternal food and water intake rather than the drug. Soon after birth, however, an interesting effect on growth was observed: whereas the bodyweights of the PF caught up to the NT controls by day 2 of life, bodyweights of both treated groups remained significantly lower. In fact, as shown in Figure 2, during the first five days of life, male pups in both dose-level groups grew at a slower rate than the controls. But beginning on day 5, the 15-mg/kg pups grew faster than the other groups

so that by day 11, they had caught up to the controls. By comparison, the 50-mg/kg pups still weighed less than all of the other groups on days 5 to 11 and did not entirely catch up in bodyweight until a month of life. By 32 days of age, there were no weight differences between any of the groups. The growth data of the female offspring are not shown here but were virtually identical to the males. Abel (1985) reviewed several rat studies from his laboratory that examined postnatal growth following prenatal exposure to cannabinoids and concluded that the results were inconsistent. But within the context of the effects found here, all suggest differential dose-response effects on growth rate — low doses produce relatively short-term growth inhibition followed by rapid catch-up, whereas high doses produce a more prolonged period of delayed growth with relatively slow catch-up.

Offspring Behavior

Intact litters from each of the treated and control groups were tested for differences in activity level at three-day intervals from birth to 32 days of age. We had previously reported that prenatally administered methadone (Hutchings, Towey & Bodnarenko, 1980) and more recently, cocaine (Hutchings, Martin et al., 1989), produces effects in the offspring on this measure. None of the THC-treated or control litters, however, showed any differences in activity level.

Pups were also tested for their ability to nipple-attach at 2, 5, 8, 11 and 14 days of age (Brake, Hutchings et al., 1987). For this, a test dam was anesthetized, placed in a test cage and two to three littermates per five-minute test period placed in proximity to her ventrum. Each pup's latency to attach was measured. As demonstrated in the group means shown in Figure 3, the 50-mg/kg pups took considerably longer to attach to the test dam's nipples on days 5 and 8. It is unlikely, however, that the drug treatment contributed to this effect as the pair-fed pups also took longer to nipple-attach on the same days. This suggests that the poor attachment behavior of the 50-mg/kg pups was probably due to the secondary effects of reduced food and water intake in the dams, particularly the severe reduction that occurred during early organogenesis.

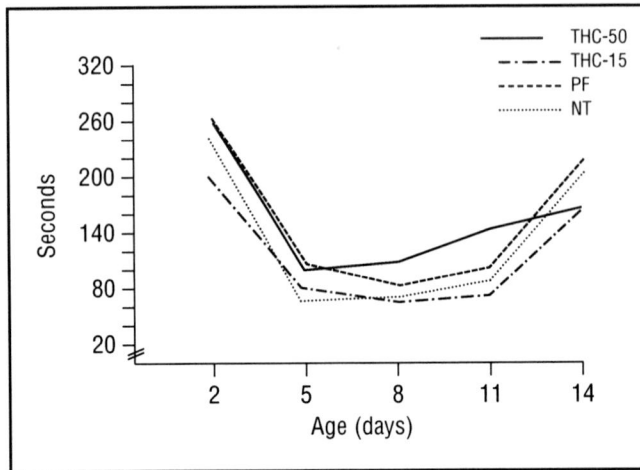

FIGURE 3.
Mean latency to attach to a nipple for THC-exposed and control pups from 2 through 14 days of age

Brain DNA, RNA and Protein

To extend the studies of prenatal THC on somatic growth to possible effects on postnatal brain growth, we analysed offspring brains at 7, 14 and 21 days of age for DNA, RNA and protein content (Morgan, Brake et al., 1988). A second problem addressed in this study is the

severe inhibition of both food and water intake produced by THC administration in the rat. In our previous studies described above we initiated THC administration on gestation day 8 so that the maximal inhibition of food and water intake occurred during the earliest development of embryonic central nervous system (CNS), on gestation days 9 to 11. In this study, drug treatment was initiated on the day after conception so that the severe THC-induced undernutrition/dehydration would be confined to the pre-implantation period (i.e., day 1 to approximately day 6), a period generally found to be refractory to teratogenic effects. Except for beginning treatment earlier, treated and control groups were prepared and fostered as described above. On postnatal days 7, 14 and 21, three treated and control pups were decapitated, brains excised and using standard procedures, analysed for total protein, DNA and RNA.

As shown in Figure 4, there was an increase in brain DNA, RNA and protein with increasing age in all groups. There were no differences among groups at any time for values of DNA or RNA. However, the brains of the non-treated, 15-mg/kg and pair-fed groups all had significantly greater amounts of total protein than the 50-mg/kg group. The difference disappeared with age so that by postnatal day 21, all of the treated and control groups yielded the same brain protein content.

In this study, no differences were observed among the non-treated and the pair-fed pups with respect to DNA and RNA, indicating that the reduced food intake of the mother during gestation had no effect on nucleic acid synthesis in the brain. Furthermore, there were no differences in RNA and DNA levels between the THC-treated pups and the pair-fed group, which suggests that RNA or DNA synthesis was not affected by THC.

Protein, however, was affected by THC. As with the nucleic acids, there were no differences

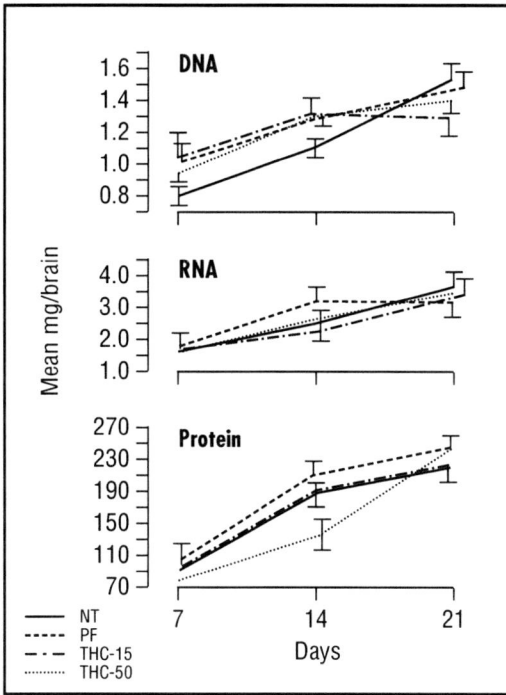

FIGURE 4.
Mean DNA, RNA and protein values for THC-exposed and control offspring. The number of pools of tissues ranged from 4 to 8 for each of the brain measures.

between the values for pair-fed and non-treated animals, indicating that the nutritional deficit in the dam was not great enough to impair protein synthesis. Neither was the 15-mg/kg dose of THC sufficient to affect protein synthesis as pups in this group showed similar protein accumulation to the non-treated and pair-fed groups. However, the 50-mg/kg pups were significantly affected. Brain protein levels were significantly lower than in the other groups at postnatal days 7 and 14, suggesting that the higher dose reduced protein synthesis for at least the first 14 days of life. Subsequently, 50-mg/kg pups rapidly caught up, increasing their brain protein by 43 per cent in the next seven days compared with only 18 per cent in the PF controls. Protein synthesis in the brain correlates with growth of axons and dendrites and the formation of synaptic connections between cells. Thus, the 50-mg/kg dose of THC appears to have inhibited

proliferation of neural processes during the first 14 days of life. Subsequently, however, they caught up to the controls by day 21.

In our findings for somatic growth, we described a dose-response relationship for THC. A dose of 15 mg/kg produced short-term growth inhibition followed by rapid catch-up whereas 50 mg/kg produced a prolonged period of delayed growth followed by gradual catch-up. Here, the 15-mg/kg dose had no observable effect on brain growth. That the lower dose was without effect on brain parallels similar studies of maternal undernutrition that find offspring CNS to be more resistant to growth deficits than other developing organ systems (Winick, 1976).

The observation that there were no differences in RNA, DNA and protein between the NT and PF controls suggests that confining the severe maternal nutrition/dehydration to the pre-implantation period spared offspring brain from growth inhibition. The decreased brain protein synthesis among the 50-mg/kg animals followed by catch-up parallels the delayed rate of somatic growth described above and suggests a transitory rather than a permanent effect of THC on both somatic and brain growth.

THC Plasma Concentrations

Because of the reported slow clearance of THC in several species (see Marijuana and Health, 1982) it was possible that this could result in the prenatal accumulation of THC in dams and fetuses followed by its postnatal persistence and slow clearance in the offspring. To study this possibility, THC was administered to pregnant dams either repeatedly throughout pregnancy or acutely, as a single dose on the last day of gestation (Hutchings, Martin et al., 1989).

For the multiple exposure, beginning on gestation day 2, either 15 or 50 mg/kg of THC suspended in sesame oil was administered to two groups of gravid dams (MULT THC-15; MULT THC-50) once daily by gastric intubation. Both MULT dose-level groups received daily drug administration through gestation day 22. For the acute exposure, the same doses, vehicle and route were used but the dams received THC only once on gestation day 22 (ACUTE THC-15; ACUTE THC-50).

Sixty minutes after the last drug administration on gestation day 22, all dams and their offspring were decapitated, blood collected and quantitative measurement of THC carried out using capillary column gas chromatography negative ion chemical ionization mass spectrometry. The mean plasma concentrations of THC found in dams and fetuses following either acute or multiple exposure are shown in Table 2.

TABLE 2.

Mean [± SEM] Concentration of Plasma THC (ng/mL)

	Acute	Subacute
Dams		
15 mg/kg	(N = 8) 98.8 ± 20.0[a,b]	(N = 10) 134.4 ± 37.7[a]
50 mg/kg	(N = 8) 132.4 ± 35.5[b]	(N = 9) 309.1 ± 59.2
Fetuses		
15 mg/kg	(N = 9) 10.2 ± 2.0[a]	(N = 10) 11.8 ± 3.7[a]
50 mg/kg	(N = 8) 18.6 ± 2.0[a]	(N = 9) 41.4 ± 6.1

[a] $p < 0.05$ compared to 50-mg/kg group
[a,b] $p < 0.05$ compared to subacute group

Among the dams, plasma concentrations co-varied with dose, and multiple dosing produced higher concentrations than acute. Although the MULT-50 dams yielded a mean plasma concentration that was nearly three times higher than the other groups, the dose × treatment statistical interaction was not significant.

Among the fetuses, plasma concentrations were approximately 10 per cent of those found for the dams and differed significantly as a function of dose and treatment. In addition, the high plasma concentrations found for the MULT-50 fetuses yielded a significant dose × treatment interaction.

It is well documented that radioactivity appears in the fetus following an acute adminis-

tration of ^{3}H-delta-9-THC to maternal mice (Kennedy & Waddell, 1972), rats (Harbison & Mantilla-Plata, 1972), and dogs (Martin, Dewey et al., 1977). Greater than 60 per cent of the radioactivity in fetal dog brain corresponded to unchanged ^{3}H-delta-9-THC, demonstrating placental transfer (Martin, Dewey et al., 1977). Bailey et al. (1987) reported that THC administered during late pregnancy in the rhesus monkey resulted in the rapid transfer of parent compound but not 11-*nor*-9-carboxy-THC to fetal tissues. All these studies demonstrated that the placenta acted to partially limit the exposure of the fetus to THC and its metabolites. The findings reported here similarly show that the concentrations of THC in fetal plasma were 10 and 7 times less than those in the plasma of dams receiving the low and high dose of THC, respectively.

Multiple dosing of THC to the dams resulted in an insignificant increase in the maternal plasma concentrations of the 15-mg/kg treatment group but a significant twofold increase in the 50-mg/kg group. A similar profile of THC concentrations in fetal plasma suggests that the maternal plasma concentration, rather than fetal tissue depots, serves as the primary source for fetal plasma levels. These findings are particularly relevant given the lack of information regarding fetal concentrations of cannabinoids following repeated exposure of dams. Additionally, most previous studies have been concerned with measurement of placental transfer of undifferentiated radioactivity following exposure to radiolabelled THC rather than the direct measurement of parent compound.

Summary: Animal Studies

These studies describe three dose-related effects in the offspring following maternal administration of THC in the rat. At birth, a dose-related increase in the sex ratio of live offspring was consistently found, suggesting that female conceptuses have greater susceptibility to THC lethality. During the postnatal period, a dose-related inhibition of both somatic growth and brain protein synthesis was found. These effects were transitory, however, and the THC-exposed animals caught up to the controls by the time of weaning. Although confirming studies are needed, both the accumulation of THC in the 50-mg/kg treatment group and the possibility that THC is persisting in pharmacologically active concentrations into the postnatal period may be important elements underlying the transitory inhibition of both body growth and brain protein synthesis. These studies found no evidence of neurobehavioral deficits in the offspring independent of maternal toxicity, findings that are consistent with other well-controlled animal studies (Abel, 1985).

If there is one major lesson to be learned from the animal research on THC it is an obvious one: poorly controlled experiments that do not adequately consider the confounding influences of maternal toxicity, both pre- and postnatally, are likely to yield a high rate of false positive results. This is well illustrated by those studies of cannabis that antedate the concern for pair-feeding and surrogate fostering. Nearly all the studies that failed to include nutritional and fostering controls found neurobehavioral effects that included changes in activity as well as impairments in learning and memory. Although these effects were assumed to represent primary effects of the compound, they were more likely secondary to maternal undernutrition and/or postnatally mediated by altered maternal behavior.

Cannabis Use and Human Pregnancy

Among illegal substances, marijuana is the drug most widely used by pregnant women (Johnston, O'Malley & Bachman, 1994a; 1994b) and yet the scientific literature dealing with the possible consequences of such use is very sparse. In considering

the relationship between marijuana use during pregnancy and the impact of such use upon the behavioral outcome of the young children of these pregnancies, the lack of objective information is striking and, from one point of view, quite surprising. Marijuana is far from being a passing fad. References have been found to its use in civilizations thousands of years ago (Abel, 1980) and it has had a role in pregnancy folklore for many centuries.

The very limited number of contemporary scientific studies that focus upon marijuana's potential long-term behavioral teratological effects on the developing fetus is of major concern in light of the number of women of reproductive age who use this drug. From a scientific point of view, the drug context in which marijuana is smoked can vary considerably. In some cases, marijuana may be the only potentially teratogenic substance used; in other cases, it may be used with legal potentially teratogenic agents (e.g., alcohol and tobacco); while in further instances, marijuana may be combined with other illegal substances that are under extensive investigation for their possible role in affecting the unborn child. For example, the majority of studies of long-term consequences of *in utero* exposure to cocaine report the use of that substance being highly correlated with marijuana (e.g., Chasnoff, Griffith et al. 1992; Frank, Zuckerman et al. 1988). Although it is possible (but not always) to control to a certain extent marijuana's impact by statistical means, knowing the singular role of cannabis upon the dependent variable in question is clearly of great importance in interpreting the nature of the contribution of other substances.

A 1991 survey conducted by the National Institutes of Health indicated that 8.5 per cent of women reported using marijuana during the previous year, while 5 per cent reported using the drug during the previous month (National Institute on Drug Abuse, 1991). Among those of reproductive age the proportion who used marijuana was considerably higher: 17.5 per cent during the previous year and 8.5 per cent during the previous month. Reports of surveys conducted in 1993 in the United States and Canada reflected an upswing in the use of marijuana by high school and college students, suggesting that use during the reproductive years is unlikely to decline in the immediate future.

In NIDA's 1994 Monitoring the Future survey (Johnston, O'Malley & Bachman, 1994b), 10.4 per cent of women between the ages of 19 and 32 reported using marijuana in the past month, in contrast to an 8.3 per cent rate among women of the same age in the 1990 survey (National Institute on Drug Abuse, 1991). Also of note is the fact that among high school seniors (those entering reproductive years) the use of marijuana during the past year increased between 1992 and 1993 from 21.9 per cent to 26.0 per cent (sexes not differentiated) reversing a previous declining trend seen since the early 1980s (Johnston, O'Malley & Bachman, 1994a).

Several reports have examined the extent of use of marijuana during pregnancy, but frequently the prevalence rates cited may not be representative of that drug's use in the general population since sampling procedures involve populations that are selectively biased towards drug use. On the basis of either interviews or urine screens conducted prenatally or postpartum, a rate of 27 per cent was reported among a high-risk, predominantly non-white, Boston inner-city sample (Zuckerman, Frank et al., 1989). In another high-risk sample in Pittsburgh (Day, Sambamoorthi et al., 1991), a random sampling of women from an outpatient prenatal clinic found a 30 per cent rate of use. At the Yale-New Haven Hospital, with a relatively low-risk sample, the rate at any time during pregnancy was found to be 10 per cent (Hatch & Bracken, 1986). In another low-risk population in the Seattle area, the rate was 17 per cent (Streissguth, Barr et al., 1989). In a comparison between public health clinics and private obstetrical offices located in Florida, the rate, based on urine screens, was quite similar with 12.4 per cent in the former and 11.3 per cent in the latter group (Chasnoff, Landres & Barrett, 1990). In contrast in Chicago, based on urine screens at the time of admission into the labor-and-delivery unit, a marked difference of marijuana rates was noted between clinic patients

(32 per cent) and private patients (7.5 per cent) (MacGregor, Sciarra et al., 1990).

In our own work in Ottawa, Canada (described in detail below), among predominantly middle-class volunteers (Fried, Barnes & Drake, 1985; Fried, Innes & Barnes, 1984), in the year before pregnancy 80 per cent did not use any marijuana, 12 per cent used the drug irregularly, 3 per cent smoked two to five joints per week, and 5 per cent smoked more than that amount. After the recognition of pregnancy, usage declined significantly, although during each of the three trimesters the percentages remained relatively constant. Approximately 6 per cent reported irregular use, 1 per cent reported smoking two to five joints per week, and 3 per cent continued to smoke a greater amount. The heaviest users were the most likely to re-establish pre-pregnancy levels of consumption in the year following the birth of the baby.

In spite of the fact that marijuana is the illicit drug most widely used by pregnant women (Day & Richardson, 1991) as mentioned at the outset of this article, there is a notable lack of information about its immediate and long-term consequences. This is particularly the case in the latter instance. The major reasons for this state of affairs lie in the ethical and practical difficulties surrounding the quasi-experimental research paradigm (Kilbey & Asghar, 1992) that is necessitated by research with human subjects in the area of potentially teratogenic illegal drugs. Clearly, drugs cannot be administered to gravid women and so the exact doses or amounts utilized and the precise timing of such use are impossible to quantify. Further, potentially confounding factors (including other drug use and socioeconomic factors) cannot be controlled by random assignment to groups. Human studies, particularly those investigating the long-term effects of *in utero* exposure, have to be based on volunteer samples with reports of drug use being gathered either before (i.e., prospectively) or after (i.e., retrospectively) birth. These limitations are severe ones and, although a degree of control can be attained with statistical procedures (but sometimes, as discussed later, statistical overcontrol may also occur), the research must be interpreted, and conclusions drawn, only with the appropriate caveats in mind.

Aside from one or two studies, all of the information pertaining to the behavioral effects of prenatal exposure to marijuana in children beyond the toddler stage is limited to the reports coming from the Ottawa Prenatal Prospective Study (Fried, Watkinson et al., 1980). Because of this, the protocol and the limitations of this Canadian work is described in some detail. Additional information can be found elsewhere (Fried, Watkinson et al., 1980).

The Ottawa Prenatal Prospective Study (OPPS)

As recently as 1980, the only information describing the effect marijuana may have upon the pregnant user and her offspring was limited to two polydrug case reports. This lack of information, the results of animal work (reviewed earlier in this article and in Fried, Watkinson & Willan, 1984; Dalterio & Fried, 1992), the extent of use among women of reproductive age, and the co-operation of the teaching hospitals in the Ottawa area combined to establish the need and set the climate and opportunity for the inception of the OPPS in 1978.

Birth data have been collected in a prospective fashion from approximately 700 women residing in the Ottawa, Canada, region. For a number of pragmatic reasons it has been feasible to have followed-up offspring of approximately 200 women of this sample, including all those who reported using marijuana during pregnancy. Pregnant women volunteered after being informed of the study by a variety of means, including their physicians, notices in the waiting rooms of obstetricians, or notices in the reception rooms of prenatal clinics in the major hospitals in Ottawa. The information that was disseminated by the various means did not, at this juncture, mention marijuana but rather discussed in general terms how lifestyle habits during pregnancy may influence the developing fetus. Upon contacting our research facility, the potential subject was given further details about the particular habits we were interested in — marijuana, alcohol and cigarettes. It was emphasized that, for purposes of comparison, it was desirable to recruit women who used any of these substances to a very small degree or not at all. After volunteering and signing an informed consent, the mother-to-be was interviewed once during each of the trimesters remaining in her pregnancy by a trained female interviewer.

This procedure of recruiting volunteers has both strengths and weaknesses that pervade the entire OPPS. The self-selection procedure limits the extent to which generalizations can be made in terms of epidemiological information collected, with the possibility of selection bias being the most obvious interpretative problem. However, as noted elsewhere (Fried, Innes & Barnes, 1984; Fried, Watkinson et al., 1980), on several key demographic variables including parity, age and family income, the volunteer sample participating in the OPPS is quite similar to non-participating women living in the Ottawa area and giving birth in the hospitals taking part in our study.

The recruitment procedure described above has the advantage of increasing the reliability of self-report (elaborated below) and of increasing the probability of a long-term commitment to the study. Aside from subjects who have moved from the Ottawa area (about a third), a retention rate of more than 95 per cent has been maintained over more than a decade.

During each of the prenatal interviews, information was collected on such variables as socioeconomic status, mother's health (both current and before pregnancy), the health history of the father, obstetrical history of previous pregnancies, a 24-hour dietary recall (including an assessment of caffeine intake), as well as past and present drug use patterns with particular detailed information being gathered with respect to marijuana, cigarettes and alcohol. Detailed information on the latter two drugs was thought desirable because of the extant literature suggesting that marijuana-using individuals also tended to use more cigarettes and alcohol. Thus, there would be a need for comparison groups just using these substances. For the establishment of the use of these three drugs, information was gathered both for the year preceding the pregnancy and for each trimester of the pregnancy. Further details of the interview and the categorization of the various drugs have been described previously (Fried, Watkinson et al.,1980). There was an extensive range of marijuana use in the sample, and the drug was not used by a similar number of subjects across the range of usage. As a result of these factors, for descriptive and some statistical purposes, the marijuana data were treated categorically. There were the non-users, irregular users (one joint or less per week), moderate users (two to five joints per week) and heavy users (more than five joints per week).

The women who smoked marijuana regularly during their pregnancy differed from the remainder of the sample on a number of factors that potentially influence the development of the offspring and were dealt with by various statistical procedures. These possible confounding factors included lower socioeconomic level, less formal education and increased cigarette smoking. Although no difference in parity was noted, the heavy users were 3.2 years younger than the non-users. In terms of nutritional adequacy and weight gain during pregnancy there were no differences among the four groups.

The self-report procedure used in the OPPS to assess drug habits raises the critical issues of validity and reliability. Despite the obvious shortcomings of this mode of assessing drug use, at the time of the collection of data (primarily between 1979 and 1983) no practical alternative was available. Today, laboratory tests can measure the presence of metabolites of marijuana up to one to two weeks from the time of use. The use of both the interview and biological assessment approaches are critically discussed in a well-reasoned paper by Day and Richardson (1991). In the OPPS, procedures were undertaken to enhance the likelihood of accurate interview data collection. A congenial relationship in a non-stressful, familiar environment (typically the mother's home) between the interviewer and the individual being interviewed has been part of

the protocol of the OPPS, and the same female interviewer "followed" the mother-to-be during her entire pregnancy. However, all testing of the children was carried out by individuals who were "blind" to the mother's prenatal drug history. A second procedure designed to enhance the accuracy of the self-reports was the number of times the same drug-related questions are asked. The questionnaire was administered once during each trimester. During each interview, the questions pertaining to drug use for each three-month period of pregnancy that had passed and for the 12 months prior to pregnancy were repeated, permitting a test-retest reliability measure.

COURSE OF PREGNANCY

Several studies have reported no effect of maternal marijuana use on neonatal growth or on the course of pregnancy (Fried, Buckingham & Von Kulmiz, 1983; Fried & O'Connell, 1987; Linn, Schoebaum et al., 1983). In the data derived from the low-risk Ottawa sample, a linear association between decreased length of gestation and marijuana use was found but no higher rate of prematurity (Fried, Watkinson & Willan, 1984). In an Australian sample, a higher rate of prematurity was noted (Gibson, Baghurst & Colley, 1983), and in women delivering at the Yale-New Haven Hospital, marijuana use was associated with prematurity but only among the offspring of white mothers (Hatch & Bracken, 1986).

In the Ottawa study (Fried, Buckingham & Von Kulmiz, 1983), there was no evidence of increased meconium staining associated with marijuana use. This observation contrasts with the first, but not the second of two reports by Greenland and associates (1982; 1983). One of the primary differences between Greenland's two studies was the greater risk status (general health and lifestyle) of the sample in the first study, whereas the women in the second report were more similar to the Ottawa sample in terms of ethnicity, education and general health.

The seemingly critical role that lifestyle and its accompanying risk factors may have in interacting with the potential teratogenic effects of marijuana has important ramifications for the interpretation of much of the data described in the remainder of this paper. An examination of one aspect of the complex issue of the interaction between risk factors and fetal marijuana exposure has been addressed using an animal model.

Pregnant rats were exposed to relatively low amounts of marijuana smoke, placebo smoke (cannabis product with the cannabinoids chemically removed), or no smoke while the diet of the animals was manipulated (Charlebois & Fried, 1980). Animals in each of the three drug conditions were subdivided into three groups so that the pregnant dams received one of three diets differing in protein content. One diet was enriched, one was the standard laboratory rat chow and the third was relatively low in protein. The drug plus diet manipulations were started 20 days before mating and were continued throughout gestation. A dramatic interaction between marijuana exposure and protein levels was seen. In the highest risk condition — marijuana smoke coupled with a low protein diet — outcomes such as still births, litter destruction and postnatal deaths were markedly higher than in all other groups. In contrast, some of the physiological and developmental milestones that were delayed in the rats given a normal diet and marijuana smoke were attenuated in the high protein/marijuana smoke condition. Thus, in this work the combination of poor diet plus marijuana considerably added to the adverse outcome whereas the enriched diet plus the drug apparently protected, to a degree, the fetus from some of the drug's effects.

These results are certainly suggestive of adverse effects from maternal marijuana use potentiated by other risk factors although, as with all animal work, the extent of extrapolation is problematic. It is not unreasonable, however, to view these results coupled with those of Greenland described earlier as indicating that marijuana's potential for teratogenicity is more likely to be manifest in an environment in which the lifestyle contains risk factors before marijuana is brought into consideration. It therefore would follow that in a relatively low-risk population (of which the Ottawa sample is a case in point), the fetus may be somewhat protected from some

of marijuana's consequences whereas in samples that are at high risk marijuana effects may be more apparent.

Certainly this argument appears congruent with a number of observations in the extant literature pertaining to the issue of marijuana and birthweight. Of the more than a dozen studies examining birthweight (reviewed in Fried & O'Connell, 1987) only four have reported a significant relationship. In a high-risk sample, women who used marijuana during pregnancy delivered babies that averaged 105 grams less than the newborns of non-users (Hingson, Alpert et al., 1982). However, in this study it was noted that maternal weight prior to pregnancy and maternal weight gain during pregnancy each had nearly three times the impact on this outcome that marijuana did. In another study (Kline, Stein & Hutzler, 1987), daily use of marijuana was related to lower birthweight but in this work the influence of demographic variables and alcohol and cigarette use was not statistically controlled and the authors conclude that the marijuana effects may have been due, in large part, to the use of other drugs such as cocaine. In a report using a high-risk sample, infants of marijuana users were found to be both lighter and shorter at birth than babies of non-users, but only if the users had been identified by positive urine analysis as opposed to self-report (Zuckerman, Frank et al., 1989). Since the urine assay only detects the metabolites of marijuana for up to 72 hours after ingestion of the drug, it is a reasonable assumption that those identified by the assay represent the heavier and more frequent users of the drug.

In a study of a sample of lower socioeconomic status women attending an inner city prenatal clinic, no significant effect of marijuana use during any of the three trimesters of pregnancy was found on head or chest circumference or birthweight, nor was there an association with small-for-gestational age babies (Day, Sambamoorthi et al., 1991). A relationship was noted between reduced infant length and marijuana use in the first two months of pregnancy but this association was not observed with later pregnancy use. Very similar findings with respect to birth-length were reported in an earlier conducted study (Tennes, Avitable et al., 1985).

The hypothesis of a drug-lifestyle inter-action may also be relevant in an examination of the relationship between physical anomalies and prenatal marijuana exposure. In the Ottawa study, after finding no evidence for major physical anomalies associated with *in utero* exposure to marijuana, an examination was undertaken to assess whether maternal use of cannabis in-creased the risk for minor physical anomalies in the offspring (O'Connell & Fried, 1984). The children of women who used marijuana on a regular basis were compared to matched controls for the presence (and degree) of over 40 types of minor anomalies. Neither the frequency of par-ticular anomalies nor their total number was significantly different between the two groups of subjects. Although no specific pattern or increased incidence of anomalies was seen among the children born to the marijuana users, two anomalies associated with the visual system were noted only among some of the offspring of the heaviest users of the drug. One anomaly noted was the presence of severe epicanthal folds (un-usual amount of skin covering the nasal portion of the eye) in three children. The other anomaly found uniquely among three other children born to heavy marijuana users was true ocular hyper-telorism (unusually wide separation of the eyes).

The lack of a clear relationship in the Ottawa sample between minor physical anom-alies and prenatal marijuana exposure is consis-tent with the findings from several other research centres (Day, Sambamoorthi et al., 1991; Linn, Schoenbaum et al., 1983; Tennes, Avitable et al., 1985). There are, however, two apparent excep-tions. One is a large study (Hingson, Alpert et al., 1982) and the other involves two reports of five individual cases (Qazi, Mariano et al., 1982; 1985). In both cases, the anomalies related to maternal marijuana use are part of the diagnostic criteria of the fetal alcohol syndrome (FAS).

In the case reports, four of the five marijuana users who had children manifesting FAS features denied the use of alcohol. This denial by 80 per cent of the subjects appears quite unusual since virtually all reports in the literature have noted a moderately high correlation between regular marijuana use and drinking. Furthermore, in the five case reports, little demographic information or medical history was provided, making it impossible to assess other risk factors. Finally, no control (matching or otherwise) was undertaken to assess the role of potentially confounding variables.

In the large study that reported an associa-tion between smoking marijuana during preg-nancy and anomalies, a fivefold increase in the probability of the offspring having FAS features was observed. The difference between this obser-vation and those noted in the OPPS could be due to a number of factors. Included among these are the sample size, the age of the subjects and as described earlier, the risk status of the mothers-to-be. The relatively small size of the Ottawa sample (25 subjects in the regular mari-juana usage category) certainly decreased the likelihood of finding a significant relationship. In the large study (Hingson, Alpert et al., 1982), the rate of occurrence of the anomalies in the marijuana-exposed offspring was 2 per cent. Applying that figure to the Ottawa study, only one child would be expected to display the FAS features. It should be noted that epicanthal folds observed in three of the children born to heavy marijuana users in the Ottawa sample (O'Connell & Fried, 1984) are consistent with FAS facial characteristics.

A second, potentially important difference between the two studies is that, in the OPPS, the assessment took place when the children were an average of 29 months of age. In the large study the children were examined in their first week after birth. As there is evidence that some of the FAS anomalies may be transient (Majewaki, 1981), the age of examination becomes a crucial factor.

Finally, and certainly not least in impor-tance, is the notion of risk factor. One compo-nent that serves as an indicator of risk is maternal weight gain. In the large study the average gain during pregnancy was 13.6 kilograms, whereas in the Ottawa sample the gain was 16 kilograms.

Additional risk factors that were more prevalent in the large study were lower socioeconomic status and more chronic maternal illnesses. The absence or presence of such risk variables may be vital factors in determining the effects of marijuana on dysmorphology in the young infant.

In the above discussion, the interaction of risk factors and the consequences of exposure to marijuana revolves primarily around risk factors present during the course of pregnancy. As will be seen later in this paper, postnatal risk factors also appear to play a significant role in affecting the consequences of *in utero* marijuana exposure.

NEUROBEHAVIORAL OBSERVATIONS

The literature pertaining to the behavioral effects of prenatal marijuana exposure is relatively sparse and, although suggestive, is far from definitive. In 1980, in the first published report, four-day-old babies born to 12 regular users in the OPPS were examined (Fried, 1980), and the findings were replicated in a subsequent, considerably larger study using the Ottawa sample (Fried & Makin, 1987). Using the Brazelton Neonatal Behavioral Assessment Scale, prenatal exposure to the drug was associated with decreased rates of visual habituation and increased tremors, frequently accompanied by exaggerated startles that were both spontaneous and in response to minimal, external stimulation. Similar observations were noted at 9 and 30 days using the Prechtl neurologic assessment (Fried, Watkinson et al., 1987). Further, at 9 days, increased hand-to-mouth behavior was found among the babies born to the marijuana users. Coles et al. (1992) noted that maternal marijuana use depressed the Orientation cluster and the Range of State cluster of the Brazelton at 14 and 30 days respectively. Further, the interaction of marijuana and cocaine and alcohol accounted for significant amounts of variance during the neonate's first month.

These possible indicators of impairments in nervous system state regulation and/or mild withdrawal were noted by some others (Chasnoff, 1990) but not by all (Richardson, Day & Taylor, 1989; Tennes, Avitable et al., 1985). Other signs of alterations in nervous system integrity have also been associated with *in utero* marijuana exposure, including alterations in the cry of newborns in a Jamaican sample (Lester & Dreher, 1989). Further, sleep cycling and motility in newborns differed between marijuana and non-marijuana babies (Scher, Richardson et al., 1988), and disturbed sleep patterns were still associated with prenatal exposure when the offspring were three years of age (Dahl, Scher et al., 1989).

In contrast to the above observations, in a recent ethnographic study based on a Jamaican sample, Dreher et al. (1994) found no differences between exposed and non-marijuana-exposed three-day-old neonates on the Brazelton and at one month, particularly among the babies born to the heavy users — the offspring of the marijuana users actually performed better on a number of cluster and supplementary scores on this scale including quality of alertness and autonomic stability. The results were attributed by the authors to more social and economic resources available in the postnatal environment of the heavy users because of a lower child/adult ratio among this portion of the sample. This interpretation of the vital role of environmental, non-drug factors on the consequences of *in utero* exposure to marijuana is consistent with the discussion earlier in this article and, as will be seen in later portions of this paper, is very relevant in the interpretation of the performance of the exposed children as they become older. The observations with the OPPS sample in the newborn period were, as will be described below, the only significant associations noted with prenatal marijuana exposure for a number of years as the children continued to be tested.

The children in the OPPS were examined at one year of age (Fried & Watkinson, 1988) using the Bayley Scales (Bayley, 1969). No adverse effects of prenatal marijuana exposure were noted. The Bayley test consists of three components. The Mental Developmental Index (MDI) assesses sensory perceptual abilities, early acquisition of object constancy, memory, problem solving, vocalization and the onset of words. The Psychomotor Developmental Index (PDI) assesses gross and fine motor movement. The

Infant Behavior Record (IBR) evaluates the infant's attitudes, interests and temperament. The failure to find a relationship between the one-year-old infant's behavior and maternal marijuana use is consistent with other reports assessing the children at the same age (Astley & Little, 1990; Tennes, Avitable et al., 1985).

Studies with their principal objective being the neurobehavioral assessment of *in utero* marijuana exposure in children older than a year are, with one exception, limited to those based on the data derived from the OPPS. At 24 months, prenatal marijuana exposure was not negatively correlated with overall scores on the Bayley test (Fried & Watkinson, 1988). At this age, using the Reynell Developmental Language Scale (Reynell, 1977) a negative association with a measure of language comprehension but not language expression was observed but this association did not persist after statistically adjusting for other variables, especially ratings of the home environment.

At three years of age, children in the Ottawa sample (Fried & Watkinson, 1990) were administered the Reynell test of language expression and comprehension as well as the McCarthy Scales of Children's Abilities (McCarthy, 1972). This latter instrument is based upon six scales: verbal, perceptual, quantitative, general cognitive (a composite of the three previous scales), memory and motor. As found when the children were a year younger, after controlling for potentially confounding variables, prenatal marijuana exposure was not significantly associated with any of the outcome variables. In a recent report from Pittsburgh based on three-year-old children born to women of generally lower social status (Day, Richardson et al., 1994), prenatal marijuana exposure was not found to have an influence on the overall composite score of the Stanford-Binet Intelligence Scale. There was, however, a significant effect on the short-term memory subscale. When the sample was broken down into white and African-American children, marijuana negative effects on verbal reasoning and short-term memory were noted in the latter group of children. Interestingly, the importance of the

postnatal environment was, once again, vividly demonstrated in this work as preschool/day-care attendance offset the marijuana-associated deficit in the white children but not in the African-American children. In a further recent study examining three-year-old children prenatally exposed to drugs, Griffith et al. (1994) reported, using the same instruments as the just described Pittsburgh work, that marijuana exposure predicted poor abstract/visual reasoning.

At four years of age, the OPPS sample were given the test battery that was administered a year earlier plus the Peabody Test (Dunn & Dunn, 1981) of receptive vocabulary and a series of motor tests (Fried & Watkinson, 1990). General, global intellectual measures were not related to prenatal cannabis exposure, congruent with the findings of another study in which alcohol rather than marijuana was the primary drug of interest (Streissguth, Barr et al., 1989). However, in the OPPS sample on tests of verbal ability (both the McCarthy subscale and the Peabody) and memory, the children of regular marijuana users were significantly inferior to other children. This relationship persisted after statistically controlling for a host of potentially confounding factors including the home environment. In terms of the neurobehavioral dimensions that appear vulnerable to prenatal marijuana exposure, the results are strikingly similar to those noted very recently in three-year-olds as described above (Day, Richardson et al., 1994). Within the OPPS, this negative relationship was the first reported association beyond the neonatal stage. The observation of a neurobehavioral significant effect at this age (and not earlier) may indicate that the degree and type of deficits noted can be identified only when normal neurological development has proceeded to a certain level of maturity and when complex behavior can be examined at a more specific, rather than global level. This maturation hypothesis reflects the notion that the effects of prenatal exposure to marijuana are subtle and that their consequences for complex behavior are not manifested and/or cannot be tested before four years. This line of thinking will be elaborated later in this paper.

The difficulty in unraveling the long-term consequences of *in utero* marijuana exposure becomes apparent when one examines the data gleaned from the cognitive and language assessment of the five- and six-year-old OPPS participants (Fried, O'Connell & Watkinson, 1992). These children were given the same battery as when they were four but, unlike the findings at 48 months, upon statistical analysis, no relationship was observed at either five or six years of age between any of the subscales of the McCarthy or the Peabody tests and maternal marijuana use.

The reason for the disparity of observations is not at all clear. One possibility may be, as discussed earlier, the effect of environmental variables. In the Ottawa sample, as the children get older, they are exposed to an increasing similarity of postnatal influences that bear on cognitive development. For example, by five years of age, 89 per cent of the non-exposed children and 87 per cent of the exposed children had a year of formal schooling. Could it be that this common feature would tend to overwhelm some of the quite subtle differences on memory and verbal abilities noted at an earlier age?

Indirect evidence of the possible influence of ubiquitous, relevant environmental factors may be seen by the age corrected "catching up" scores of the marijuana children. The McCarthy verbal and memory age-adjusted scores at four and five years of age were essentially unchanged for the non-exposed children. At both ages these children scored 1 to 1.5 [SD] above-age norms. On the same subscales, the marijuana children improved their scores by approximately half a standard deviation between the ages of four and five to 1 [SD] above the age norm at 60 months. Thus, the postnatal influence of school may have served to overcome the marijuana-associated observations noted at four years. This would certainly be entirely consistent with the findings from Pittsburgh described earlier (Day, Richardson et al., 1994) in which the negative association with prenatal marijuana exposure in the verbal and memory domains were attenuated by attendance at preschool or day care in the white children of the sample.

Instruments that provide a general description of cognitive abilities may not be capable of identifying nuances in neurobehavior that may discriminate between the marijuana and non-marijuana-exposed children. However, tests that examine specific characteristics that may underlie cognitive performance may be more appropriate and successful. This approach to assessing the consequences of prenatal marijuana exposure was examined in a study (Fried, Watkinson & Gray, 1992) in which impulse control and sustained attention was examined in six-year-olds and in a study assessing specific aspects of cognitive performance (O'Connell & Fried, 1991).

The children were assessed using two forms of a computerized vigilance task involving a one-button solid-state console (McClure & Gordon, 1983). In order to examine the child's ability to withhold responding, a six-second DRL (differential reinforcement of low rate responding) schedule was employed. Under this regimen a reinforcement (points displayed on a screen) would be obtained when a button press occurred six seconds after the emission of a previous response. Responses that occurred prior to the termination of this six seconds were not reinforced and served to reset the timer so that six seconds of no button pressing would have to elapse before the next button press would result in a reinforcement. Thus, on this DRL six-second schedule, a child would receive a reinforcement for every button press emitted after an interval of six seconds.

Three sets of data were obtained: the absolute number of responses, the total number of rewarded responses and an efficiency ratio that was determined by dividing the number of rewarded responses by the total number of responses.

The same apparatus was used to examine sustained attention. A series of single-digit numbers was shown on the screen at a rate of one per second. They were displayed for 200 milliseconds with an 800-millisecond interval between each signal. Each subject was asked to press a button whenever the target stimulus appeared on the display screen among a series of randomly presented numbers. The scores were the number of correct responses, the number of omissions (missed target stimuli) and the number of commissions (button press to non-target stimuli or false alarms). The scores were computed for each of three-minute blocks and then totalled for the overall nine-minute trial.

As an additional facet in this work, parents assessed the child's impulsivity/inattention at home by using portions of the Conners' Parent Rating Scale-48 (CPRS-48) (Conners, 1989). This 48-item behavioral symptom checklist was completed by the child's mother at the time of testing using a four-point rating system. The scale yields six behavioral clusters, one of which — the Impulsive-Hyperactive Scale — was used for this assessment. The four items that enter into this scale include excitable, impulsive; restless or "squirmy"; wants to run things; and restless, always on the go.

In the vigilance task the commission errors were very similar among all three marijuana groups, but the omission errors and the number correct were differentiated, in a dose-related fashion, among the children of the various marijuana groups. Further, across temporal epochs within the vigilance task, only the children in the heavy marijuana category increased their omission errors. The overall increase in omission errors and the greater number towards the end of the vigilance task may reflect a deficit in sustained attention.

There was a significant tendency for the women who used marijuana heavily during pregnancy to rate their children as being more impulsive/hyperactive. The nature of the scale emphasizes overall activity rather than attention behavior. Although consistent with the more objective measurements, there is a difficulty in interpreting these results. The fact that women in the heavy marijuana group tended to identify their children as more problematic in this domain may be an accurate reflection of the child's behavior or it may represent the mother's perception and attitude towards this behavior. Do the present observations indicate a true behavioral difference in the attention-related domain or is there a lowered parental tolerance? Ratings by other observers such as teachers and additional assessments

of maternal parenting attitudes and expectations might help to clarify this issue.

In a preliminary report, O'Connell and Fried (1991) examined the school-aged (six to nine years of age) offspring of regular marijuana users and matched (in terms of alcohol and cigarette use during pregnancy) controls participating in the OPPS school age on a battery of neurobehavioral tests. These included assessment of intellectual abilities, visual perceptual skills, distractibility, memory, language comprehension, academic achievement, visual motor skills and parental rating of behavior.

Measures that discriminated between the study groups and on which the children of the marijuana users scored more poorly included parental behavior ratings (particularly conduct problems), visual perceptual and visual memory tasks, language comprehension and distractibility. It is striking that these behaviors are ones that have cropped up in our work with these children at earlier ages and in the report on three-year-olds from the Pittsburgh sample (Day, Richardson et al., 1994). On the other hand, the data from the OPPS work are not without interpretative complications. For the measure of visual memory and language comprehension, the mother's age at the child's birth potentiated the effect of cannabis use to produce lowered scores for children of young, cannabis-using mothers relative to children of young, non-using mothers. Further, when controlling for the influence of the mother's age at delivery, mother's self-rated personality — the marijuana cohort being higher on neuroticism and lower on agreeableness and conscientiousness — and the home environment in which greater aggression and less supervision was present in the marijuana homes, the discriminating variables were no longer statistically significant.

Whether the inclusion of the personality and home environment variables as statistical controls is appropriate is a difficult issue and has been discussed elsewhere (Fried & Watkinson, 1988; O'Connell & Fried, 1991). The important question is whether this inclusion results in a too conservative approach to the data analysis. The finding of differing personality and home environment ratings between the users and non-users of marijuana may well be viewed in a trans-actional framework (Sameroff & Chandler, 1975). This model states that the developmental outcomes are the product of both maternal and child characteristics and the relationship between the mother and child characteristics is a recipro-cal one. Thus home environment measures and personality characteristics may be an outcome in themselves arising from interactions with a behaviorally altered child.

Recently, data was reported on cognitive function in 9- to 12-year-old children participat-ing in the OPPS (Fried, Watkinson & Gray, in press). The assessment battery at this age included the Wechsler Intelligence Scale for Children (WISC-III) and a series of tests examining aspects of cognition subsumed under the rubric of executive function. This function is the cogni-tive ability to maintain an appropriate problem-solving set for the attainment of a future goal and involves the integration of cognitive processes.

There was no association between the Full Scale IQ derived from the WISC and *in utero* marijuana exposure. However, using discrimi-nant function analysis (DFA), both the Block Design and the Picture Completion subtests of the WISC were negatively discriminated among the marijuana children, suggesting that *in utero* marijuana exposure affects particular rather than global aspects of intelligence.

In the Block Design subtest, subjects are directed to assemble blocks to form a design iden-tical to one presented in a picture. This non-verbal concept formation task requires the ability of perceptual organization, spatial visualization and abstract conceptualization. The Picture Completion subtest requires the subject to identify a missing portion of an incompletely drawn picture and tests the ability to differentiate essential from non-essential details.

The marijuana findings on the two WISC subtests persisted after statistically controlling for underlying, basic spatial and motor abilities, thus supporting the interpretation that the impact of prenatal marijuana exposure on these WISC sub-tests is on "higher-order" cognitive processes.

The negative relationship between these two subtests and maternal marijuana use in the present work is consistent with the finding of poorer abstract/visual reasoning in three-year-olds exposed *in utero* to marijuana (Griffith, Azuma & Chasnoff, 1994).

The results of the non-WISC outcome measures that assessed aspects of executive func-tion in the 9- to 12-year-olds in the OPPS sam-ple were consistent with the observations for the marijuana groups gleaned from the WISC tasks. The primary variables (in addition to the Block Design and Picture Completion subtests of the WISC) that were associated with the composite score that maximally discriminated among the marijuana groups, were two tests. One required the subject to visually identify abstract categories and shift cognitive sets as response criteria changes. The other involved a test of the ability to inhibit a prepotent response.

The common elements that underlie the WISC subtests and the non-WISC measures that discriminate among marijuana groups appear to be a facet of executive function that involves visual analysis, hypothesis testing and inhibition of prepotent responses. This type of integrative, "top-down" behavior (Denckla, 1996) is consid-ered to be an important facet of the neurocogni-tive domain of executive function (e.g., Welsh, Pennington & Groisser, 1991).

The finding that only particular facets of executive function appear to be associated with maternal marijuana use can be interpreted as consistent with substantial evidence suggesting that behaviors predicated upon successful execu-tive functioning are not of a singular nature. One such report that appears relevant to the findings reported above is the study of Welsh, Pennington and Groisser (1991). These authors reported that, in a battery of tests examining the construct of executive function, when administered to a normative sample of children from 3 to 12 years, three independent factors were revealed. One factor was labelled Hypothesis Testing and Impulse Control. This identified a convergence of cognitive processes that were strikingly similar to those associated with prenatal marijuana exposure in the present work with the factor being defined by requiring visual analysis and inhibition of prepotent responses.

One of the dilemmas in making conclusions about the consequences of drug exposure during fetal development is that the effects noted in the offspring are, in fact, not only due to the drug in question but also to the lifestyle and parent-child interaction that are often concomitant of a particular drug habit. Looking for the statistically unique contribution of a drug after controlling for so-called confounding factors may well obscure the reality of the drug effect(s). Furthermore, there is a reciprocal relationship between the offspring's behavior and the parent's interaction with their child. This transactional state of affairs (Sameroff & Chandler, 1975) may well serve to exacerbate particular *in utero* effects. For example, if an infant tends to be hypertonic and less cuddly, the parents may respond by less physical contact with the baby which, in turn may decrease the baby's relaxation when held.

Although statistically a significant amount of variance may be accounted for by the drug(s) in question, the amount of the variability attributable to the drug(s) is relatively small compared to other factors and decreases as the child gets older. In our own work spanning more than a decade, non-drug lifestyle habits account for up to 35 per cent of the cognitive outcome variability, but the behavioral effects uniquely associated with maternal drug use (tobacco or alcohol or marijuana) only ranges from 1.5 to 8 per cent after the variance due to other potentially confounding factors is partialled out. In other laboratories the figure can be less. This low proportion of unique, explained variance should not be interpreted as indicating that maternal drug use is of little significance. Far from it. Not only does it have real, measurable effects as described above, but it is also one of the few variables that can realistically be modified — more so than other lifestyle factors such as socioeconomic status that impinge on the mother and child. Furthermore, rarely does a drug act in isolation or in a, statistically speaking, unique fashion. It interacts with a host of other factors including

other drugs, as well as other environmental and genetic risk factors.

In other publications (e.g., Fried & Watkinson, 1988) arising from the OPPS, it has been argued that it is more likely that the drug's real association with the behavioral outcomes in question may lie between the drug's unique contribution (after potential confounds are considered) and its zero-order correlation (with no potential confounds considered). In the latter approach, variance attributable to drugs may be as high as 12 per cent, whereas, as stated earlier, the unique contribution is often in the region of 1 or 2 per cent. The likely contribution or influence of the drug may well fall between these two sets of figures.

The small proportion of unique variance attributable to maternal drug use, however, does lead to a variety of interpretative problems and emphasizes the importance of longitudinal investigations in which suspected drug effects from maternal usage can be examined across many ages. If one notes effects in the very young infant along particular dimensions of behavior and continues to see effects in related spheres as the offspring gets older, more confidence can be had in attributing some of the findings to the *in utero* exposure.

In interpreting the evidence presented in this chapter, this interactional state of affairs must not be forgotten and should be an integral part in drawing conclusions about marijuana's effects on the mother, fetus and child. Two additional points have to be kept in mind in interpreting the findings with respect to prenatal marijuana exposure described in this chapter. The women in the Ottawa work represent a very low-risk sample. There is a considerable body of literature (animal and human) to suggest that the drug's effect is potentiated in a higher-risk environment (reviewed in Fried, 1993) and thus one must be very cautious in extrapolating the present observations to other marijuana-using populations. There is also the concern that the potency of marijuana preparations, in terms of THC content, has increased several fold (ElSohly & ElSohly, 1989) since the entrance of pregnant women into the Ottawa study in the late seventies and early eighties. This increase in potency adds to the importance of interpreting the present results as representing conservative observations.

ATTEMPT AT A SYNTHESIS

What can one determine from the material, based on human subjects, described up to this point? On the surface it appears that the only conclusive statement would be that, if there are long-term consequences of prenatal exposure to marijuana, such effects are very subtle. However, the data may allow conclusions that go somewhat further.

The marijuana findings may be summarized in the following manner. In the newborn and neonate, although far from definitive, there appears to be an association between nervous system state regulation and prenatal exposure to marijuana. However, between six months and three years of age no neurobehavioral consequences of marijuana have been reported, although at two years of age language comprehension was lower among the children of cannabis users prior to statistical control for the home environment. At four years, tests of verbal ability and memory statistically discriminated between the offspring of regular marijuana users and the remainder of the children in the OPPS sample. The same domains of vulnerability were noted in three-year-olds in the high-risk Pittsburgh sample (Day, Richardson et al., 1994). At five and six years of age, prenatal marijuana exposure was not associated with global tests of cognition and language after statistically controlling for potentially confounding data. However, at approximately these ages and slightly older, tests that examined more specific aspects of behavior did appear to suggest a relationship between performance and *in utero* exposure to marijuana. In school-aged children, a deficit in sustained attention was noted on a task that differentiated between impulsivity and vigilance. Further, parental ratings of behavior indicated greater problems (particularly in the area of inattention and conduct) among the children of cannabis users. Visual perceptual, visual memory, language comprehension and distractibility discriminated

between the six- to nine-year-old offspring of marijuana and non-marijuana users. The latter findings did not remain statistically significant upon the inclusion of maternal personality and home environment conditions as potential confounds, although this statistical control (as discussed above) may be inappropriate. Finally, the most recent findings with the OPPS sample suggest that whereas overall IQ in offspring is not associated with prenatal marijuana exposure, certain types of integrative cognitive functions may be affected by such exposure.

Two issues that arise from this data are the seeming absence of prenatal marijuana-related cognitive effects prior to four years of age and the question of whether there is any common theme among the effects and trends noted at four years and beyond. Dealing with the latter issue first, the areas of vulnerability that have emerged over the course of the OPPS (as well as the finding at three years of age in the two other samples, Day, Richardson et al., 1994; Griffith, Azuma & Chasnoff, 1994) are ones that are quite consistent with the cognitive construct that several authors have termed executive function (Duncan, 1986; Luria, 1966; Welsh & Pennington, 1988). The executive function behaviors noted to be negatively associated with prenatal marijuana exposure include those that involve self-regulatory abilities (the dysfunction possibly manifesting itself in the form of behavioral problems), the ability to maintain attention (noted as impairments in vigilance and distractibility) and the ability to act on accumulated knowledge (poorer performance on facets of language, memory and abstract/visual reasoning).

Executive function is thought to serve as a marker of prefrontal lobe function and thus it may be that this part of the central nervous system may be particularly vulnerable to prenatal marijuana exposure. Frontal lobe development is not an all-or-none phenomenon but appears to be a multistage process, as is executive functioning (Welsh & Pennington, 1988). Although aspects of executive functioning are present in infants and toddlers (e.g., object permanence behavior) many aspects of prefrontal functioning are not apparent or are difficult to test until children approach or reach school age. This is certainly congruent with the OPPS results.

An important further property of executive functioning is that it is disassociated from measures of global intelligence. This is consistent with the observation of the sparing of IQ after frontal lobe damage (Damasio, 1979) and may reflect the fact that traditional, global intelligence tests evaluate overlearned information and established cognitive sets. One of the consistent findings noted among the children in the OPPS (and in the Pittsburgh sample, Day, Richardson et al., 1994) was that prenatal marijuana exposure was not associated with a lowering of general IQ.

Recent observations from diverse fields within the general marijuana literature also implicate the frontal lobes in that drug's effects. The discovery of receptors for cannabinoid substances in the mammalian brain (including humans) provides very convincing evidence for the direct action of marijuana on certain mental processes (e.g., Herkenham, Lynn et al., 1990; 1991; Matsuda, Lolait et al., 1990). In long-term, chronic adult users these include fragmentation of thought, difficulty in short-term memory tasks, disturbances in attention, concentration and judgment — tasks that are associated with frontal lobe functioning. Recently, Australian researchers (Solowij, Michie & Fox, 1993) have reported that among chronic users the ability to evaluate stimuli and reject irrelevant stimuli is impaired and these alterations in cognitive ability do not reverse themselves even after five years of abstinence (Solowij, personal communication, October 1993).

In the rat, within different regions of the cortex, the frontal area has been reported to contain the highest density of binding sites (Herkenham, Lynn et al., 1991). In nine chronic adult users, Tunving et al. (1986) reported reduced blood flow throughout the cerebral cortex. Intriguingly, only two of the users were not polydrug users and in these cases in which marijuana was the drug uniquely used, the prefrontal area was the most affected (Lundqvist, personal

communication, July 1993). Finally, Struve and colleagues (1989; 1993) have recently reported that chronic, daily use of marijuana results in a marked alteration in alpha activity primarily in the frontal region even after prolonged cessation of use.

At this stage, then, a suggestive but highly speculative picture is beginning to emerge. The behavioral evidence gathered primarily from the children participating in the OPPS over the past years, the delayed temporal appearance of the observed effects, and the recent findings linking altered frontal lobe functioning with chronic marijuana exposure is certainly compatible with the notion that prenatal marijuana exposure may result in altered frontal lobe functioning in the offspring. One of the next steps in clarifying this picture is to examine the children in the OPPS in tasks that are thought to be particularly sensitive to frontal lobe dysfunction. These include tests of problem solving that require cognitive flexibility, route finding tasks, and measures of distractibility, attention and working memory. These assessments are presently underway.

Conclusion

There are a number of dilemmas for researchers interested in the developmental toxicity of cannabis. Basic to an understanding of the pharmacology and toxicity of a compound is knowledge of how much active substance is delivered to biological tissues. In animal studies, it is possible to administer specified quantities of a compound in order to describe precisely dose-response effects. Nearly all of the developmental animal studies have investigated THC, which is only one — albeit the major — psychoactive constituent of cannabis. On the other hand, human reproductive studies typically investigate the effects of smoked cannabis, and dosage can only be estimated by the user. These facts constrain the interpretation, comparison and extrapolation of cannabis research data.

Animal Studies

In 1985, Abel pointed out the serious methodological and interpretive flaws that characterized the early literature of animal studies on the developmental toxicity of THC. Adverse effects observed in the offspring may not have been produced by direct drug effects on the embryo and fetus but instead were secondary to THC-induced maternal toxicity. THC substantially inhibits food and water intake in rats, with consequent poor maternal nutrition and dehydration. THC can also disrupt normal maternal care at parturition and, through hormonal effects, inhibit milk production and let-down, all having possible adverse consequences for the neurobehavioral development of the offspring (Hutchings, 1985).

Several dose-related effects have been found in rat offspring following administration of THC to the pregnant dam in studies using appropriate controls for maternal nutrition and fostering. At birth, a dose-related increase in the sex ratio of live offspring was consistently found, suggesting that female conceptuses have greater susceptibility to THC lethality (Hutchings, Brake et al., 1987; Morgan, Brake et al., 1988). During the postnatal period, a dose-related inhibition of both somatic growth and brain protein synthesis was found. These effects were transitory, however, and the THC-exposed animals caught up to the controls by the time of weaning (Hutchings, Brake et al., 1987). Hutchings found no evidence of neurobehavioral deficits in the offspring independent of maternal toxicity, results that are consistent with those of other well-controlled animal studies (Abel, 1985).

Human Studies

EPIDEMIOLOGICAL STUDIES

Epidemiological studies of the prevalence of drug use in pregnant women are often complicated by sampling procedures that involve populations that are selectively biased towards drug use. Besides the difficulty in estimating very well the prevalence of marijuana use in this population, there are other factors complicating the interpretation of drug studies. The exact doses or amounts of THC utilized and the time of such use are impossible to quantify. Other drug use and socioeconomic factors cannot be controlled by random assignment to groups. Human studies must be based on volunteer samples, with reports of drug use being gathered either before (i.e., prospectively) or after (i.e., retrospectively) birth.

NEUROBEHAVIORAL STUDIES

Fried and his colleagues have undertaken a large-scale prospective study of maternal marijuana use, the Ottawa Prospective Prenatal Study. From these data, it appears that if there are long-term consequences to the child of prenatal exposure to marijuana, such effects are very subtle. In the newborn and neonate, there appears to be an association between nervous system state regulation and prenatal exposure to marijuana. However, between six months and three years of age, no neurobehavioral consequences of maternal marijuana use have been reported. At four years, tests of verbal ability and memory discriminate between offspring of regular marijuana users and other children. Similar deficits were seen in school-aged children as well. In sum, these results suggest that the domains affected, even if to a rather small extent, by *in utero* exposure to marijuana have the potential to affect the capabilities of the growing child. For example, the child's ability to attend to critical stimuli, to refrain from impulsive and intrusive behavior, and to retain and recall material may be affected. Thus, the impairments suggested by the data have clear implications for performance in the classroom.

Acknowledgments

The animal research reported here was supported by grant DA03544 from the National Institute on Drug Abuse to D. Hutchings. Portions of the human research reviewed here were presented at a National Institute on Drug Abuse technical review on "Behaviors of Drug-Exposed Offspring: Research Update" held in Washington, DC, July 1993. The OPPS has been supported in the past by grants from the National Research Council of Canada, National Health and Welfare Canada and a Carleton University Social Science Research Grant. In recent years and presently, the work is supported by a National Institute on Drug Abuse grant DA04874. The work described could not have been carried out without the continuing and ongoing assistance of my long-time associates over the years, including B. Watkinson, H. Linttell and R. Gray, and the enduring patience of the mothers and their children during the past decade.

References

Abel, E.L. (1980). *Marijuana: The First Twelve Thousand Years*. New York: Plenum Press.

Abel, E.L. (1985). Effects of prenatal exposure to cannabinoids. In T.M. Pinkert (Ed.), *Current Research on the Consequences of Maternal Drug Abuse* (NIDA Research Monograph No. 59, pp. 20–35) (DHHS Publication No. 85-1400). Washington, DC: U.S. Government Printing Office.

Abood, M.E. & Martin, B.R. (1992). Neurobiology of marijuana abuse. *Trends in Pharmacological Sciences*, *13*, 201–206.

Astley, S. & Little, R. (1990). Maternal marijuana use during lactation and infant development at one year. *Neurotoxicology and Teratology*, *12*, 161–168.

Bailey, J.R., Cunny, H.C., Paule, M.G. & Slikker, W., Jr. (1987). Fetal disposition of delta-9-tetrahydrocannabinol (THC) during late pregnancy in the rhesus monkey. *Toxicology and Applied Pharmacology*, *90*, 315–321.

Barr, H.M., Streissguth, A.P., Martin, D.C. & Hermes, C.S. (1984). Infant size at 8 months of age: Relationship to maternal use of alcohol, nicotine, and caffeine during pregnancy. *Pediatrics*, *74*, 336–341.

Bayley, N. (1969). *Bayley Scales of Infant Development*. New York: Psychological Corporation.

Belue, R.C., Howlett, A.C., Westlake, T.M. & Hutchings, D.E. (1995). The ontogeny of cannabinoid receptors in the brain of postnatal and aging rats. *Neurotoxicology and Teratology, 17*, 25–30.

Bornstein, M.H. & Sigman, M.D. (1986). Continuity in mental development from infancy. *Child Development, 57*, 251–274.

Brake, S.C., Hutchings, D.E., Morgan, B., Lasalle, E. & Shi, T. (1987). Delta-9-tetrahydrocannabinol during pregnancy in the rat: II. Effects on ontogeny of locomotor activity and nipple attachment in the offspring. *Neurotoxicology and Teratology, 9*, 45–49.

Charlebois, A.T. & Fried, P.A. (1980). The interactive effects of nutrition and cannabis upon rat perinatal development. *Developmental Psychobiology, 13*, 591–605.

Chasnoff, I.J. (1990). *Cocaine use in pregnancy: Effect on infant neurobehavioural functioning.* Paper presented at the American Society for Pharmacology and Experimental Therapeutics, Washington, DC.

Chasnoff, I.J., Griffith, D.R, Freier, C. & Murray, J. (1992). Cocaine/polydrug use in pregnancy: Two-year follow-up. *Pediatrics, 89*, 284–289.

Chasnoff, I.J., Landres, H.J. & Barrett, M.E. (1990). The prevalence of illicit drug or alcohol use during pregnancy and discrepancies in mandatory reporting in Pinellas county, Florida. *New England Journal of Medicine, 322*, 1202–1206.

Coles, C.D., Platzman, K.A., Smith, I., James, M.E. & Falek, A. (1992). Effects of cocaine, alcohol, and other drug use in pregnancy on neonatal growth and neurobehavioral status. *Neurotoxicology and Teratology, 14*, 22–33.

Conners, C.K. (1989). *Manual for Conners' Rating Scales.* Toronto: Multi Health Systems.

Dahl, R.E., Scher, M.S., Day, N.L., Richardson, G., Klepper, T. & Robles, N. (1988). The effects of prenatal marijuana exposure: Evidence of EEG-sleep disturbances. *Journal of Developmental and Behavioral Pediatrics, 9*, 333–339.

Dalterio, S.L. & Fried, P.A. (1992). The effects of marijuana use on offspring. In T.B. Sonderegger (Ed.), *Perinatal Substance Abuse Research Findings and Clinical Implications* (pp. 161–183). Baltimore: The Johns Hopkins University Press.

Damasio, A. (1979). The frontal lobes. In K.M. Heilman & E. Valenstein (Eds.), *Clinical Neuropsychology* (pp. 360–412). New York: Oxford University Press.

Day, N. & Richardson, G.A. (1991). Prenatal marijuana use: Epidemiology, methodological issues and infant outcome. In I. Chasnoff (Ed.), *Clinics in Perinatology* (pp. 77–92). Philadelphia: W.B. Saunders.

Day, N., Richardson, G.A., Goldschmidt, L., Robles, N., Taylor, P.M., Stoffer, D.S., Cornelius, M.D. & Geva, D. (1994). The effect of prenatal marijuana exposure on the cognitive development of offspring at age three. *Neurotoxicology and Teratology, 16*, 169–176.

Day, N., Sambamoorthi, U., Taylor, P., Richardson, G., Robles, N., Jhon, Y., Scher, M., Stoffer, D. & Cornelius, M. (1991). Prenatal marijuana use and neonatal outcome. *Neurotoxicology and Teratology, 13*, 329–334.

Denckla, M.B. (1996). A theory and model of executive function. In G.R. Lyon & N.A. Krasnegor (Eds.), *Attention, Memory and Executive Function* (pp. 263–278). Baltimore: Paul H. Brookes.

Dewey, W.L. (1986). Cannabinoid pharmacology. *Pharmacological Reviews, 38*, 151–178.

Dreher, M.C., Nugent, K. & Hudgins, R. (1994). Prenatal marijuana exposure and neonatal outcomes in Jamaica: An ethnographic study. *Pediatrics, 93*, 254–260.

Duncan, J. (1986). Disorganization of behaviour after frontal lobe damage. *Cognitive Neuropsychology, 3*, 271–290.

Dunn, L.M. & Dunn, L.M. (1981). *Peabody Picture Vocabulary Test — Revised.* Circle Pines, MN: American Guidance Service.

ElSohly, M.A. & ElSohly, H.N. (1989). Marijuana: Analysis and detection of use through urinalysis. In K. Redda, C. Walker & G. Barnett (Eds.), *Cocaine, Marihuana and Designer Drugs: Chemistry, Pharmacology, and Behaviour* (p. 145). Boca Raton, FL: CRC Press.

Frank, D.A., Zuckerman, B.S., Amaro, H. et al. (1988). Cocaine use during pregnancy: Prevalence and correlates. *Pediatrics, 82*, 888–895.

Fried, P.A. (1976). Short and long-term effects of pre-natal cannabis inhalation upon rat offspring. *Psychopharmacology (Berl), 50*, 285–291.

Fried, P.A. (1980). Marijuana use by pregnant women: Neurobehavioral effects in neonates. *Drug and Alcohol Dependence, 6*, 415–424.

Fried, P.A. (1984). Prenatal and postnatal consequences of marijuana use during pregnancy. In J. Yanai (Ed.), *Neurobehavioural Teratology* (pp. 275–285). New York: Elsevier.

Fried, P.A. (1993). Prenatal exposure to tobacco and marijuana: Effects during pregnancy, infancy, and early childhood. *Clinical Obstetrics and Gynecology, 36*, 319–337.

Fried, P.A., Barnes, M.V. & Drake E.R. (1985). Soft drug use after pregnancy compared to use before and during pregnancy. *American Journal of Obstetrics and Gynecology, 151*, 787–792.

Fried, P.A., Buckingham, M. & Von Kulmiz, P. (1983). Marijuana use during pregnancy and perinatal risk factors. *American Journal of Obstetrics and Gynecology, 146*, 992–994.

Fried, P.A., Innes, K.E. & Barnes, M.V. (1984). Soft drug use prior to and during pregnancy: A comparison of samples over a four-year period. *Drug and Alcohol Dependence, 13*, 161–176.

Fried, P.A. & Makin, J.E. (1987). Neonatal behavioural correlates of prenatal exposure to marijuana, cigarettes, and alcohol in a low risk population. *Neurotoxicology and Teratology, 9*, 1–7.

Fried, P.A. & O'Connell, C.M. (1987). A comparison of the effects of prenatal exposure to tobacco, alcohol, cannabis and caffeine on birth size and subsequent growth. *Neurotoxicology and Teratology, 9*, 79–85.

Fried, P.A., O'Connell, C.M. & Watkinson, B. (1992). 60- and 72-month follow-up of children prenatally exposed to marijuana, cigarettes, and alcohol: Cognitive and language assessment. *Journal of Developmental and Behavioral Pediatrics, 13*, 383–391.

Fried, P.A. & Watkinson, B. (1988). 12- and 24-month neurobehavioral follow-up of children prenatally exposed to marijuana, cigarettes, and alcohol. *Neurotoxicology and Teratology, 10*, 305–313.

Fried, P.A. & Watkinson, B. (1990). 36- and 48-month neurobehavioural follow-up of children prenatally exposed to marijuana, cigarettes and alcohol. *Journal of Developmental and Behavioral Pediatrics, 11*, 49–58.

Fried, P.A., Watkinson, B., Dillon, R.F. & Dulberg, C.S. (1987). Neonatal neurological status in a low-risk population after prenatal exposure to cigarettes, marijuana and alcohol. *Journal of Developmental and Behavioral Pediatrics, 8*, 318–326.

Fried, P.A., Watkinson, B., Grant, A. & Knights, R.M. (1980). Changing patterns of soft drug use prior to and during pregnancy: A prospective study. *Drug and Alcohol Dependence, 6*, 323–343.

Fried, P.A., Watkinson, B. & Gray, R. (1992). A follow-up study of attentional behaviour in 6-year-old children exposed prenatally to marijuana, cigarettes, and alcohol. *Neurotoxicology and Teratology, 14*, 299–311.

Fried, P.A., Watkinson, B. & Gray. R. (in press). Differential effects on cognitive functioning in 9 to 12 year olds prenatally exposed to cigarettes and marihuana. *Neurotoxicology and Teratology.*

Fried, P.A., Watkinson, B. & Willan, A. (1984). Marijuana use during pregnancy and decreased length of gestation. *American Journal of Obstetrics and Gynecology, 150*, 23–27.

Gibson, G.T., Baghurst, P.A. & Colley, D.P. (1983). Maternal alcohol, tobacco and cannabis consumption and the outcome of pregnancy. *Australian and New Zealand Journal of Obstetrics and Gynaecology, 23*, 15–19.

Gordon, M. & McClure, D.F. (1984). *Gordon Diagnostic System: Interpretive Supplement.* Goldon, CO: Clinical Diagnostics.

Greenland, S., Staisch, K., Brown, N. & Gross, S. (1982). The effects of marijuana use during pregnancy: I. A preliminary epidemiological study. *American Journal of Obstetrics and Gynecology, 143*, 408–413.

Greenland, S., Staisch, K., Brown, N. & Gross, S. (1983). Effects of marijuana on human pregnancy, labor and delivery. *Neurobehavioral Toxicology and Teratology, 4*, 447–450.

Griffith, D.R., Azuma, S.D. & Chasnoff, I.J. (1994). Three-year outcome of children exposed prenatally to drugs. *Journal of the American Academy of Child and Adolescent Psychiatry, 33*, 20–27.

Harbison, R.D. & Mantilla-Plata, B. (1972). Prenatal toxicity, maternal distribution and placental transfer of tetrahydrocannabinol. *Journal of Pharmacology and Experimental Therapeutics, 180*, 446–453.

Hatch, E.E. & Bracken, M.B. (1986). Effect of marijuana use in pregnancy on fetal growth. *American Journal of Epidemiology, 124*, 986–993.

Herkenham, M., Lynn, A.B., Johnson, M.R., Melvin, L.S., De Costa, B.R. & Rice, K.C. (1991). Characterization and localization of cannabinoid receptors in rat brain: A quantitative in vitro autoradiographic study. *Journal of Neuroscience, 11*, 563–583.

Herkenham, M., Lynn, A.B., Little, M.D., Johnson, M.R., Melvin, L.S., De Costa, B.R. & Rice, K.C. (1990). Cannabinoid receptor localization in brain. *Proceedings of the National Academy of Sciences of the United States of America, 87*, 1932–1936.

Hingson, R., Alpert, J., Day, N., Dooling, E., Kayne, H., Morelock, S., Oppenheimer, E. & Zuckerman, B. (1982). Effects of maternal drinking and marijuana use on fetal growth and development. *Pediatrics, 70*, 539–546.

Hutchings, D.E. (1985). Issues of methodology and interpretation in clinical and animal behavioral teratology studies. *Neurobehavioral Toxicology and Teratology, 7*, 639–642.

Hutchings, D.E. (1987). Drug abuse during pregnancy: Embryopathic and neurobehavioral effects. In M.C. Braude & A.M. Zimmerman (Eds.), *Genetic and Perinatal Effects of Abused Substances* (pp. 131–151). New York: Academic Press.

Hutchings, D.E., Brake, S.C., Shi, T. & Lasalle, E. (1987). Delta-9-tetrahydrocannabinol during pregnancy in the rat: I. Differential effects on maternal nutrition, embryotoxicity and growth in the offspring. *Neurotoxicology and Teratology, 9*, 39–43.

Hutchings, D.E., Fico, T.A. & Dow-Edwards, D.L. (1989). Prenatal cocaine: Maternal toxicity, fetal effects and motor activity in the offspring. *Neurotoxicology and Teratology, 11*, 65–69.

Hutchings, D.E., Martin, B.R., Gamagaris, Z., Miller, N. & Fico, T. (1989). Plasma concentrations of delta-9-tetrahydrocannabinol in dams and fetuses following acute or multiple prenatal dosing in rats. *Life Sciences, 44*, 697–701.

Hutchings, D.E., Towey, J.P. & Bodnarenko, S.R. (1980). Effects of prenatal methadone on activity level in the preweanling rat. *Neurobehavioral Toxicology, 2*, 231–235.

Johnston, L., O'Malley, P. & Bachman, J. (1994a). *National Survey Results on Drug Use from Monitoring the Future Study, 1975–1993: Vol. 1. Secondary School Study* (NIH Publication No. 94-3809). Rockville, MD: National Institute on Drug Abuse.

Johnston, L., O'Malley, P. & Bachman, J. (1994b). *National Survey Results on Drug Use from Monitoring the Future Study, 1975–1993: Vol. 2. College Students and Young Adults* (NIH Publication No. 94-3809). Rockville, MD: National Institute on Drug Abuse.

Jones, R.T. (1980). Human effects: An overview. In R.C. Petersen (Ed.), *Marijuana Research Findings: 1980* (NIDA Research Monograph No. 31, pp. 54–80) (DHHS Publication No. ADM 80-1001). Washington, DC: U.S. Government Printing Office.

Keith R.W. (1986). *SCAN — A Screening Test for Auditory Processing Disorders.* San Antonio, TX: The Psychological Corporation, Harcourt Brace Jovanovich.

Kennedy, J.S. & Waddell, W.J. (1972). Whole-body autoradiography of the pregnant mouse after administration of ^{14}C-delta-9-THC. *Toxicology and Applied Pharmacology, 22*, 252–258.

Kilbey, M.M. & Asghar, K. (Eds.). (1992). *Methodological Issues in Epidemiological, Prevention, and Treatment Research on Drug-Exposed Women and Their Children* (NIDA Research Monograph No. 117) (DHHS Publication No. ADM 92-1881). Washington, DC: U.S. Government Printing Office.

Kline, J., Stein, Z. & Hutzler, M. (1987). Cigarettes, alcohol and marijuana: Varying associations with birthweight. *International Journal of Epidemiology, 16*, 44–51.

Lester, B. & Dreher, M. (1989). Effects of marijuana use during pregnancy on newborn cry. *Child Development, 60*, 765–771.

Linn, S., Schoenbaum, S.C., Monson, R.R., Rosner, R., Stubblefield, P.C. & Ryan, K.J. (1983). The association of marijuana use with outcome of pregnancy. *American Journal of Public Health, 73*, 1161–1164.

Luria, A.R. (1966). *Higher Cortical Functions in Man.* New York: Basic Books.

MacGregor, S.N., Sciarra, J.C., Keith, L. & Sciarra, J.J. (1990). Prevalence of marijuana use during pregnancy: A pilot study. *Journal of Reproductive Medicine, 23,* 1147–1149.

Majewaki, F. (1981). Alcohol embryopathy: Some facts and speculations about pathogenesis. *Neurobehavioral Toxicology and Teratology, 3,* 129–144.

Marijuana and Health. (1982). *Report of a Study by the Committee of the Institute of Medicine, Division of Health Sciences Policy.* Washington, DC: National Academy Press.

Martin, B.R. (1986). Cellular effects of cannabinoids. *Pharmacological Reviews, 38,* 45–74.

Martin, B.R., Dewey, W.L., Harris, L.S. & Beckner, J.S. (1977). ^{3}H-delta-9-tetrahydro-cannabinol distribution in pregnant dogs and their fetuses. *Research Communications in Chemical Pathology and Pharmacology, 17,* 457–470.

Matsuda, L.A., Lolait, S.J., Brownstein, M.J., Young, A.C. & Bonner, T.I. (1990). Structure of a cannabinoid receptor and functional expression of the cloned cDNA. *Nature, 346,* 561–564.

McCarthy, P. (1972). *McCarthy Scales of Children's Abilities.* New York: The Psychological Corporation, Harcourt Brace Jovanovich.

McClure, F.D. & Gordon, M. (1983). Performance of disturbed hyperactive and non-hyperactive children on an objective measure of hyperactivity. *Journal of Abnormal Child Psychology, 168,* 26–33.

Morgan, B., Brake, S.C., Hutchings, D.E., Miller, N. & Gamagaris, Z. (1988). Delta-9-tetra-hydrocannabinol during pregnancy in the rat: Effects on development of RNA, DNA, and protein in offspring brain. *Pharmacology, Biochemistry and Behavior, 31,* 365–369.

National Institute on Drug Abuse. (1991). *National Household Survey on Drug Abuse: Main Findings 1990* (DHHS Publication No. ADM 91-1788). Rockville, MD: U.S. Department of Health and Human Services.

NIDA Marijuana Project. (1988). *Quarterly Report: Potency Monitoring Project* (Report No. 26, Research Institute of Pharmaceutical Sciences). Oxford, MS: The University of Mississippi.

O'Connell, C.M. & Fried, P.A. (1984). An investigation of prenatal cannabis exposure and minor physical anomalies in a low risk population. *Neurotoxicology and Teratology, 6,* 345–350.

O'Connell, C.M. & Fried, P.A. (1991). Prenatal exposure to cannabis: A preliminary report of postnatal consequences in school-age children. *Neurotoxicology and Teratology, 13,* 631–639.

Qazi, Q.H., Mariano, E., Bellar, E., Milman, D. & Crumbleholme, W. (1982). Is marijuana smoking fetotoxic? *Pediatric Research, 16,* 272A.

Qazi, Q.H., Mariano, E., Bellar, E., Milman, D. & Crumbleholme, W. (1985). Abnormalities associated with prenatal marijuana exposure. *Developmental Pharmacology and Therapeutics, 8,* 141–148.

Reynell, J. (1977). *Reynell Developmental Language Scales — Revised.* Windsor, UK: NFER Publishing.

Richardson, G.A., Day, N.L. & Taylor, P.M. (1989). The effect of prenatal alcohol, marijuana and tobacco exposure on neonatal behaviour. *Infant Behavior and Development, 12,* 199–209.

Sameroff, A. & Chandler, M. (1975). Reproductive risk and the continuum of caretaking causality. In F. Horwitz, E. Hetherington, S. Scarr-Salaptek & G. Siegal (Eds.), *Review of Child Development Research* (Vol. 4) (pp. 187–243). Chicago: University of Chicago Press.

Scher, M.S., Richardson, G.A., Coble, P.A., Day, N.L. & Stoffer, D. (1988). The effects of prenatal alcohol and marijuana exposure: Disturbances in sleep cycling and arousal. *Pediatric Research, 24,* 101–105.

Solowij, N., Michie, P.T. & Fox, A.M. (1993). Differential impairments of selective attention due to frequency and duration of cannabis use. Paper presented at the International Cannabis Research Society, Toronto, Canada.

Streissguth, A.P., Barr, H.M., Sampson, P.D., Darby, B.L. & Martin, D.C. (1989). IQ at age 4 in relation to maternal alcohol use and smoking during pregnancy. *Developmental Psychology, 25,* 3–11.

Struve, F., Straumanis, J., Patrick, G., Norris, G., Nixon, F., Fitz-Gerald, M., Manno, J., Leavitt, J. & Webb, P. (1993). Topographic quantitative EEG sequelae of chronic cumulative THC exposure: Recent and continuing studies. Paper presented at the International Cannabis Research Society, Toronto, Canada.

Struve, F.A., Straumanis, J.J., Patrick, G. & Price, L. (1989). Topographic mapping of quantitative EEG variables in chronic heavy marijuana users: Empirical findings with psychiatric patients. *Clinical Electroencephalography, 20,* 6–23.

Tennes, K., Avitable, N., Blackard, C., Boyles, C., Hassoun, B., Holmes, L. & Kreye, M. (1985). Marihuana: Prenatal and postnatal exposure in the human. In T.M. Pinkert (Ed.), *Current Research on the Consequences of Maternal Drug Abuse* (NIDA Research Monograph No. 59, pp. 48–60) (DHHS Publication No. 85-1400). Washington, DC: U.S. Government Printing Office.

Tunving, K., Thulin, S.O., Risberg, J. & Warkentin, S. (1986). Regional cerebral blood flow in long-term heavy cannabis use. *Psychiatry Research, 17,* 15–21.

Welsh, M.C. & Pennington, B.F. (1988). Assessing frontal lobe functioning in children: Views from developmental psychology. *Developmental Neuropsychology, 4*, 199–230.

Welsh, M.C., Pennington, B.F. & Groisser, D.B. (1991). A normative-developmental study of executive function: A window on prefrontal function in children. *Developmental Neuropsychology, 7*, 131–149.

Winick, M. (1976). Malnutrition and prenatal growth. In M. Winick (Ed.), *Malnutrition and Brain Development* (pp. 98–127). New York: Oxford University Press.

Zuckerman, B., Frank, D., Hingson, R., Amaro, H., Levenson, S., Kayne, H., Parker, S., Vinci, R., Aboagye, K., Fried, L., Cabral, H., Timperi, R. & Bauchner, S. (1989). Effects of maternal marijuana and cocaine use on fetal growth. *New England Journal of Medicine, 320*, 762–768.

Effects of Cannabis on the Cardiovascular and Gastrointestinal Systems

Effects of Cannabis on the Cardiovascular and Gastrointestinal Systems

GREGORY CHESHER AND WAYNE HALL

This chapter deals with the effects of Ø-tetrahydrocannabinol (THC) and cannabis on the cardiovascular and gastrointestinal systems. Much of the research reported in it is based on animal and human experimental studies. Clinical evidence is scant and epidemiological evidence largely non-existent, reflecting a lack of concern about the effects of cannabis on these body systems by comparison with concerns about its effects on the central nervous system (CNS). In each case we begin with a review of animal and human experimental evidence before discussing the limited clinical evidence that is available. The possible clinical significance of the findings in the available literature is also briefly discussed.

Cardiovascular Effects of Cannabis

The cardiovascular effects of cannabis were extensively researched in the 1970s and early 1980s. This literature has been reviewed within the last decade or so (Coper, 1981; Dewey, 1986; Huber, Griffith & Langsjoen, 1988; Jones, 1984) and very little new information has appeared since these publications. None of it substantially changes their conclusions. Further reviews will be required within the next few years as more is revealed about the role in cardiovascular function of the recently discovered endogenous "anandamide" system. As will be described, on the basis of available evidence, the cardiovascular effects of the cannabinoids appear to be entirely central in origin. The only data on peripheral cannabinoid receptors concerns components of the immune system. There also appears to be no evidence for specific THC binding in the heart (Lynn & Herkenham, 1994).

Studies conducted earlier this century indicated that cannabis use produced tachycardia but only a slight increase, if at all, in blood pressure. These included studies conducted for the Panama Canal Zone (Siler, Sheep & Bates, 1933) and the LaGuardia committee (Allentuck & Bowman, 1942). Another important early study was that of Williams et al. (1946) who gave either cannabis or the synthetic cannabinoid, pyrahexyl, and obtained the first indication that tolerance might develop to the cardiovascular effects of cannabis. All this work was done before the identification of the cannabinoids and therefore the relationship of these effects to the dose of THC could not be determined. The subsequent isolation, identification and synthesis of the active cannabinoids greatly facilitated research on the cardiovascular effects of cannabis (Gaoni & Mechoulam, 1964). Because there are as yet unexplained differences in the cardiovascular responses to cannabis between humans and other species, only the effects in humans will be emphasized here.

Heart Rate in Humans

The most consistent and reproducible of the human effects of cannabis is an increase in heart rate. The effect is dose-dependent, both in terms of peak rate, and when heart rate is measured over time and expressed as area under the curve (AUC) (Beaconsfield, Ginsburg & Rainsbury, 1972; Johnson & Domino, 1971; Perez-Reyes, 1990; Perez-Reyes, Lipton et al., 1973). The changes in heart rate were found to mimic in all respects the subjective ratings of "high" (Perez-Reyes, 1990). In addition, mean peak heart rates and AUC (0 to 35') have been shown to increase in proportion to the magnitude of the THC plasma concentrations. Group data have not revealed a significant correlation between peak heart rate and peak THC plasma concentrations, presumably because of the very large individual differences in these measures and in the manner of smoking (Perez-Reyes, 1990).

An interaction between marijuana and task performance on the effects on heart rate and mean arterial blood pressure was demonstrated in a study involving 10 healthy volunteers by Capriotti et al. (1988). Performance of a 10-minute serial acquisition task increased heart rate by four beats per minute (bpm) and blood pressure by 5 mm Hg. Marijuana used alone (1.8 per cent THC cigarette) increased these measures by 18 bpm and 3 mm Hg. The combination of marijuana and task performance resulted in changes of heart rate to 29 bpm and blood pressure increase of 15 mm Hg. These results suggest that marijuana may increase cardiovascular responsivity.

Similar results were found in a study that examined the interaction between marijuana, cocaine and performance of a learning task (Foltin & Fischman, 1990). Increases in resting heart rate

were: 15 bpm for cocaine (up to 96 milligrams, snorted); 27 bpm for marijuana (a 1-gram cigarette of 2.9 per cent THC); and 5 bpm for the learning task alone. Cocaine and marijuana used together produced the same effect as marijuana used alone, but when marijuana and cocaine were combined with the task performance heart rate increased to 37 bpm. The largest increases in blood pressure resulted when the two drugs were combined with task performance.

Both sympathetic and parasympathetic mechanisms seem to be involved in cannabis-induced tachycardia. This is indicated by the fact that cannabis-induced tachycardia is abolished by β adrenoceptor blockade alone and together with atropine (Beaconsfield, Ginsburg & Rainsbury, 1972; Benowitz, Rosenberg et al., 1979; Kanakis, Pouget & Rosen, 1976; Martz, Brown et al., 1972; Perez-Reyes, Lipton et al., 1973; Sulkowski, Vachon & Rich, 1977). Gash et al. (1978) have also reported increases in plasma levels of noradrenaline while studying the effects of cannabis on heart rate and left ventricular performance. However, this increase was not observed until some 30 minutes after the onset of the tachycardia. The delayed increase in plasma levels of noradrenaline was confirmed by Maddock et al. (1979) who described the marked changes in skin temperature which reached a peak at about 40 to 50 minutes after the administration of cannabis or THC. These effects were found to be dose-related, could be as much as 7 degrees C and paralleled the increase in noradrenaline concentration.

Peripheral Resistance

Increases in heart rate lead to increases in cardiac output, but the extent of the effect on blood pressure depends on peripheral resistance. Cannabis-induced increase in heart rate may increase cardiac output as much as 30 per cent, yet increases in supine blood pressure are usually less than 10 per cent. Cannabis has been shown to increase limb blood flow (Beaconsfield, Ginsburg & Rainsbury, 1972; Benowitz, Rosenberg et al., 1979; Kanakis, Pouget &

Rosen, 1976; Weiss, Watanabe et al., 1972). Weiss et al. reported that the increased limb blood flow did not occur when subjects were standing. Indeed, the postural (orthostatic) blood pressure fall can be considerably exaggerated after cannabis (Benowitz & Jones, 1975).

Vascular Reflexes

Some vascular reflexes are reduced by THC. For example, THC can suppress the cardiac slowing after the Valsalva manoeuvre (Renault, Schuster et al., 1971), attenuate the reduction in hand blood flow in response to cold (Beaconsfield, Ginsburg & Rainsbury, 1972), and can impair reflex vasoconstriction produced by deep breathing (Weiss, Watanabe et al., 1972). Davidoff (1973) suggested that the β adrenergically mediated effects of cannabis might account for increased heat loss because of increased muscle blood flow. Indeed, as pointed out by Maddock (Maddock, Farrell et al., 1979), a drop in skin temperature is accompanied by central changes in thermoregulation and leaves the cannabis user more thermolabile. As a consequence, cannabis users may respond with increases in body temperature in a hot climate. Decreases in exercise tolerance under cannabis have been reported (Renaud & Cormier, 1986; Shapiro, Reiss et al., 1976).

In summary, the described effects of an acute cannabis exposure appear to be centrally mediated via sympathomimetic and parasympatholytic (vagal inhibitory) mechanisms. The ways in which the cannabinoids induce these responses remain to be demonstrated. These questions are likely to be answered as research on the anandamide pathways is pursued.

Cardiovascular Effects of Chronic Cannabis Use

Tachycardia is characteristic of cannabis intoxication in both occasional and experienced users. However, the degree of tachycardia is less in those whose exposure to the drug is more frequent, probably because of the development of tolerance to THC.

A great deal of the pharmacology of chronic exposure to cannabis has been described from the studies of Jones and Benowitz (1975; 1976; 1977) in which normal, healthy, paid volunteers, all of whom were experienced cannabis users, were hospitalized for the period of study. The volunteers were dosed on a four-hourly schedule of 70 milligrams of THC per day and some increased to 210 milligrams per day over a period of between 5 and 20 days. This dose schedule maintained a continuous and moderately steady plasma THC concentration similar to that achieved by a smoked dose of 10 milligrams of THC (Jones, 1984).

Tolerance to many of the cardiovascular effects developed rapidly, within 24 hours for some volunteers. In some subjects, tolerance to the tachycardia was nearly complete (Benowitz & Jones, 1975). Marked weight gain was observed in all subjects, an effect that has been shown to be related to fluid retention and plasma volume expansion. Possibly because of plasma volume expansion, tolerance developed to orthostatic hypotension, but not to the supine hypotensive effects.

After such a dose schedule had continued for about 8 to 10 days, the characteristic acute tachycardia response and the slight increase in supine blood pressure changed to one of bradycardia and a decrease in supine blood pressure. These changes were accompanied by impaired circulatory responses to standing, exercise, Valsalva manoeuvre, and cold pressor testing — all of which suggest a state of sympathetic insufficiency and/or increased parasympathetic activity. This hypotensive response resembles that seen with antihypertensive drugs such as guanethidine. It occurs in the absence of hypovolaemia and it is associated with a submaximal compensatory heart rate increase but with little or no change in peripheral resistance.

Electrocardiograph

Even in large doses, cannabis produces minimal effects on the electrocardiograph in normal healthy volunteers (Beaconsfield, Ginsburg &

Rainsbury, 1972; Benowitz & Jones, 1975; Benowitz, Rosenberg et al., 1979; Clark, Greene et al., 1974; Hollister, Richards & Gillespie, 1968; Johnson & Domino, 1971; Weiss, Watanabe et al., 1972). Miller et al. (1977) used recordings from the bundle of His to show that THC markedly enhanced sinus automaticity and facilitated sinoatrial and atrioventricular (A-V) nodal conduction. The clinical significance of these effects needs further evaluation in terms of potential therapeutic benefit and harm. As noted by Jones (1984), all the effects of cannabis on the electrocardiogram have been collected on relatively short-term recordings. The cardiovascular effects of longer sessions of use should be assessed using recording monitors.

Clinical Implications

Young, healthy hearts are likely to be only mildly stressed by the acute cardiovascular effects of cannabis (Tennant, 1983). The clinical significance of the repeated occurrence of these effects in chronic, heavy cannabis users remains uncertain because there is clinical and experimental evidence that tolerance develops to the acute cardiovascular effects of cannabis (Benowitz & Jones, 1975; Jones & Benowitz, 1976; Nowlan & Cohen, 1977) (see above).

The field studies of chronic, heavy cannabis users in Costa Rica (Carter, Coggins & Doughty, 1980), Greece (Stefanis, Dornbush & Fink, 1977) and Jamaica (Rubin & Comitas, 1975) failed to disclose any evidence of cardiac toxicity related to their cannabis use, even in those subjects with heart disease. The findings of the field studies have been supported by the fact that electrocardiographic studies of acute and prolonged administration have rarely revealed pathological changes (Benowitz & Jones, 1975; Jones, 1984). It seems reasonable to conclude then that among healthy young adults who use the drug intermittently, cannabis is not a major risk factor for life-threatening cardiovascular events in the way that the use of cocaine and other psychostimulants can be (Gawin & Ellinwood, 1988). This statement has to be qualified by the fact that there

have been a number of case reports of myocardial infarction in young men who were heavy cannabis smokers and who had no personal history of heart disease (Choi & Pearl, 1989; Pearl & Choi, 1992; Podczeck, Frohmer & Steinbach, 1990; Tennant, 1983). Such cases deserve closer investigation to exclude the role of other cardiotoxic drugs.

The possibility remains that chronic heavy cannabis smoking may have more subtle effects on the cardiovascular system. Jones (1984) suggested, for example, that after years of repeated exposure there may be persistent alterations of cardiovascular system function. By analogy with the long-term cardiotoxic effects of tobacco smoking, he argued that there were "enough similarities between THC and nicotine cardiovascular effects to make the possibility plausible." Moreover, since many cannabis smokers are also cigarette smokers, there is the possibility that there may be adverse interactions between nicotine and cannabinoids in their effects on the cardiovascular system.

Effects on Patients with Cardiovascular Disease

There are a number of concerns about the potentially deleterious effects of cannabis use on patients with ischaemic heart disease, hypertension, and cerebrovascular disease (Jones, 1984; Institute of Medicine, 1982). First, THC appears to increase the production of catecholamines that stimulate the activity of the heart, thereby increasing the risk of cardiac arrhythmias in susceptible patients. Second, THC increases heart rate, thereby producing chest pain (angina pectoris) in patients with ischaemic heart disease, and perhaps increasing the risk of a myocardial infarction. Third, THC also has analgesic properties that may attenuate chest pain, delaying treatment seeking, and thereby perhaps increase the risk of fatal arrhythmias. Fourth, marijuana smoking increases the level of carboxyhemoglobin, thereby decreasing oxygen delivery to the heart, increasing the work of the heart and, perhaps, the risk of atheroma formation.

Moreover, the reduced delivery of oxygen to the heart is compounded by a concomitant increase in the work of the heart — and therefore its oxygen requirements — because of the tachycardia induced by THC. Fifth, patients with cerebrovascular disease may be put at risk of experiencing strokes by unpredictable changes in blood pressure, and patients with hypertension may experience exacerbations of their disease for the same reason.

After considering the known cardiovascular effects of THC, and their likely interactions with cardiovascular disease, the Institute of Medicine (1982) concluded that it: "seems inescapable that this increased work, coupled with stimulation by catecholamines, may tax the heart to the point of clinical hazard" (p. 70). Despite the plausibility of the reasoning, there is very little direct evidence of the adverse effects of cannabis on persons with heart disease (Jones, 1984).

Among the few relevant pieces of research evidence are several laboratory studies of the acute cardiovascular effects of smoking marijuana cigarettes on patients with occlusive heart disease. Aronow and Cassidy (1974) conducted a double-blind placebo-controlled study comparing the effect on heart rate and the time required to induce chest pain during an exercise tolerance test of smoking a single marijuana cigarette containing 20 milligrams of THC with the effect of a placebo marijuana cigarette. Heart rate by 43 per cent, and the time taken to produce chest pain was approximately halved after smoking a marijuana cigarette. It appeared that cannabis increased the myocardial oxygen demand while reducing the amount of oxygen delivered to the heart (Aronow & Cassidy, 1974).

Aronow and Cassidy (1975) compared the effects of smoking a single marijuana cigarette and a high-nicotine tobacco cigarette in 10 men with occlusive heart disease, all of whom were 20-a-day cigarette smokers. A 42 per cent increase in heart rate was observed after smoking the marijuana cigarette compared with a 21 per cent increase after smoking the tobacco cigarette. Exercise tolerance time was halved (49 per cent) after smoking a marijuana cigarette by

comparison with a 23 per cent decline after smoking a tobacco cigarette.

Gottschalk et al. (1977) examined the effects of cannabis on cardiovascular function and on the cognitive and emotional states of 10 male patients with angina. In addition to confirming the cardiovascular effects of the drug (a marijuana cigarette containing 18 milligrams of THC), these authors described an increase in cognitive impairment of their patients and concluded that "for anginal patients marijuana is more a medical hazard than a help." These reports are not surprising in view of the fact that the cannabis-induced increase in heart rate will increase the heart's demand for oxygen. After the smoking of a cannabis cigarette there is also an increase in carboxyhemoglobin concentration in the blood, the effect of which is to reduce the oxygen carrying capacity of the blood. Therefore, smoking cannabis decreases the delivery of oxygen to the heart in the face of an increase in oxygen demand.

Apart from these studies, there is very little direct evidence on the risks of cannabis use by persons with cardiovascular disease. The reasons for the absence of adverse effects of chronic cannabis use on diseased cardiovascular systems are unclear. It should not be assumed in the absence of evidence, however, that such effects do not exist. The absence of evidence may simply reflect the lack of systematic study. It may be that the development of tolerance to the cardiovascular effects with chronic heavy dosing has protected the heaviest users from experiencing such effects; it may be that there has been an insufficient exposure to cannabis smoking of a sufficiently large number of vulnerable individuals for any such effects to be noticed (Institute of Medicine, 1982); or it may be that cardiologists have missed any evidence because they have not inquired about cannabis use among their patients.

Public Health Significance of Cardiovascular Effects

The possibility of many current cannabis smokers developing clinically detectable heart disease may seem remote. Most cannabis users are healthy, young adults who smoke intermittently, most discontinue their use by their late twenties (Bachman, Wadsworth et al., 1997; Kandel, 1984); and very few of the minority who become heavy cannabis users are likely to have clinical occlusive heart disease or other atherosclerotic disease. But the possibility of such adverse effects occurring in a minority of chronic cannabis users may be of public health significance.

First, any such effects would contraindicate the therapeutic uses of cannabinoids among patients with cancer and glaucoma, who are at higher risk because of their age of having significant heart disease (Jones, 1984). Second, the chronic heavy cannabis users who were initiated in cannabis use in the late 1960s and early 1970s are now entering the period in which that minority who have continued to smoke cannabis will be at risk of experiencing symptoms of clinical heart disease. Among this group, cannabis use may produce an earlier expression of heart disease, especially if they have also been heavy cigarette smokers. Because of the high rates of cessation of cannabis use with age, however, this may be such a small number of persons that the effect is difficult to detect clinically. Our ability to detect it will be further reduced if cannabis use is not considered to be a risk factor about which cardiologists should systematically inquire. It may be worth exploring this possibility by including questions on cannabis use in case-control studies of cardiovascular disease among middle-aged adults.

On the available evidence, it is still appropriate to endorse the conclusion reached by the expert committee appointed by the Institute of Medicine in 1982. This was that although the smoking of marijuana "causes changes to the heart and circulation that are characteristic of stress ... there is no evidence ... that it exerts a permanently deleterious effect on the normal cardiovascular system" (p. 72). The situation may be less benign for those with "abnormal heart or circulation" since there is evidence that marijuana poses "a threat to patients with hypertension, cerebrovascular disease and coronary atherosclerosis" (p. 72) by increasing the work of the heart.

The "magnitude and incidence" of the threat remains to be determined as the cohort of chronic cannabis users of the late 1960s enters the age of maximum risk for complications of atherosclerosis of the cardiac, brain and peripheral vessels. In the interim, because any such effects could be life-threatening in patients with significant occlusion of the coronary arteries or other cerebrovascular disease, such persons should be advised not to smoke cannabis (Tennant, 1983).

Effects of Cannabinoids on the Liver and the Gastrointestinal Tract

The Liver

Studies in experimental animals have not reported any evidence of liver damage, although decreases in liver weight and glycogen levels have been recorded (Ham & De Jon, 1975; Lukas & Temple, 1974; Sprague, Rosenkrantz & Braude, 1973; Thompson, Rosenkrantz et al., 1975). Reduction in liver weight was associated with anorexia, as animals reduced their food consumption (Thompson, Mason et al., 1973). The consensus was that this response was attributable to a generalized stress reaction or a need for oxidizable substrate for cannabinoid metabolism and detoxification. The doses of cannabinoids used in these studies were also very high.

There is little evidence to suggest that the chronic use of cannabis by humans produces disturbances in liver function. The few references to the possible liver toxicity of cannabinoids in humans were dated in the early 1970s or earlier. Kew and colleagues (1969), for example, reported on 12 young, heavy cannabis users, 3 of whom showed abnormalities in liver function tests, and 8 of whom showed "mild liver dysfunction." Complicating the interpretation of this report was the fact that many had used other drugs. Six users had also used amphetamines and 3 drank alcohol.

Similar observations were made by Hochman and Brill (1971) in a study of 50 randomly selected cannabis users. Although 10 subjects had disturbed liver function, a more detailed drug-taking history revealed that they had all used alcohol heavily and for a long period before using cannabis. Abstention from alcohol (but not from cannabis) for at least one month resulted (with one exception) in the return of their liver function to normal. A study of 31 heavy hashish users by Tennant et al. (1971) found no evidence for liver abnormalities while Boulougouris et al. (1976) found enlarged livers in 8 of 44 hashish users and in 2 of 38 controls. Subsequent analysis revealed that the latter cases were associated with alcohol rather than cannabis use.

The Gastrointestinal Tract

Among the early studies of the cannabinoids were those that examined their effects on intestinal motility. It was observed, for example, that THC reduced defecation in a dose-dependent way in rats that had previously been found to have a high index of defecation (Drew, Miller & Wikler, 1972; Masur, Martz et al., 1971). Other researchers studied the effects of the cannabinoids on the rate of passage of a charcoal meal in mice (Anderson, Jackson & Chesher, 1974; Chesher, Dahl et al., 1973; Dewey, Harris & Kennedy, 1972) and found that THC reduced the passage of the meal in a dose-dependent manner. Cannabinol was approximately eight times less potent than THC, and cannabidiol was found to be inactive at doses up to 50 mg/kg (Anderson, Jackson & Chesher, 1974). However, a greater depressant effect was observed when THC and cannabidiol were orally administered together (by gavage). Morphine on this measure was found to be approximately five times more potent than THC and it was reversed by nalorphine (Chesher, Dahl et al., 1973).

Tolerance to the effect of THC on the passage of a charcoal meal developed after two doses at 24-hour intervals and was almost complete after the third dose. Five days after cessation of dosage, the response to an acute dose of THC had returned to about 70 per cent of the initial acute effect, but it did not return to the level of the acute dose in non-tolerant animals even after 19 dose-free days. This duration of tolerance was considerably longer than that recorded to other effects of THC, including locomotor activity (which returned within four days) and hypothermia (which returned in less than 12 dose-free days) (Anderson, Jackson et al., 1975).

A more recent study confirmed the effect of THC on intestinal motility and also reported a delay of gastric emptying in rats and mice. These effects were examined with the hypothesis that the anti-nausea and anti-emetic effects of this cannabinoid might be due to an effect on the gastrointestinal tract at a peripheral site (Shook & Burks, 1989; Shook, Dewey & Burks, 1986). These authors demonstrated that the effect of THC was greater on gastric emptying and small intestine transit than on large bowel transit, suggesting a selective effect for the proximal parts of the gastrointestinal tract.

Shook and Burks administered THC both intravenously and directly into the brain (intracerebroventricular; icv). They found that the intestinal transit was inhibited after icv injection, but only at doses that were active when given intravenously. This implies a peripheral site of activity of THC in the gastrointestinal tract. Shook and Burns speculated that such studies may not only identify alternative ways to treat nausea and vomiting and relieve diarrhea without constipation but they may also reveal more about the relationship between GI motility and nausea. An alternative possibility is that the rate of diffusion of the icv-administered THC to the central cannabinoid receptors may be slow. The possible peripheral effects of cannabinoids on the intestine are considered further below. Furthermore, the doses employed were equivalent to or lower than those reported to produce central effects in rodents. The effect of this cannabinoid on the gastrointestinal tract of rodents was not antagonized by the opioid antagonist, naloxone.

Clinical Significance of the Effects of Cannabinoids on Intestinal Motility

The slowing of gastric emptying and of intestinal activity produced by the cannabinoids would be expected to produce constipation. Yet Shook and Burks (1989) failed to observe cannabis-induced constipation. They attributed this to their finding that THC had only a minimal effect on the large bowel.

Similarly, the intestinal effects of the cannabinoids would be expected to affect the absorption of alcohol. The delay in gastric emptying would delay alcohol absorption, but the cannabinoid effect on the small intestine would not be expected to affect alcohol, as it is rapidly absorbed at this site. Surprisingly, the results of studies of the interaction of cannabinoids and alcohol have conflicted as to the effect of cannabis use on blood alcohol concentration. Most studies have reported no difference in the blood alcohol concentration in the presence of cannabis (oral or smoked) when compared with drinking of alcohol alone or with a cannabis placebo.

A series of studies of the interaction of alcohol (0.57 g/kg) with THC by mouth (140, 215 and 320 µg/kg) undertaken by Chesher and colleagues has also produced conflicting findings (Belgrave, Bird et al., 1979a; Chesher, Franks et al., 1976; 1977). A double-blind cross-over design was used in each study. Blood alcohol concentration (BAC) was measured approximately 40 minutes after each volunteer began drinking alcohol. Further measures of BAC were made 100 and 160 minutes after the beginning of drinking. Only with the lowest dose was there a higher blood alcohol concentration in those who received the active dose of THC. In the other studies, with 15 and 25 volunteers (respectively), there were no significant differences in the BAC with or without THC.

In further studies, this group reported the interactions between alcohol and cannabidiol (320 µg/kg; n = 15, design double-blind cross-over) (Belgrave, Bird et al., 1979b), and between alcohol and all combinations of THC (215 µg/kg), cannabidiol and cannabinol (both

320 µg/kg; n = 161, each volunteer being used only once) (Bird, Boleyn et al., 1980). The time courses for drinking and measurement of BAC were the same as the above. In all of these cases, there were no significant differences in the BAC with or without the cannabinoids.

Chesher and colleagues have also reported an interaction study involving 320 volunteers. It used alcohol doses of 0.0, 0.25, 0.5 and 0.75 g/kg, and cannabis was smoked to provide THC at doses of 0.0, 2.5, 5.0 and 10.0 mg. Blood alcohol concentrations were measured at 40 minutes and again 190 minutes after drinking began. There were no significant differences between these groups.

A clearer picture of the effect of smoked marijuana on the absorption of alcohol can be seen in a study by Perez-Reyes et al. (1988). This study involved six male volunteers who were tested in a latin square cross-over design involving six combinations of marijuana (2.4 per cent THC) or placebo and three doses of alcohol (placebo, low dose [0.42 g/kg] and high dose [0.85 g/kg]). Blood samples were collected over a period of six hours at regular intervals at 0, 30, 45, 60, 75, 90, 120, 150, 180, 210 and 360 minutes after beginning to drink the alcohol. Marijuana (or placebo) smoking began 15 minutes after the completion of drinking. The mean blood alcohol concentrations across time for each dose indicated that there were no differences among the groups. However, the mean values did obscure individual results. For the low alcohol dose, the peak BAC varied between 46 and 96 mg/dL with placebo marijuana and between 29 and 90 mg/dL with "active" marijuana. For the high-dose alcohol, the peak values were 76 to 140 mg/dL with placebo marijuana and 77 to 140 mg/dL with the "active" marijuana. In this study, the extent of the individual differences in the absorption of alcohol with and without the active cannabinoids can be seen to be quite small, although they were more obvious with the low alcohol dose.

A study by Lukas et al. (1992) clarifies the marijuana-alcohol interaction and possibly explains the different findings of the studies reviewed above. Lukas et al. very carefully controlled the rate of administration of both alcohol and marijuana. Alcohol was administered in orange juice via a peristaltic pump delivering 23 mL/min on a schedule of three minutes of drinking followed by one minute of rest. Even though the fluid was delivered continuously during the three minutes, subjects swallowed at 20- to 30-second intervals. Marijuana cigarettes (smoked through a smoking device) were smoked according to a schedule of "inhale" for three seconds; "hold" for five seconds; then "exhale." This process was repeated every 30 seconds until only 10 millimetres of the cigarette remained. Adherence to the smoking schedule was checked by a vacuum-driven pen recorder. Marijuana smoking began 30 minutes after drinking began. This degree of control over the administration of the two drugs was much greater than that in the other studies reviewed here. It is also much greater than that encountered in a social setting.

Using this technique, Lukas et al. (1992) were able to demonstrate in 15 volunteers that marijuana produced a significant and dose-dependent attenuation of the rise in plasma alcohol concentration after the ingestion of 0.7 g/kg alcohol. With this dose of alcohol and three doses of marijuana (placebo, 1.26 and 2.53 per cent THC), peak plasma levels of alcohol were: (1) with placebo marijuana, 78.25 ± 4.95 mg/dL (reached at 50 minutes after drinking); (2) with 1.26 per cent marijuana, 60.50 ± 10.60 mg/dL (reached at 85 minutes); and (3) with 2.53 per cent marijuana, 54.80 ± 8.32 mg/dL (reached at 105 minutes).

It may be concluded that marijuana does affect the rate of absorption of alcohol when the administration of these two drugs is controlled in an optimal way. Since, however, these conditions are rarely met under ordinary conditions of social cannabis use, this interaction is unlikely to be as striking as that demonstrated by Lukas et al. (1992).

Appetite and Weight Gain with Cannabis

Anecdotal accounts of a cannabis-induced increase in appetite ("the munchies" or "hash hungries") have been reported by several authors (Allentuck & Bowman, 1942; Haines & Green, 1970; Siler, Sheep & Bates, 1933; Snyder, 1970; Tart, 1970). Contrary to this effect in humans, the cannabinoids in experimental animals reduce food and water intake. Studies in the rat (Abel & Schiff, 1969; Fujimoto, Morrill et al., 1982; Hanasono, Sullivan et al., 1987; Manning, McConough et al., 1971; Morrill, Kostellow et al., 1983; Phillips, Brown et al., 1972; Sjoden, Järbe & Henrikksson, 1973; Thompson, Mason et al., 1973), the rabbit (Thompson, Rosenkrantz et al., 1975), the dog (Hanasono, Sullivan et al., 1987), and the monkey (Thompson, Fleischman et al., 1974) all report a reduction in food intake after ingestion of cannabinoids.

Experimental evidence in humans provides some support for the anecdotal reports of appetite stimulant effects of cannabinoids. Abel (1971) reported that volunteers who had smoked cannabis consumed significantly more marshmallows than did the control subjects. Similarly, Hollister (1971), in two separate experiments, showed that the total intake of chocolate milkshakes was increased after the oral administration of cannabis. Responses to questionnaires also indicated a cannabis effect on perception of hunger and appetite.

An increase in bodyweight of volunteers during a period of continued administration of cannabis has been described (Jones & Benowitz, 1976; Mendelson, 1976; Williams, Himmelsbach et al., 1946). Jones and Benowitz reported that the volunteers in a 30-day study involving the daily intake of THC by mouth increased their bodyweight by an average of 3.4 kilograms. However, within 48 hours of cessation of THC, their bodyweight had fallen to near predrug levels, suggesting that the weight increase was due to body fluid shifts.

Mendelson (1976) reported an increased caloric intake and weight gain in a study of more than 70 chronic marijuana users in a research ward setting over a period of 31 days. The weight gain was in part attributable to water retention. Greenberg et al. (1976) studied volunteers, also in a research ward setting, and recorded significant increases in both bodyweight and daily caloric intake during the period of cannabis use. These authors concluded, however, that water retention was not a major factor in these weight gains. Although both the caloric intake and the body-weight of the drug-using groups fell significantly in the postdrug period of the study, urine output actually decreased, particularly among the heavy cannabis users. Also, during the period of mari-juana use, the urine output was increased when compared with the predrug measurements.

When the THC preparation dronabinol (Marinol™) was introduced for the treatment of nausea and vomiting associated with patients undergoing cancer chemotherapy, clinical observers reported weight gain (Carey, Burish & Brenner, 1983; Levitt, 1986; Nelson, Walsh et al., 1994; Regelson, Butler et al., 1976). Using doses similar to those employed in the earlier studies with cancer patients, Plasse et al. (1991) reported weight gain among patients with HIV infection. Similar findings have been reported by Struwe and colleagues (1993).

Further clinical investigation of the appetite-enhancing effect of THC in such condi-tions must face several problems, the first of which is the pharmacokinetics of this substance. The only preparation currently available legally for clinical use and/or study, Marinol™ (drona-binol), is orally administered. The oral absorp-tion of THC is erratic (Agurell, Halldin et al., 1986; Shaw, Edling-Owens & Mattes, 1991). For example, Shaw et al. administered THC (15 milligrams for males and 10 milligrams for females) as Marinol™ to 57 healthy adults and measured the area under the curve (AUC) for six hours after oral administration. The mean AUC for THC was 3.13 + 4.74 [SD]. These low con-centrations and enormous variability reflect the finding that a large proportion of this population did not have measurable concentrations of THC in plasma at two, four and six hours post dosing. Wall et al. (1983) previously reported that the bioavailability of THC was only 10 to 20 per cent in healthy adults. For this reason, alternative routes of administration of this substance are necessary to achieve a higher bioavailability for

clinical studies. A preparation of THC hemi-succinate for rectal administration has been described by ElSohly et al. (1991) and was further demonstrated by Mattes et al. (1993) to provide much higher, sustained and much less erratic plasma concentrations of THC than after oral administration (Mattes, Shaw et al., 1993).

It is also important that the clinical end-point be defined. Is the end-point a measure of the acute stimulation of appetite or is it weight gain? Mattes et al. (1994) conducted a series of experiments, both acute and chronic (only three days of drug administration and food intake measures). The acute study involved drug administration by the oral and sublingual routes (15 milligrams for males and 10 milligrams for females) and by inhalation, using a controlled smoking schedule of marijuana (2.57 per cent THC in a 710- to 795-milligram cigarette). The chronic study involved oral THC or a rectal sup-pository at the lower dose of 2.5 milligrams twice per day for three days. The acute studies failed to reveal a significant effect of THC on total ener-gy intake or energy derived from different food groups or items with various taste qualities. The same wide variability of plasma concentration of THC was recorded after oral or sublingual administration. The examination of food intake in subjects with a measurable plasma THC failed to reveal treatment effects. On the other hand, the inhalation of THC led to higher and more consistent THC levels in plasma and tended to increase intake, although not significantly. Daily energy intakes were higher with chronic dosing. This was statistically significant for administra-tion by suppository compared to all acute dosing except when the drug was inhaled. The hemisuc-cinate ester of THC is still an experimental preparation so it may be some time before it is available for therapeutic use. Similarly, the data from Mattes et al. (1994) suggest that inhalation of THC as a mode of drug delivery requires experimental confirmation. Although smoking a crude preparation of vegetable leaf is not the ideal means for the delivery of any drug (nicotine included), it is quite possible to prepare a smok-able preparation of pure THC which is devoid of vegetable material. In the meantime, it has been argued that clinical studies in terminally ill patients (with wasting syndrome of AIDS or cancer) may determine whether or not further efforts are required to provide a more realistic inhalation method for the delivery of THC.

The studies reviewed above have used only THC (dronabinol) or placebo. To date, there is only one comparative study of dronabinol with another appetite-stimulating agent. This study involved dronabinol and the synthetic progestin, megestrol acetate. In a very careful study, Timpone et al. (1997) compared the safety and feasibility of using dronabinol and the synthetic progestin, megestrol acetate, alone and in combination, to treat patients with AIDS wasting syndrome. As the two drugs exert their action by different mechanisms, the authors wished to determine if there were any adverse effects from the combination and if there was an additive interaction effect on appetite and weight gain.

There were four drug groups: dronabinol 2.5 mg twice per day; megestrol acetate 750 mg per day; megestrol acetate 750 mg per day + dronabinol 2.5 mg twice per day; megestrol acetate 250 mg per day + dronabinol 2.5 mg twice per day. Fifty-two patients (mean CD4+ count, 59 cells/μL) were randomized to one of the four groups, and 39 completed the planned 12-week study.

The authors stressed that their purpose was primarily to study the pharmacokinetics and safety of the drug combination. The interpretation of the efficacy is limited by several factors. These included: the relatively small sample size; the fact that the weight measures did not include the pre-study data to calculate percentage weight loss; the fact that weight measures were collected by standard clinical methods rather than by methods with rigorous controls, such as monitoring scale calibration; and weight measurements were not controlled for time of day, time from last meal time, and the amount of clothing worn. Notwithstanding these limitations, the data did show statistically significant weight gain in the two treatment groups that included megestrol acetate at the dose of 750 mg/day.

This result is of considerable interest, but some possibilities should be considered before the efficacy of dronabinol is dismissed. The problems indicated earlier with the bioavailability of dronabinol (THC) after oral administration must be considered. The authors indicated that some problems were encountered in their study of the pharmacokinetics of dronabinol. Of the 37 patients who began treatment with dronabinol, 31 participated in the pharmacokinetic sessions. Data from 11 of these patients were excluded from analysis. The authors reported that: "three patients (one from each arm) had incomplete datasets and eight patients (dronabinol alone = 3 patients; megestrol 750 + dronabinol = 2 patients; and megestrol 250 + dronabinol = 3) had inadequate adherence to protocol." The terms *incomplete datasets* and *inadequate adherence to protocol* are not explained. It is possible that it might relate to the finding discussed earlier that a large proportion of a population dosed with dronabinol may be without measurable concentrations of the drug some two, four and six hours post dosing (Agurell, Halldin et al., 1986; Shaw, Edling-Owens & Mattes, 1991; Wall, Sadler et al., 1983). The determination of the pharmacokinetics of megestrol acetate was without these problems as 34 of the 37 patients who initiated therapy with this drug participated in the pharmacokinetic sessions, and data from all 34 patients were included in the analysis.

The data on weight change were collected from all 37 of the patients whose dose schedule included dronabinol. It is possible, therefore, that many of these patients did not efficiently absorb the administered dronabinol. There is no doubt that some patients absorbed an active concentration of dronabinol because adverse reactions consistent with this drug were reported. Indeed, the authors considered that of the 37 patients who received dronabinol (alone or in combination with megestrol acetate) 5 reported side effects that were considered attributable to dronabinol. As good as this initial comparative study was, the caveats and cautions mentioned by the authors indicate that there is a need to examine the efficacy of cannabinoids in AIDS wasting syndrome and to compare this agent with other drugs.

The Isolated Intestine as a Model for Central Activity of Drugs

The possibility that the cannabinoids act on GI motility at a peripheral rather than a central site was discussed above in describing the work of Shook and Burks (1989). This possibility implies that cannabinoid receptors exist in the enteric nervous system which may or may not differ from those in the CNS. Although these possibilities await further research, it is pertinent to draw attention briefly to the studies of centrally acting drugs which have been conducted on isolated *(in vitro)* tissues.

Studies of the enteric system revealed an immensely complex peripheral nervous system involving, at present knowledge, some 30 functional types of neurone and about 25 different possible neurotransmitters (McConalogue & Furness, 1994).

The isolated guinea-pig ileum is considered by Collier and Tucker (1984) to provide a model of drug dependence. According to these authors, the characteristics of opioid dependence in the ileum closely resemble those of dependence in whole animals (Collier & Tucker, 1984). Preparations of isolated ileum electrically stimulated by coaxially placed electrodes respond with a twitchlike contraction. Opioids depress the amplitude of this response in a dose-dependent manner (Paton, 1957), and the ileum can be made tolerant to the morphine-induced reduction of electrically initiated contractures. When the "morphine-tolerant" ileum is exposed to naloxone, a sustained contraction ensues — an effect considered by Hammond et al. (1976) to be a "withdrawal effect," suggesting that dependence as well as tolerance had developed. Dewey et al. (1976) also reported that methionine enkephalin was more potent than morphine in inhibiting the contraction of the coaxially stimulated guinea-pig ileum. The enteric nervous system therefore provides a model for the study of the central effects of the opioids.

Prostaglandin E_1 (PGE_1) given intraperitoneally to mice produces a dose-dependent decrease in intestinal motility as measured by the passage of a charcoal meal (Jackson, Malor et al., 1976). The cannabinoids THC and cannabinol, but not cannabidiol, antagonize the effect of PGE_1 (Jackson, Malor et al., 1976). Kinetic analysis of the data *(in vivo* data from whole animal experiments) suggested that PGE_1 and THC act on the same receptor site.

In the light of the recent discovery of the THC receptor as a G-protein-linked receptor (Houston & Howlett, 1993; Howlett, Qualy & Khachatrian, 1986), these findings suggest the presence in the guinea-pig ileum of a THC receptor. Pertwee et al. (1992) also described the activity of cannabinoids to reduce the twitch resulting from the electrical stimulation of the vas deferens preparation of the mouse. It was on this preparation that the activity of the newly isolated endogenous cannabinoid neuromodulator, "anandamide" from pig brain, was tested (Devane, Hanus et al., 1992). Later, Pertwee et al. (1996a) further suggested that these cannabis receptors were of the CB_1 type, those found in the CNS. It is of interest, therefore, that $\varnothing$-THC and $\varnothing$-THC inhibited the response of the stimulated guinea pig ileum, an effect that was considered to be presynaptic (Pertwee, Stevenson et al., 1992; Rosell & Agurell, 1975). Cannabinol and cannabidiol were found to be inactive in this preparation.

Pertwee et al. (1996b) described the effects of THC and several cannabinoid agonists and antagonists on the electrically evoked contractions of the myenteric plexus–longitudinal muscle preparation of the guinea pig. The reduction in the electrically evoked twitch response was accompanied by a reduction in the release of acetylcholine, supporting the hypothesis that the cannabinoid agonists act at a prejunctional site. What is more, the activity of a cannabinoid (CB_1) antagonist (SR141716A) reduced the agonist-induced inhibition of the twitch, as well as the release of acetylcholine. The potency of the various cannabinoid agonists in reducing the twitch response correlated well with their potency for their activity (displacement of a radiolabelled probe from cannabinoid binding sites) in brain tissue (Herkenham, Lynn et al., 1990).

Given these observations, and those of Shook and Burks (1989), further attention needs to be given to the possibility that the anti-nausea and anti-emetic effects of cannabinoids might be a peripheral effect on the gastrointestinal tract. In this context, the effect of cannabis on appetite might be considered as either a peripheral effect on the gastrointestinal tract, or the activity of cannabinoids on the enteric system may serve as a model for the central action of the cannabinoids. Perhaps cannabis researchers might direct their attention to this already very productive technique, to differentiate the peripheral and central cannabinoid receptors.

Summary of Cannabinoid Effects on Liver and Gastrointestinal Tract

There appears to be little or no human or animal evidence that cannabinoids affect liver function, whether used acutely or chronically. There is reasonable animal evidence that cannabinoids affect intestinal motility and delay gastric emptying. The clinical significance of this effect seems minimal. There does not appear to be any evidence of significant symptoms of constipation as a consequence, and under most conditions of use it has minimal effect on the absorption of alcohol.

The most interesting aspects of the gastrointestinal effects of cannabis are theoretical and therapeutic. The site of action of the anti-nausiant and anti-emetic effects, and also the appetite-stimulant effects of the cannabinoids, remain to be described clearly. As with studies of the opioids, the isolated intestine preparation may serve as a useful model for the central cannabinoid receptors, and may provide the opportunity to differentiate central and peripheral receptors.

References

Abel, E.L. (1971). Effects of marijuana on the solution of anagrams, memory and appetite. *Nature, 231,* 260–261.

Abel, E.L. & Schiff, B.B. (1969). Effects of the marihuana homologue, Pyrahexyl, on food and water intake and curiosity in the rat. *Psychonomic Science, 16,* 38.

Agurell, S., Halldin, M., Lindgren, J.-E., Ohlsson, A., Widman, M., Gillespie, H. & Hollister, L. (1986). Pharmacokinetics and metabolism of $\varnothing$-tetrahydrocannabinol and other cannabinoids with emphasis on man. *Pharmacological Reviews, 38,* 21–43.

Allentuck, S. & Bowman, K.M. (1942). The psychiatric aspects of marihuana intoxication. *American Journal of Psychiatry, 99,* 248–251.

Anderson, P.F., Jackson, D.M. & Chesher, G.B. (1974). Interaction of delta-9-tetrahydrocannabinol and cannabidiol on intestinal motility in mice. *Journal of Pharmacy and Pharmacology, 26,* 136–137.

Anderson, P.F., Jackson, D.M., Chesher, G.B. & Malor, R. (1975). Tolerance to the effect of delta-9-tetrahydrocannabinol in mice on intestinal motility, temperature and locomotor activity. *Psychopharmacologia, 43,* 31–36.

Aronow, W.S. & Cassidy, J. (1974). Effect of marihuana and placebo marihuana smoking on angina pectoris. *New England Journal of Medicine, 291,* 65–67.

Aronow, W.S. & Cassidy, J. (1975). Effect of smoking marihuana and of a high nicotine cigarette on angina pectoris. *Clinical Pharmacology and Therapeutics, 17,* 549–554.

Bachman, J.G., Wadsworth, K.N., O'Malley, P.M., Johnston, L.D. & Schulenberg, J.E. (Eds.). (1997). *Smoking, Drinking and Drug Use in Young Adulthood.* Mahwah, NJ: Erlbaum.

Beaconsfield, P., Ginsburg, J. & Rainsbury, R. (1972). Marihuana smoking: Cardiovascular effects in man and possible mechanisms. *New England Journal of Medicine, 287,* 209–212.

Belgrave, B.E., Bird, K.D., Chesher, G.B., Jackson, D.M., Lubbe, K.E., Starmer, G.A. & Teo, R.K.C. (1979a). The effect of (–) trans delta-9-tetrahydrocannabinol, alone and in combination with ethanol, on human performance. *Psychopharmacology, 62,* 53–60.

Belgrave, B.E., Bird, K.D., Chesher, G.B., Jackson, D.M., Lubbe, K.E., Starmer, G.A. & Teo, R.K.C. (1979b). The effect of cannabidiol, alone and in combination with ethanol on human performance. *Psychopharmacology, 64,* 243–246.

Benowitz, N.L. & Jones, R.T. (1975). Cardiovascular effects of prolonged delta-9-tetra-hydrocannabinol ingestion. *Clinical Pharmacology and Therapeutics, 18,* 287–297.

Benowitz, N.L. & Jones, R.T. (1977). Prolonged delta-9-tetrahydrocannabinol ingestion: Effects of sympathomimetic amines and autonomic blockades. *Clinical Pharmacology Therapeutics, 21,* 336–342.

Benowitz, N.L., Rosenberg, J., Rogers, W., Bachman, J. & Jones, R.T. (1979). Cardiovascular effects of intravenous delta-9-tetrahydrocannabinol: Autonomic nervous mechanisms. *Clinical Pharmacology Therapeutics, 25,* 440–446.

Bird, K.D., Boleyn, T., Chesher, G.B., Jackson, D.M., Starmer, G.A. & Teo, R.K.C. (1980). Intercannabinoid and cannabinoid-ethanol interactions and their effects on human performance. *Psychopharmacology, 71,* 181–188.

Boulougouris, J.C., Panayiotopoulos, C.P., Antypas, E., Liakos, A. & Stefanis, C. (1976). Effects of chronic hashish use on medical status in 44 users compared with 38 controls. *Annals of the New York Academy of Sciences, 282,* 168–172.

Capriotti, R.M., Foltin, R.W., Brady, J.V. & Fischman, M.W. (1988). Effects of marijuana on the task-elicited physiological response. *Drug and Alcohol Dependence, 21,* 183–187.

Carey, M.P., Burish, T.G. & Brenner, D.E. (1983). Delta-9-tetrahydrocannabinol in cancer chemotherapy: Research problems and issues. *Annals of Internal Medicine, 99,* 106–114.

Carter, W.E., Coggins, W. & Doughty, P.L. (1980). *Cannabis in Costa Rica: A Study of Chronic Marihuana Use.* Philadelphia: Institute for the Study of Human Issues.

Chesher, G.B., Dahl, C., Everingham, M., Jackson, D.M., Marchant-Williams, H. & Starmer, G.A. (1973). The effects of cannabinoids on intestinal motility and their antinociceptive effect in mice. *British Journal of Pharmacology, 49,* 588–594.

Chesher, G.B., Franks, H.M., Hensley, V.R., Hensley, W.J., Jackson, D.M. & Starmer, G.A. (1976). The interaction of ethanol and delta-9-tetrahydrocannabinol in man: Effects on perceptual, cognitive and motor functions. *Medical Journal of Australia, 2,* 159–163.

Chesher, G.B., Franks, H.M., Jackson, D.M. & Starmer, G.A. (1977). Ethanol and delta-9-tetrahydrocannabinol: Interactive effects on human perceptual, cognitive and motor functions. *Medical Journal of Australia, 1,* 478–481.

Choi, Y.S. & Pearl, W.R. (1989). Cardiovascular effects of adolescent drug abuse. *Journal of Adolescent Health Care, 10,* 332–337.

Clark, S.C., Greene, C., Karr, G.W., MacCannell, K.L. & Milstein, S.L. (1974). Cardiovascular effects of marihuana in man. *Canadian Journal of Physiology and Pharmacology, 52,* 706–719.

Collier, H.O. & Tucker, J.F. (1984). Sites and mechanisms of dependence in the myenteric plexus of guinea pig ileum. (NIDA Research Monograph No. 54, pp. 81–94). Washington, DC: Government Printing Office.

Coper, H. (1981). Pharmacology and toxicology of cannabis. In F. Hoffmeister & G. Stille (Eds.), *Handbook of Experimental Pharmacology* (pp. 135–158). Berlin: Springer-Verlag.

Davidoff, I.G. (1973). Marihuana not for skiers. *New England Journal of Medicine, 288*, 52.

Devane, W.A., Hanus, L., Breuer, A., Pertwee, R.G., Stevenson, L.A., Griffin, G., Gibson, D., Mandelbaum, A., Etinger, A. & Mechoulam, R. (1992). Isolation and structure of a brain constituent that binds to the cannabinoid receptor. *Science, 258*, 1946–1949.

Dewey, W.L. (1986). Cannabinoid pharmacology. *Pharmacological Reviews, 38*, 151–178.

Dewey, W.L., Chau-Pham, T.T., Day, A., Lujan, M., Harris, L.S. & Freer, R.J. (1976). The effects of enkephalins on the isolated guinea pig ileum: Stereospecific binding of dihydromorphine and antinociception in mice. In H.W. Kosterlitz (Ed.), *Opiates and Endogenous Opioid Peptides* (pp. 103–110). Amsterdam: North Holland.

Dewey, W.L., Harris, L.S. & Kennedy, J.S. (1972). Some pharmacological and toxicological effects of 1-trans-8 and 1-trans-9-tetrahydrocannabinol in laboratory rodents. *Archives Internationales de Pharmacodynamie et de Therapie, 196*, 133–145.

Drew, W.G., Miller, L.L. & Wikler, A. (1972). Effects of delta-9-THC on the open field activity of the rat. *Psychopharmacology, 23*, 289–299.

ElSohly, M.A., Stanford, D.F., Harland, E.C., Hikal, A.H., Walker, L.A., Little, T.J., Rider, J.N. & Jones, A.B. (1991). Rectal bioavailability of delta-9-tetrahydrocannabinol from the hemisuccinate ester in monkeys. *Journal of Pharmacological Science, 80*, 942–945.

Foltin, R.W. & Fischman, M.W. (1990). The effects of combinations of intranasal cocaine, smoked marijuana, and task performance on heart rate and blood pressure. *Pharmacology, Biochemistry and Behavior, 36*, 311–315.

Fujimoto, G.I., Morrill, G.A., O'Connell, M.E., Kostellow, A.B. & Retura, G. (1982). Effects of cannabinoids given orally and reduced appetite on the male rat reproductive system. *Pharmacology, 24*, 303–313.

Gaoni, Y. & Mechoulam, R. (1964). Isolation, structure, and partial synthesis of an active constituent of hashish. *Journal of American Chemical Society, 8*, 1646–1647.

Gash, A., Karliner, J.S., Janowsky, D. & Lake, C.R. (1978). Effects of smoking marihuana on left ventricular performance and plasma norepinephrine: Studies in normal men. *Annals of Internal Medicine, 89*, 448–452.

Gawin, F.H. & Ellinwood, E.H. (1988). Cocaine and other stimulants: Actions, abuse and treatment. *New England Journal of Medicine, 318*, 1173–1182.

Gottschalk, L.A., Aronow, W.S. & Prakash, R. (1977). Effect of marijuana and placebo-marijuana smoking on psychological state and on psychophysiological cardiovascular functioning in anginal patients. *Biological Psychiatry, 12*, 255–266.

Greenberg, I., Kuehnle, J., Mendelson, J.H. & Bernstein, J.G. (1976). Effects of marihuana use on body weight and caloric intake in humans. *Psychopharmacology (Berl), 49*, 79–84.

Haines, L. & Green, W. (1970). Marijuana use patterns. *British Journal of Addictions, 65*, 347–362.

Ham, M.T. & De Jon, J. (1975). Effects of delta-9-tetrahydrocannabinol and cannabidiol on blood glucose concentrations in rabbits and rats. *Pharmaceutisch Weekblad, 110*, 1157–1161.

Hammond, M.D., Schneider, C. & Collier, H.O. (1976). Induction of opiate tolerance in isolated guinea pig ileum and its modification by drugs. In H.W. Kosterlitz (Ed.), *Opiates and Endogenous Opioid Peptides* (pp. 169–176). Amsterdam: North Holland.

Hanasono, G.K., Sullivan, H.R., Gries, C.L., Jordan, W.H. & Emmerson, J.L. (1987). A species comparison of the toxicity of nabilone, a new synthetic cannabinoid. *Fundamental and Applied Toxicology, 9*, 185–197.

Herkenham, M., Lynn, A.B., Little, M.D., Johnson, M.R., Melvin, L.S., De Costa, B.R. & Rice, K.C. (1990). Cannabinoid receptor localization in brain. *Proceedings of the National Academy of Sciences of the United States of America, 87*, 1932–1936.

Hochman, J.S. & Brill, N.Q. (1971). Chronic marihuana usage and liver function. *Lancet, 2*, 818–819.

Hollister, L.E. (1971). Hunger and appetite after single doses of marijuana, alcohol, and dextroamphetamine. *Clinical Pharmacology and Therapeutics, 12*, 44–49.

Hollister, L., Richards, R.K. & Gillespie, H.K. (1968). Comparison of tetrahydrocannabinol and synhexyl in man. *Clinical Pharmacology and Therapeutics, 9*, 783–791.

Houston, D.B. & Howlett, A.C. (1993). Solubilization of the cannabinoid receptor from rat brain and its functional interaction with guanine nucleotide-binding proteins. *Molecular Pharmacology, 43*, 17–22.

Howlett, A.C., Qualy, J.M. & Khachatrian, L.L. (1986). Involvement of Gi in the inhibition of adenylate cyclase by cannabimimetic drugs. *Molecular Pharmacology, 29*, 307–313.

Huber, G.L., Griffith, D.E. & Langsjoen, P.M. (1988). The effects of marijuana on the respiratory and cardiovascular systems. In G. Chesher, P. Consroe & R. Musty (Eds.), *Marijuana: An International Research Report* (National Campaign Against Drug Abuse Monograph No. 7, pp. 1–18). Canberra: Australian Government Publishing Service.

Institute of Medicine. (1982). *Marijuana and Health*. Washington, DC: National Academy Press.

Jackson, D.M., Malor, R., Chesher, G.B., Starmer, G.A., Welburn, P.J. & Bailey, R. (1976). The interaction between prostaglandin E1 and delta-9-tetrahydrocannabinol on intestinal motility and on the abdominal constriction response in the mouse. *Psychopharmacologia*, *47*, 187–193.

Johnson, S. & Domino, E.F. (1971). Some cardiovascular effects of marihuana smoking in normal volunteers. *Clinical Pharmacology and Therapeutics*, *12*, 172–176.

Jones, R.T. (1984). Cardiovascular effects of cannabinoids. In D.J. Harvey, W. Paton & G.G. Nahas (Eds.), *Marihuana '84: Proceedings of the Oxford Symposium on Cannabis* (pp. 325–334). Oxford: IRL Press.

Jones, R.T. & Benowitz, N. (1976). The 30-day trip — Clinical studies of cannabis tolerance and dependence. In M.C. Braude & S. Szara (Eds.), *Pharmacology of Marihuana* (Vol. 2, pp. 627–642). New York: Academic Press.

Kanakis, C.J., Pouget, J.M. & Rosen, K.M. (1976). The effects of delta-9-tetrahydrocannabinol (cannabis) on cardiac performance with and without beta blockade. *Circulation*, *53*, 703–707.

Kandel, D.B. (1984). Marijuana users in young adulthood. *Archives of General Psychiatry*, *41*, 200–209.

Kew, M.C., Bershon, I. & Siew, S. (1969). Possible hepatotoxicity of cannabis. *Lancet*, *1*, 578–579.

Levitt, M. (1986). Cannabinoids as antiemetics in cancer chemotherapy. In R. Mechoulam (Ed.), *Cannabinoids as Therapeutic Agents* (pp. 71–103). Boca Raton, FL: CRC Press.

Lukas, M.C. & Temple, D.M. (1974). Some effects of chronic cannabis treatment. *Australian Journal of Pharmaceutical Sciences*, *NA3*, 20–22.

Lukas, S.E., Benedikt, R., Mendelson, J.H., Kouri, E., Sholar, M. & Amass, L. (1992). Marihuana attenuates the rise in plasma ethanol levels in human subjects. *Neuropsychopharmacology*, *7*, 77–81.

Lynn, A. & Herkenham, M. (1994). Localization of cannabinoid receptors and nonsaturable high-density cannabinoid binding sites in peripheral tissues of the rat: Implications for receptor-mediated immune modulation by cannabinoids. *Journal of Pharmacology and Experimental Therapeutics*, *268*, 1612–1623.

Maddock, R., Farrell, T.R., Herning, R. & Jones, R.T. (1979). Marijuana and thermoregulation in a hot environment. In B. Cox, P. Lomax, A.S. Milton & E. Schonbaum (Eds.), *Thermoregulatory Mechanisms and Their Therapeutic Implications* (pp. 62–64.) Basel: Karger.

Manning, F.J., McConough, J.H., Jr., Elsmore, T.F., Saller, C. & Sodetz, F.J. (1971). Inhibition of normal growth by chronic administration of delta-9-tetrahydrocannbinol. *Science, 174*, 424–426.

Martz, R., Brown, D.J., Forney, R.B., Bright, T.P. & Kiplinger, G.F. (1972). Propranolol antagonism of marihuana induced tachycardia. *Life Sciences, 11*, 999–1005.

Masur, J., Martz, R.M.W., Korte, F.J. & Bieniek, D. (1971). Influence of (–) delta-9-trans-tetrahydrocannabinol and mescaline on the behavior of rats submitted to food competition situations. *Psychopharmacologia, 22*, 187–194.

Mattes, R.D., Engelman, K., Shaw, L.M. & ElSohly, M. (1994). Cannabinoids and apppetite stimulation. *Pharmacology, Biochemistry and Behavior, 49*, 187–195.

Mattes, R.D., Shaw, L.M., Edling, O.J., Engelman, K. & ElSohly, M.A. (1993). Bypassing the first-pass effect for the therapeutic use of cannabinoids. *Pharmacology, Biochemistry and Behavior, 44*, 745–747.

McConalogue, K. & J. B. Furness. (1994). Gastrointestinal neurotransmitters. *Baillieres Clinical Endocrinology & Metabolism, 8*, 51–76.

Mendelson, J.H. (1976). Marihuana use: Biologic and behavioral aspects. *Postgraduate Medicine, 60*, 111–115.

Miller, R.H., Dhingra, R.C. & Kanakis, C. (1977). The electrophysiological effects of delta-9-tetrahydrocannabinol (cannabis) on cardiac conduction in man. *American Heart Journal, 94*, 740–747.

Morrill, G.A., Kostellow, A.B., Ziegler, D.H. & Fujimoto, G.I. (1983). Effects of cannabinoids on function of testis and secondary sex organs in the Fischer rat. *Pharmacology, 26*, 20–28.

Nelson, K., Walsh, D., Deeter, P. & Sheehan, F. (1994). A phase II study of delta-9-tetrahydrocannabinol for appetite stimulation in cancer-associated anorexia. *Journal of Palliative Care, 10*, 14–18.

Nowlan, R. & Cohen, S. (1977). Tolerance to marijuana: Heart rate and subjective "high." *Clinical Pharmacology and Therapeutics, 22*, 550–556.

Paton, W.D.M. (1957). The action of morphine and related substances on contraction and on acetylcholine output of coaxially stimulated guinea-pig ileum. *British Journal of Pharmacology and Chemotherapy, 11*, 119–127.

Pearl, W. & Choi, Y.S. (1992). Marijuana as a cause of myocardial infarction. *International Journal of Cardiology, 34*, 353–354.

Perez-Reyes, M. (1990). Marijuana smoking: Factors that influence the bioavailabililty of tetrahydrocannabinol. In C.N. Chiang & R.L. Hawks (Eds.), *Research Findings on Smoking of Abused Substances* (NIDA Research Monograph No. 99, pp. 42–62). Washington, DC: U.S. Government Printing Office.

Perez-Reyes, M., Hicks, R.E., Bumberry, J., Jeffcoat, A.R. & Cook, C.E. (1988). Interaction between marihuana and ethanol: Effects on psychomotor performance. *Alcoholism: Clinical and Experimental Research, 12*, 268–276.

Perez-Reyes, M., Lipton, M.A., Timmons, M.C., Wall, M.E., Brine, D.R. & Davis, K.H. (1973). Pharmacology of orally admininstered delta-9-tetrahydrocannabinol. *Clinical Pharmacology Therapeutics, 14*, 48–55.

Pertwee, R., Fernando, J., Nash, A. & Coutts, A. (1996a). Further evidence for the presence of cannabinoid CD1 receptors in guinea pig small intestine. *British Journal of Pharmacology, 118*, 2199–2205.

Pertwee, R., Joe-Adigwe, G. & Hawksworth, G. (1996b). Further evidence for the presence of cannabinoid CB1 receptors in the mouse vas deferens. *European Journal of Pharmacology, 296*, 169–173.

Pertwee, R.G., Stevenson, L.A., Elrick, D.B., Mechoulam, R. & Corbett, A.D. (1992). Inhibitory effects of certain enantiomeric cannabinoids in the mouse vas deferens and the myenteric plexus preparation of guinea-pig small intestine. *British Journal of Pharmacology, 105*, 980–984.

Phillips, R.N., Brown, D.J., Martz, R.C., Hubbard, H.D. & Forney, R.B. (1972). Subacute toxicity of aqueous-suspended delta-9-tetrahydrocannabinol in rats. *Toxicology and Applied Pharmacology, 25*, 45–49.

Plasse, T.F., Gorter, R.W., Krasnow, S.H., Lane, M., Shepard, K.V. & Wadleigh, R.G. (1991). Recent clinical experience with dronabinol. *Pharmacology, Biochemistry and Behavior, 40*, 695–700.

Podczeck, A., Frohmer, K. & Steinbach, K. (1990). Acute myocardial infarction in juvenile patients with normal coronary arteries. *International Journal of Cardiology, 30*, 359–361.

Regelson, W., Butler, J., Schulz, J., Kirk, T., Peek, L., Green, M. & Zalsi, M. (1976). Delta-9-tetrahydrocannabinol as an effective antidepressant and appetite stimulating agent in advanced cancer patients. In M.C. Braude & S. Szara (Eds.), *Pharmacology of Marijuana: A Monograph of the National Institute on Drug Abuse* (pp.763–776). New York: Raven Press.

Renaud, A.M. & Cormier, Y. (1986). Acute effects of marihuana smoking on maximal exercise performance. *Medicine and Science in Sports and Exercise, 18*, 685–689.

Renault, P.F., Schuster, C.R., Heinrich, R. & Freedman, D.X. (1971). Marihuana: Standardised smoke administration and dose effect on heart rate in humans. *Science*, *174*, 589–591.

Rosell, S. & Agurell, S. (1975). Effects of 7-OH-delta-6-tetrahydrocannabinol and some related cannabinoids on the Guinea Pig Isolated Ileum. *ACTA Physiologica Scandinavica*, *94*, 142–144.

Rubin, V. & Comitas, L. (1975). *Ganja in Jamaica: A Medical Anthropological Study of Chronic Marihuana Use*. The Hague: Mouton.

Shapiro, B.J., Reiss, S., Sullivan, S.F., Tashkin, D.P., Simmons, M.S. & Smith, R.T. (1976). Cardiopulmonary effects of marijuana smoking during exercise. *Chest*, *70*, 441.

Shaw, L.M., Edling-Owens, J. & Mattes, R. (1991). Ultrasensitive measurement of delta-9-tetrahydrocannabinol with a high energy dynode detector and electron-capture negative chemical-ionization mass spectrometry. *Clinical Chemistry*, *37*, 2062–2068.

Shook, J.E. & Burks, T.F. (1989). Psychoactive cannabinoids reduce gastrointestinal propulsion and motility in rodents. *Journal of Pharmacology and Experimental Therapeutics*, *249*, 444–449.

Shook, J.E., Dewey, W.L. & Burks, T.F. (1986). *The Central and Peripheral Effects of Delta-9-tetrahydrocannabinol on Gastrointestinal Transit in Mice* (NIDA Research Monograph No. 6, pp. 222–227). Washington, DC: Government Printing Office.

Siler, J.F., Sheep, W.L. & Bates, L.B. (1933). Marijuana smoking in Panama. *Military Surgery*, *73*, 269–280.

Sjoden, P., Järbe, T. & Henrikksson, B. (1973). Influence of tetrahydrocannabinol (delta-8-THC and delta-9-THC) on body weight, food and water intake in rats. *Pharmacology, Biochemistry and Behavior*, *1*, 395–399.

Snyder, S. (1970). *Use of Marijuana*. New York: Oxford University Press.

Sprague, R.A., Rosenkrantz, H. & Braude, M.C. (1973). Cannabinoid effects on liver glucogen stores. *Life Sciences*, *12*, 409–416.

Stefanis, C., Dornbush, R. & Fink, M. (Eds.). (1977). *Hashish: Studies of Long-Term Use*. New York: Raven Press.

Struwe, M., Kaempfer, S., Geiger, C., Pavia, A., Plasse, T., Shepard, K., Ries, K. & Evans, T. (1993). Effect of dronabinol on nutritional status in HIV infection. *Annals of Pharmacotherapy*, *27*, 827–831.

Sulkowski, A., Vachon, L. & Rich, E., Jr. (1977). Propranolol effects on acute marihuana intoxication in man. *Psychopharmacology (Berl)*, *52*, 47–53.

Tart, C.T. (1970). Marijuana intoxication common experiences. *Nature, 226*, 701–704.

Tennant, F.S. (1983). Clinical toxicology of cannabis use. In K.O. Fehr & H. Kalant (Eds.), *Cannabis and Health Hazards* (pp. 69–90). Toronto: Addiction Research Foundation.

Tennant, F.S., Preble, M., Prendergast, T.J. & Ventry, P. (1971). Medical manifestations associated with hashish. *Journal of American Medical Association, 216*, 1965–1969.

Thompson, G.R., Fleischman, R.W., Rosenkrantz, H. & Braude, M.C. (1974). Oral and intravenous toxicity of delta-9-tetrahydrocannabinol in rhesus monkeys. *Toxicology and Applied Pharmacology, 27*, 648–665.

Thompson, G.R., Mason, M.M., Rosenkrantz, H. & Braude, M.C. (1973). Chronic oral toxicity of cannabinoids in rats. *Toxicology and Applied Pharmacology, 25*, 373–390.

Thompson, G.R., Rosenkrantz, H., Fleischman, R.W. & Braude, M.C. (1975). Effects of delta-9-tetrahydrocannabinol administered subcutaneously to rabbits for 28 days. *Toxicology, 4*, 41–51.

Timpone, J., Wright, D., Li, N., Egorin, M., Enama, M., Mayers, J. & Galetto, G. (1997). The safety and pharmacokinetics of single-agent and combination therapy with megestrol acetate and dronabinol for the treatment of HIV wasting syndrome. *AIDS Research and Human Retroviruses, 13*, 305–315.

Wall, M.E., Sadler, B.M., Brine, D., Taylor, H. & Perez-Reyes, M. (1983). Metabolism, disposition and kinetics of $\varnothing^9$-tetrahydrocannabinol in men and women. *Clinical Pharmacology and Therapeutics, 34*, 352–363.

Weiss, J.L., Watanabe, A.M., Lemberger, L., Tamarkin, N.R. & Cardon, P.V. (1972). Cardiovascular effects of delta-9-tetrahydrocannabinol in man. *Clinical Pharmacology and Therapeutics, 13*, 671–684.

Williams, E.G., Himmelsbach, C.K., Wikler, A., Ruble, D.C. & Lloyd, B.J. (1946). Studies on marihuana and pyrahexyl compound. *Public Health Report, 61*, 1059–1085.

Therapeutic Uses of Cannabis and Cannabinoids

Therapeutic Uses of Cannabis and Cannabinoids

CHRISTINE R. HARTEL

History of Marijuana as Medicine

The first written record of marijuana being used for therapeutic purposes comes from a Chinese text on pharmacy written about 2800 B.C. Physical evidence of its medical use is almost ancient: Nerlich et al. (1995) found significant depositions of $\varnothing$-tetrahydrocannabinol (THC), nicotine and cocaine in the organs of an Egyptian mummy dating from approximately 950 B.C. Zias et al. (1993) analysed materials found in an ancient family tomb near Jerusalem, and discovered that cannabis had been administered to a young girl, apparently to facilitate the birth process, about A.D. 400. Cannabinoids have many physical and psychological effects described elsewhere in this volume; in this chapter, we will focus on their actual and potential therapeutic effects, including analgesia and sedation, and the anticonvulsant and anti-emetic properties. These have long been exploited throughout India, Turkey and other parts of the Middle East (Mechoulam, 1986). Cannabis came to the attention of Western medicine during the middle of the 19th century, when the British in

India began to study its medicinal properties intensively. They acclaimed its utility in the treatment of the spasms and convulsions of rabies, tetanus and epilepsy, and as an analgesic for rheumatism (Nahas, 1984). As a consequence, use of various preparations of the plant became popular in Western medicine during the middle and latter parts of the 19th century (Reynolds, 1890).

Marijuana fell out of favor, however, because the potency of the preparations was often unreliable, resulting in lack of efficacy. Even when potency was known, patients frequently had variable responses to the same dosage. Finally, the advent of new, pharmaceutically purer drugs such as the opiates, aspirin, chloral hydrate, and the barbiturates, which could be given in standard doses with reliable efficacy, resulted in less interest in the medical use of the cannabis plant or its extracts in Britain and the United States. Social and legal sanctions against its use further inhibited the development of its medical utility.

The recently revived interest in the medical uses of marijuana arose at least partly from its popularity as a recreational drug in the 1960s and 1970s. Young cancer patients who used marijuana reported that it relieved the nausea and vomiting caused by their cancer chemotherapy treatments.

Modern chemistry also brought about increased interest in the use of at least one of the constituents of marijuana. In 1964, Goani and Mechoulam isolated and synthesized delta-9-tetrahydrocannabinol (THC), the principal psychoactive chemical in marijuana. This made possible the clinical testing of THC during the 1970s and 1980s, and eventually the official approval and marketing of prescription capsules of THC in sesame oil (dronabinol, Marinol™) in 1986. The chemical synthesis of THC also made possible the synthesis and clinical testing of an entirely new class of pharmaceutical compounds, the synthetic cannabinoids.

At the time, it was generally assumed that THC capsules, with their known, standardized dosage, stability, and purity were the obvious candidates for medical use, rather than the tar-laden smoke of marijuana cigarettes, with its uncontrolled dosage, dubious purity and potency, and its complex of more than 40 cannabinoid-related compounds. The psychoactive and physiological effects of THC are the same whether the THC is synthetically produced as dronabinol, or whether the THC occurs naturally in plant material. However, smoking marijuana is quite different from taking oral THC capsules because of the complex mixture of cannabinoids and other compounds that occur in each plant, and because the onset of THC effects is much more rapid with smoked marijuana than with oral THC administration. The subjective effects also differ in intensity depending on the dose and on the expectations of the user. Hence, the subjective effect of smoked THC may be perceived by the experienced, "recreational" marijuana smoker as desirable, relaxing and euphoria-inducing, while the older chemotherapy patient who has never used marijuana and is now taking dronabinol may perceive the same effects as undesirable, sedating, anxiety-inducing and dysphoric. Physiological side effects include changes in blood pressure and tachycardia, which are usually undesirable in older patients.

As a result, there have been few trials of the efficacy of crude cannabis in Western clinical medicine. In the United States, this is due at least as much to a scientific distrust of herbal medicine, with its many interacting compounds and unspecified potency and purity, as it is to concern over the psychoactive effects of THC. Many medical scientists favor (or at least do not oppose) the clinical testing of pharmaceutically pure cannabinoids as therapeutic agents in a variety of disorders. They also perceive many practical and scientific barriers to the conduct of clinical trials of a smoked plant material and to the interpretation of the resulting data. These issues are discussed at length in the report made by the Expert Panel on the Possible Medical Uses of Marijuana to the Director of the U.S. National Institutes of Health (NIH) (1997, pp. 8–12).

In addition to these significant scientific barriers, there are political and economic barriers to the testing of smoked cannabis for therapeutic purposes in the United States. Approval and funding for a clinical trial of marijuana is difficult to obtain because of lack of interest in cannabis drug development by government health agencies and pharmaceutical companies, which have strong scientific and economic incentives to develop pure pharmaceuticals rather than to test the potential of herbal medications. Although these attitudes are beginning to change (see the NIH report cited above), the practical and scientific difficulties in carrying out cannabis research have resulted in almost all the literature reviewed here being from the testing of synthetic THC rather than from clinical trials of smoked cannabis.

Many controlled drugs have therapeutic uses and are available as medicines, distributed under appropriate diversion control measures. Likewise, cannabinoids, if proven useful for therapeutic purposes, can be used medically, although some regulatory adjustments will be necessary to enable cannabinoids other than THC to be made available for medical use. It should be emphasized that therapeutic use of a controlled

Chapter 14

substance under appropriate diversion control measures is a quite separate issue from its legalization for non-medical use.

THC as an Anti-emetic in Cancer Chemotherapy

In response to anecdotal reports by cancer patients that smoking marijuana alleviated the nausea and vomiting caused by powerful chemotherapeutic agents, synthetic THC capsules (dronabinol) were widely distributed in the United States in the 1970s and tested for efficacy. Sallan et al. proved in randomized, double-blind, placebo-controlled trials that dronabinol was more effective than placebo (1975) or even prochlorperazine (1980), a commonly prescribed phenothiazine, in controlling nausea and vomiting resulting from chemotherapy. Results were mixed, however. For example, Gralla et al. (1984) found that dronabinol was less effective and caused more side effects than metoclopramide in a randomized double-blind trial in patients given cisplatin. Still, dronabinol was approved by the U.S. Food and Drug Administration for this indication in 1985, under the trade name Marinol™. Other cannabinoids, nabilone and levonantradol, were synthesized and tested successfully (Levitt, 1986; Pomeroy, Fennelly et al., 1986). Nabilone is marketed under the trade name Cesamet™ in the United Kingdom, Canada and Austria for the control of nausea induced by cancer chemotherapy. Once marketed in the United States, Cesamet™ is no longer available there.

A review of the literature on control of nausea induced by cancer chemotherapy (Grunberg & Hesketh, 1993) concludes that today dronabinol is used principally as an adjunctive therapy in the United States, because of dysphoric reactions, although the addition of a low dose of prochlorperazine to a cannabinoid regimen reduces the incidence of this effect (Lane, Vogel et al., 1991). Dronabinol remains a useful part of the oncologist's armamentarium in controlling the effects of chemotherapeutic agents that create mild to moderate nausea in some cancer patients.

More recently, Abrahamov and colleagues (1995) successfully treated young children (aged 3 to 13 years) with delta-8-tetrahydrocannabinol, a cannabinoid with fewer psychotropic effects than THC, during their cancer chemotherapy. The drug was administered in an edible oil and prevented nausea and vomiting in most cases. Further controlled studies are necessary to prove its long-term efficacy and safety.

Only two published studies have examined cannabis (in contrast to dronabinol) as an anti-emetic in cancer chemotherapy patients (Levitt, Faiman et al., 1984; Vinciguerra, Moore & Brennan, 1988). Vinciguerra and colleagues looked at self-rated marijuana efficacy in 56 cancer patients in an open label trial. Some 34 per cent of the patients rated the drug as very effective, 44 per cent found it moderately effective, and 22 per cent found no benefit. Levitt et al. (1984) conducted a randomized double-blind comparison of dronabinol and marijuana for the treatment of chemotherapy-induced nausea and vomiting in 20 patients. They found that while 75 per cent of patients in both groups suffered significant nausea and vomiting, among the 11 patients who found relief and expressed a preference, 7 preferred dronabinol. These results do not argue convincingly for the superiority of smoked cannabis over oral THC in treating nausea induced by cancer chemotherapy.

Advocates of the use of smoked cannabis point out that there are considerable differences in effect between oral THC and use of the plant material: the speed of drug delivery and its absorption because of the route of administration, and the possible interactions of other compounds in the cannabis in achieving an anti-emetic effect.

There is no doubt that smoking is an effective and rapid means of drug delivery, and many patients who are experienced smokers find they can titrate a dose of cannabis to fit their needs.

However, the smoke itself irritates the respiratory system and contains tars, carbon monoxide, hydrogen cyanide and nitrosamines. This is enough to keep many non-smokers from attempting to use this route of THC administration.

The pharmacokinetics of THC are known to vary with the route of administration; the differences in pharmacokinetics between smoked and oral administration have been well documented for many years (Institute of Medicine, 1982, pp. 20–23). Smoking and intravenous injection result in plasma concentrations that rapidly reach a high peak and then fall steadily. Oral doses achieve a steadier, lower blood level that does not peak in the same way as that achieved with smoking or intravenous administration. Clinical effects (reddened conjunctivae and tachycardia) have a much slower onset, occur at much lower blood levels, and last longer with oral doses than with smoked doses (Ohlsson, Lindgren et al., 1980). There is considerable variability in absorption through the gastric route, but, as just noted, blood levels need not be as high as those achieved by smoking for clinical effects. Subjective effects (the "high") are not in phase with blood levels, but since the desired therapeutic effect (control of nausea) is achieved orally with doses of dronabinol, it appears that the peak in blood level achieved by smoking is not necessary for therapeutic efficacy.

Introducing smoke of any sort into the lungs of patients with suppressed immune systems, like AIDS and cancer chemotherapy patients, is less than optimal. Cannabis plant material is subject to contamination by salmonella (Schrader, Steris et al., 1981) and aspergillus, a common fungus. Marijuana smoking is a risk factor for pulmonary aspergillosis in AIDS patients (Denning, Follansbee et al., 1991). Contamination of marijuana with herbicides and pesticides (and even other drugs) is probably more common, at least with "street" material. Finally, the variable potency of cannabis plant material and the difficulty in administering standard doses cannot be ignored. After a series of experiments, Perez-Reyes concluded that even when using cigarettes of known and standard potency, "marijuana smoking is a complex process that does not permit controlled dosing" (1990, p. 61). The U.S. NIH Expert Panel also describes the challenges of controlling the dosage of smoked marijuana (1997, pp. 10–11). These difficulties make many clinical pharmacologists doubt the practicality and value of comparative testing of cannabis and dronabinol.

As chemists synthesize new cannabinoid compounds, the hope remains that it might be possible to develop new cannabinoids with fewer and less severe side effects. For example, in 1989, Feigenbaum et al. found that an isomer of the synthetic cannabinoid, 7-hydroxy-delta-6-tetrahydrocannabinol, which has no psychoactive effects, showed anti-emetic effectiveness in animals. It is likely, however, that this research has not been confirmed or expanded because of the development of a new class of medications, the serotonin receptor antagonists, which are the current anti-emetic drugs of choice. One of the several subtypes of serotonin receptors, $5-HT_3$, appears to have a pivotal role in emesis (Tyers, 1990); blockade of this receptor type results in complete prevention of emesis in approximately 80 per cent of patients receiving certain types of chemotherapy (Italian Group for Antiemetic Research, 1995). The side effects of this class of drugs, which includes ondansetron, are minor and transient (Grunberg, Stevenson et al., 1989; Kris, Gralla et al., 1988).

In addition to the drug-induced nausea and vomiting of cancer chemotherapy, patients with cancer in its advanced stages frequently suffer from anorexia. Because of the moderate success of THC in stimulating appetite in AIDS patients, Nelson et al. (1994) tested its utility in cancer patients in an open trial. Thirteen of 18 patients given low does of dronabinol reported an improved appetite.

THC and AIDS Wasting Syndrome

In the United States, approximately 16 per cent (about 14,000 people) of the total AIDS population suffers from the progressive anorexia and weight loss known as AIDS wasting syndrome. The pathophysiology of this condition is unknown, but undoubtedly many factors contribute to its etiology. Through malnutrition, wasting exacerbates the primary illness; wasting syndrome is associated with a poor prognosis. There are only a few therapeutic options available for this condition, including the use of invasive nutritional procedures, which have not proven effective, and pharmacological treatments, such as the use of Megace™ or Marinol™.

Megace™ is the trade name for megestrol acetate, a synthetic hormone originally developed for the treatment of advanced breast and ovarian carcinomas. Two double-blind, randomized, placebo-controlled studies of the efficacy of Megace™ in patients with HIV-associated wasting syndrome showed statistically significant improvement in weight gain and increased appetite (Dickmeyer, Brown et al., 1991; Von Roenn, Armstrong et al., 1994; Von Roenn, Roth et al., 1991).

Dronabinol (Marinol™) was approved in 1992 by the U.S. Food and Drug Administration as a stimulant of food intake for AIDS patients suffering from wasting syndrome. The approval was based in part on an uncontrolled clinical study (Plasse, Gorter et al., 1991), in which it was found that AIDS patients demonstrated improved appetite at a dose that was tolerated during chronic administration. Subsequent studies (Beal, Olson et al., 1995; 1997; Gorter, Seifried & Volberding, 1992) have shown that dronabinol does improve appetite in some patients with AIDS-related wasting syndrome, but the resulting weight gain is usually water or fat, not the more desirable lean body mass. The mechanism for these effects is unknown (see chapter 13 in this volume).

An open-labelled, randomized trial comparing the efficacy of dronabinol and megestrol acetate in treating the wasting syndrome found that daily doses of 750 milligrams megestrol resulted in significant weight gain, but 2.5 milligrams of dronabinol twice a day did not (Timpone, Wright et al., 1997).

There are many early studies with animals (Munson & Fehr, 1983) that demonstrate the compromise of immune functions by cannabinoids. While there is little evidence that effects of THC on the immune system are clinically significant in healthy young people, its effects on the compromised immune systems of HIV-infected individuals or AIDS patients are unknown.

The smoking of marijuana to obtain THC for treating wasting syndrome is problematic. Kaslow et al. (1989) found that use of illegal drugs of abuse did not hasten the progression from HIV infection to AIDS. More recently, though, Nieman et al. (1993) have shown that cigarette smoking by HIV seropositive individuals is associated with a more rapid development of AIDS because smoking increases the incidence of *Pneumocystis carinii* pneumonia (PCP). Furthermore, the use of smoke to deliver medication of any sort is clearly a poor choice in those with impaired pulmonary function (see chapter 9 in this volume).

Marijuana, THC and Glaucoma

Glaucoma is a disease of the eye characterized by a chronic increase in pressure in the anterior chamber of the eye. This increased intraocular pressure is caused by failure of the aqueous humor to drain properly from the anterior chamber of the eye. The rise in pressure causes progressive destruction of nerves essential for vision.

THC has long been known to reduce intraocular pressure transiently (Hepler & Petrus, 1971). In one of the few clinical studies conducted with inhaled marijuana smoke, Merritt et al. (1980) found decreased intraocular and blood pressure in 18 subjects with heterogeneous glaucomas. However, the psychoactive side effects of the drug were so frequent and severe as to militate against its routine use in the general glaucoma population. In addition, physiological side effects of THC (dry eye and changes in blood pressure) are particularly undesirable for glaucoma patients.

These findings were substantiated in other studies using oral and intravenous routes of THC administration. However, in no case was intraocular pressure lowered long enough by THC to prevent optic nerve damage from glaucoma. Research with other drugs used in glaucoma treatment has shown that simply lowering intraocular pressure transiently does not control the disease; it must be lowered far enough and for a long period of time, in most cases, for life. This means that the glaucoma patient would have to take THC several times a day to keep intraocular pressure low; furthermore, it is not known whether tolerance develops to this effect of THC. There is sufficient concern over the long-term ocular and systemic effects of THC and marijuana use, especially in older individuals who are the most frequent victims of glaucoma, that THC and marijuana are not considered candidates for drug development for this indication.

Colasanti (1990) has reported that cannabigerol, a THC homologue with little psychoactivity, causes a two- to threefold increase in the outflow of aqueous humor, an action that might have therapeutic potential for the treatment of glaucoma. Further testing is indicated for this substance, but has not been undertaken.

Cannabinoids as Analgesics

There is considerable evidence that cannabinoids produce significant analgesia in experiments using animal models (Lichtman & Martin, 1991; Welch & Stevens, 1992; Zeltzer, 1991); this appears to be true in humans, as well (Martin, 1995). In early studies, cannabinoids were no more effective than other drugs used as analgesics, such as opiates, and relief of pain was achieved only at doses that induce severe side effects, including sedation, dizziness, ataxia and

blurred vision (Noyes, Brunk et al., 1975a; 1975b; Raft, Gregg et al., 1977). There is also a report from China (Wu, 1992) that THC was effective in relieving the moderate to severe pain caused by cancer in 51 patients in an open trial. Side effects were sedation, nausea, dizziness, heart palpitation, anorexia and constipation.

The newest synthetic cannabinoids are extremely potent analgesics, but again there is no separation between analgesic and side effects in laboratory animals. Testing of these compounds in humans remains to be done.

The mechanisms of action underlying pain relief by cannabinoids seem to be different from those of other drugs (Martin, 1995). Further experiments with cannabinoids are necessary because they not only illuminate the mechanisms of action of the drugs, but they also elucidate the body's multiple mechanisms of pain reception and blockade. It may be possible to develop cannabinoids that are both therapeutically useful and free of side effects, but this is a challenge for the future.

The Anti-convulsant and Anti-spasmodic Effects of the Cannabinoids

As mentioned above, one of the traditional uses of cannabis was to control the convulsions of epilepsy, rabies and tetanus (Nahas, 1984). The U.S. Institute of Medicine report on *Marijuana and Health* summarizes the early animal studies on cannabinoids by stating that there is "substantial evidence" that cannabinoids block most types of induced seizures or reduce the severity of the convulsions (1982, pp. 145–146). Cannabidiol (CBD), a naturally occurring cannabinoid without psychoactivity, is particularly potent (Consroe & Snider, 1986).

Cunha et al. (1980) conducted the only double-blind study examining the effects of CBD on human epileptic patients. They found

Chapter 14

that the drug had considerable efficacy in enhancing the effects of conventional anti-epileptic drugs that were taken together with CBD. Nevertheless, there has been no further research on CBD for this indication, which is surprising considering its lack of psychoactivity.

Evidence for the use of cannabinoids in multiple sclerosis or movement disorders such as Huntington's disease and Parkinson's disease consists of single case studies (e.g., Maurer, 1990; Meinck, Schonle et al., 1989) and anecdotal reports (e.g., Grinspoon & Bakalar, 1993). Clifford (1983) found some objective evidence that THC reduced tremor in two of eight cases of multiple sclerosis in which the patients had ataxia and tremor. More recently, Consroe et al. (1997) surveyed 112 patients with multiple sclerosis who reported some alleviation of their symptoms with cannabis use.

In an open label study, Consroe et al. (1986) reported that CBD reduced dystonia in five patients. However, there was an increase in resting tremor in two patients with Parkinson's disease in this preliminary study. These results stimulated additional animal research (Consroe, Musty & Conti, 1988; Conti, Johannesen et al., 1988) and another successful open label clinical trial of CBD with four patients with Huntington's chorea (Sandyk, Consroe et al., 1988). However, the authors were not able to replicate their results in a double-blind, controlled trial with 19 Huntington's disease patients (Consroe, Laguna et al., 1991). Clearly, further controlled research is indicated before conclusions can be drawn about the efficacy of the cannabinoids in spasticity or movement disorders.

Use of THC in Asthma

Because marijuana causes bronchodilatation, it was thought that either marijuana or an aerosol form of THC might be useful in treatment of asthma (Tashkin, Shapiro et al., 1975). Enthusiasm for the latter route of administration waned rapidly, however, when it was found that the irritating properties of the inhalant mist caused a reflex bronchoconstriction (Tashkin, Calverses et al., 1978). Newer aerosol technology may reduce the irritating properties of cannabinoid inhalant preparations, but these remain to be developed and tested. Smoking marijuana clearly has many respiratory disadvantages for asthmatics, and oral THC has a smaller bronchodilatory effect with a delayed onset that is not acceptable for asthmatic patients.

Basic Research

The characterization and cloning of the receptor for the THC molecule (Matsuda, Lolait et al., 1990) and the isolation of at least three endogenous cannabinoid ligands (Devane, Hanus et al., 1992; Hanus, Gopher et al., 1993) suggest several new pathways for research on the therapeutic potential of the cannabinoids. The distribution of the receptors is widespread in brain, with heavy concentrations in the basal ganglia, hippocampus and cerebellum (Herkenham, Lynn et al., 1990). The synthesis of specific cannabinoid receptor antagonists is also opening new vistas for clinical research with cannabinoids (Compton, Aceto et al., 1996). As the functions of receptor agonists and antagonists, both endogenous and synthetic, are delineated, it may become possible to separate the unwanted side effects of cannabinoids (psychoactivity, blood pressure changes, etc.) from their clinically desirable effects.

Research on the sites of action of THC will undoubtedly reveal the complex and redundant systems that mediate pain, appetite and motor control. This should lead to the development of ever safer and more effective medications, some of which are likely to be based on cannabinoid receptor and ligand chemistry. It is also likely that the risks and the benefits of cannabinoid therapeutics will be weighed carefully in each individual case.

Summary

Although people have used marijuana for therapeutic purposes for thousands of years, it is only
in the last 30 that its chemical constituents have
become known and its pharmacological actions
characterized. The broad range of potential
therapeutic applications of cannabinoids reflects
the widespread distribution of cannabinoid
receptors throughout the brain and other parts of
the body. Current therapeutic applications
include the use of THC as an anti-emetic agent
and appetite stimulator in cancer chemotherapy
and in the stimulation of food intake in AIDS
patients with wasting syndrome. Areas of therapeutic potential for synthetic cannabinoids
include analgesia and the treatment of convulsant or movement disorders, and possibly glaucoma and asthma. These roles for cannabinoids
remain to be determined, as more potent
cannabinoid compounds with fewer side effects
are synthesized, and as new routes of administration are developed.

References

Abrahamov, A., Abrahamov, A. & Mechoulam, R. (1995). An efficient new cannabinoid antiemetic in pediatric oncology. *Life Sciences, 56,* 2097–2102.

Adams, I.B. & Martin, B.R. (1996). Cannabis: Pharmacology and toxicology in animals and humans. *Addiction, 91,* 1585–1614.

Beal, J.E., Olson, D.O., Laubenstein, L., Morales, J.O., Bellman, P., Yangco, B., Lefkowitz, L., Plasse, T.F. & Shepard, K.V. (1995). Dronabinol as a treatment for anorexia associated with weight loss in patients with AIDS. *Journal of Pain and Symptom Management, 10,* 89–97.

Beal, J.E., Olson, D.O., Lefkowitz, L., Laubenstein, L., Bellman, P., Yangco, B., Morales, J.O., Murphy, R., Powderly, W., Plasse, T.F., Mosdell, W.W. & Shepard, K.V. (1997). Long-term efficacy and safety of dronabinol for acquired immunodeficiency syndrome-associated anorexia. *Journal of Pain and Symptom Management, 14,* 7–14.

Clifford, D.B. (1983). Tetrahydrocannabinol for tremor in multiple sclerosis. *Annals of Neurology, 13,* 669–671.

Colasanti, B.K. (1990). A comparison of the ocular and central effects of delta-9-tetra-hydrocannabinol and cannabigerol. *Journal of Ocular Research, 6,* 259–269.

Compton, D.R., Aceto, M.D., Lowe, J. & Martin, B.R. (1996). In vivo characterization of a specific cannabinoid receptor antagonist (SR141716A): Inhibition of delta-9-tetrahydrocannabinol-induced responses and apparent agonist activity. *Journal of Pharmacology and Experimental Therapeutics, 277,* 586–594.

Consroe, P., Laguna, J., Allender, J., Snider, S., Stern, L., Sandyk, R., Kennedy, K. & Schram, K. (1991). Controlled trial of cannabidiol in Huntington's disease. *Pharmacology, Biochemistry and Behavior, 40,* 701–708.

Consroe, P., Musty, R. & Conti, L. (1988). Effects of cannabidiol in animal models of neurological dysfunction. In G. Chesher, P. Consroe & R. Musty (Eds.)., *Marijuana: An International Research Report* (National Campaign Against Drug Abuse Monograph No. 7, pp. 147–152). Canberra: Australian Government Publishing Service.

Consroe, P., Musty, R., Rein, J., Tillery, W. & Pertwee, R. (1997). The perceived effects of smoked cannabis on patients with multiple sclerosis. *European Neurology, 38,* 44–48.

Consroe, P., Sandyk, R. & Snider, S.R. (1986). Open label evaluation of cannabidiol in dystonic movement disorders. *International Journal of Neuroscience, 30,* 277–282.

Consroe, P. & Snider, S.R. (1986). Therapeutic potential of cannabinoids in neurological disorders. In R. Mechoulam (Ed.), *Cannabinoids as Therapeutic Agents* (pp. 21–50). Boca Raton, FL: CRC Press.

Conti, L.S., Johannesen, J., Musty, R. & Consroe, P. (1988). Anti-dyskinetic effects of cannabidiol. In G. Chesher, P. Consroe & R. Musty (Eds.), *Marijuana: An International Research Report* (National Campaign Against Drug Abuse Monograph No. 7, pp. 153–156). Canberra: Australian Government Publishing Service.

Cunha, J.M., Carlini, E.A., Pereira, A.E., Ramos, O.L., Pimentel, C., Gagliardi, R., Sanvito, W.L., Lander, N. & Mechoulam, R. (1980). Chronic administration of cannabidiol to healthy volunteers and epileptic patients. *Pharmacology, 21,* 175–185.

Denning, D.W., Follansbee, S.E., Scolaro, M., Norris, S., Edelstein, H. & Stevens, D.A. (1991). Pulmonary aspergillosis in the acquired immunodeficiency syndrome. *New England Journal of Medicine, 324,* 654–662.

Devane, W.A., Hanus, L., Breuer, A., Pertwee, R.G., Stevenson, L.A., Griffin, G., Gibson, D., Mandelbaum, A., Etinger, A. & Mechoulam, R. (1992). Isolation and structure of a brain constituent that binds to the cannabinoid receptor. *Science, 258,* 1946–1949.

Dickmeyer, M.S., Brown, S., Pursell, K., Thaler, H. & Armstrong, D. (1991, June). Improved appetite and weight gain in patients with Acquired Immunodeficiency Syndrome treated with megestrol acetate. *International Conference on AIDS, 1,* 231 (Abstract M.B. 2198).

Expert Panel on the Possible Medical Uses of Marijuana. (1997). Report to the Director, U.S. National Institutes of Health. Workshop on the Medical Utility of Marijuana, February 19–20, 1997 [Online]. Retrieved March 25, 1998 from the World Wide Web: http://www.nih.gov/news/medmarijuana/MedicalMarijuana.htm

Feigenbaum, J.J., Richmond, S.A., Weissman, Y. & Mechoulam, R. (1989). Inhibition of cisplatin-induced emesis in the pigeon by a non-psychotropic synthetic cannabinoid. *European Journal of Pharmacology, 169,* 159–165.

Goani, Y. & Mechoulam, R. (1964). Isolation, structure and partial synthesis of an active constituent of hashish. *Journal of the American Chemical Society, 86,* 1646–1647.

Gorter, R., Seifried, M. & Volberding, P. (1992). Dronabinol effects on weight in patients with HIV infection. *AIDS, 6,* 127.

Gralla, R.J., Tyson, L.B., Bordin, L.A., Clark, R.A., Kelsen, D.P., Kris, M.G., Kalman, L.B. & Groshen, S. (1984). Antiemetic therapy: A review of recent studies and a report of a random assignment trial comparing metoclopramide with delta-9-tetrahydro-cannabinol. *Cancer Treatment Reports, 68,* 163–172.

Grinspoon, L. & Bakalar, J.B. (1993). *Marijuana, the Forbidden Medicine.* New Haven: Yale University Press.

Grunberg, S.M. & Hesketh, P.J. (1993). Control of chemotherapy-induced emesis. *New England Journal of Medicine, 329,* 1790–1796.

Grunberg, S.M., Stevenson, L.L., Russell, C.A. & McDermed, J.E. (1989). Dose ranging phase I study of the serotonin antagonist GR38032F for prevention of cisplatin-induced nausea and vomiting. *Journal of Clinical Oncology, 7*, 1137–1141.

Hanus, L., Gopher, A., Almog, S. & Mechoulam, R. (1993). Two new unsaturated fatty acid ethanolamides in brain that bind to the cannabinoid receptor. *Journal of Medicinal Chemistry, 36*, 3032–3034.

Hepler, R.S. & Petrus, R.J. (1971). Marihuana smoking and intraocular pressure. *Journal of the American Medical Association, 217*, 1392.

Herkenham, M., Lynn, A.B., Little, M.D., Johnson, M.R., Melvin, L.S., De Costa, B.R. & Rice, K.C. (1990). Cannabinoid receptor localization in brain. *Proceedings of the National Academy of Sciences of the United States of America, 87*, 1932–1936.

Institute of Medicine. (1982). *Marijuana and Health*. Washington, DC: National Academy Press.

Italian Group for Antiemetic Research. (1995). Ondansetron versus granisetron, both combined with dexamethasone, in the prevention of cisplatin-induced emesis. *Annals of Oncology, 6*, 805–810.

Kaslow, R.A., Blackwelder, W.C., Ostrow, D.G., Yerg, D., Palenick, J., Coulson, A.H. & Valdiserri, R.O. (1989). No evidence for a role of alcohol or other psychoactive drugs in accelerating immunodeficiency in HIV-1-positive individuals: A report from the Multicenter AIDS Cohort Study. *Journal of the American Medical Association, 261*, 3424–3429.

Kris, M.G., Gralla, R.J., Clark, R.A. & Tyson, L.B. (1988). Dose-ranging evaluation of the serotonin antagonist GR-C507/75 (GR38032F) when used as an antiemetic in patients receiving anticancer chemotherapy. *Journal of Clinical Oncology, 6*, 659–662.

Lane, M., Vogel, C.L., Ferguson, J., Krasnow, S., Saiers, J.L., Hamm, J., Salva, K., Wiernik, P.H., Holroyde, C.P., Hammill, S., Shepherd, K. & Plasse, T. (1991). Dronabinol and prochlorperazine in combination for treatment of cancer. *Journal of Pain and Symptom Management, 6*, 352–359.

Levitt, M. (1986). Cannabinoids as antiemetics in cancer chemotherapy. In R. Mechoulam (Ed.), *Cannabinoids as Therapeutic Agents* (pp. 71–103). Boca Raton, FL: CRC Press.

Levitt, M., Faiman, C., Hawks, R. & Wilson, A. (1984). Randomized double blind comparison of delta-9-tetrahydrocannabinol (THC) and marijuana as chemotherapy antiemetics. *Proceedings of the meeting of the American Society of Clinical Oncology, 3*, 91 (ASCO Abstract C-354).

Lichtman, A.H. & Martin, B.R. (1991). Spinal and supraspinal mechanisms of cannabinoid-induced antinociception. *Journal of Pharmacology and Experimental Therapeutics, 258*, 517–523.

Martin, B.R. (1995). Marijuana. In F.E. Bloom & C. Kupfer (Eds.), *Psychopharmacology: Fourth Generation of Progress* (pp. 1757–1765). New York: Raven Press.

Matsuda, L.A., Lolait, S.J., Brownstein, M.J., Young, A.C. & Bonner, T.I. (1990). Structure of a cannabinoid receptor and functional expression of the cloned cDNA. *Nature, 346*, 561–564.

Maurer, M., Henn, V., Dittrich, A. & Hofmann, A. (1990). Delta-9-tetrahydrocannabinol shows antispastic and analgesic effects in a single case double-blind trial. *European Archives of Psychiatry and Clinical Neuroscience, 240*, 1–4.

Mechoulam, R. (1986). The pharmacohistory of cannabis sativa. In R. Mechoulam (Ed.), *Cannabinoids as Therapeutic Agents* (pp. 1–20). Boca Raton, FL: CRC Press.

Meinck, H.M., Schonle, P.W. & Conrad, B. (1989). Effect of cannabinoids on spasticity and ataxia in multiple sclerosis. *Journal of Neurology, 236*, 120–122.

Merritt, J.C., Crawford, W.J., Alexander, P.C., Anduze, A.L. & Gelbart, S.S. (1980). Effect of marihuana on intraocular and blood pressure in glaucoma. *Ophthalmology, 87*, 222–228.

Munson, A.E. & Fehr, K.O. (1983). Immunological effects of cannabis. In K.O. Fehr & H. Kalant (Eds.), Cannabis and health hazards. *Proceedings of an ARF/WHO Scientific Meeting on Adverse Health and Behavioral Consequences of Cannabis Use* (pp. 257–354). Toronto: Addiction Research Foundation.

Nahas, G.G. (1984). The medical use of cannabis. In G.G. Nahas (Ed.), *Marijuana in Science and Medicine* (pp. 247–262). New York: Raven Press.

Nelson, K., Walsh, D., Deeter, P. & Sheehan, F. (1994). A phase II study of delta-9-tetrahydrocannabinol for appetite stimulation in cancer-associated anorexia. *Journal of Palliative Care, 10*, 14–18.

Nerlich, A.G., Parsche, F., Wiest, I., Schramel, P. & Lohrs, U. (1995). Extensive pulmonary haemorrhage in an Egyptian mummy. *Virchows-Archives, 7*, 423–429.

Nieman, R.B., Fleming, J., Coker, R.J., Harris, J.R. & Mitchell, D.M. (1993). The effect of cigarette smoking on the development of AIDS in HIV-1-seropositive individuals. *AIDS, 7*, 705–710.

Noyes, R., Jr., Brunk, F., Avery, D.H. & Canter, A. (1975a). The analgesic properties of delta-9-tetrahydrocannabinol and codeine. *Clinical Pharmacology and Therapeutics, 18* (1), 84–89.

Noyes, R., Jr., Brunk, S.F., Baram, D.A. & Canter, A. (1975b). Analgesic effect of delta-9-tetrahydrocannabinol. *Journal of Clinical Pharmacology, 15* (2–3), 139–143.

Ohlsson, A., Lindgren, J.-E., Wahlen, A., Agurell, S., Hollister, L.E. & Gillespie, H.K. (1980). Plasma delta-9-tetrahydrocannabinol concentrations and clinical effects after oral and intravenous administration and smoking. *Clinical Pharmacology and Therapeutics, 28*, 409–416.

Perez-Reyes, M. (1990). Marijuana smoking: Factors that influence the bioavailability of tetrahydrocannabinol. In C.N. Chiang & R.L. Hawks (Eds.), *Research Findings on Smoking of Abused Substances* (NIDA Research Monograph No. 99, pp. 42–62). Washington, DC: U.S. Government Printing Office.

Plasse, T.F., Gorter, R.W., Krasnow, S.H., Lane, M., Shepard, K.V. & Wadleigh, R.G. (1991). Recent clinical experience with dronabinol. *Pharmacology, Biochemistry and Behavior, 40*, 695–700.

Pomeroy, M., Fennelly, J.J. & Towers, M. (1986). Prospective randomized double-blind trial of nabilone versus domperidone in the treatment of cytotoxic-induced emesis. *Cancer Chemotherapy and Pharmacology, 17*, 285–288.

Raft, D., Gregg, J., Ghia, J. & Harris, L. (1977). Effects of intravenous tetrahydrocannabinol on experimental and surgical pain. *Clinical Pharmacology and Therapeutics, 21*, 26–33.

Reynolds, J.R. (1890). Therapeutic uses and toxic effects of cannabis indica. *Lancet, 1*, 637–638.

Sallan, S.E., Cronin, C., Zelen, M. & Zinberg, N.E. (1980). Antiemetics in patients receiving chemotherapy for cancer: A randomized comparison of delta-9-tetrahydrocannabinol and prochlorperazine. *New England Journal of Medicine, 302*, 135–138.

Sallan, S.E., Zinberg, N.E. & Frei, E., III. (1975). Antiemetic effect of delta-9-tetrahydrocannabinol in patients receiving cancer chemotherapy. *New England Journal of Medicine, 293*, 795–797.

Sandyk, R., Consroe, P., Stern, L., Snider, S.R. & Bliken, R. (1988). Preliminary trial of cannabidiol in Huntington's Disease. In G. Chesher, P. Consroe & R. Musty (Eds.), *Marijuana: An International Research Report* (National Campaign Against Drug Abuse Monograph No. 7, pp. 157–162). Canberra: Australian Government Publishing Service.

Schrader, J., Steris, C. & Halpin, T. (1981). Salmonellosis traced to marijuana. Ohio, Michigan. *Morbidity and Mortality Weekly Report, 30*, 77–79.

Tashkin, D.P., Calverses, B.M., Simmons, M.S. & Shapiro, B.J. (1978). Respiratory status of 74 habitual marijuana smokers. Paper presented at the annual meeting of the American Thoracic Society, Boston.

Tashkin, D.P., Shapiro, B.J., Lee, Y.E. & Harper, C.E. (1975). Effects of smoked marijuana in experimentally induced asthma. *American Review of Respiratory Disease, 112*, 377–386.

Timpone, J.G., Wright, D.J., Li, N., Egorin, M.J., Enama, M.E., Mayers, J. & Galetto, G. (1997). The safety and pharmacokinetics of single-agent and combination therapy with megestrol acetate and dronabinol for the treatment of HIV wasting syndrome. *AIDS Research and Human Retroviruses, 13,* 305–315.

Tyers, M.B. (1990). 5-HT3 receptors. *Annals of the New York Academy of Sciences, 600,* 194–202.

Vinciguerra, V., Moore, T. & Brennan, E. (1988). Inhalation of marijuana as an antiemetic for cancer chemotherapy. *New York State Journal of Medicine, 88,* 525–527.

Von Roenn, J.H., Armstrong, D., Kotler, D.P., Cohn, D.L., Klimas, N.G., Tchekmedyian, N.S., Cone, L., Brennan, P.J. & Weitzman, S.A. (1994). Megestrol acetate in patients with AIDS-related cachexia. *Annals of Internal Medicine, 121,* 393–399.

Von Roenn, J., Roth, E., Murphy, R., Weitzman, S., Armstrong, D. & the U.S. Megestrol Acetate Study Group. (1991, June). Controlled trial of megestrol acetate for the treatment of AIDS related anorexia and cachexia. *International Conference on AIDS, 1,* 280 (Abstract W.B. 2392).

Welch, S.P. & Stevens, D.L. (1982). Antinociceptive activity of intrathecally administered cannabinoids alone, and in combination with morphine in mice. *Journal of Pharmacology and Experimental Therapeutics, 262,* 10–18.

Wu, G.Q. (1992). Pain-relief effect of tramadol HCL capsule for moderate and severe cancer pain. (English abstract). *Chung-Hua-Chung-Liu-Tsa-Chih, 14,* 219–221.

Zeltser, A., Seltzer, Z., Eisen, A., Feigenbaum, J.J. & Mechoulam, R. (1991). Suppression of neuropathic pain behavior in rats by a non-psychotropic synthetic cannabinoid with NMDA receptor-blocking properties. *Pain, 47,* 95–103.

Zias, J., Stark, H., Sellgman, J., Levy, R., Werker, E., Breuer, A. & Mechoulam, R. (1993). Early medical use of cannabis (letter). *Nature, 363,* 215.

CHAPTER 15

Comparing the Health and Psychological Risks of Alcohol, Cannabis, Nicotine and Opiate Use

Comparing the Health and Psychological Risks of Alcohol, Cannabis, Nicotine and Opiate Use

WAYNE HALL, ROBIN ROOM AND SUSAN BONDY

This chapter compares the nature and extent of harm attributable to cannabis with the magnitude of harmful health consequences of other commonly used psychoactive substances in Western societies, namely, alcohol and tobacco. We have also included some comparisons with the health effects of opiates to calibrate the health risks of cannabis against those of a drug that is widely regarded as a major public health concern even though it is not widely used. Our purpose in making these comparisons is not to promote one drug over another, but rather to apply to cannabis the same standards that have been used to appraise the health effects of these other drugs.

Challenges in Making Cross-Drug Comparisons of Harm

There are a number of issues that arise in comparing the direct public health impact of cannabis with these other drugs. The first are difficulties in making causal inferences about the connections between cannabis use and the adverse health and psychological consequences which have been attributed to it (see chapter 1). The second set of issues concerns lack of information about the quantitative risk or seriousness of the risks of cannabis use for users. Both of these problems relate to the scarcity of epidemiological studies of cannabis use by comparison with epidemiological studies of alcohol and tobacco use. In some instances, estimates of the magnitude of the association between cannabis use and some health consequences are derived from evidence on the magnitude of similar risks of tobacco (e.g., respiratory disease) and alcohol use (e.g., motor vehicle accidents).

A third set of issues concerns the difficulties in making comparative appraisals of the public health significance of identified risks. This requires that different types of consequences be explicitly or implicitly weighted according to their perceived importance for the community as well as the individual. The methods used to date have typically involved comparisons of the numbers of deaths, person years of life lost, or hospital bed days attributable to each type of drug (e.g., English, Holman et al., 1995).

A fourth complication in comparative assessment is that different drugs are used in different ways. In contemporary developed societies, cannabis and tobacco are typically smoked, that is, used by inhaling the smoke of a smouldering preparation containing the drug. In pharmaceutical use, opiates are administered orally or by injection, while non-medical use is primarily by injection, snorting or smoking. Alcohol is consumed orally, although in combination with a wide variety of other substances. The route of administration of a drug can change over time in a given society. For instance, in North America tobacco was primarily chewed or sniffed in the late 19th century. In Europe, there is evidence of a recent shift from injecting to smoking heroin (Grund, 1993). In this analysis, we have focused on predominant routes of administration in developed societies.

A final issue is the difficulty in predicting the public health consequences of changes in prevalence of use and route of administration of these drugs. Changes in either or both of these would substantially change the size and profile of adverse effects in ways that are difficult to predict.

Our Approach

The approach we have adopted in addressing each of these issues is as follows. First, we have identified the most probable causal relationships between cannabis use and specific health effects. In doing so, we have used standard criteria for assessing the strength of evidence for causal relationships, although we have had to relax the degree of confidence required so that some provisional conclusions can be drawn as to the most probable health risks of cannabis use.

Second, in so far as it is possible, we have attempted to quantify the severity of personal and public health risk for each adverse health effect that can be reasonably attributed to cannabis. We have attempted to estimate the probable relative risk, and the prevalence of the relevant pattern of use.

Third, we have compared these estimates with the best estimates of the mortality and morbidity burden of alcohol, opiates and tobacco. This has been done initially in a qualitative way by indicating whether or not particular adverse health effects that may reasonably be attributed to cannabis have also been attributed to alcohol, nicotine and opiates. This is followed by a discussion of the probable quantitative risks of cannabis by comparison with those of alcohol and nicotine. Finally, we consider some direct comparative evidence on consequences reported by users of the three drugs.

In making these comparisons, we have relied on epidemiological evidence on the health and psychological consequences of cannabis use which is largely based on studies conducted in the English-speaking countries, and most particularly the United States. Unfortunately, countries with a long tradition of heavy cannabis use are not well represented in the research literature. The conduct of research on cannabis use in developing countries should be a priority, especially those countries that have a long history of traditional use, including very heavy use among some subpopulations. These subpopulations are the ones most likely to show any adverse health effects of chronic heavy cannabis use.

Our comparisons of health effects are also largely confined to the effects on the health of users. We have said little about the effects of cannabis use on the health and well-being of other persons who do not use cannabis. Such indirect health effects have not been well studied for most drugs, with the limited exceptions of motor vehicle accidents, violence for alcohol and passive smoking in the case of tobacco. Such effects deserve more attention than they have hitherto received, but in the absence of the necessary research we are unable to address them in this review.

It should be noted that our comparisons are confined to the *adverse* health and psychological effects of the different drugs. There are also potential or established positive health effects of some drugs, a few of which are mentioned briefly in the present analysis.

The Probable Health Effects of Cannabis Use

Acute Psychological and Health Consequences

The acute toxicity of cannabis is very low. There are no confirmed cases of human deaths from cannabis poisoning in the world medical literature. Animal studies indicate that the dose of $\varnothing^9$-tetrahydrocannabinol (THC) required to produce 50 per cent mortality in rodents is extremely high by comparison with other commonly used pharmaceutical and recreational drugs (Rosenkrantz, 1983).

DYSPHORIC EFFECTS

The most common unpleasant acute psychological effects of cannabis use are anxiety, panic and depressive feelings (Weil, 1970). These effects are most often reported by naive users who are unfamiliar with the drug's effects, and by patients who have been given oral THC for therapeutic purposes. More experienced users may occasionally report these effects after receiving a much larger than intended dose of THC. These effects can usually be prevented by adequate preparation of users about the type of effects they may experience, or they can be managed by reassurance and support.

MOTOR VEHICLE ACCIDENTS

The major potential health risks from the acute use of cannabis arise from its effects on cognitive and psychomotor performance. Intoxication produces dose-related impairments in a wide range of cognitive and behavioral functions that are relevant to a skilled performance such as driving an automobile or operating machinery. These include: slowed reaction time and information processing; impaired perceptual-motor co-ordination and motor performance; impaired short-term memory, signal detection and tracking behavior; and slowed time perception (Chait & Pierri, 1992).

The negative effect of cannabis on the performance of psychomotor tasks is almost always related to dose (Chait & Pierri, 1992). The effects are generally larger, more consistent and persistent in tasks that involve sustained attention. The acute effects of "recreational" doses of cannabis on driving performance in laboratory simulators and over standardized driving courses are similar to those of doses of alcohol that achieve blood alcohol contents (BACs) between 0.07 per cent and 0.10 per cent (Smiley, 1986).

Although cannabis impairs performance in laboratory and simulated driving settings, studies of the effects of cannabis on on-road driving performance have found, at most, modest impairments (e.g., Robbe, 1994). Cannabis-intoxicated persons drive more slowly, perhaps because they are more aware of their level of psychomotor impairment, than alcohol-intoxicated drinkers who generally drive at faster speeds (Smiley, 1986; see also chapter 5 in this volume).

MORTALITY

There are two epidemiological studies of mortality among cannabis users. A prospective Swedish study of mortality over 15 years among military conscripts found an increased risk of premature mortality among men who had smoked cannabis 50 or more times by age 18. Violent deaths were the major contributor to this excess, of which 26 per cent were motor vehicle and 7 per cent other accidents (e.g., drownings and falls). The increased risk disappeared, however, after multivariate statistical adjustment for confounding variables such as alcohol and other drug use (Andreasson & Allebeck, 1990).

Sidney et al. (1997) reported a 10-year study of mortality in cannabis users among 65,171 Kaiser Permanente Medical Care Program members aged between 15 and 49. The sample comprised 38 per cent who had never used cannabis, 20 per cent who had used less than six times, 20 per cent who were former users and 22 per cent who were current cannabis users. They found that regular cannabis use had a small impact on mortality (RR = 1.33). This was wholly explained by increased AIDS mortality among men, probably because marijuana use was a marker for male homosexual behavior in this cohort. It is too early, however, to conclude that marijuana use does not increase mortality because the average age at follow-up was only 43 years, and cigarette smoking and alcohol use were also only modestly associated with premature mortality in the cohort.

The Health Effects of Chronic Cannabis Use

The Immune System

There is reasonably consistent evidence that THC can produce cellular changes such as alterations in cell metabolism and DNA synthesis *in vitro* (Bloch, 1983). There is even stronger evidence that cannabis smoke is mutagenic *in vitro* and *in vivo,* and hence, that it is potentially carcinogenic for the same reasons as tobacco smoke (Leuchtenberger, 1983).

As well, there is reasonably consistent evidence that cannabinoids impair both the cell-mediated and humoral immune systems in rodents (Munson & Fehr, 1983). These changes have decreased resistance to infection by bacteria and viruses. There is also evidence that the non-cannabinoid components of cannabis smoke impair the functioning of alveolar macrophages, the first line of the body's defence system in the lungs (Baldwin, Tashkin et al., 1997; Munson & Fehr, 1983).

To date, there has been no epidemiological evidence of increased rates of disease among chronic heavy cannabis users. There is one large prospective study of HIV-positive homosexual men which indicates that continued cannabis use did not increase the risk of progression to AIDS (Kaslow, Blackwelder et al., 1989). There are a number of studies, however, which suggest that cannabis smoking increases susceptibility to infectious disease, such as pneumonia, in HIV-infected patients (Baldwin, Tashkin et al., 1997).

An epidemiological study by Polen et al. (1993), which compared health service utilization by non-smokers and daily cannabis-only smokers, has provided the first suggestive evidence of an increased rate of presentation for respiratory conditions among cannabis smokers. This remains suggestive, however, because infectious and non-infectious respiratory conditions were not separated.

The Respiratory System

Chronic heavy cannabis smoking impairs the functioning of the large airways and probably causes symptoms of chronic bronchitis such as coughing, sputum and wheezing (Bloom, Kaltenborn et al., 1987; Huber, Griffith & Langsjoen, 1988; Tashkin, Wu et al., 1988). Cannabis smoke is qualitatively very similar to tobacco smoke (Tashkin, 1993; Wu, Tashkin et al., 1988) and there is evidence that chronic cannabis smoking may produce histopathological changes in lung tissues of the kind that precede the development of lung cancer (Fligiel, Beals et al.,1988; Fligiel, Roth et al., 1997).

More recently, concern about respiratory cancers has been heightened by a series of case reports of cancers of the aerodigestive tract in young adults who have a history of heavy cannabis use (e.g., Caplan & Brigham, 1990; Donald, 1991; Taylor, 1988). Although these reports were uncontrolled, and many of the cases used alcohol and tobacco, such cancers are rare in adults under the age of 60, even among those who smoke tobacco and drink alcohol (Tashkin, 1993). Smoking cannabis may also pose an acute risk to individuals with respiratory diseases such as asthma, since evidence linking tobacco smoke to asthma and asthmatic symptoms is increasing.

Reproductive Effects

Chronic cannabis use probably disrupts the male and female reproductive systems in animals, reducing the secretion of testosterone, and sperm production, motility and viability in males, and disrupting the ovulatory cycle in females (Bloch,

1983; Institute of Medicine, 1982). It is uncertain whether it causes these effects in humans, given the inconsistency in the limited literature on human males (Mendelson & Mello, 1984), and the lack of research in the case of human females (Hollister, 1986). There is uncertainty about the clinical significance of these effects in normal healthy young adults.

Cannabis smoking during pregnancy probably impairs fetal development (Gibson, Baghurst & Colley, 1983; Hatch & Bracken, 1986; Tennes, Avitable et al., 1985; Zuckerman, Frank et al., 1989), leading to a reduction in birthweight (Abel, 1985). This may be a consequence of a shorter gestation period, and probably occurs by the same mechanism as cigarette smoking, namely, fetal hypoxia. There is uncertainty about whether cannabis use during pregnancy produces a small increase in the risk of birth defects as a result of exposure of the fetus *in utero*. There is animal evidence of such effects although these studies have usually involved very high oral doses of THC (Abel, 1985). The limited studies in humans have generally, but not always, produced null results (Gibson, Baghurst & Colley, 1983; Hatch & Bracken, 1986; Hingson, Alpert et al., 1982; Zuckerman, Frank et al., 1989).

There is not a great deal of evidence that cannabis use can produce chromosomal or genetic abnormalities in either parent, which could be transmitted to offspring. The animal and *in vitro* evidence suggests that the mutagenic capacities of cannabis smoke are greater than those of THC and of greater relevance to the risk of developing cancer than to the transmission of genetic defects to children (Bloch, 1983; Hollister, 1986).

There is evidence that infants exposed *in utero* to cannabis may experience behavioral and developmental effects during the first few months after birth and detectable later in childhood (e.g., Fried et al., 1985; 1989; 1990; 1992; 1996). There are several case-control studies which suggest that there is an increased risk of certain childhood cancers (namely, astrocytomas and leukemia) among children born to women who reported that they had used cannabis during their pregnancies (Kuijten, Bunin et al., 1990; Robinson, Buckley et al., 1989). None of these studies was planned as an investigation of the carcinogenicity of cannabis, so purposive replication is a research priority.

POSSIBLE HEALTH EFFECTS OF CONTAMINANTS IN CANNABIS

Because cannabis is an illegal drug, its cultivation, harvesting and distribution are not subject to quality control mechanisms to ensure the reliability and safety of the product used by consumers. It is well recognized in developing countries, such as Kenya, that illicit alcohol production can result in contamination with toxic by-products or adulterants that can kill or seriously affect the health of users. The same may be true of illicit drugs such as opiates, cocaine and amphetamine in developed societies.

There is no evidence that contaminants in cannabis produce comparable health effects, although there have been concerns about the possible effects of using cannabis contaminated by herbicides, such as paraquat, that were used to control illicit cannabis cultivation in the United States in the 1970s. These concerns have proved unfounded (Hollister, 1986). There have also been concerns about microbial or fungal contamination of cannabis leaf, and there are a number of reports of *Pneumocystis carinii* pneumonia and invasive pulmonary aspergillosis in cannabis smokers whose immune systems have been impaired by AIDS or by immunosuppressant drugs (Caiaffa, Vlahov et al., 1994; Denning, Follansbee et al., 1991; Hamadeh, Ardehali et al., 1988; Marks, Florence et al., 1996; Sutton, Lum & Torti, 1986).

Psychological Effects of Chronic Cannabis Use

Adult Motivation

A major concern about the psychological effects of chronic heavy cannabis use has been that it impairs adult motivation. Evidence for an "amotivational syndrome" among adults consists largely of case histories (e.g., Kolansky & Moore, 1971). The small number of controlled field and laboratory studies have not found compelling evidence for such a syndrome (Hollister, 1986), but these have been limited by their small sample sizes, and the restricted sociodemographic characteristics of their samples. The laboratory studies have involved short periods of sustained cannabis use, and made minimal demands on the healthy young volunteers (Cohen, 1982).

Some regular cannabis users report a loss of ambition and impaired school and occupational performance as adverse effects of their use (e.g., Hendin, Haas et al., 1987). Some heavy cannabis users have given impaired motivation and occupational performance as reasons for stopping (Jones, 1984). Nonetheless, it is doubtful that cannabis use produces a well-defined amotivational *syndrome*. It may be more parsimonious to regard the impaired motivation as a symptom of chronic cannabis intoxication (Hall, Solowij & Lemon, 1994).

Adolescent Development

In the United States in the 1970s and 1980s, cannabis use was associated with an increased risk of discontinuing a high school education and of experiencing job instability in young adulthood (e.g., Friedman, Granick et al., 1996; Newcombe & Bentler, 1988). These relationships are stronger in cross-sectional studies (e.g., Kandel, 1984) because those adolescents who are most likely to use cannabis have lower academic aspirations and poorer high school performance prior to using cannabis than peers who do not use cannabis (Fergusson & Horwood, 1997; Newcombe & Bentler, 1988). Although it remains possible that factors other than the marijuana use account for the relationship, a small association remains after controlling for pre-existing risk factors (Fergusson & Horwood, 1997).

A major finding of research on adolescent cannabis use has been the regular sequence of initiation into the use of illicit drugs among American adolescents in the 1970s (Donovan & Jessor, 1983; Kandel, 1984; Yamaguchi & Kandel, 1984a; 1984b) and the 1980s (Kandel & Yamaguchi, 1993). In this sequence, alcohol and tobacco use preceded cannabis use, which in turn preceded involvement with "harder" drugs such as stimulants and opioids.

The causal significance of this sequence of initiation into drug use remains controversial. The hypothesis that the sequence reflects a direct effect of cannabis use on the use of the later drugs in the sequence is the least compelling. There is better support for two other hypotheses which are not mutually exclusive. The first is that there is a selective recruitment into early cannabis use of non-conforming adolescents who have a propensity to use other illicit drugs. The second is that once recruited to cannabis use, social interaction with other drug-using peers and exposure to other drugs when purchasing cannabis on the black-market, increases the opportunity to use other illicit drugs (Baumrind, 1983; Fergusson & Horwood, 1997).

A Dependence Syndrome

A cannabis dependence syndrome can occur in heavy chronic users of cannabis (American Psychiatric Association, 1994). There is good experimental evidence that chronic heavy cannabis users can develop tolerance to its subjective and cardiovascular effects (Compton, Dewey & Martin, 1990). There is also suggestive evidence that some users may experience a withdrawal syndrome on the abrupt cessation of cannabis use, although one that is much milder and less marked than that experienced when withdrawing from alcohol or opiates (Compton, Dewey & Martin, 1990). The *Diagnostic and Statistical Manual of Mental Disorders, Fourth Edition*, notes that "symptoms of possible cannabis withdrawal (e.g., irritable or anxious mood accompanied by physical changes such as tremor, perspiration, nausea and sleep disturbances) have been described in association with the use of very high doses, but their clinical significance is uncertain" (*DSM-IV*, p. 215).

There is clinical and epidemiological evidence that some heavy cannabis users experience problems in controlling their cannabis use and continue to use the drug despite experiencing adverse personal consequences of use (Jones, 1984; Roffman, Stephens et al, 1988; Stephens & Roffman, 1993). There is also evidence for a cannabis dependence syndrome analogous to the alcohol dependence syndrome (Kosten, Rounsaville et al., 1987). Epidemiological surveys of the prevalence of drug dependence in the general population (e.g., Anthony & Helzer, 1991; Anthony, Warner & Kessler, 1994) indicate that cannabis dependence, as defined in the diagnostic manuals, is among the most common forms of drug dependence in Western societies by virtue of its high prevalence of use. On the other hand, relatively few users seek treatment for cannabis dependence (*DSM-IV,* pp. 220–221).

Cognitive Effects

The available evidence suggests that long-term heavy use of cannabis does not produce any severe or grossly debilitating impairment of cognitive function (Carter, Coggins & Doughty, 1980; Fehr & Kalant, 1983; Rubin & Comitas, 1975; Wert & Raulin, 1986). If it did, research to date should have detected it (Hall, Solowij & Lemon, 1994).

There is some clinical and experimental evidence, however, that the long-term use of cannabis may produce more subtle cognitive impairment in the higher cognitive functions of memory, attention and organization, and the integration of complex information (Fletcher, Page et al., 1996; Pope & Yurgelun-Todd, 1996; Solowij, Michie & Fox, 1991; 1995) (see chapter 6 in this volume). While subtle, these impairments may affect everyday functioning, particularly among individuals in occupations that require high levels of cognitive capacity. The evidence suggests that the longer the period that cannabis has been used, the more pronounced is the cognitive impairment (Solowij, Michie & Fox, 1991; 1995). It remains to be seen whether

the impairment can be reversed by an extended period of abstinence from cannabis.

Brain Damage

A suspicion that chronic heavy cannabis use may cause gross structural brain damage was prompted by a poorly controlled study which reported that cannabis users had enlarged cerebral ventricles (Campbell, Evans et al., 1971). Since then, a number of better-controlled studies using more sophisticated methods of investigation have consistently failed to demonstrate evidence of structural change in the brains of heavy long-term cannabis users (e.g., Co, Goodwin et al., 1977; Kuehnle, Mendelson & David, 1977). These negative results are consistent with the evidence that any cognitive effects of chronic cannabis use are subtle, and hence unlikely to be manifest as gross structural changes in the brain.

Psychoses

There is clinical evidence that large doses of THC can produce an acute psychosis in which confusion, amnesia, delusions, hallucinations, anxiety, agitation and hypomanic symptoms predominate. The evidence comes from laboratory studies of the effects of THC on normal volunteers and clinical observations of psychotic symptoms in heavy cannabis users which remit rapidly following abstinence (Chopra & Smith, 1974) (see chapter 7 in this volume).

There is less support for the hypothesis that cannabis use can cause either an acute or a chronic functional psychosis (Thornicroft, 1990). Such possibilities are difficult to study because of the rarity of such psychoses and because of the near impossibility of distinguishing them from schizophrenia and manic depressive psychoses occurring in individuals who also use cannabis (Ghodse, 1986).

There is evidence from a prospective study that heavy cannabis use may precipitate schizophrenia in vulnerable individuals (Andreasson, Allebeck et al., 1987; Schneier & Siris, 1987; Thornicroft, 1990). This relationship is still only strongly suggestive because the use of cannabis was not documented at the time of diagnosis, there was a possibility that cannabis use was confounded by amphetamine use, and there are doubts about whether the study could reliably distinguish between schizophrenia and acute cannabis, or other drug-induced, psychoses (Negrete, 1989; Thornicroft, 1990). There is good evidence that cannabis use can adversely affect the course of schizophrenia in affected individuals who continue to use it (Cleghorn, Kaplan et al., 1991; Jablensky, Sartorius et al., 1991; Linszen, Dingemans et al., 1994; Martinez-Arevalo, Calcedo-Ordonez & Varo-Prieto, 1994; Negrete, Knapp et al., 1986).

A Qualitative Comparison of the Health Risks of Alcohol, Cannabis, Nicotine and Opiate Use

In undertaking these qualitative comparisons we have avoided the necessity to review comprehensively the vast literature on the health effects of alcohol and tobacco by using the following authorities for our assertions about their health risks: the analysis of the health effects of alcohol, tobacco and illicit drugs by English et al. (1995); the Institute of Medicine (1982); the International Agency for Research into Cancer (1990); the Royal College of Physicians (1987); the U.S. Department of Health and Human Services (1989; 1997).

In the absence of an authoritative current review of the health effects of the opioids, it was necessary to use several sources. General pharmacological texts, and other reviews, were used to describe the pharmacological effects of the opioids (e.g., Belkin & Gold, 1991; Duggan & North, 1983; Jacobs & Fehr, 1987). Information on the chronic health effects and social consequences of illicit opiates (injectable and non-

injectable) and of methadone was taken from reports of several longitudinal studies of opioid users (e.g., Joe & Simpson, 1987; 1990; Maddux & Desmond, 1981; O'Donnell, 1969; Simpson, Joe et al., 1986; Vaillant, 1973). These cohort studies typically involve populations in contact with drug treatment services rather than representative samples of users.

Acute Effects

ALCOHOL

The major risks of acute cannabis use show some parallels with the acute risks of alcohol intoxication. First, both drugs produce psychomotor and cognitive impairment, especially of memory and planning. The impairment produced by alcohol increases risks of various kinds of accident. It may also increase the likelihood of engaging in risky behavior, such as dangerous driving, and unsafe sexual practices. While cannabis intoxication increases the risks of casualties in hazardous situations, it remains to be determined to what extent it increases the likelihood of engaging in risky behavior.

Alcohol and cannabis intoxication appear to differ in their relation to intentional rather than accidental casualties. Alcohol intoxication is strongly associated with aggressive and violent behavior. The relationship is complex, and the nature and extent of drinking's causal effect remains controversial at the level of the individual drinker (Martin, 1993; Pernanen, 1991; Pohorecky, Brick & Milgram, 1993). But there is good causal evidence to show that changes in the level of alcohol consumption affect the incidence of violent crime, at least in some populations (Cook & Moore, 1993; Lenke, 1990; Room, 1983). There is also increasing evidence that alcohol may play a role in suicide (Edwards, Ferrence et al., 1994). There is little to suggest a causal relationship of cannabis use to aggression or violence, at least in present-day developed societies.

Second, there is a major health risk of acute alcohol use that is not shared with cannabis. In large doses, alcohol can cause death by asphyxiation, alcohol poisoning, cardiomyopathy and cardiac infarct, whereas there are no recorded cases of overdose fatalities attributed to cannabis.

TOBACCO

The major acute health risks that cannabis shares with tobacco are the irritant effects of smoke upon the respiratory system, and the stimulating effects of THC and nicotine on the cardiovascular system that can be detrimental to persons with cardiovascular and respiratory diseases. For both drugs, the respiratory effects do not apply to oral ingestion.

OPIOIDS

Some of the opioids share with alcohol and cannabis an acute intoxicating effect, although the sedative effect is more pronounced. Acute administration of heroin causes euphoria in many users, although other opioids, such as methadone, do not have this effect in tolerant individuals. The extent of euphoria is also affected by route of administration. As is found with cannabis, some naive users report unpleasant feelings with opiate use, specifically nausea and dysphoria. All opioids are central nervous system depressants and as such can reduce level of consciousness and cause sleep.

The literature on the effects of opiates on driving and other exacting skills is not well developed. A maintenance dose in a tolerant user may produce little psychomotor or cognitive impairment. A heroin user who has reached a stage of "nodding" is in no condition to drive a car, but will probably have little inclination to do so. As with cannabis, there is little direct epidemiological evidence of opiate-induced casualties. One study showed that the driving-related skills of persons maintained on stable doses of methadone were not impaired when assessed on a laboratory task that is sensitive to the effects of alcohol (Chesher, Lemon et al., 1989).

While there is no risk of overdose associated with cannabis, use of illicit opioids carries a real risk of overdose. High doses of most opioids can lead to depression of breathing rate and blood pressure and cause respiratory arrest. The risk of overdose is worsened by use in combination with alcohol, cannabis or other drugs, and is thought to be worsened by variations in the potency of opiates obtained illegally (Darke & Zador, 1996).

Chronic Effects

ALCOHOL

There are a number of risks of heavy chronic alcohol use, some of which may be shared by chronic cannabis use. First, heavy use of either drug increases the risk of developing a dependence syndrome in which users experience difficulty in stopping or controlling their use. There is strong evidence of such a syndrome in the case of alcohol and reasonable evidence in the case of cannabis. A major difference between the two is that withdrawal symptoms are either absent or mild after dependent cannabis users abruptly stop their cannabis use. By contrast, the abrupt cessation of alcohol use in severely dependent drinkers produces a well-defined withdrawal syndrome which can be fatal in a small proportion of cases (Hall & Zador, 1997).

Second, there is reasonable clinical evidence that the chronic heavy use of alcohol can produce psychotic symptoms and psychoses in some individuals, either during acute intoxication or during the process of withdrawal in dependent drinkers. There is some clinical evidence that chronic heavy cannabis use may produce a toxic psychosis, prospective epidemiological evidence that heavy cannabis use may precipitate schizophrenia in individuals with a personal or a family history of psychiatric disorder, and stronger evidence that continued cannabis use may worsen the course of schizophrenia.

Third, there is good evidence that chronic heavy alcohol use can indirectly cause brain injury — the Wernicke-Korsakov syndrome — with symptoms of severe memory defect and an impaired ability to plan and organize. With continued heavy drinking, and in the absence of vitamin supplementation, this injury may produce severe irreversible cognitive impairment. There is good reason for concluding that chronic cannabis use does not produce cognitive impairment of comparable severity. There is suggestive evidence that chronic cannabis use may produce subtle defects in cognitive functioning, which may or may not be reversible after abstinence.

Fourth, there is reasonable evidence that chronic heavy alcohol use generally impairs occupational performance in adults and educational achievements in adolescents. There is suggestive evidence that chronic heavy cannabis use produces similar, albeit more subtle, impairments in the occupational and educational performance of adults (Kandel, Davies et al., 1986; Newcombe & Bentler, 1988).

Fifth, there is good evidence that chronic heavy alcohol use increases the risk of premature mortality from accidents, suicide and violence. There is no comparable evidence for chronic cannabis use, although it is likely that dependent cannabis users who frequently drive while intoxicated with cannabis would increase their risk of accidental injury or death.

Sixth, alcohol use has been accepted as a contributory cause of cancer in various tissues and organs of the digestive system and of female breast cancer. There is suggestive clinical evidence that chronic cannabis smoking may also be a contributory cause of cancers of the aerodigestive tract.

Seventh, alcohol use is a major cause of liver cirrhosis. Heavy drinking is also implicated in gastritis, high blood pressure, stroke, cardiac arrhythmias, cardiomyopathy, pancreatitis and polyneuropathy. On the other hand, regular light alcohol use is associated with a reduction in the risk of heart disease that is of considerable public health significance in societies with high rates of heart disease. No equivalent adverse or protective effects have been reported for cannabis. There is some evidence that some cannabinoids may be therapeutically useful for appetite stimulation and as anti-emetics in patients undergoing cancer therapy (Hall, Solowij & Lemon, 1994) (see chapter 14 in this volume).

Eighth, there is good evidence that substantial doses of alcohol taken during pregnancy can produce a fetal alcohol syndrome. There is suggestive but far from conclusive evidence that cannabis can also adversely affect the development of the fetus, when used during pregnancy. A clear equivalent for cannabis of the fetal alcohol syndrome has not been established.

TOBACCO

The major adverse health effects shared by chronic cannabis and tobacco smokers are chronic respiratory diseases, such as chronic bronchitis, and probably, cancers of the aerodigestive tract (i.e., the mouth, tongue, throat, esophagus, lungs). The increased risk of cancer in the aerodigestive tract is a consequence of the shared route of administration by smoking. It is possible that chronic cannabis smoking also shares the cardiotoxic properties of tobacco smoking, although this possibility remains to be investigated. These respiratory risks could be avoided by a change to the oral route of administration, which would also reduce but not eliminate the cardiovascular risks.

Tobacco smoking is associated with a wide variety of other chronic health conditions for which cannabis smoking has not so far been implicated. These include cancer of the cervix, stomach, bladder and kidney, coronary heart disease, peripheral vascular disease and stroke, as well as cataracts and osteoporosis.

OPIOIDS

The specific health effects of opioid use largely depend on the route of administration. The use of injectable opiates carries risks not common to alcohol, tobacco or cannabis, especially when associated with illegally obtained injectables and shared needles. Injecting heroin or morphine can lead to trauma, inflammation and infection at the site of administration. Liver damage in opiate addicts may be caused by viral hepatitis contracted through needle sharing or from chronic alcohol abuse. Serious infection such as endocarditis is also possible. Local tissue and organ damage may also result from the adulterants in injection drugs obtained on the street (Belkin & Gold, 1991). Intravenous drug use is a major concern for the transmission of communicable diseases such as viral hepatitis and AIDS.

Chronic use of non-injected opioids appears to carry little risk of adverse health effects other than a modest effect on endocrine activity, some suppression of the immune system which has similar implications to the immune suppression associated with cannabis use, and chronic constipation.

While it is unclear that a withdrawal syndrome exists for cannabis, physical dependence on opiates has been recognized for centuries. Opiate withdrawal is associated with considerable discomfort but is rarely life-threatening. Despite the low risk, avoidance of withdrawal appears to be a powerful motive for continued use of opiates among very heavy users (Mattick & Hall, 1996).

Chronic opioid users may experience instability of mood, anorexia, lethargy and depression, which are related to acute drug effects. Opioids have not been causally linked to chronic psychiatric disorders, but street addicts have a shortened life expectancy and experience social and emotional problems more frequently. This is in part due to their exposure to infection, violence and poor living conditions rather than their drug use.

Opioids, like cannabis, cause some suppression of hormone levels. These decreased hormonal levels, however, do not necessarily result in infertility in men or women using opioids for extended periods (Belkin & Gold, 1991; Duggan & North, 1983; Martin & Martin, 1980). Like alcohol, tobacco and cannabis, the opiates have been associated with miscarriage, fetal death and low birthweight. There is no clear relationship with an identifiable syndrome of fetal defects from opioids that parallels fetal alcohol syndrome. Although poor nutrition and prenatal care clearly contribute to the risk of adverse outcomes in pregnant women addicted to street drugs, even methadone maintenance has been found to result in higher rates of pregnancy problems. Methadone and other orally administered opioids have been shown to cause fetal death and low birthweight in laboratory animals (Caviston, 1987; Martin & Martin, 1980; Woody & O'Brien, 1991).

Summarizing the Effects

Table 1 is an attempt to summarize in rough form our assessment of the main adverse affects of regular heavy use of the most harmful form of each type of drug, as commonly used for non-medical purposes in developed societies. For tobacco and marijuana, this means the smoked form; for alcohol, distilled spirits; for opiates, injected heroin. By "heavy use," we are referring to regular use of substantial doses, within the general limits of *present levels of use* in developed societies. The table does not consider potential beneficial health effects of each drug.

The table distinguishes in rough terms between effects that are important (marked **) in terms of the numbers of heavy users who are

TABLE 1.

Comparing Adverse Effects on Health for Heavy Users of the Most Harmful Common Form of Each Substance: A First Approximation

	Marijuana	Alcohol	Tobacco	Heroin
Traffic and other accidents	*	**		*
Violence and suicide		**		
Overdose death		*		**
HIV and liver infections		*		**
Liver cirrhosis		**		
Heart disease		*	**	
Respiratory diseases	*		**	
Cancers	*	*	**	
Mental illness	*	**		
Dependence/addiction	**	**	**	**
Lasting effects on the fetus	*	**	*	*

* less common or less well-established effect
** important effect

affected, and effects that are less well established or less important numerically (marked *).

The entries in the table are necessarily a matter of judgment, and expert opinions differ on some of them. We present the table as a first approximation and as a stimulus to further epidemiological work and analyses to put such comparisions on a firmer basis in the future.

Clearly, a heavy user of each of the four compared drug categories risks harm to his or her health on multiple fronts, but there are differences in the profiles of health harm for the different drugs. Whole categories of health harm that are important for some drugs are not important for others.

All four of the drugs were judged to produce dependence or addiction to some degree. More detailed judgments can be made on the psychoactive and addictive effects of different drugs, drawing on experimental and other data. Table 2 shows the rankings made by two U.S. experts, Neal Benowitz and Jack Henningfield, on five dimensions relevant to the capacity of each drug to produce addiction and casualties (Hilts, 1995). These are *comparative* ratings so a lower ranking in the table does not necessarily mean that the drug has no significant effects on that dimension.

As we have noted above, for instance, all four drugs have important effects on the "dependence" dimension. Again, experts differ with the rankings in the table, which is offered simply as a stimulus to further research and analysis.

Comparing the Magnitude of Risks

The standard measures of the magnitude of health risks are relative risk and population attributable risk (which is a function of the relative risk and the prevalence of drug use). An appraisal of the personal and public health importance of cannabis and other drug use must take account of the relative risk of harm, the prevalence of use and the base rate of the adverse effect.

The Relative Risks of Adverse Health Effects of Cannabis Use

Many of the quantitative risks of cannabis use can only be guessed at in the absence of studies of the dose-response relationship between cannabis use and the various adverse health effects.

TABLE 2.
Comparative Ratings of the Dependence Potential of Marijuana, Alcohol, Tobacco and Heroin: The Opinions of Two Experts (Hilts, 1995)

	Marijuana	Alcohol	Tobacco	Heroin
Withdrawal: presence and severity of withdrawal symptoms	4	1	3	2
Reinforcement: capacity to get human or animal users to use again and again, in preference to other substances	4	2	3	1
Tolerance: how much more needed by a regular user to get the same effect	4	3*	2*	1
Dependence: difficulty quitting and avoiding relapse, perceived need to use; use persisting despite harm	4	3	1	2
Intoxication: impairment of motor abilities, distortion of thinking and mood	3	1	4	2

Note: These rankings are the opinions of Neal Benowitz and Jack Henningfield and do not represent a consensus of expert opinion.
* minor disagreement in rankings

The following are our own rough estimates of the risks of cannabis use for the most probable adverse health effects. When in doubt we have assumed that the relative risks of cannabis use are comparable to the relevant risks of alcohol or tobacco.

MOTOR VEHICLE ACCIDENTS

If we assume that driving while intoxicated with cannabis produces a comparable increase in the risk of accidents to that produced by driving while intoxicated with alcohol (say with a blood alcohol level of 0.05 per cent to 0.10 per cent), then the relative risk (RR) of an accident while intoxicated would be in the range of 2 to 4. The fact that alcohol and cannabis are often used in combination complicates the task of estimating the relative risk of cannabis use alone to motor vehicle accidents.

RESPIRATORY DISEASES

If we assume that a daily cannabis user who smokes five or more joints per day faces a comparable risk of respiratory disease to that of a 20-a-day tobacco smoker, then the RR of developing chronic bronchitis would be 6 or greater for those who had ever smoked cannabis, and substantially higher among those who had been daily cannabis smokers over many years and those who also smoked tobacco (English, Holman et al., 1995).

RESPIRATORY TRACT CANCERS

If we make the same worst case assumptions about daily cannabis smoking, then the relative risks of various cancers of the respiratory tract would be of the order of: 4.6 for oropharangeal cancer, 4 for esophageal cancer, and 7 for lung cancer (English, Holman et al., 1995). Again, these risks would be substantially higher among cannabis smokers who also smoked tobacco, but would be minimal for ingested cannabis use.

LOW BIRTHWEIGHT BABIES

Making a worst case assumption in the absence of good data, a woman who smokes cannabis during pregnancy approximately doubles her chance of giving birth to a low birthweight baby (English, Holman et al., 1995).

SCHIZOPHRENIA

This is one of the few health consequences for which there is quantitative estimate of relative risk. If we use the estimated RR from the study by Andreasson et al. (1987) after adjustment for confounding variables, then an adolescent who had smoked cannabis 50 or more times by age 18 would have approximately a two to three times higher risk of developing schizophrenia than an adolescent who had not been a cannabis smoker.

DEPENDENCE

Since cannabis use is a necessary condition of developing dependence, the best way of quantifying the risk of dependence is to estimate the proportion of those who have ever used cannabis, or those who have had a history of daily use who become dependent on the drug. A variety of estimates have been derived from U.S. studies in the late 1970s and early 1980s, which defined cannabis use and dependence in a variety of ways. These studies suggested that between 10 and 20 per cent of those who have ever used cannabis, and between 33 and 50 per cent of those who have had a history of daily cannabis use, showed symptoms of cannabis dependence (see Hall, Solowij & Lemon, 1994). A more recent and better estimate of the risk of meeting *DSM-III-R* criteria for cannabis dependence was obtained from data collected in the National Comorbidity Study (Anthony, Warner & Kessler, 1994). This indicated that 9 per cent of lifetime cannabis users met *DSM-III-R* criteria for dependence at some time in their life, compared to 32 per cent of tobacco users, 23 per cent of opiate users and 15 per cent of alcohol users.

SUMMARY

From the perspective of the individual cannabis user, the major health risks of cannabis use are, with one exception, most likely to be experienced by those who smoke the drug daily over a period of years. These are in probable order of decreasing prevalence: developing a cannabis dependence syndrome, developing chronic bronchitis, and being involved in a motor vehicle accident if driving while intoxicated. In all these cases, the risk will be increased if cannabis is combined with either alcohol or tobacco or both. The risk most likely to be experienced by the occasional user is an increased risk of a motor vehicle accident if used when driving a car, especially if cannabis is combined with alcohol.

Public Health Significance

MOTOR VEHICLE ACCIDENTS

An assessment of the public health significance of motor vehicle accidents caused by cannabis is made difficult by the strong association between cannabis and alcohol use. The epidemiological studies indicate that in its own right, cannabis makes at most a very small contribution to motor vehicle accidents, and so, on the whole, it may seem to be a minor road safety problem by comparison with alcohol. Its major public health significance for road safety may be in amplifying the adverse effects of alcohol in the majority of drivers who drive when intoxicated by alcohol and cannabis.

RESPIRATORY DISEASES

The public health significance of respiratory diseases caused by cannabis smoking is probably greater than that for respiratory cancers. This is for two reasons. First, respiratory cancers require a greater length of exposure to cigarette smoke (15 to 20 years) than is required to develop chronic bronchitis. Second, as few as 7 per cent of cannabis users use daily for more than five years (Kandel & Davies, 1992). "Spells of near daily use" were reported by 44 per cent of young American marijuana users, usually beginning around age 19 and continuing into their early twenties. By age 29, 85 per cent of those who have ever been near-daily marijuana users had not used daily for six years on average (Kandel & Davies, 1992). The exposure period required to develop chronic bronchitis is probably shorter among those cannabis smokers who also smoke tobacco, since concurrent tobacco and cannabis smoking appear to have additive adverse effects on the respiratory system. On current patterns of use, the contribution that cannabis makes to respiratory diseases is more likely to be reflected in morbidity than mortality.

RESPIRATORY TRACT CANCERS

If we make the worst case assumption that the risks of cancer are comparable among daily tobacco and cannabis smokers, then cannabis smoking will make at most a small contribution to the occurrence of these cancers, at least on the basis of current patterns of use in developed societies. This is because only a minority of those who ever use cannabis become daily users, and a much smaller proportion of these daily users persist in smoking cannabis beyond their middle twenties by comparison with the proportions of tobacco smokers who do so (Bachman, Wadsworth et al., 1997). Among this minority, concurrent cannabis and tobacco use may amplify each other's adverse respiratory effects.

LOW BIRTHWEIGHT BABIES

Again making a worst case assumption, cannabis smoking during pregnancy may double the risks of a woman giving birth to a low birthweight baby. The public health significance is likely to be much lower than that of tobacco smoking during pregnancy, because the prevalence of cannabis use is likely to be much lower. Although fetal exposure to cannabis smoke may be relatively low, the risks of a low birthweight baby will be even higher among those women who also smoke tobacco, as do most of those who smoke cannabis during pregnancy.

SCHIZOPHRENIA

As argued elsewhere, there is uncertainty about whether the association observed between cannabis use and schizophrenia reflects a causal relationship (Hall, Solowij & Lemon, 1994). If we assume that the relationship is causal, on the data of Andreasson et al., cannabis use would account for a little less than 10 per cent of new cases of schizophrenia. Even this figure seems unlikely, however, since the incidence of schizophrenia has probably declined during the period when cannabis use among adolescents and young adults has increased (Der, Gupta & Murray, 1990).

DEPENDENCE

Cannabis dependence is potentially a more prevalent outcome than any of the other potentially adverse health effects of cannabis. On the epidemiological catchment area (ECA) estimates, approximately 4 per cent of the adult U.S. population met diagnostic criteria for cannabis abuse or dependence, as against 14 per cent who met diagnostic criteria for alcohol abuse and dependence. This is a non-trivial proportion of the population, although its consequences are somewhat ameliorated because there is probably a high rate of remission of symptoms in the absence of treatment.

OVERALL PUBLIC HEALTH SIGNIFICANCE

Overall, in our view most of these risks are small to moderate in size. In aggregate they are unlikely to produce public health problems comparable in scale to those currently produced by alcohol and tobacco. This is largely because on current patterns of use in developed societies, the proportion of the population that uses cannabis heavily over a period of years is much smaller than the proportions that use alcohol or tobacco in a comparable way (Hall, 1995).

A direct estimation of the contribution to the global burden of disease from 10 major risk factors, including alcohol, tobacco and all illicit drugs together, has been made by Murray and Lopez (1996). Of the total global loss of disability-adjusted life-years (DALYs) due to disease and injury, the study estimated that 3.5 per cent was due to alcohol, 2.6 per cent to tobacco, and 0.6 per cent to all illicit drugs (p. 311). In six of the eight world regions used in the study's analysis, both tobacco and alcohol outranked illicit drugs in DALYs. Illicit drugs outranked alcohol in the Middle Eastern region, and outranked tobacco in the Latin American region (pp. 312–315). However, the authors caution that "because of

the great difficulty in reliably estimating prevalence of illicit drug use, and of reliably quantifying its health effects, the estimates for this risk factor may well be too low" (p. 310).

A comparative estimate of the health costs from alcohol, tobacco and marijuana has been made for the Canadian province of Ontario in 1992. In a study of the economic costs of alcohol, tobacco and illicit drug abuse in Ontario, the direct health care costs attributable to alcohol were estimated at $442 million, while those attributable to tobacco were $1,073 million, and those to *all* illicit drugs were $39 million (Xie, Rehm et al., 1996). The portion of the illicit drug costs attributable to marijuana was $8 million (Addiction Research Foundation, 1997). Such analyses leave little doubt that on current patterns of use, alcohol and tobacco cause much more public health harm in developed societies than marijuana.

Studies like these strongly suggest that alcohol and tobacco presently far outrank marijuana in terms of their contribution to the global burden of disease, death and disability.

Predicting the Effects of Changes in the Prevalence of Cannabis Use

The comparison of the public health impacts of cannabis with those of alcohol, opiates and tobacco was based upon existing patterns of use of each of these drugs. This analysis cannot be used to predict what would happen if there was a major change in the prevalence of cannabis use, as may happen if existing criminal penalties were replaced with civil penalties, or if cannabis were to become as freely available and as heavily promoted as alcohol and tobacco.

In principle, it would seem a simple matter to estimate what the health risks of cannabis use would be if its prevalence of use were to approach that of alcohol or tobacco. Although conceptually a simple matter, a number of questionable assumptions would have to be made. The most questionable assumption would be that the public health consequences of increased cannabis use would simply be the product of the current patterns of use multiplied by the ratio of the new to old users. Such a calculation would assume that the risks were the same regardless of the characteristics of the user or the legal regime under which the drug was used.

These assumptions may be unreasonable. Cannabis may be used by a different population when its prevalence of use is low than when it is high. This phenomenon has been reported with alcohol, for example, with different patterns of alcohol consumption and problems in "dry" and "wet" cultures (Mäkelä, Room et al., 1981). If adult use were legalized, it might also be easier to reduce some of these health risks, for example, by encouraging cannabis users to ingest rather than to smoke the drug, or by increasing the THC content and reducing the tar content of marijuana, for those who continue to smoke. Decriminalizing cannabis for adult use would also increase use by adolescents, the health effects of which would be very difficult to predict. Estimating the net effects of harm reduction efforts in adults and increased adolescent use would be difficult.

For these reasons, we have not attempted to provide quantitative estimates of the health risks of cannabis if its prevalence of use were to approach those of alcohol and tobacco. All that can be said with confidence is that if the prevalence of cannabis use increased to the levels of cigarette smoking and alcohol use, its public health impact would increase. It is impossible to say by how much with any precision.

The reasons for this uncertainty operate in both directions. On the one hand, unlike alcohol, cannabis does not produce cirrhosis, and in developed societies it appears to play little role in injuries caused by violence, as does alcohol. Unlike tobacco, all the evidence suggests that the proportion of cannabis smokers who become daily smokers is substantially less than the proportion of tobacco smokers who do so. It is unlikely that the proportion of cannabis users who become very heavy users would ever be as high in industrial societies as it is for tobacco, since the heavy use of tobacco fits more easily

into the rhythms of daily life than heavy alcohol or cannabis use. On the other hand, it is unlikely that *all* the adverse health effects of cannabis use have been identified, and so far there is no evidence that cannabis has the protective cardiovascular benefits that moderate alcohol use appears to have.

Some Direct Comparative Evidence on Consequences: What Users Report

To a limited extent, epidemiological data are available on the adverse consequences that users attribute to their drug use. Since this data has not been collated and reviewed, we summarize some of it here. These data should be interpreted with caution. And it should be recognized that the range of consequences considered here reaches far beyond the bounds of the clinically significant physical and mental illnesses that are our focus elsewhere in this chapter.

In a large sample of U.S. men, aged 20 to 30 years, interviewed in 1974 (see Table 3), a higher proportion of tobacco smokers rated the effects of their use as bad, and more drinkers of alcohol gave a bad than a good rating. Good ratings outweighed bad for marijuana users. In a survey of Ontario adults in 1994 (see Table 3), current users aged 18 to 34 gave a similarly negative weighting to tobacco, but gave alcohol a relatively more favorable weighting. Again, marijuana users were the most likely to give a favorable rating.

In another Ontario survey in 1992, current users were asked whether their use of a drug had a harmful effect on different aspects of their life in the past 12 months. Table 4 shows the results for users of alcohol, tobacco and marijuana, and also for heavier or more frequent users of each drug: drinkers who drank five or more drinks on an occasion at least once a month, marijuana users who smoked at least once a month and tobacco smokers who smoked at least 11 cigarettes a day. Tobacco smokers were more likely than marijuana or alcohol users to report harm to their physical health, to their finances and to

TABLE 3.

Summary of Ratings of Overall Effect of Drug Use by Current Users (%)

United States 1974: Males aged 20–30
O'Donnell et al. (1976)

Ontario 1994: Both sexes aged 18–34
Retabulated data from study reported in Paglia (1995)

	Lifetime users of:				Current users of:		
Responses	Alcohol	Tobacco	Marijuana or hashish	Responses	Alcohol	Tobacco	Marijuana or hashish
Total N	(2434)	(2211)	(1382)	Total N	(601)	(256)	(121)
"Very good" or "more good than bad"	33	12	45	More good than harm	19	3	29
No effect	21	22	22	Harm and good about equal	70	47	59
"More bad than good" or "very bad"	46	66	33	More harm than good	11	50	12

TABLE 4.

Types of Problems Reported in the Past 12 Months by Current Users Age 18–34 (Ontario 1992)

[In the past 12 months] Was there ever a time that your use of ____ had a harmful effect on your...?	ALCOHOL			TOBACCO			CANNABIS		
		Frequency 5+			Cigs/day			Frequency of use	
	Total	0–11	12+ times in year	Total	0–11	11+	Total	less than monthly	1+ times per month
Total N	338	255	77	126	44	82	42	19	24
Friendship or social life	5	3	11	18	20	17	7	–	12
Physical health	10	4	21	58	60	56	11	1	20
Home life or marriage	4	1	9	10	8	10	11	2	18
Work, studies or employment opportunities	4	1	8	7	8	6	7	–	12
Financial situation	6	3	12	43	26	52	14	–	24
One or more	17	9	35	69	63	72	28	4	47
Two or more	6	2	18	39	26	47	8	–	14

Note: Retabulated data from study by Ferris et al. (1993).
0 indicates a percentage between .1 and .4. Cells that actually had no responses are indicated as "–".

their friendships or social life, among both lighter and heavier users. The small number of regular marijuana users seemed more likely than heavier drinkers to report harm to their home life or marriage and to their finances. On other comparisons, the proportions reporting harm were fairly similar.

In the 1991 U.S. National Household Survey on Drug Abuse, large samples of current tobacco, alcohol and marijuana users were asked comparable questions about 11 consequences of use. Marijuana users were a little more likely to report consequences (15.5 per cent reporting any of the 11 consequences) than alcohol users (11.4 per cent) or cigarette smokers (11.2 per cent). If these rates are multiplied by the prevalence of use of each drug, then 1.9 per cent of the population reported consequences of marijuana use, 7.2 per cent reported consequences of drinking and 3.4 per cent reported consequences of cigarette smoking. Marijuana users reported noticeably higher rates on four items: "became depressed or lost interest in things," "found it difficult to think clearly," "got less work done than usual at school or on the job," and "felt suspicious and mistrustful of people." Drinkers reported higher rates of "arguments and fights with family or friends" and "found it difficult to think clearly." Cigarette smokers reported higher rates of "felt very nervous and anxious" and "had health problems" (SAMHSA, 1993, Table 9.2).

Great caution must be used in interpreting such comparisons. In the first place, the base of users is different for each drug. Those using a widely used drug are likely to differ on salient characteristics from those using a more rarely used drug. Second, the reported consequence may not be seen by the respondents themselves as adverse. For instance, if the purpose of use is intoxication, it may not be seen as a problem that the respondent "found it difficult to think clearly." Third, responses are likely to be influenced by cultural beliefs about causal connections. The high proportion of young adult smokers who reported that smoking has harmed their health may reflect acceptance of conventional wisdom as much as personal experience. Fourth and most important, the connection between drug use and adverse consequences will be influenced by a variety of factors applying differentially to different drugs. In particular, a drug's illegal status can create adverse consequences for the user, not only directly, through arrest, but also indirectly, in the form of "harm to home life" from the adverse reactions by others to the drug use that involves a risk of arrest.

Keeping these caveats in mind, it is clear that a minority of marijuana users do report harm from their smoking, and some would be likely to do so even if cannabis were legalized. In an era where the health consequences of tobacco smoking are well recognized, tobacco smokers seem to be more likely than users of either cannabis or alcohol to regard their use as doing more harm than good in their lives, and the good is seen as outweighing the bad more often by cannabis smokers than by drinkers or tobacco smokers. In the present-day North America, cannabis smokers are at least as likely as alcohol drinkers to report adverse consequences of their use. But the higher rate for alcohol of "arguments and fights with family or friends" reminds us of the special potential alcohol consumption has to have harmful effects on others. Given current patterns of use, when rates of consequences are projected to the proportion of the whole population that use each drug, the consequences of alcohol and tobacco use are clearly of greater public health significance than the consequences of marijuana use.

Conclusion

There are health risks of cannabis use, especially when it is used daily over a period of years or decades. Considerable uncertainty remains about whether these effects are attributable to cannabis use alone, and about the quantitative relationship between frequency, quantity and duration of cannabis use, and the risk of experiencing these effects. Using estimates of the magnitude of the known effects of alcohol and tobacco, the most probable of the health risks of chronic heavy cannabis use over a period of years are: the development of a dependence syndrome; an increased risk of being involved in motor vehicle accidents; an increased risk of developing chronic bronchitis; an increased risk of respiratory cancers; an increased risk of giving birth to low-birthweight babies when used during pregnancy; and perhaps, an increased risk of developing schizophrenia among those who are vulnerable. Many of these risks are shared with alcohol and tobacco, which is not surprising given that cannabis is an intoxicant like alcohol, and is typically smoked like tobacco.

On *current patterns of use,* cannabis appears to pose a much less serious public health problem than is currently posed by alcohol and tobacco in Western societies. This is no cause for complacency, however, as the public health significance of alcohol and tobacco are major, and the public health significance of cannabis would undoubtedly increase if the prevalence of its heavy daily use were to approach that of heavy alcohol use among young adults, or the prevalence of daily cigarette smoking among adults.

This comparative analysis, which was undertaken at the request of the WHO Committee on the Health Implications of Cannabis Use, proved difficult and controversial. The analysis was hindered by a dearth of epidemiological studies of the health consequences of cannabis use that would permit quantitative comparisons. Our approach was perforce primarily qualitative. The comparisons also identified gaps in the literature, and hence priorities for further research. We expect that our analysis will be transcended by new and more exact comparative analyses, in the normal way of science, as better data become available.

References

Abel, E.L. (1985). Effects of prenatal exposure to cannabinoids. In T.M. Pinkert (Ed.), *Current Research on the Consequences of Maternal Drug Abuse* (NIDA Research Monograph No. 59, pp. 20–35). Washington, D.C.: U.S. Government Printing Office.

Addiction Research Foundation. (1997). *Cannabis, Health and Public Policy*. Toronto: Addiction Research Foundation.

American Psychiatric Association. (1987). *Diagnostic and Statistical Manual of Mental Disorders* (3rd ed., rev.). Washington, DC: American Psychiatric Association.

American Psychiatric Association. (1994). *Diagnostic and Statistical Manual of Mental Disorders* (4th ed.). Washington, DC: American Psychiatric Association.

Andreasson, S. & Allebeck, P. (1990). Cannabis and mortality among young men: A longitudinal study of Swedish conscripts. *Scandinavian Journal of Social Medicine, 18*, 9–15.

Andreasson, S., Allebeck, P., Engstrom, A. & Rydberg, U. (1987). Cannabis and schizophrenia: A longitudinal study of Swedish conscripts. *Lancet, 2*, 1483–1486.

Andreasson, S., Allebeck, P. & Rydberg, U. (1989). Schizophrenia in users and nonusers of cannabis. *Acta Psychiatrica Scandinavica, 79*, 505–510.

Anthony, J.C. & Helzer, J.E. (1991). Syndromes of drug abuse and dependence. In L.N. Robins & D.A. Regier (Eds.), *Psychiatric Disorders in America* (pp. 116–154). New York: Free Press.

Anthony, J.C., Warner, L.A. & Kessler, R.C. (1994). Comparative epidemiology of dependence on tobacco, alcohol, controlled substances and inhalants: Basic findings from the National Comorbidity Study. *Clinical and Experimental Psychopharmacology, 2*, 244–268.

Bachman, J.G., Wadsworth, K.N., O'Malley, P.M., Johnston, L.D. & Schulenberg, J.E. (Eds.). (1997). *Smoking, Drinking and Drug Use in Young Adulthood*. Mahwah, NJ: Erlbaum.

Baldwin, G.C., Tashkin, D.P., Buckley, D.M., Park, A.N., Dubinett, S.M. & Roth, M.D. (1997). Habitual smoking of marijuana and cocaine impairs alveolar macrophage function and cytokine production. *American Journal of Respiratory and Critical Care Medicine, 156*, 1606–1613.

Baumrind, D. (1983). Specious causal attribution in the social sciences: The reformulated stepping stone hypothesis as exemplar. *Journal of Personality and Social Psychology, 45*, 1289–1298.

Belkin, B.M. & Gold, M.S. (1991). Opioids. In N.S. Miller (Ed.), *Comprehensive Handbook of Drug and Alcohol Addiction* (pp. 537–547). New York: Marcel Dekker.

Bloch, E. (1983). Effects of marijuana and cannabinoids on reproduction, endocrine function, development and chromosomes. In K.O. Fehr & H. Kalant (Eds.), *Cannabis and Health Hazards* (pp. 355–432). Toronto: Addiction Research Foundation.

Bloom, J.W., Kaltenborn, W.T., Paoletti, P., Camilli, A. & Lebowitz, M.D. (1987). Respiratory effects of non-tobacco cigarettes. *British Medical Journal, 295*, 1516–1518.

Caiaffa, W.T., Vlahov, D., Graham, N.M., Astemborski, J., Solomon, L., Nelson, K.E. & Muñoz, A. (1994). Drug smoking, Pneumocystis carinii pneumonia, and immuno-suppression increase risk of bacterial pneumonia in human immuno-deficiency virus-seropositive injection drug users. *American Journal of Respiratory and Critical Care Medicine, 150*, 1493–1489.

Campbell, A.M.G., Evans, M., Thomson, J.L.G. & Williams, M.J. (1971). Cerebral atrophy in young cannabis smokers. *Lancet, 2*, 1219–1224.

Caplan, G.A. & Brigham, B.A. (1990). Marijuana smoking and carcinoma of the tongue. Is there an association? *Cancer, 66*, 1005–1006.

Carter, W.E., Coggins, W. & Doughty, P.L. (1980). *Cannabis in Costa Rica: A study of chronic marihuana use*. Philadelphia: Institute for the Study of Human Issues.

Caviston, P. (1987). Pregnancy and opiate addiction. *British Medical Journal, 295*, 285–286.

Chait, L.D. & Pierri, J. (1992). Effects of smoked marijuana on human performance: A critical review. In L. Murphy & J. Bartke (Eds.), *Marijuana/Cannabinoids: Neurobiology and Neurophysiology* (pp. 387–423). Boca Raton, FL: CRC Press.

Chesher, G., Lemon, J., Gomel, M. & Murphy, G. (1989). *The Effects of Methadone, as Used in a Methadone Maintenance Program, on Driving-related Skills* (National Drug and Alcohol Research Centre Technical Report No. 3). Sydney: National Drug and Alcohol Research Centre.

Chopra, G.S. & Smith, J.W. (1974). Psychotic reactions following cannabis use in East Indians. *Archives of General Psychiatry, 30*, 24–27.

Cleghorn, J.M., Kaplan, R.D., Szechtman, B., Szechtman, H., Brown, G.M. & Franco, S. (1991). Substance abuse and schizophrenia: Effect on symptoms but not on neurocognitive function. *Journal of Clinical Psychiatry, 52*, 26–30.

Co, B.T., Goodwin, D.W., Gado, M., Mikhael, M. & Hill, S.Y. (1977). Absence of cerebral atrophy in chronic cannabis users: Evaluation by computerized transaxial tomography. *Journal of the American Medical Association, 237*, 1229–1230.

Cohen, S. (1982). Cannabis effects upon adolescent motivation. In *Marijuana and Youth: Clinical Observations on Motivation and Learning* (pp. 2–10). Rockville, MD: National Institute on Drug Abuse.

Compton, D.R., Dewey, W.L. & Martin, B.R. (1990). Cannabis dependence and tolerance production. *Advances in Alcohol and Substance Abuse, 9*, 128–147.

Cook, P.J. & Moore, M.J. (1993). Economic perspectives on reducing alcohol-related violence. In S.E. Martin (Ed.), *Alcohol and Interpersonal Violence: Fostering Multidisciplinary Perspectives* (NIAAA Research Monograph No. 24, pp. 193–212) (NIH Publication No. 93-3496). Rockville, MD: Department of Health and Human Services.

Darke, S., & Zador, D. (1996). Fatal heroin overdose: A review. *Addiction, 91*, 1757–1764.

Denning, D.W., Follansbee, S.E., Scolaro, M., Norris, S., Edelstein, H. & Stevens, D.A. (1991). Pulmonary aspergillosis in the acquired immunodeficiencey syndrome. *New England Journal of Medicine, 324*, 654–662.

Der, G., Gupta, S. & Murray, R.M. (1990). Is schizophrenia disappearing? *Lancet, 1*, 513–516.

Donald, P.J. (1991). Marijuana and upper aerodigestive tract malignancy in young patients. In G. Nahas & C. Latour (Eds.), *Physiopathology of Illicit Drugs: Cannabis, Cocaine, Opiates*. Oxford: Pergamon Press.

Donovan, J.E. & Jessor, R. (1983). Problem drinking and the dimension of involvement with drugs: A Guttman Scalogram analysis of adolescent drug use. *American Journal of Public Health, 73*, 543–552.

Duggan, A.W. & North, R.A. (1983). Electrophysiology of opioids. *Pharmacologic Reviews, 35*, 219–282.

Edwards, G., S., Ferrence, R., Giesbrecht, N. & Room, R. (1994). *Alcohol Policy and the Public Good*. Oxford: Oxford University Press.

English, D., Holman, C.D.J., Milne, E., Winter, M.G., Hulse, G.K., Codde, J.P., Corti, B., Dawes, V., de Klerk, N., Knuiman, M.W., Kurinczuk, J.J., Lewin, G.F. & Ryan, G.A. (1995). *The Quantification of Drug-Caused Morbidity and Mortality in Australia, 1995 edition*. Canberra: Commonwealth Department of Human Services and Health.

Fehr, K.O. & Kalant, H. (Eds.). (1983). *Cannabis and Health Hazards*. Toronto: Addiction Research Foundation.

Fergusson, D. & Horwood, J.L. (1997). Early onset cannabis use and psychosocial development in young adults. *Addiction, 92*, 279–296.

Ferris, J., Templeton, L. & Wong, S. (1993). *Alcohol, Tobacco and Marijuana: Use Norms, Problems and Policy Attitudes among Ontario Adults: A Report of the Ontario Alcohol and Other Drug Opinion Survey, 1992* (ARF Research Document No. 118). Toronto: Addiction Research Foundation.

Fletcher, J.M., Page, J.B., Francis, D.J., Copeland, K., Naus, M.J., Davis, C.M., Morris, R. Krauskopf, D. & Satz, P. (1996). Cognitive correlates of long-term cannabis use in Costa Rican men. *Archives of General Psychiatry, 53,* 1051–1057.

Fligiel, S.E.G., Beals, T.F., Venkat, H., Stuth, S., Gong, H. & Tashkin, D.P. (1988). Pulmonary pathology in marijuana smokers. In G. Chesher, P. Consroe & R. Musty (Eds.), *Marijuana: An International Research Report* (National Campaign Against Drug Abuse Monograph No. 7, pp. 43–48). Canberra: Australian Government Publishing Service.

Fligiel, S.E.G., Roth, M.D., Kleerup, E.C., Barsky, S.H., Simmons, M.S. & Tashkin, D.P. (1997). Tracheobronchial histopathology in habitual smokers of cocaine, marijuana and/or tobacco. *Chest, 112,* 319–326.

Fried, P.A. (1985). Postnatal consequences of maternal marijuana use. In T.M. Pinkert (Ed.), *Current Research on the Consequences of Maternal Drug Abuse* (NIDA Research Monograph No. 59, pp. 61–72) (DHHS Publication No. 85-1400). Washington, DC: U.S. Government Printing Office.

Fried, P.A. (1989). Postnatal consequences of maternal marijuana use in humans. *Annals of the New York Academy of Sciences, 562,* 123–132.

Fried, P.A. (1993). Prenatal exposure to tobacco and marijuana: Effects during pregnancy, infancy, and early childhood. *Clinical Obstetrics and Gynecology, 36,* 319–337.

Fried, P.A. (1996). Behavioral outcomes in preschool-aged children exposed prenatally to marijuana: A review and speculative interpretation. In C.L. Wetherington, C.L. Smeriglio & L. Finnegan (Eds.), *Behavioral Studies of Drug Exposed Offspring: Methodological Issues in Human and Animal Research* (NIDA Research Monograph No. 164, pp. 242–260). Washington, DC: U.S. Government Printing Office.

Fried, P.A., O'Connell, C.M. & Watkinson, B. (1992). 60- and 72-month follow-up of children prenatally exposed to marijuana, cigarettes, and alcohol: Cognitive and language assessment. *Journal of Developmental and Behavioral Pediatrics, 13,* 383–391.

Fried, P.A. & Watkinson, B. (1990). 36- and 48-month neurobehavioral follow-up of children prenatally exposed to marijuana, cigarettes and alcohol. *Journal of Developmental and Behavioral Pediatrics, 11,* 49–58.

Friedman, A.S., Granick, S., Bransfield, S., Kreisher, C. & Schwartz. A. (1996). The consequences of drug use/abuse for vocational career: A longitudinal study of a male urban African-American sample. *American Journal of Drug and Alcohol Abuse, 22,* 57–73.

Ghodse, A.H. (1986). Cannabis psychosis. *British Journal of Addiction, 81*, 473–478.

Gibson, G.T., Baghurst, P.A. & Colley, D.P. (1983). Maternal alcohol, tobacco and cannabis consumption and the outcome of pregnancy. *Australian and New Zealand Journal of Obstetrics and Gynaecology, 23*, 15–19.

Grund, J.P. (1993). *Drug Use as a Social Ritual: Functionality, Symbolism, Determinants of Self-Regulation* (IVO Series No. 4). Rotterdam: Addiction Research Institute.

Hall, W. (1995). The public health implications of cannabis use. *Australian Journal of Public Health, 19*, 235–242.

Hall, W., Solowij, N. & Lemon, J. (1994). *The Health and Psychological Consequences of Cannabis Use* (National Drug Strategy Monograph No. 25). Canberra: Australian Government Publication Services.

Hall, W. & Zador, D. (1997). The alcohol withdrawal syndrome. *Lancet, 349*, 1857–1860.

Hamadeh, R., Ardehali, A., Locksley, R.M. & York, M.R. (1988). Fatal aspergillosis associated with smoking contaminated marijuana, in a marrow transplant recipient. *Chest, 94*, 432–433.

Hatch, E.E. & Bracken, M.B. (1986). Effect of marijuana use in pregnancy on fetal growth. *American Journal of Epidemiology, 124*, 986–993.

Hendin, H., Haas, A.P., Singer, P., Eller, M. & Ulman, R. (1987). *Living High: Daily Marijuana Use Among Adults.* New York: Human Sciences Press.

Hilts, P.J. (1995). Rating addictiveness. *The Journal* (Toronto), *24*, 12.

Hingson, R., Alpert, J., Day, N., Dooling, E., Kayne, H., Morelock, S., Oppenheimer, E. & Zuckerman, B. (1982). Effects of maternal drinking and marijuana use on fetal growth and development. *Pediatrics, 70*, 539–546.

Hollister, L.E. (1986). Health aspects of cannabis. *Pharmacological Reviews*, 38, 1–20.

Huber, G.L., Griffith, D.E. & Langsjoen, P.M. (1988). The effects of marihuana on the respiratory and cardiovascular systems. In G. Chesher, P. Consroe & R. Musty (Eds.), *Marijuana: An International Research Report* (National Campaign Against Drug Abuse Monograph No. 7, pp. 1–18). Canberra: Australian Government Publishing Service.

Institute of Medicine. (1982). *Marijuana and Health.* Washington, DC: National Academy Press.

International Agency on Research into Cancer. (1990). In L. Tomatis (Ed.), *Cancer: Causes, Occurrence and Control.* Lyon: International Agency on Research into Cancer.

Jablensky, A., Sartorius, N., Ernberg, G., Anker, M., Korten, A., Cooper, J.E., Day, R. & Bertelsen, A. (1991). *Schizophrenia: Manifestations, Incidence and Course in Different Cultures. A World Health Organization Ten-Country Study* (Psychological Medicine Monograph Supplement No. 20).

Jacobs, M.R. & Fehr, K. O'B. (1987). *Drugs and Drug Abuse: A Reference Text.* Toronto: Addiction Research Foundation.

Joe, G.W. & Simpson, D.D. (1987). Mortality rates among opioid addicts in a longitudinal study. *American Journal of Public Health, 77*, 347–348.

Joe, G.W. & Simpson, D.D. (1990). Death rates and risk factors. In S.B. Sells & B.S. Brown (Eds.), *Opioid Addiction and Treatment: A 12-year Follow-up* (pp. 193–202). Malabar FL: Robert E. Krieger.

Jones, R.T. (1984). Marijuana: Health and treatment issues. *Psychiatric Clinics of North America, 7*, 703–712.

Kandel, D.B. (1984). Marijuana users in young adulthood. *Archives of General Psychiatry, 41*, 200–209.

Kandel, D.B. (1988). Issues of sequencing of adolescent drug use and other problem behaviors. *Drugs and Society, 3*, 55–76.

Kandel, D.B. & Davies, M. (1992). Progression to regular marijuana involvement: Phenomenology and risk factors for near daily use. In M. Glantz & R. Pickens (Eds.), *Vulnerability to Drug Abuse* (pp. 211–253). Washington, DC: American Psychological Association.

Kandel, D.B., Davies, M., Karus, D. & Yamaguchi, K. (1986). The consequences in young adulthood of adolescent drug involvement. *Archives of General Psychiatry, 43*, 746–754.

Kandel, D. & Faust, R. (1975). Sequence and stages in patterns of adolescent drug use. *Archives of General Psychiatry, 32*, 923–932.

Kandel, D. & Yamaguchi, K. (1993). From beer to crack: Developmental patterns of drug involvement. *American Journal of Public Health, 83*, 851–855.

Kaslow, R.A., Blackwelder, W.C., Ostrow, D.G., Yerg, D., Palenick, J., Coulson, A.H. & Valdiserri, R.O. (1989). No evidence for a role of alcohol or other psychoactive drugs in accelerating immunodeficiency in HIV-1-positive individuals: A report form the Multicenter AIDS Cohort Study. *Journal of the American Medical Association, 261*, 3424–3429.

Kolansky, H. & Moore, R.T. (1971). Effects of marihuana on adolescents and young adults. *Journal of the American Medical Association, 216*, 486–492.

Kosten, T.R., Rounsaville, B.J., Babor, T.F., Spitzer, R.L. & Williams, J.B.W. (1987). Substance-use disorders in *DSM-III-R*. *British Journal of Psychiatry, 151*, 834–843.

Kuehnle, J., Mendelson, J.H. & David, K.R. (1977). Computed tomographic examination of heavy marijuana users. *Journal of the American Medical Association, 237*, 1231–1232.

Kuijten, R.R., Bunin, G.R., Nass, C.C. & Meadows, A.T. (1990). Gestational and familial risk factors for childhood astrocytoma: Results of a case-control study. *Cancer Research, 50*, 2608–2612.

Lenke, L. (1990). *Alcohol and Criminal Violence —Time Series Analyses in a Comparative Perspective*. Stockholm: Almqvist and Wiksell.

Leuchtenberger, C. (1983). Effects of marihuana (cannabis) smoke on cellular biochemistry of *in vitro* test systems. In K.O. Fehr & H. Kalant (Eds.), *Cannabis and Health Hazards* (pp. 177–223). Toronto: Addiction Research Foundation.

Linszen, D.H., Dingemans, P.M. & Lenior, M.E. (1994). Cannabis abuse and the course of recent-onset schizophrenic disorders. *Archives of General Psychiatry, 51*, 273–279.

Maddux, J.F. & Desmond, D.P. (1981). *Careers of Opioid Users*. New York: Praeger.

Mäkelä, K., Room, R., Single, E., Sulkunen, P. & Walsh, B., with 13 others. (1981). *Alcohol, Society, and the State: A Comparative Study of Alcohol Control*. Toronto: Addiction Research Foundation.

Marks, W.H., Florence, L., Lieberman, J., Chapman, P., Howard, D., Roberts, P. & Perkinson, D. (1996). Successfully treated invasive pulmonary aspergillosis associated with smoking marijuana in a renal transplant recipient. *Transplantation, 61*, 1771–1774.

Martin, C.A. & Martin, W.R. (1980). Opiate dependence in women. In O. Kalant (Ed.), *Alcohol and Drug Problems in Women: Research Advances in Alcohol and Drug Problems* (Vol. 5) (pp. 465–486). New York: Plenum Press.

Martin, S.E. (Ed.). (1993). *Alcohol and Interpersonal Violence: Fostering Multidisciplinary Perspectives* (NIAAA Research Monograph No. 24) (NIH Publication No. 93-3496). Rockville, MD: Department of Health and Human Services.

Martinez-Arevalo, M.J., Calcedo-Ordonez, A. & Varo-Prieto, J.R. (1994). Cannabis consumption as a prognostic factor in schizophrenia. *British Journal of Psychiatry, 164*, 679–681.

Mattick, R.P. & Hall, W. (1996). Is detoxification effective? *Lancet, 347*, 97–100.

Mendelson, J.H. & Mello, N.K. (1984). Effects of marijuana on neuroendocrine hormones in human males and females. In M.C. Braude & J.P. Ludford (Eds.), *Marijuana Effects on the Endocrine and Reproductive Systems*. (pp. 97–114). Rockville, MD: National Institute on Drug Abuse.

Munson, A.E. & Fehr, K.O. (1983). Immunological effects of cannabis. In K.O. Fehr & H. Kalant (Eds.), *Cannabis and Health Hazards* (pp. 257–354). Toronto: Addiction Research Foundation.

Murray, C.J.L. & Lopez, A.D. (1996). Quantifying the burden of disease and injury attributable to ten major risk factors. In C.J.L. Murray & A.D. Lopez (Eds.), *The Global Burden of Disease: A Comprehensive Assessment of Mortality and Disability from Diseases, Injuries, and Risk Factors in 1990 and Projected to 2020* (pp. 295–324). Cambridge, MA: Harvard School of Public Health.

Negrete, J.C. (1989). Cannabis and schizophrenia. *British Journal of Addiction, 84*, 349–351.

Negrete, J.C., Knapp, W.P., Douglas, D. & Smith, W.B. (1986). Cannabis affects the severity of schizophrenic symptoms: Results of a clinical survey. *Psychological Medicine, 16*, 515–520.

Newcombe, M.D. & Bentler, P. (1988). *Consequences of Adolescent Drug Use: Impact on the Lives of Young Adults*. Newbury Park, CA: Sage.

O'Donnell, J.A. (1969). *Narcotic Addicts in Kentucky* (U.S. Public Health Service Publication No. 1881). Washington, DC: U.S. Government Printing Office.

O'Donnell, J., Voss, H., Clayton, R., Slatin, R. & Room, R. (1976). *Young Men and Drugs: A Nationwide Survey* (NIDA Research Monograph No. 5). Washington, DC: U.S. Government Printing Office.

Page, J.B., Fletcher, J. & True, W.R. (1988). Psychosociocultural perspectives on chronic cannabis use: The Costa Rican follow-up. *Journal of Psychoactive Drugs, 20*, 57–65.

Paglia, A. (1995). *Alcohol, Tobacco, and Drugs: Dependence, Problems, and Consequences of Use: A Report of the 1994 Ontario Alcohol and Other Drug Opinion Survey* (ARF Research Document No. 121). Toronto: Addiction Research Foundation.

Peck, R.C., Biasotti, A., Boland, P.N., Mallory, C. & Reeve, V. (1986). The effects of marijuana and alcohol on actual driving performance. *Alcohol, Drugs and Driving, 2*, 135–154.

Pernanen, K. (1991). *Alcohol in Human Violence*. New York: Guilford.

Pohorecky, L.A., Brick, J. & Milgram, G.G. (Eds.). (1993, September). Alcohol and aggression. *Journal of Studies on Alcohol* (Suppl. 11).

Polen, M.R., Sidney, S., Tekawa, I.S., Sadler, M. & Friedman, G.D. (1993). Health care use by frequent marijuana smokers who do not smoke tobacco. *Western Journal of Medicine, 158*, 596–601.

Pope, H.G. & Yurgelun-Todd, D. (1996). The residual cognitive effects of heavy marijuana use in college students. *Journal of the American Medical Association, 275*, 521–527.

Robbe, H.W.J. (1994). *Influence of Marijuana on Driving*. Maastricht: Institute for Human Psychopharmacology, University of Limberg.

Robinson, L.I., Buckley, J.D., Daigle, A.E., Wells, R., Benjamin, D., Arthur, D.C. & Hammond, G.D. (1989). Maternal drug use and the risk of childhood nonlymphoblastic leukemia among offspring: An epidemiologic investigation implicating marijuana. *Cancer, 63*, 1904–1911.

Roffman, R.A., Stephens, R.S., Simpson, E.E. & Whitaker, D.L. (1988). Treatment of marijuana dependence: Preliminary results. *Journal of Psychoactive Drugs, 20*, 129–137.

Room, R. (1983). *Alcohol and crime: Behavioral aspects*. In S.H. Kadish (Ed.), *Encyclopaedia of Crime and Justice* (Vol. 1) (pp. 35–44). New York: Free Press.

Rosenkrantz, H. (1983). Cannabis, marihuana, and cannabinoid toxicological manifestations in man and animals. In K.O. Fehr & H. Kalant (Eds.), *Cannabis and Health Hazards: Proceedings of an ARF/WHO Scientific Meeting on Adverse Health and Behavioral Consequences of Cannabis Use* (pp. 91–175). Toronto: Addiction Research Foundation.

Royal College of Physicians of London. (1987). *A Great and Growing Evil?: The Medical Consequences of Alcohol Abuse*. London: Tavistock.

Rubin, V. & Comitas, L. (1975). *Ganja in Jamaica: A Medical Anthropological Study of Chronic Marihuana Use*. The Hague: Mouton.

Schneier, F.R. & Siris, S.G. (1987). A review of psychoactive substance use and abuse in schizophrenia: Patterns of drug choice. *Journal of Nervous and Mental Disorders, 175*, 641–652.

Sidney, S., Beck, J.E., Tekawa, I.S., Quesenberry, C.P. & Friedman, G.D. (1997). Marijuana use and mortality. *American Journal of Public Health, 87*, 585–590.

Simpson, D.D., Joe, G.W., Lehman, W.E.K. & Sells, S.B. (1986). Addiction careers: Etiology, treatment and 12 year follow-up outcomes. *The Journal of Drug Issues, 16*, 107–121.

Smiley, A. (1986). Marijuana: On-road and driving simulator studies. *Alcohol, Drugs and Driving, 2*, 121–134.

Solowij, N., Michie, P.T. & Fox, A.M. (1991). Effects of long-term cannabis use on selective attention: An event-related potential study. *Pharmacology, Biochemistry and Behavior, 40*, 683–688.

Solowij, N., Michie, P.T. & Fox, A.M. (1995). Differential impairments of selective attention due to frequency and duration of cannabis use. *Biological Psychiatry, 37*, 731–739.

Stephens, R.S. & Roffman, R.A. (1993). Adult marijuana dependence. In J.S. Baer, G.A. Marlatt & R.J. MacMahon (Eds.), *Addictive Behaviors Across the Lifespan: Prevention, Treatment and Policy Issues* (pp. 202–218). Newbury Park, CA: Sage.

Substance Abuse and Mental Health Services Administration (SAMHSA). (1993). *National Household Survey on Drug Abuse: Main Findings, 1991* (DHHS Publication No. SMA 93-1980). Rockville, MD: U.S. Department of Health and Human Services.

Sutton, S., Lum, B.L. & Torti, F.M. (1986). Possible risk of invasive pulmonary aspergillosis with marijuana use during chemotherapy for small cell lung cancer. *Drug Intelligence and Clinical Pharmacy, 20*, 289–291.

Tashkin, D.P. (1993). Is frequent marijuana smoking harmful to health? *Western Journal of Medicine, 158*, 635–637.

Tashkin, D.P., Fligiel, S., Wu, T.-C., Gong, H., Jr., Barbers, R.G., Coulson, A.H., Simmons, M.S. & Beals, F. (1990). Effects of habitual use of marijuana and/or cocaine on the lung. In C.N. Chiang & R.L. Hawks (Eds.), *Research Findings on Smoking of Abuse Substances* (NIDA Research Monograph No. 99, pp. 63–87) (DHHS Publication No. ADM 90-1690). Washington, DC: U.S. Government Printing Office.

Tashkin, D.P., Wu, T.-C., Djahed, B. & Rose, J.E. (1988). Smoking topography and delivery of insoluble particulates and carbon monoxide to the lung during the smoking of tobacco and marihuana of varying potency in habitual smokers of both substances. In G. Chesher, P. Consroe & R. Musty (Eds.), *Marijuana: An International Research Report* (National Campaign Against Drug Abuse Monograph No. 7, pp. 31–36). Canberra: Australian Government Publishing Service.

Taylor, F.M. (1988). Marijuana as a potential respiratory tract carcinogen: A retrospective analysis of a community hospital population. *Southern Medical Journal, 81*, 1213–1216.

Tennes, K., Avitable, N., Blackard, C., Boyles, C., Hassoun, B., Holmes, L. & Kreye, M. (1985). Marihuana: Prenatal and postnatal exposure in the human. In T.M. Pinkert (Ed.), *Current Research on the Consequences of Maternal Drug Abuse* (NIDA Research Monograph No. 59, pp. 48–60) (DHHS Publication No. 85-1400). Washington, DC: U.S. Government Printing Office.

Thornicroft, G. (1990). Cannabis and psychosis: Is there epidemiological evidence for association. *British Journal of Psychiatry, 157*, 25–33.

U.S. Department of Health and Human Services. (1989). *Reducing the Health Consequences of Smoking: 25 Years of Progress. A Report of the Surgeon General.* Washington, DC: U.S. Department of Health and Human Services, Public Health Service, Centers for Disease Control, Center for Chronic Disease Prevention, Office on Smoking and Health.

U.S. Department of Health and Human Services. (1997). *Ninth Special Report to the U.S. Congress on Alcohol and Health from the Secretary of Health and Human Services.* Washington, DC: U.S. Department of Health and Human Services, Public Health Service, National Institutes of Health, National Institute on Alcohol Abuse and Alcoholism.

Vaillant, G.E. (1973). A 20-year follow-up of New York narcotic addicts. *Archives of General Psychiatry, 29,* 237–241.

Weil, A. (1970). Adverse reactions to marihuana. *New England Journal of Medicine, 282,* 997–1000.

Weller, R.A., Halikas, J. & Morse, C. (1984). Alcohol and marijuana: Comparison of use and abuse in regular marijuana users. *Journal of Clinical Psychiatry, 45,* 377–379.

Wert, R.C. & Raulin, M.L. (1986). The chronic cerebral effects of cannabis use: II. Psychological findings and conclusions. *The International Journal of the Addictions, 21,* 629–642.

Woody, G.E. & O'Brien, C.P. (1991). Update of methadone maintenance. In N.S. Miller (Ed.), *Comparison Handbook of Drug and Alcohol Addiction* (pp. 1113–1125). New York: Marcel Dekker.

Wu, T.-C., Tashkin, D.P., Djahed, B. & Rose, J.E. (1988). Pulmonary hazards of smoking marijuana as compared with tobacco. *New England Journal of Medicine, 318,* 347–351.

Xie, X., Rehm, J., Single, E. & Robson, L. (1996). *The Economic Costs of Alcohol, Tobacco and Illicit Drug Abuse in Ontario: 1992* (Research Document No. 127). Toronto: Addiction Research Foundation.

Yamaguchi, K. & Kandel, D.B. (1984a). Patterns of drug use from adolescence to adulthood: II. Sequences of progression. *American Journal of Public Health, 74,* 668–672.

Yamaguchi, K. & Kandel, D.B. (1984b). Patterns of drug use from adolescence to adulthood: III. Predictors of progression. *American Journal of Public Health, 74,* 673–681.

Zuckerman, B., Frank, D., Hingson, R., Amaro, H., Levenson, S., Kayne, H., Parker, S., Vinci, R., Aboagye, K., Fried, L., Cabral, H., Timperi, R. & Bauchner, H. (1989). Effects of maternal marijuana and cocaine use on fetal growth. *New England Journal of Medicine, 320,* 762–768.

INDEX

A

abstinence, 205, 215, 216, 221, 225, 233–237, 274, 276, 282, 424, 483, 486
accidents, 98–100, 271, 479, 484, 486
    fatalities, 173, 485
    motor vehicle, 11, 43–44, 47, 89, 98–100, 173, 179, 477–479, 484, 489–490, 495
acetylcholine, 28, 32, 198, 199, 200, 448
acids. *See* amino acids; arachidonic acid; carboxy acids; fatty acids; gamma-aminobutyric acid; nucleic acids
addiction, 270, 488. *See also* dependence
Addiction Research Foundation, x, xi
adenylyl cyclase, 26, 27–28, 30, 31, 50, 354
adolescence, 89, 97, 99, 106. *See also* children
    and cannabis use, 8, 9, 11, 71, 73, 75, 76, 78, 96, 215, 232–233, 271, 279
    and decriminalization, 492
    and delinquency, 86, 89–90
    development and cannabis use, 84–90, 213, 232, 482
    and income, 82
    and learning, 134
    and non-conformity, 86, 89, 97, 225
    peer disapproval of cannabis use, 76
    sexual behavior, 86, 88
administration, of cannabis. *See* route of administration
    rate, 444–445
adrenocorticotropic hormone (ACTH), 27, 30, 32, 201, 209, 381–382, 384, 386
aerodigestive tract. *See* cancer
affect, 129, 273, 275
Africa, 80, 481
African-Americans, x, 83, 86, 418
age, 43, 73, 77, 78, 82, 93, 151, 160, 244
    and rates of cannabis use, 173
aging, 198, 209, 212, 213, 246
agonists, 22, 23, 29, 31–32, 211–212, 362, 384, 448
    cholinergic, 32
    GABA, 32
AIDS, 100–101, 106–107, 329, 334, 335, 360, 447, 464, 465, 479–481, 487
    wasting syndrome, 464–465, 468
airways
    hyperresponsiveness (AHR), 324, 336
    injury, 326–329, 335
    obstruction, 101–102, 321–324
Alberta, 95, 278

alcohol
    adverse effects, 3, 5, 99–100, 484–488
    and aggressive behavior, 158
    benefits, 492
    in the brain, 207–208
    and cancer, 102
    and cannabis use, 11–14, 40, 42–44, 48, 72, 83, 85, 94, 102, 140, 144–146, 173–188, 207, 244, 247, 269, 281, 332, 413–418, 443, 444, 477–495
    and driving, 39–44, 99
    health effects, 4, 5, 13, 484–488
    industry, 3
    and pregnancy, 103, 405
    quantification of use, 11
alveolar macrophages. *See* macrophages
Alzheimer's disease, 212
amino acids, 27, 32, 50, 362, 363
aminoalkylindoles, 23–24, 28
Ammons Full-Range Picture Vocabulary Test, 218
amnesia, 274, 275, 277, 282
amotivational syndrome, 90–91, 98, 146, 199, 224, 269, 276–277, 281, 482
amphetamines, 10, 11, 85, 97, 98, 156, 207, 208, 210, 277, 279, 282, 443, 484
amygdala, 201, 207, 208
analgesics, 22, 23, 440, 461, 466, 468
anandamide, xi, 28, 32, 50, 198–199, 202, 211, 247, 381, 384, 439, 448
    metabolism, 30–31, 198
    pharmacological properties, 23–25, 49
    synthesis, 30–31
    system, 32–33, 437
    THC-like properties, 29–31, 198
androgen, 384
anhedonia, 96
animal research, cannabis, 6
    analgesics, 466
    anti-convulsant drugs, 467
    anti-emetic drugs, 464
    behavioral studies, 195–202
    brain morphology and histology, 207–211
    cannabinoid studies, 23–33, 246
    cardiovascular and gastrointestinal effects, 437, 442, 445
    and central nervous system, 49
    developmental toxicity, 404–411, 424–425
    experiments, 6, 7, 10, 11, 13
    extrapolating to humans, 13, 196, 213, 314, 405, 415
    and hunger, 136–137

immunoglobin levels, 351
limb blood flow, 438–439
muscle blood flow, 439
pressure, 437–439, 462, 465–466, 485, 486
blurred vision, 466
bodyweight, 406, 407, 445–447
Boston, 412
bowels, 443–444
brain. *See also* cognitive function; cortex; memory
atrophy, 208, 210–211, 215
cannabinoids in, 25–28, 29, 467
CAT scans, 206, 208, 210, 211
and cerebral blood flow, 204–205
"damage," 195, 206, 213, 215, 223, 225, 483, 485
electrophysiology, 201–204
histology, 196, 206–211, 214
and long-term cannabis use, 215–247
metabolism, 206, 213
morphology, 196, 206–209, 213
MRI scans, 206
and neurotoxicity, 195–214
and PET, 205–207
protein synthesis, 408–409, 411
structure, 196, 206
ultrastructure, 208–210, 213, 214
Wernicke-Korsakov syndrome, 485
brainstem, 25, 50, 200
Brazelton Neonatal Behavioral Assessment Scale, 104, 417
breast feeding, 104, 385
milk production and let-down, 405, 425
breathing, 326, 485
Britain, ix, 461, 463
bronchial alveolar lavage (BAL), 328–330, 350
bronchial cytology, 330
bronchitis, chronic, 101–102, 106, 313, 316–318, 322, 336, 480, 486, 489, 490, 495
Buschke's Verbal Selective Reminding Test, 220, 223, 233, 235

C

caffeine, 413
calcium, 28–31, 50, 360, 362, 363
California, 99–100, 173, 181
California Verbal Learning Test (CVLT), 238–239, 241
cAMP, 26, 28, 29, 30, 211, 350, 351, 354, 362
Canada, 77–78, 82, 95, 224–230, 411–412, 463, 491

cancer, 6, 8, 10, 106–107, 294–295, 298–304, 329, 334, 447, 466
aerodigestive tract, 101–102, 106, 332, 333, 336, 362, 480, 486
astrocytoma, 302, 481
bladder, 302, 304
breast, 465, 486
childhood, 104–105, 107, 301, 481
digestive system, 486
esophagus, 301, 304
leukemia, 104–106, 302, 361, 481
lung, 303, 330, 332
mouth and tongue, 301, 303, 304, 332
ovarian, 465
and prenatal cannabis exposure, 301
respiratory tract, 6, 106, 301, 303–304, 318, 327, 331, 489, 490, 495
rhabdomyosarcoma, 105, 302
Candida albicans, 328, 335, 354
cannabidiol, 22, 203, 294, 296, 354, 357, 379, 403, 443, 444, 448, 466, 467
cannabigerol, 466
cannabimimetic effect, 356, 363
cannabinoid(s), 6, 21–50, 209, 313, 334. *See also* receptors, cannabinoid; THC
and accidents, 44, 99, 105
behavioral effects, 21, 22, 25, 33, 49, 129–161, 196–199, 269–282
bicyclic and tricyclic, 23, 24
binding, 23, 25–27, 31, 50, 200
in the brain, 25–29, 195–214, 232, 237, 245, 377, 382, 384, 386
cardiovascular effects, 437–442
and chromosomes, 296–300
defined, 403
exogenous, 246
gastrointestinal effects, 443–445
immunological effects, 100–101, 349–364
mechanisms of action, ix, 25–53, 377, 382–385, 466
molecules, 21
neurochemistry, 29, 32–33, 199–201
as neuromodulators, 28, 31, 32, 200
pharmacological effects, 25, 28, 50, 299
physicochemical properties, 21, 29
and reproduction, 103, 377–386
synthetic, ix, 462, 464, 468
toxicity, 25, 48–50, 160, 195–214, 404
cannabinol, 294, 296, 354, 357, 379, 403, 443, 444, 448, 466

cannabis, health effects, 3–17, 98–107, 403, 477–495. *See also* animal research, cannabis; cannabis, use; cannabis, users; cognitive function; human research, cannabis; marijuana; memory; studies, cannabis use
acute, 3, 10, 14, 38, 84, 127–161, 195–247, 479–480
adverse, x, xi, 3–17, 76, 84, 101–105, 295, 297, 325, 377, 415, 477–495
assessing, 3–14
benefits, ix, xi, 84, 442, 461–468, 479
cardiovascular, 92, 207, 270, 437–442, 482, 485, 486, 492
chronic, 3, 4, 10–11, 14, 38, 480–484
compared to other drugs, 484–494
immunological, 11, 26, 50, 98, 100–101, 105, 333, 334, 349–364, 437, 464, 465, 480, 481, 487
positive, 478
psychological, 3–14, 76, 83–98, 106–107, 159, 479–484
ratings, user, 492–494
reproductive, 8, 98, 103–106, 323, 377–386, 405–425, 480–481
respiratory, 101–103, 106–107, 215, 313–336, 480
therapeutic uses, ix, xi, 84, 442, 461–468, 479
"cannabis psychosis," 273–275, 281
cannabis, use. *See also* cannabis, health effects; cannabis, users; cognitive function; marijuana
availability, 77, 78, 83, 85–87
and ceremony, ix
cessation, 92, 245–246, 270, 320, 424, 442, 482
chronic, 4, 8, 11, 71, 82, 84, 89–90, 92, 97, 98, 100–101, 106, 199, 207, 208, 212–214, 216, 217, 226, 247, 270, 274, 276, 316, 319, 385, 478, 481, 495
daily, 3, 75, 82, 203–204, 275, 281, 294, 317, 322, 380, 415, 424
decline, 76–78
detecting time of, 33–35, 47–48
discontinuation, 73–78, 84, 215
and environment, 160–161
and ethnicity, 82
frequent/infrequent, 48
heavy, 11, 71, 89–90, 92, 98, 100, 101, 239, 271, 273–274, 276, 316, 317, 319–321, 324–325, 329, 335, 420, 478, 480–481, 483, 485

and history, ix–xi, 160–161
and income, 82
initiation, 71, 78, 82, 85, 89, 482
lifetime, 72, 73, 75–76, 78–82, 323
long-term, 11, 38, 98, 102, 195–247, 483
moderate, 152
near-daily, 79
opponents/proponents, 5, 12
patterns of, 71–83, 495
prevalence of, 77–83, 478, 488, 491–492
quantification, 11, 231
and religion, 81, 227
rise, 76–78
self-reported, 71–73, 83, 90, 96, 97, 99, 278, 279, 379, 380, 413
and social behavior, 129, 156–161
as a "special drug," 5–6, 12
weekly, 73–74, 78, 91
cannabis, users. *See also* cannabis, health effects; cannabis, use; cognitive function; marijuana
chronic, 91, 102, 105, 204, 205, 210, 213, 217, 219, 276, 317, 327, 331, 379, 424, 440, 442, 480, 482
daily, 83, 88, 92, 94, 102, 221, 270, 273, 329, 489
experienced, 35, 38, 84, 131, 136, 138, 145, 152, 160, 177, 203–205, 217–221, 235–236, 242, 317
ex-users, 237, 277
heavy, 38, 46, 87, 91, 205, 208, 220, 222, 225, 237, 238, 269, 270, 277, 298, 303, 318, 323, 326, 327, 331, 332, 333, 414, 417, 440, 442, 480, 482, 483
inexperienced, 38, 39, 204–205
light, 38, 46, 215, 237–239, 298, 323
long-term, 91–92, 94, 203, 214, 270, 271, 333, 380
naive, 48, 84, 97, 160, 479, 485
near-daily, 94, 271, 273, 329, 490
non-users, 91, 145, 203, 217–218, 220–228, 235, 236, 242, 318–331, 380, 385, 478, 480
short-term, 203, 224
Cannabis sativa, 293, 403
carbon dioxide, 316, 326
carbon monoxide, 142, 143, 199, 204, 205, 325–326, 336
carboxy acids, 33
carcinogenicity, 293–304, 313, 333–334, 336, 480, 481
polycyclic hydrocarbons (PAHs), 331

carcinomas, 327, 465

cardiac output, 438–439

cardiovascular effects, 92, 107, 270, 437–442, 482, 485, 486, 492

card-sorting tasks, 132, 144, 149

Caribbean, the, x, 80–81, 90, 273, 276

catalepsy, 25, 27, 30, 31, 32, 50

cats, 201

caudate-putamen, 32, 200

causality, 3, 6–10, 12–14, 216

    cannabis use and health effect, 477–478

    consistency of association, 9, 14

    criteria, 6, 8, 9–14, 478

    excluding chance, 7–8, 13

    temporal order, 8, 10, 12, 482

CB_1 cannabinoid receptor, 27, 29, 31, 32, 50, 207, 448

CB_2 cannabinoid receptor, 27, 29, 31, 50, 364

cells, 10, 11, 26–31, 198, 202, 209, 211, 301, 318, 333, 350, 356, 409

    alveolar macrophage, 314–315, 320, 335

    B, 363

    CD4/CD8, 330, 352, 359, 363

    CHO, 27–28, 29, 30, 362–363

    dendritic, 332

    dysplastic, 330

    epithelial, 301, 313, 318, 321, 330

    glioma, 30

    killer, 352–358

    lymphoid, 353

    lymphoma, 27

    marijuana effects on, 293–304, 480

    metaplastic, 330

    neuroblastoma, 27, 28, 29, 30

    nucleus, 294

    SRBC, 354–355, 357

    T, 332, 352, 354, 363

    tumor, 332, 357

cDNA, 26, 27, 362–363

central nervous system, 31, 44, 45, 49, 50, 129–161, 485

    cannabinoids in, 32–33, 50, 160, 200, 382, 437

    depression, 39

    development in children, 240, 408

    and EEG, 202, 213

    long-term cannabis effects, 195–247

Centre for Addiction and Mental Health, xi

cerebellum, 25, 28–31, 50, 211, 212, 467

cerebral blood flow (CBF), 204–207, 213, 243, 424

cerebrospinal fluid (CSF), 201

Cesamet™, 463

chemistry, cannabis, ix, 21–33, 293–294

chemotherapy, 329, 334, 442, 446, 461–462, 464, 468, 486

Chicago, 412

children, 239–242, 302, 304, 411, 413–425. *See also* adolescence

Chile, 81

chromatography

    GC/MS, 34, 35, 36, 38, 410

    HPLC, 34

    TLC, 34

chromosome(s), 299

    aberrations, 295–297, 300, 333, 481

chronic obstructive pulmonary disease (COPD), 313, 319, 321, 322, 323

cigarettes. *See also* cannabis, use; cannabis, users; smoke

    herbal, 140

    joints, 199, 208, 209, 210, 217, 218, 230, 240, 320, 326, 327, 332, 405, 412

    marijuana, 35, 38–39, 91, 102, 130–160, 293, 313–336, 440, 445

    placebo, 130–160, 176–184

    tobacco, 12, 85, 100, 101, 157, 293, 295, 301, 304, 313–336, 440, 441, 442

circling, 32

circular-lights task, 39, 141, 142, 144, 150

clastogens, 296–298

cocaine, 11, 84–85, 94, 97, 147, 207, 277, 302, 332, 405, 407, 411, 415, 416, 440, 461

    crack cocaine, 323, 405

    and marijuana, 438

cognitive function, 50, 71, 84, 106, 144, 160, 205, 214–247, 273, 421–422, 479. *See also* brain; cortex; memory

    and cardiovascular function, 441

    carry-over effects, 230–242

    and chronic cannabis use, 214–247, 483

    complex reasoning, 241–243, 271

    development, 419

    dysfunction, 216, 231, 236, 244

    executive function, 241–242, 421, 423, 424

    and exposure to cannabis, 421–423

    information processing, 231, 233, 236–238, 244, 479, 483

    intelligence, 8, 95, 219, 222, 223, 228

    and neurotoxicity, 195, 214

    visual reasoning, 421

coherence, 10, 14

color cancellation test, 222

comorbidity, 277–281

flashbacks, 10, 14, 277, 282

flexible fibre optic bronchoscopy (FFB), 326, 328

Florida, 412

flying, 41–43, 129, 140, 151, 230

follicle-stimulating hormone (FSH), 377–379

food
- chemical residues, 4
- chemicals, 293
- deprivation, 153
- intake, 134–137, 157, 159–160, 446, 468
- maternal intake, 405–409, 425
- snacks, 135

forensics, 34, 47–48

forgetting, 198, 246

forskolin, 26, 29, 30

France, ix, 79

frequency, of drug use, 5, 11, 72, 95, 215, 218, 223, 224, 228, 231, 236–239, 243

frogs, 30

frontal lobes, 30, 234, 237–247, 423–424

fruit fly, 196

functional psychosis, 275–276

G

Gambia, 275

gamma-aminobutyric acid (GABA), 28, 29, 32, 199, 200, 202, 209

ganja, 90–91, 222, 226, 317

gas exchange, 316, 321, 324

gastrointestinal effects, 437, 442–449

gastrointestinal tract, 443

gateway drugs, 85–87

gender, 43, 73, 75–82, 85, 93, 99–100, 103, 151, 238, 244, 246, 272
- in drug-exposed offspring, 407
- and lung function, 323
- and neurochemical differences, 200
- and rates of cannabis use, 173
- and reproductive hormones, 379–381

gene expression, 200, 294–295, 363

General Aptitude Test Battery, 222

generational forgetting, 77

genes, 333, 362, 481

genotoxicity, 293–304
- tests, 295–296

glaucoma, 442, 465–466, 468

glucose, 205–207

gonatropins, 377–380, 382, 386

government, x, 83, 462

Greece, 71, 79, 94–95, 100, 203, 217, 219–220, 223, 316–317, 440

growth hormone, 381–383, 386

Guatemala, 81

Guilford Number Facility, 225

guinea pigs, 26, 361
- isolated ileum, 448

H

hallucinations, 84, 273, 274, 275, 278, 280, 483

hallucinogens, 11, 86, 97, 202, 277

Halstead-Reitan Battery, 225–226, 228, 229

hamsters, 318

hand-pat test, 140

handwriting, 141

hangover, 138, 230

hashish, ix, 79, 210, 213, 215, 217, 219, 270, 299, 317, 318, 385, 443
- charas, 221–222
- defined, 403

Health and Welfare Canada, 77, 173

health service use, 99–100, 106, 480

heart rate. *See* THC

heel-to-toe test, 140

herbicides, 4

heritable genetic effects, 296–298

heroin, 84–87, 90, 94, 97, 207, 297, 300, 323, 478, 485

herpes simplex virus, 351, 356, 360, 361

"high." *See* subjective report of drug effects; THC

Hill equation, 45

hippocampus, 25, 30, 32, 50, 197–203, 207–213, 232, 467

Hispanics, 83

histamine, 200

histology, 196, 206–211, 214

histopathology, 101, 102, 106
- airway, 317–318
- pulmonary, 313–314, 319, 324, 326–327, 330, 331, 335, 480

history, ix–xi, 10, 160–161

HIV, 101, 106, 329, 336, 465, 480

homicide, 43, 48

homosexuals, 100–101, 105, 106, 480

Hooper Visual Organization Test, 227

hormones, 377–386, 487

HU-210, 198, 356

HU-211, 356

HU-243, 22

O

obsessive-compulsive disorder, 207
offspring, drug-exposed, 405–425
    behavior, 407
    growth, 407
    mortality, 406
    physical anomalies, 416, 481
    sex ratio, 407, 411, 425
one-foot balance test, 140
Ontario, x, 77–78, 492–493
    health care costs, 491
opiates, 466
    and cannabis, 477
opioid(s), 23, 31, 50, 92, 94, 196, 200, 383, 405,
    448, 482, 484–487. *See also* heroin; hydro-
    morphone; nalorphine; methadone; mor-
    phine
    intravenous drug use, 486
    overdose, 485
    peptides, x, 200
organ transplantation, 329
Ottawa Prospective Prenatal Study, 104, 412,
    413–424, 425
ovulation, 103, 378, 385, 480
oxygen, 205, 316, 440–441
oxytocin, 381

P

Paced Auditory Serial Addition Test (PASAT),
    241, 242
paid participation, 134, 142, 146–149, 151, 152,
    159, 160, 230, 439
pain, 161, 440, 441, 466
paired-associate learning, 132–133, 134
Paired-Associate Learning Test, 233
pancreatic islets, 29
panic, 10, 84, 97, 275, 479
paranoia, 274, 276
parent-child interaction, 420–422
Parkinson's disease, 467
Peabody test, 240, 418–419
peer disapproval of drug use, 76–77
pentobarbital, 144
peptides, 27, 247, 383
perception, 42, 84, 95, 129, 177, 183, 205, 224,
    229. *See also* time perception
    perceptual speed and accuracy tasks, 217, 222
    visuomotor tasks, 217, 219, 222, 479
    visuoperceptual tasks, 240, 420

Performance Assessment Battery (PAB), 150
perseverative responding, 239
personal relationships, 158, 271, 483
personality, 160, 215, 217, 244, 273, 420, 423
pertussis toxin, 28, 29, 30, 362
pesticides, 4, 104
Peterson-Peterson Memory Paradigm, 226, 233
Peyer's patches, 26
PGI Memory Scale, 222
phagocytosis, 350, 363
pharmaceutical companies, 462
pharmacodynamics, 38–46
pharmacokinetic/pharmacodynamic (PK/PD)
    models, 34, 37–38, 44–46
pharmacology, ix, 5, 21, 23, 33–48, 199, 231,
    439
phencyclidine, 234, 323, 405
pigs, 29, 50, 448
"pills," 85, 86, 97
Pittsburgh, 412, 418–420, 423, 424
placenta, 410
plant, marijuana, 293, 403, 446–447, 461–462
    chemistry, 403
    contamination, 361, 464, 481
    destruction, 334
placebo, 8, 42, 43, 130–160, 174, 180, 230, 315,
    316, 320, 380, 441, 447, 463, 465. *See also*
    cigarettes
plasma, 439
    FSH levels, 378
    LH levels, 379, 380
    prolactin levels, 141
    THC levels, 34, 38–40, 45, 48, 133, 204, 206,
    319, 409–410, 438, 446, 464
Pneumocystis carinii pneumonia, 465, 481
pneumothorax, 334
politics, xi, 3, 4, 5, 216, 462
    conservatism, 4, 77
    radicalism, 4
Pompidou Group, 78
popcorn reaction, 196, 200
Portugal, 79
positron emission tomography (PET), 205–207,
    213
postnatal development, 104, 196, 407, 417, 419,
    481
pravadoline, 23
Prechtl neurologic assessment, 417
prefrontal cortex, 197, 200, 206, 207, 212, 213.
    See also frontal lobes
    prefrontal syndrome, 216

pregnancy, 88, 103–104, 106, 196, 240, 294, 297, 385, 403–425, 495
  and cancer, 302
  and cannabis use, 411–425, 481, 490
  and diet, 415
  nutrition and fostering, 406, 411
  THC plasma levels, 409–410
prenatal exposure to cannabis, 196, 200, 239–240, 297, 301, 385, 386, 403–425, 487
prevalence, 8, 12, 14, 43, 48, 72, 73, 75–83, 478, 488, 491–492
primates, 196, 320. *See also* monkeys
problem deflation/problem inflation, 3–4, 12, 13
progesterone, 378, 386
prohibition, 4, 5, 12
prolactin, 377–380, 382, 383, 386
propranolol, 138
prostaglandins, 132–133, 139, 200, 350–351, 383
  PGE$_1$, 448
prostanoids, 24
protein, 208, 293, 294, 320, 350–351, 359
  in the brain, 408–409
psychiatric disorders, 89, 90, 93, 215, 244, 269–282, 485, 487. *See also* psychoses; schizophrenia
psychological effects, 3–14, 71, 83–98, 106–107, 159
psychology, 231–232, 241, 244
psychometric testing, 228, 230, 232
psychomotor performance. *See also* driving
  and ability tests, 230
  and alcohol, 484
  and anandamide, 246
  and cannabinoids, 25, 39–44, 84, 129, 443
  carry-over effects, 230
  and charas, 222
  and cognitive impairment, 223
  cross-cultural studies, 95, 217
  and dose, 98–99, 479
  experimental studies, 135, 140–151, 159–160
psychoses, ix, 10, 14, 84, 89, 95–96, 202, 215, 244, 269–282, 483
  acute, 483
  alcohol, 485
  "cannabis psychosis," 273–275, 281
  chronic, 276
  functional, 275–276, 483
  toxic, 273–276, 279, 485
psychotomimetic effects, 25, 49, 277, 316
public health, 5, 12, 490–491, 495

and cardiovascular effects, 441–442
  and drug use, 12, 477–478
  harm to, 491
Puerto Rico, 334
pulmonary effects, 320–334, 465
pyrolysis, 21, 38, 199, 222, 293, 304, 404

R

rabbits, 378, 445
rabies, 461, 466
randomization, 8, 9, 13, 73
rat(s), 8, 23, 25, 27, 30, 196–201, 240, 294, 314, 319, 350, 356, 357, 377–379, 383, 384, 386, 405, 410, 415, 443, 445
  brain, 24–28, 32, 49, 200, 209, 211, 212, 295, 362, 379, 380, 384, 406, 424
Raven's Progressive Matrices, 219, 221, 227
reaction-time tasks, 132, 140, 144, 146–150, 158, 180, 217, 222, 223, 235, 241, 479
  visual-choice reaction-time subsidiary task, 176–177, 180, 183, 185–186
recall tasks, 130–132, 242
  arithmetic, 225–226
  free recall, 129, 133, 134, 230, 232
  number, 151, 231
  short story, 133, 134
  word, 132, 225–226, 232, 239
receptors, cannabinoid, 21–32, 49–50, 129–161, 196–199, 206, 207, 232, 237, 243, 294, 354, 362, 377, 381, 424, 443, 448, 449
  alterations, 211–214
  binding, 23–26, 209, 211, 247, 384, 424, 437
  in the brain, x, 25–28, 29, 195–214, 232, 237, 245, 377, 382, 384, 386, 467
  cloning, 26–27, 28, 49–50
  down-regulation, 211–212
  G-protein-coupled, 26, 27, 28, 30, 50, 362, 448
  and immunity, 349
  melanocortin, 27
  opioid, 27
  orphan, 26
  in the periphery, x, 26, 437, 443, 449
  peptide, 27
  and pregnancy, 406
recognition tasks, 129–130
recruitment, 86–87, 98, 413
"red eye," 205, 464
reinforcing effects of cannabis, 129, 151–156, 160, 206

Reitan Modification of the Aphasia Screening Test, 218
relaxation, 10, 83, 84
Rey Auditory Verbal Learning Test (RAVLT), 227, 239
Rey-Davis Test, 220
Rey-Osterrieth Complex-Figure Test, 220, 233, 238, 241
Reynell Developmental Language Scale, 240, 418
roadside sobriety tests, 46
Romberg test, 46, 140, 144
repeated-acquisition task, 133–134, 149
reproduction, 8, 98, 103–106, 323, 377–386, 405–425, 480–481
research. *See* animal research, cannabis; human research, cannabis; studies, cannabis use
residual effects, 149, 150–151, 214, 225, 230
respiratory system, 98, 480
 and cannabis, 101–103, 106–107, 215, 313–336, 349–350, 480
 and tobacco, 101–102, 293, 313–336, 350, 480, 485
response bias, 72, 105
risk, 4, 5, 8
 attributable risk, 12, 14, 280, 488
 health risk, of cannabis, 477–495
 magnitude of risk, 11–13, 14, 488–494
 odds ratio, 8, 105
 public health significance of, 477
 quantitative, 477, 478
 relative risk, 8, 11–12, 14, 96, 97, 99, 278, 280, 478, 488–489
 risk-taking behavior, 176–177, 183, 184–185, 187
rodents, 28, 49, 197, 212, 213, 297, 299, 349–358, 380, 443, 479, 480
route of administration, 3, 5, 48, 159, 195, 199, 381
 and cancer, 486
 compared, 462–464, 478
 intracerebral, 198
 intracerebroventricular, 30, 380, 381, 382, 443
 intramuscular, 379
 intraperitoneal, 31, 378, 379
 of opioids, 485
 oral, 9, 13, 31, 33, 36–38, 84, 103, 134, 135, 149, 151, 154, 197, 199, 201, 204, 247, 274, 315, 378–380, 443, 446–447, 466
 parenteral, 9, 13
 rectal, 135, 446
 smoked, 9, 12, 13, 33, 35, 37, 38, 293

subcutaneous, 379
sublingual, 446
rural areas, 80, 81, 95, 217, 218
RNA, 200, 294, 408–409

S

saline, 138
salivation, 32, 34
Salmonella muenchen, 361, 464
sampling, 11, 72, 77, 81, 82, 95, 103–104, 215, 217, 218, 223, 227, 231, 240, 243, 317, 323, 412, 415, 425
schizophrenia, 8, 89, 95–98, 106, 202, 269–282, 483, 485, 489, 490, 495
school performance, 8, 9, 77, 84, 87–88, 98, 106, 159, 224, 232, 233, 277, 482, 486
 drop-outs, 84, 86, 87, 224
Seashore Rhythm Test, 229
Seattle, 412
secobarbital, 156
sedation, 196, 461, 462, 466, 485
selective recruitment hypothesis, 86–87, 98
Self-Paced Continuous Performance and Underlining Tests, 220–221
septum, 201, 207, 208, 232
serial acquisition task, 438
serotonin, 32, 199, 200, 201, 383
Sinsemilla, 403
shock-intensity choice, 158
single photo emission computerized tomography (SPECT), 207
sister chromatid exchanges (SCE), 297
size-estimation task, 222
skin conductance, 140
skin-painting, 297, 302, 304
sleep, 201–202, 240, 246
slow-wave sleep, 201–202
smoke
 cannabis, 6, 100, 101, 294, 295, 304, 313–336
 chemistry, 404–405
 condensates, 295, 299, 300, 301, 302, 318
 marijuana, 35, 48, 143, 148, 150, 199, 201, 207–208, 293, 296, 298, 301, 303, 349–350, 415, 465, 480
 placebo, 208, 357, 415
 sham, 319
 tar, 318, 331–332, 334, 462, 464, 492
 tobacco, 6, 101, 293, 313–336, 350, 480, 485

smoking. *See* cannabis, use; cannabis, users; cigarettes; smoke; studies, cannabis use
social behavior, and cannabis use, 129, 156–161
societal issues, 3–13, 71
 disapproval of drug use, 72, 76–77, 85, 461
socioeconomic status, 415
South Africa, 80
specificity, 9, 14, 228, 231, 236–239, 245
speech, 215
sperm, 103, 299, 384, 480
spinal cord, 29
spleen, 26, 27, 31, 50, 362
splenocytes, 350, 356, 357, 361, 363
spontaneous activity, 27, 30
sputum, 102, 320, 321, 322, 330, 480
SR141716A, 29, 31, 50, 197, 198, 202, 207, 384, 448
standard of proof, 4, 6, 12, 13
Standard Progressive Matrices, 222
standing-on-one-foot test, 46
standing steadiness task, 147–148, 149
Stanford-Binet Intelligence Scale, 104, 418
Staphylococcus aureus, 314, 329, 335, 360
startle, 104, 240, 417
stereoisomer, 22
stereoselectivity, 22, 26, 29, 363
steroids, 209, 384
 sex, 379
strength of association, 9, 14
striatum, 25, 30, 50, 139, 211, 212. *See also* basal ganglia
Stroop test, 238
structure–activity relationships (SARs), 21, 24, 25, 49, 363
students, and cannabis use
 7th grade, 77
 8th grade, 75, 76
 9th grade, 77
 10th grade, 75, 76
 11th grade, 77
 12th grade, 75–76, 82, 85, 88, 89, 92
 13th grade, 77
 college, 73, 75, 88, 95, 224–228, 238–239, 412
 high school, 71–78, 87–88, 94, 98, 235, 412, 482
 medical, 225
studies, cannabis use
 autoradiographic, 25, 49, 384
 case, 273, 279, 480
 case-control, 6, 7, 8, 13, 72, 98, 99, 102–107,

275, 277, 301, 302, 333, 442, 481
case-series, 273, 274, 282, 302, 336, 337
clinical, ix, 6, 48, 72, 90, 92, 97, 100, 154, 214–216, 224–227, 232, 269–282, 314, 331, 332, 437, 440, 444, 446, 447, 462, 467, 483, 485
cohort, 7, 8, 13, 72, 82, 90, 239, 245, 270, 324, 333, 484
controlled, 71–72, 92, 99, 101, 134, 135, 144, 151, 154, 160, 202, 203, 214–224, 228–230, 241, 243, 276
controlled-dosing, 46, 47
cross-cultural, 94–95
cross-sectional, 7, 8, 13, 72, 84, 87–90, 95, 98, 101, 106, 317, 482
culture-specific, 216–224, 227
epidemiological, 6, 11–14, 43, 69–107, 173, 272–273, 277, 281, 282, 303, 329, 333, 335, 336, 413, 425, 437, 477–480, 483, 485, 488, 490, 495
experimental, 6, 7, 8, 11, 13, 72, 156–161, 174–188, 303, 482
field, 90–91, 100, 216, 217, 276–277, 440, 482
in utero, 411, 412, 416–419, 421, 423, 425, 481
in vitro, 6, 10, 26, 28, 31, 200, 296, 314, 320, 331, 332, 350–351, 353–354, 357–360, 363, 382, 383, 480, 481
in vivo, 25, 31, 50, 207, 296, 349–357, 383, 448, 480
laboratory, 90–91, 99, 155, 174, 223, 273, 315, 405, 441, 482, 483
longitudinal, 9, 85, 87, 88, 89, 98, 228, 239, 245, 279, 322, 324, 422, 484
postmortem, 213
residential laboratory, 135, 146, 150, 152, 153, 155, 157, 228–230, 352–253, 439
subjective report of drug effects, 38–40, 43–46, 130, 133, 136, 138–145, 147, 150, 154, 155, 157, 178, 182, 186–187, 270
suicide, 89, 484, 486
surveys, cannabis use, 71–83, 245
 of driving, 173
 face-to-face, 302
 household, 72, 74, 78, 80, 321
 interviews, 412, 414
 school, 78
 telephone, 78–79, 302
Sweden, 79, 96–97, 99–100, 270, 278, 279, 479
Symbol-Digits Modalities Test, 227

U

CPSIA information can be obtained at www.ICGtesting.com
Printed in the USA
LVOW052151140212

268740LV00003B/3/P